Transcultural Concepts in Nursing Care

Eighth Edition

Margaret M. Andrews, PhD, RN, FAAN

Dean and Professor
School of Nursing
University of Michigan-Flint
Flint, Michigan

Joyceen S. Boyle, PhD, RN, FAAN

Adjunct Professor of Nursing, College of Nursing
University of Arizona, Tucson, Arizona
Adjunct Professor of Nursing, College of Nursing
Augusta University, Augusta, Georgia

John W. Collins, PhD, RN

Project Director, Veterans to BSN Program
School of Nursing
University of Michigan-Flint
Flint, Michigan

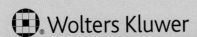 Wolters Kluwer

Philadelphia • Baltimore • New York • London
Buenos Aires • Hong Kong • Sydney • Tokyo

Vice President and Publisher: Julie K. Stegman
Executive Editor/Acquisitions Editor: Christina C. Burns
Director of Product Development: Jennifer K. Forestieri
Associate Development Editor: Rebecca J. Rist
Editorial Coordinator: David Murphy
Marketing Manager: Brittany Clements
Editorial Assistant: Kate Campbell
Design Coordinator: Teresa Mallon
Art Director, Illustration: Jennifer Clements
Production Project Manager: Marian Bellus
Manufacturing Coordinator: Karin Duffield
Prepress Vendor: SPi Global

8th edition

Cataloging-in-Publication Data available on request from the Publisher

ISBN: 978-1-9751-1067-3

RRS1907

Contributors to the Eighth Edition

Margaret M. Andrews, PhD, RN, FAAN
Dean and Professor
School of Nursing
University of Michigan-Flint
Flint, Michigan

Martha B. Baird, PhD, RN, ARNP, CTN-A
Clinical Assistant Professor
Kansas University Medical Center
The University of Kansas
Kansas City, Kansas

Joyceen S. Boyle, PhD, RN, FAAN
Adjunct Professor of Nursing
College of Nursing
University of Arizona
Tucson, Arizona
Adjunct Professor of Nursing
College of Nursing
Augusta University
Augusta, Georgia

John W. Collins, PhD, RN
Project Director, Veterans to BSN Program
School of Nursing
University of Michigan-Flint
Flint, Michigan

Melva Craft-Blacksheare, DNP, CNM
Associate Professor
School of Nursing
University of Michigan-Flint
Flint, Michigan

Joanne T. Ehrmin, PhD, RN, CNS
Professor
College of Nursing
University of Toledo
Toledo, Ohio

Marilyn K. Eipperle, DNP, RN, FNP-BC, CTN-A
Lecturer
School of Nursing
University of Michigan-Flint
Flint, Michigan

Patricia A. Hanson, PhD, RN, APRN-BC, GNP
Professor
College of Nursing and Health
Madonna University
Livonia, Michigan

Patti A. Ludwig-Beymer, PhD, RN, CTN-A, NEA-
 BC, CPPS, FAAN
Associate Professor
College of Nursing
Purdue University Northwest
Hammond, Indiana

Margaret A. McKenna, PhD, MPH, MN
Clinical Associate Professor
Department of Health Services
University of Washington
Seattle, Washington

Dula F. Pacquiao, EdD, RN, CTN-A, TNS
Professor
School of Nursing
Rutgers University
Newark, New Jersey

Contributors to the Seventh Edition

Martha B. Baird, PhD, RN, ARNP, CTN-A
Clinical Associate Professor
Kansas University Medical Center
The University of Kansas
Kansas City, Kansas

Joanne T. Ehrmin, PhD, RN, CNS
Professor
College of Nursing
University of Toledo
Toledo, Ohio

Patricia A. Hanson, PhD, RN, APRN-BC, GNP
Professor
College of Nursing and Health
Madonna University
Livonia, Michigan

Patti A. Ludwig-Beymer, PhD, RN, CTN-A,
  NEABC, CPPS, FAAN
Associate Professor
College of Nursing
Purdue University Northwest
Hammond, Indiana

Margaret A. McKenna, PhD, MPH, MN
Clinical Associate Professor
Department of Health Services
University of Washington
Seattle, Washington

Dula F. Pacquiao, EdD, RN, CTN-A, TNS
Professor
School of Nursing
Rutgers University
Newark, New Jersey

List of Reviewers to the Eight Edition

Catherine Bailey, DNP, RN, CNE
Associate Professor
Department of Nursing
Shawnee State University
Portsmouth, Ohio

Vera C. Brancato, EdD, MSN, BSN, RN, CNE
Professor
Department of Nursing
Alvernia University
Reading, Pennsylvania

Lori L. Cronin, DNP, RN, CNE
Clinical Associate Professor
Columbia College of Nursing
Glendale, Wisconsin

Michele Dickens, PhD, RN
Associate Dean, Online Nursing Programs
School of Nursing
Campbellsville University
Campbellsville, Kentucky

Peggy Fossen, DNP, RN
Associate Professor
Department of Nursing
St. Cloud State University
St. Cloud, Minnesota

Bonnie Fuller, PhD, RN, CNE
Assistant Professor
Department of Nursing
Towson University
Towson, Maryland

Laura Grunin, RN, MSN
Adjunct Faculty
School of Nursing
Kean University
Union, New Jersey

Souzan Hawala-Druy, MPH, BSN
Instructor
College of Nursing & Allied Health Sciences
Howard University
Washington, District of Columbia

P. Lee Monahan, PhD, RN
Professor, Director
School of Nursing
Western Illinois University
Macomb, Illinois

Rosa Rousseau, MSN, RNC-NIC, NPT
Associate Dean of Nursing
School of Science
St. Thomas University
Miami, Florida

Debra A. Simons, PhD, RN, CNE, CCM
Associate Dean, Associate Professor
School of Nursing and Healthcare Professions
College of New Rochelle
New Rochelle, New York

Deborah Stone, PhD, MS, RN
Assistant Professor
Fitchburg State University
Fitchburg, Massachusetts

Munira Wells, PhD, RN
Assistant Professor
College of Nursing
Seton Hall University
South Orange, New Jersey

List of Reviewers to the Seventh Edition

Angeline Bushy, PhD, RN, PHCNS-BC, FAAN
Professor and Bert Fish Chair
College of Nursing
University of Central Florida
Daytona Beach, Florida

Kevin Callaway, MSN
Adjunct Instructor
College of Nursing
Jacksonville State University
Jacksonville, Alabama

Jolyn Cooke, MN
Instructor
Mississippi University for Women
Tupelo, Mississippi

Betty B. Daniels, PhD, RN
Assistant Professor
Brenau University
Gainesville, Georgia

Debbi DelRe, MSN, RN
Director, RN-BSN Program
College of Nursing
University of St. Francis
Joliet, Illinois

Frank Druse III, MSN, MHA, CEN, CPEN, RN
Instructor
Mohawk Valley Community College
Utica College
Utica, New York

Michelle Eaton, DNP, RN
Clinical Instructor
College of Nursing
New York University
New York, New York

Susan Berry Imes, PhD, MSN, RN
Associate Professor
School of Nursing
College of Health Professions
Marshall University
Huntington, West Virginia

Patricia Joffe, PhD, APN/CNS–BC, CSN
Professor
New Jersey City University
Jersey City, New Jersey

Norma Kiser-Larson, PhD, RN
Associate Professor and MS Nurse Educator
Program Director
North Dakota State University
Fargo, North Dakota

Cathy Konrad, PhD, RNC
Professor
Trinity College of Nursing and Health Sciences
Rock Island, Illinois

Louisana Louis, DNP, RN
Professor, College of Nursing
St. Petersburg College
Pinellas Park, Florida

Pamela Y. Mahon, PhD, RN, CNE, NEA-BC, ANEF
Associate Dean and Professor, College of Nursing
SUNY Upstate Medical University
Syracuse, New York

Kim V. McCarron, MS, RN, CRNP
Clinical Associate Professor
Towson University
College of Health Professions
Towson, Maryland

Jenny Radsma, PhD, RN
Professor
University of Maine at Fort Kent
Fort Kent, Maine

Judith G. Ruvalcaba, MSN, RN
Clinical Instructor of Nursing
Clayton State University
Morrow, Georgia

Crystal Shannon, PhD, MBA, RN
Assistant Professor
School of Nursing
Indiana University Northwest
Gary, Indiana

Julie Slade, DNP, RN
RN-BSN Program Coordinator
Assistant Professor, Nursing
Chatham University
Pittsburgh, Pennsylvania

Barbara E. Stanley, MD
Clinical Assistant Professor
University of Massachusetts
Amherst, Massachusetts

Haley Strickland, EdD, RN, CNL
Assistant Professor
University of Alabama
Tuscaloosa, Alabama

Ardith Sudduth, PhD
Associate Professor
University of Louisiana at Lafayette
Lafayette, Louisiana

Laura Pruitt Walker, DHEd, MSN, RN, COI
Assistant Professor of Nursing
Jacksonville State University
Jacksonville, Alabama

Margaret Winter, MS, EdD, RN
Associate Professor of Nursing
Huntington University
Huntington, Indiana

Foreword

I am pleased for the opportunity to write the Foreword once again, this time, for the eighth edition of the *Transcultural Concepts in Nursing Care* book by Margaret Andrews, Joyceen Boyle, and John Collins. I am following in the footsteps of the founder of transcultural nursing, the late Dr. Madeleine Leininger and Dr. JoAnn Glittenberg Hinrichs, the mentor of Dr. Joyceen Boyle. Joyceen and I were classmates in the first transcultural nursing PhD program at the University of Utah College of Nursing in 1977 where we were challenged by Dr. Leininger to study the substantive knowledge and create new knowledge through research of the discipline of transcultural nursing. Dr. Andrews later was also a student at the University of Utah. Joyceen and Margaret saw the need to advance transcultural concepts in nursing care and wrote the first edition along with chapter contributions written by other authors of this book in 1989. Subsequent editions of this book have provided the foundation to study transcultural concepts related to diverse cultures of individuals, groups, and communities and is used widely in Schools of Nursing across the United States and in other nations. Their book meets the essentials and current directives of the American Association of Colleges of Nursing (AACN), the National League for Nursing (NLN), and the American Nurses Association (ANA) and other organizations for preparation of nurses in transcultural nursing to provide culturally competent care to people.

Joining Drs. Andrews and Boyle for the eighth edition as a contributing author is Dr. John Collins. John has research interests in end-of-life care and community-based nursing as well as serves as a Project Director of the Health Resources and Services Administration (HRSA)-funded Veteran Bachelor of Science in Nursing (BSN) Program at the University of Michigan-Flint. He has identified and educated others about the unique culture of persons transitioning from military service (active duty) to veteran status, increased opportunities for veteran nursing education, and made available important cultural information for the profession of nursing within the Veterans Administration. As a retired USAF Colonel and veteran myself, and a contributor to another HRSA grant proposal for Veteran BSN education in primary care for rural and underserved populations at Florida Atlantic University, John's knowledge of transcultural veteran nursing education is invaluable. In this new eighth edition, another scholar Dr. Melva Craft-Blacksheare, a certified nurse-midwife from the University of Michigan-Flint has contributed in the areas of transcultural maternal-child care and environmental science and social justice. She helped to change and/or improve water quality and policy and ultimately health care by her advocacy in the recent Flint, Michigan water crisis. This new eighth edition edited by Andrews, Boyle and Collins with contributing chapters by talented transcultural nurses illuminates critical elements of the changing health care system in the United States and the world. The chapters address historical and current trends in transcultural knowledge for national and international communities, new approaches in primary and preventive care, and immigrant and refugee care with a focus on public health and policy. A most important element of this book is the Andrews/Boyle Transcultural Interprofessional Practice Model (TIP), a transcultural nursing/health care theory that speaks to the need for a conceptual framework to guide transcultural nursing education, research, administration, and practice. I recently attended the Nursing

Theory Conference, Nursing Theory: A 50 Year Perspective: Past and Future at Case Western Reserve University in Cleveland, Ohio, where 50 years ago, Dr. Leininger and other scholars met to address the state of nursing theory and find ways to create paradigms and synthesize important concepts for the practice of nursing. Leininger already had developed a transcultural nursing theory and soon thereafter published her Culture Care Diversity and Universality Theory, represented in this book. She also encouraged those of us in graduate programs to advance transcultural nursing theory from philosophy and/or research. At the conference in Cleveland, select nurse leaders stated that all research should culminate in nursing theory. My memory helped realize the creativity of Madeleine Leininger and what an effective mentor she was. One motto articulated at the outset of the initiation of the Transcultural Nursing Society, "the cultural needs of people in the world would be met by nurses prepared in transcultural nursing," triggered thoughts within me. Although this is a crucial maxim, at this latest 2019 theory conference, references to transcultural nursing scholarship were not identified by the leaders and left me feeling very disappointed. Therefore, I think that creating and publishing transcultural nursing theory has become more critical than ever. As a nursing theorist myself, a Fellow of different organizations, especially a Fellow of the National Academies of [Interprofessional] Practice, I am particularly supportive of the Andrews/Boyle Transcultural Interprofessional Practice Model (TIP Theory) that highlights what is necessary interprofessionally to care for diverse people today. Their theory illuminates transcultural communication, team work, collaboration, and culturally competent skills that are built upon a transcultural care philosophy and contemporary research to improve the care of patients, families, groups, communities, and institutions in national and global communities. Their person-centered, communicative and collaborative nursing and health care theoretical approach includes not only communication about interactional concepts to improve

transcultural practice with professionals from all health care disciplines but also the importance of folk, indigenous, and religious healer knowledge and skill in care plans. As a person-centered theory, it focuses on consideration of the contributions of persons who are being served transculturally to participate in sharing their views of their own cultural care practices with the health care team. In a culturally diverse world and as the need for transcultural nursing becomes even more relevant, the reinforcement of theories or the emergence of new theories will continue to improve the practice of person-centered care and ultimately enhance the discipline of transcultural nursing and contribute to the legacy created by Leininger in the 1950s.

Because of their long history of knowledge generation in transcultural nursing, this work of Andrews, Boyle, and Collins is very comprehensive and shows the depth of their scholarship in terms of culture, theoretical applications, research and evidence-based/informed practice, case study presentations for cultural clarity and explanation, and summaries. This work also illuminates a response to understanding the United Nations Sustainable Millennium Development Goals 2030, which show that most of the goals relate to the need for transcultural health care. As such, the eighth edition will inspire the nurse as a self-reflective professional who can engage with clients, families, and team members through thoughtful and knowledgeable transcultural interaction. Along with the application of the Andrews/Boyle Transcultural Interprofessional Practice Model (the TIP theory) as a framework for cross-cultural communication, team work, and interprofessional collaborative practice, each chapter consists of Key Terms, Learning Objectives, and an analysis of the major concerns and issues of transcultural nursing care including an understanding of complementary disciplines in the sciences and humanities for transcultural care of individuals, families, groups, communities, and institutions. Review Questions, Critical Thinking Activities, and Instructor Resources complete the process. Part One focuses on

Foundations of Transcultural Nursing. Andrews, Boyle, and Collins hold the view that rather than focusing on culture groups per se, they advocate a focus on cultural groups and how their transcultural nursing TIP theoretical concepts emanate from the study of the groups. Part Two of the book focuses on the Life Span. Given the importance of understanding transcultural care from childhood to adulthood, their approach with contributors shows the depth of the need to understand transcultural perspectives at each stage of life. Part Three addresses organizations as living and dynamic organizations. As a transcultural nurse and theorist of transcultural care in complex organizations and committed to research in these dynamic systems myself, Part three responds to that call to create culturally competent care in these environments that also includes mental health care settings. Part four considers how religion, spirituality, and ethics play a significant role in providing culturally competent care. In my own transcultural caring scholarship, I have found that the study of universal sources is a main component of transcultural nursing for awareness, understanding, and choice-making for persons in any health care environment.

As we witness, rapid changes in science, technology, genetics, genomics, health care, economics, geopolitics, transportation, demographics, migration and immigration, including refugee challenges, religious ideologies, wars, and global issues including human rights and social justice nurses are challenged to understand new ways of engaging with persons and professional colleagues transculturally. Complexity sciences and the generation of enormous quantities of research of every affiliation and diverse philosophical, political, and religious perspectives, we can see the interconnectedness of everything in the universe and the necessity for discernment and evaluation of what is really happening in the world. Theoretical and experiential knowledge about our responsibilities to one another thus is growing and impacts the need for intense communication to examine and solve problems both locally and globally. Continuing

to identify relevant issues to promote health, human safety, and improve the quality of life of all people is a major goal of thoughtful transcultural health care professionals. These developments have shaped Andrew, Boyle, and Collins' paradigmatic and theoretical thinking in the eighth edition. Their interest in addressing the challenges of the interconnectedness of all by their Transcultural Interprofessional Practice Model (TIP Theory) illuminates the necessity for increased collaboration and communication with patients and health care and "folk" participants to address complex approaches in the digital age to appreciate transcultural issues in the provision of culturally congruent, safe, and competent care. The key concepts identified in the TIP model are *context, interprofessional health care team, communication, and problem-solving process.* The cultural *context* (health-related beliefs and practices that weave together environmental, economic, social, religious, moral, legal, political, educational, biophysical, genetic, and technological factors), the *interprofessional health care team* (nurses, physicians, social workers, therapists, pharmacists, and others), *cross-cultural communication* among clients, families, and significant others, and members of the interprofessional health care team including "folk" and traditional healers, and religious and spiritual healers facilitate the foundation of the problem-solving process that has five steps. These five steps include comprehensive holistic patient/client assessment, mutual goal setting, planning, implementation of the plan of action and interventions, and evaluation of the plan for effectiveness to achieve the stated goals, and desired outcomes; provide culturally congruent and competent care; deliver quality care that is safe and affordable; and ensure that the care is evidence-based with best practices.

As I reflect on the work of my colleagues, Margaret Andrews, Joyceen Boyle, and John Collins, not only within the pages of this book but also what each of them has accomplished over many years as leaders, teachers, researchers, on-line educators, and Margaret and Joyceen as

Presidents of the Transcultural Nursing Society, what comes to mind is their *deep dedication and devotion* to the discipline and profession of Transcultural Nursing. Through their intellectual astuteness and creative actions, they are role models and mentors to students and other leaders who can enlighten and broaden transcultural care knowledge worldwide. They are committed to the primary goal of transcultural nursing to facilitate culturally congruent knowledge and care so that people of the world are understood, and their health care needs can be met within the dynamics of their cultures and cultural understanding. An eighth edition of a book attests to the fact that students, faculty, and other practitioners will find within its pages relevant and challenging information and a theory to learn about and apply to diverse culture groups, know how to relate and serve them, conduct research, and facilitate the solving of problems. Today, *interprofessional collaboration and communication* are the key to change and effective transcultural care. The authors have captured that essence in

their Transcultural Interprofessional Practice (TIP) theory and model presented in this work. I wholeheartedly endorse this new edition. I am most proud to call these authors not only my colleagues but also my friends as they move forward in the evolution of what can be termed authentic transcultural nursing by means of collaboration and interprofessionalism. Nursing students, faculty, other health care professionals, and practitioners of every health care and anthropological/sociological discipline will be stimulated by the theory and the content expressed by the authors and the many contributors in this new edition to improve the health of and help people of diverse cultures worldwide.

Marilyn A. Ray, RN, PhD, CTN-A, FSfAA, FAAN, FESPCH (hon), FNAP
Colonel (Retired), United States Air Force, Nurse Corps
Professor Emeritus and Adjunct Professor
The Christine E. Lynn College of Nursing
Florida Atlantic University
Boca Raton, Florida

Preface

Given the large number of cultures and subcultures in the world, it's impossible for nurses to know everything about them all; however, it is possible for nurses to develop excellent cultural assessment and cross-cultural communication skills and to follow a systematic, orderly process for the delivery of culturally competent care.

The Andrews/Boyle Transcultural Interprofessional Practice (TIP) Model, which we introduced in the seventh edition of *Transcultural Concepts in Nursing Care,* has been well received at national and international conferences and by readers. Chapters 1 and 2 emphasize the need for effective communication, efficient client- and patient-centered teamwork, teambuilding, and collaboration among members of the interprofessional health care team.

The TIP Model has a theoretical foundation in transcultural nursing that fosters communication and collaboration between and among all members of the team and enables multiple team members to manage complex, frequently multifaceted transcultural care issues, moral and ethical dilemmas, challenges, and care-related problems in a collegial, respectful, synergistic manner. The process used in the TIP Model is an adaptation and application of the classic scientific problem-solving method. The model has application in the care of people from different national origins, ethnicities, races, socioeconomic backgrounds, religions, genders, marital statuses, sexual orientations, ages, abilities/disabilities, sizes, veteran status, and other characteristics used to compare one group of people to another.

The Commission on Collegiate Nursing Education, the American Association of Colleges of Nursing's Essentials of Baccalaureate Education for Professional Nursing Practice, Accreditation Commission for Education in Nursing, most state boards of nursing, and other accrediting and certification bodies require or strongly encourage the inclusion of cultural aspects of care in nursing curricula. This, of course, underscores the importance of the purpose, goal, and objectives for *Transcultural Concepts in Nursing Care, Eighth Edition.*

Purpose: To contribute to the development of theoretically based transcultural nursing knowledge and the advancement of transcultural nursing practice.

Goal: To increase the delivery of culturally competent care to individuals, families, groups, communities, and institutions.

Objectives:

1. To apply a transcultural nursing framework to guide nursing practice in diverse health care settings across the life span.
2. To analyze major concerns and issues encountered by nurses in providing transcultural nursing care to individuals, families, groups, communities, and institutions.
3. To expand the theoretical basis for using concepts from the natural and behavioral sciences and from the humanities to provide culturally competent nursing care.
4. To provide a contemporary approach to transcultural nursing that includes effective cross-cultural communication, team work, and interprofessional collaborative practice.

We believe that cultural assessment skills, combined with the nurses' critical thinking abilities, will provide the necessary knowledge on which to base transcultural nursing care. Using this approach, nurses have the ability to provide culturally competent and contextually meaningful care for clients—individuals, groups, families, communities, and institutions.

The editors and chapter authors share a commitment to:

- Foster the development and maintenance of a disciplinary knowledge base and expertise in culturally competent care.
- Synthesize existing theoretical and research knowledge regarding nursing care of different ethnic/minority/marginalized and other disenfranchised populations.
- Identify and describe evidence-based practice and best practices in the care of diverse individuals, families, groups, communities, and institutions.
- Create an interdisciplinary and interprofessional knowledge base that reflects heterogeneous health care practices within various cultural groups.
- Identify, describe, and examine methods, theories, and frameworks appropriate for developing knowledge that will improve health and nursing care to minority, underserved, underrepresented, disenfranchised, and marginalized populations.

Recognizing Individual Differences and Acculturation

We believe that it is tremendously important to recognize the myriad of health-related beliefs and practices that exist within population categories. For example, differences are rarely recognized among people who identify themselves as Hispanic/Latino yet this group includes people from along the United States–Mexico border, Mexican Americans, Puerto Ricans, Guatemalans, Cubans (such as those living in "little Havana" in Miami), as well as other Central and South American countries. These individuals may share some similarities (e.g., speaking Spanish) but also have distinct cultural differences. It should be noted that people from Spain do not necessarily culturally self-identify with individuals from the cultural groups previously cited; rather, they take pride in being Spanish and speaking Castilian Spanish. Spanish or Castilian Spanish, is a Western Romance language that originated in the Castile region of Spain and today has hundreds of millions of native speakers in the Americas and Spain. It is usually considered a global language and the world's second-most spoken native language, after Mandarin Chinese.

We would like to comment briefly on the terms *minority* and *ethnic minorities*. These terms are perceived by some to be offensive because they connote inferiority and marginalization. Although we have used these terms occasionally, we prefer to make reference to a specific culture or subculture whenever possible. We refer to categorizations according to race, ethnicity, religion, or a combination, such as ethnoreligion, but we make every effort to avoid using any label in a pejorative manner. We do believe, however, that the concepts or terms *minority* or *ethnicity* are limiting, not only for those to whom the label perhaps applies but also for nursing theory and practice. We believe the concept of *culture* is richer and has more theoretical usefulness. In addition, we all have cultural attributes while not all are from a minority group or claim a particular ethnicity.

Critical Thinking Linked to Delivering Culturally Competent Care

We believe that nurses' critical thinking, cultural assessment, and clinical problem-solving abilities will provide the necessary knowledge and skills on which to base transcultural nursing care. Using this approach, we believe that nurses will be able to provide culturally competent and contextually meaningful care for clients from a wide variety of cultural backgrounds, rather than simply memorizing the esoteric health beliefs and practices of any specific cultural group. We believe that nurses must acquire the skills needed to assess clients from virtually any and all groups they encounter throughout their professional life.

Many educational programs in nursing are now teaching transcultural nursing content across the curriculum. We suggest that *Transcultural Concepts in Nursing Care* be used by faculty members to integrate transcultural content across the curriculum in the following manner:

- Chapters 1 to 4 should be used in the first clinical courses when students are learning how to conduct health histories, health assessments, and physical examinations.
- Chapters 5 to 8 include nursing care across the life span and are particularly useful in courses that focus on the nursing care of:
  - The childbearing family
  - Children
  - Adults and older adults
- Chapter 9 examines approaches for creating and maintaining culturally competent health care organizations and is useful in courses that focus on nursing leadership and management.
- Chapters 10 and 11 align with mental health nursing and family and community nursing in the appropriate specialty nursing courses.
- Chapter 12 explores the interconnections between religion, culture, and nursing, including health-related beliefs and practices of selected religions.
- Chapter 13 focuses on competence in ethical decision-making.

New to the Eighth Edition

All content in this edition was reviewed and updated to capture the nature of the changing health care delivery system, new research studies and theoretical advances, emphasis on effective communication, team work, and collaboration, and to explain how nurses and other health care providers can use culturally competent skills to improve the care of clients, families, groups, and communities. In writing the eighth edition, we have been impressed with the developments in the field of transcultural nursing and included current trends and issues in this edition. The Andrews/Boyle Transcultural Interprofessional Practice Model provides a contemporary framework for putting the client or patient first and expanding the traditional notion of those who

should be included as members of the health care team. While credentialed healers such as nurses, physicians, pharmacists, social workers, interpreters, and therapists remain key to health, wellness, and healing, the team also includes others whom the clients or patients believe contribute to their care, such as folk, indigenous, spiritual, and religious healers. This expansion of the team membership requires openness by credentialed healers to those with different scopes of practices, health belief systems, and healing practices. Clients or patients should always be included as integral members of the health care team here as their understanding, acceptance, and cooperation are essential to the delivery of culturally competent health care. Similarly, the conceptualization of family and/or significant other has expanded to include the needs of those with diverse sexual orientations (LGBTQ), reflecting changing norms in some cultures, societies, and nations. Lastly, the Andrews/Boyle TIP Practice Model includes service animals, pets, and other sentient beings that clients and patients find therapeutic and might request as part of their plan of care.

New Contributors

We welcome Dr. John Collins as a contributing editor to the book. Dr. Collins is a long-standing colleague and friend from the University of Michigan-Flint School of Nursing. Dr. Collins is currently the Project Director of the Health Resources and Services Administration (HRSA)–funded Veterans to BSN Program Bachelor of Nursing program at University of Michigan-Flint School of Nursing and has a long history with transcultural nursing initiatives. He served with Dr. Andrews on another HRSA-funded grant as Program Manager on the Cultural Competence for Nurses project, and was the Data Evaluator on the Nursing Workforce Diversity program University of Michigan-Flint Initiatives in Nursing Diversity. Dr. Collins' clinical and research interests include care of the adult patient particularly at End-of-Life, as well as community health nursing and the cultural factors that influence health care decisions and practices. Likewise, Dr. Collins is passionate about nursing education, specifically in reducing the challenges facing nontraditional populations including military veterans.

We are very pleased that Dr. Melva Craft-Blacksheare has joined us as the author of Chapter 5, Transcultural Perspectives on Childbearing. A Certified Nurse Midwife, Dr. Craft-Blacksheare is associate professor of nursing University of Michigan-Flint School of Nursing. During the community crisis that ensued as a result of contaminated Flint (Michigan) River water, Dr. Craft-Blacksheare was a champion for pregnant teens and women and their newborns. She fought against environmental injustice and advocated for parents and newborns who were exposed to toxic lead levels and respiratory distress caused by Legionella (Legionnaire's disease) in newborns exposed to the contaminated water. As a nursing faculty member, Dr. Craft-Blacksheare has created an interdisciplinary blueprint to foster a more diverse nursing workforce to improve health care to clients and patients from culturally diverse backgrounds.

Chapter Pedagogy

Learning Activities

All of the chapters include review questions and learning activities to promote critical thinking. In addition, learning objectives and key terms are included at the beginning of each chapter to help readers understand the purpose and intent of the content.

Evidence-Based Practice Features

Current research studies related to the content of the chapter are presented as Evidence-Based Practice boxes. We have included a section in each box describing clinical implications of the research.

Case Studies

Case studies based on the authors' actual clinical experiences and research findings are presented

to make conceptual linkages and to illustrate how concepts are applied in health care settings. Case studies are oriented to assist the reader to begin to develop cultural competence with selected cultures.

Text Organization

Part One: Foundations of Transcultural Nursing

This first section focuses on the foundational aspects of transcultural nursing. The development of transcultural nursing frameworks that include concepts from the natural and behavioral sciences is described as they apply to nursing practice. Because nursing perspectives are used to organize the content in *Transcultural Concepts in Nursing Care*, the reader will not find a chapter purporting to describe the nursing care of a specific cultural group. Instead, the nursing needs of culturally diverse groups are used to illustrate cultural concepts used in nursing practice. Chapter 1 provides an overview of the theoretical foundations of transcultural nursing, and Chapter 2 introduces key concepts associated with cultural competence using the Andrews/Boyle Transcultural Interprofessional Practice Model as the organizing framework. In Chapter 3, we discuss the domains of cultural knowledge that are important in cultural assessment and describe how this cultural information can be incorporated into all aspects of care. Chapter 4 provides a summary of the major cultural belief systems embraced by people of the world with special emphasis on their health-related and culturally based values, attitudes, beliefs, and practices.

Part Two: Life Span

Chapters 5 through 8 use a developmental framework to discuss transcultural concepts across the life span. The care of childbearing women and their families, children, adolescents, middle-aged adults, and the elderly is examined, and information about cultural groups is used to illustrate common transcultural nursing issues, trends, and concerns. Chapter 7, "Transcultural Perspectives in the Nursing Care of Adults," is the collaborative effort of Drs. Boyle, Baird, and Collins. Originally developed and written by Drs. Boyle and Baird, eighth edition content has been updated with new references, new insights, and more contemporary examples.

Part Three: Health Care Settings

In the third section of the text (Chapters 9 through 12), we explore the components of cultural competence in mental health and in family and community health care settings. We also examine cultural competence in health care organizations and cultural diversity in the health care workforce, two very critical and current topics of concern. The clinical application of concepts throughout this section uses situations commonly encountered by nurses and describes how transcultural nursing principles can be applied in diverse settings. The chapters in this section are intended to illustrate the application of transcultural nursing knowledge to nursing practice.

Part Four: Other Considerations in Culturally Competent Care

In the fourth section of the text, Chapters 12 and 13, we examine selected contemporary issues and challenges that face nursing and health care. In Chapter 12, we review major religious traditions of the United States and the interrelationships among religion, culture, and nursing. Recognizing the numerous moral and ethical challenges in contemporary health care as well as within transcultural nursing, Chapter 13 discusses cultural competence in ethical and moral dilemmas from a transcultural perspective.

Resources for Instructors

Tools to assist you with teaching your course are available upon adoption of this text on thePoint® at https://thePoint.lww.com/Andrews8e.

- The **Test Generator** lets you generate new tests from a bank of NCLEX-style questions to help you assess your students' understanding of the course material.
- **PowerPoint Presentations** provide an easy way for you to integrate the textbook with your students' classroom experience, either via slide shows or handouts.
- **Case Studies** bring the content to life through real-world situations with these scenarios that can be used in class activities or group assignments.
- Plus **Assignments** and **Discussion Topics**.

Resources for Students

An exciting set of resources is available on thePoint® to help students review material and become even more familiar with vital concepts. Students can access all these resources at https://thePoint. lww.com/Andrews8e using the codes printed in the front of their text.

- **Review Questions** help students master important concepts and practice for exams.
- **Journal Articles** corresponding to book chapters offer access to current research available in Wolters Kluwer journals.
- Plus **Learning Objectives** from each chapter.

Lippincott® CoursePoint

The same trusted solution, innovation and unmatched support that you have come to expect from *Lippincott CoursePoint* is now enhanced with more engaging learning tools and deeper analytics to help prepare students for practice. This powerfully integrated, digital learning solution combines learning tools, real-time data, and the most trusted nursing education content on the market to make curriculum-wide learning more efficient and to meet students where they're at in their learning. And now, it's easier than ever for instructors and students to use, giving them everything they need for course and curriculum success!

Lippincott CoursePoint includes:

- Engaging course content provides a variety of learning tools to engage students of all learning styles.
- Interactive learning activities help students learn the critical thinking and clinical judgment skills needed to help them become practice-ready nurses.

- Unparalleled reporting provides in-depth dashboards with several data points to track student progress and help identify strengths and weaknesses.
- Unmatched support includes training coaches, product trainers, and nursing education consultants to help educators and students implement CoursePoint with ease.

Acknowledgments

We are pleased to acknowledge the assistance and support of our families, friends, and colleagues in once again making this book possible. We also appreciate the help of the many nursing faculty members, practitioners, and students who have offered helpful comments and suggestions. We have found it very gratifying to be able to call upon many of our colleagues for help and advice in this new edition.

We would like to gratefully acknowledge and thank Rebecca "Beck" Rist, Development Editor, Wolters Kluwer Health, for her insightful, creative, constructive, helpful, recommendations on ways to update and strengthen the content of the eighth edition. We highly value her professionalism, flexibility, and the long hours that she spent reviewing and rereviewing the chapters and appendices. We also thank David Murphy, Jr., for his valuable help throughout the process. We would also like to thank all of the other behind-the-scene members of the editorial and production team for their roles in bringing this text to publication.

We deeply appreciate the support of our friends, too numerous to list by name, who wrote encouraging e-mails, texts, or phoned to express their interest and encouragement. We thank all of our colleagues who have purchased our book in the past and the many who have expressed interest in the eighth edition. We are always appreciative of their support.

With this edition, we are pleased to have Dr. John Collins as an integral part of the project. He has brought a fresh perspective to the book, and we have enjoyed working with him. Through it all, we have found our professional endeavors in transcultural nursing and the friends that we have made along the way to be both satisfying and rewarding.

Margaret M. Andrews, PhD, RN, FAAN
Joyceen S. Boyle, PhD, RN, FAAN
John W. Collins, PhD, RN

Contents

Contributors to the Eighth Edition   iii
Contributors to the Seventh Edition   iv
List of Reviewers to the Eight Edition   v
List of Reviewers to the Seventh Edition   vi
Foreword   viii
Preface   xii
Acknowledgments   xviii

PART ONE Foundations of Transcultural Nursing   1

Chapter 1   **Theoretical Foundations of Transcultural Nursing**   3
Margaret M. Andrews and Joyceen S. Boyle

Chapter 2   **Culturally Competent Nursing Care**   31
Margaret M. Andrews

Chapter 3   **Cultural Competence in the History and Physical Examination**   55
Margaret M. Andrews

Chapter 4   **Influence of Cultural and Health Belief Systems on Health Care Practices**   105
Marilyn K. Eipperle and Margaret M. Andrews

PART TWO Lifespan   125

Chapter 5   **Transcultural Perspectives in Childbearing**   127
Melva Craft-Blacksheare

Chapter 6   **Transcultural Perspectives in the Nursing Care of Children**   173
Margaret M. Andrews

Chapter 7   **Transcultural Perspectives in the Care of Adults**   209
Joyceen S. Boyle and John W. Collins

Chapter 8   **Transcultural Perspectives in the Care of Older Adults**   237
Margaret A. McKenna

PART THREE Health Care Settings 263

Chapter 9   **Creating Culturally Competent Health Care Organizations** 265
Patti A. Ludwig-Beymer

Chapter 10   **Transcultural Perspectives in Mental Health Nursing** 299
Joanne T. Ehrmin

Chapter 11   **Culture, Family, and Community** 333
Joyceen S. Boyle, Martha B. Baird, and John W. Collins

PART FOUR Other Considerations in Culturally Competent Care 371

Chapter 12   **Religion, Culture, and Nursing** 373
Patricia A. Hanson and Margaret M. Andrews

Chapter 13   **Cultural Competence in Ethical Decision-Making** 416
Dula F. Pacquiao

Appendix A   Transcultural Nursing Assessment Guide for Individuals and Families 429
Joyceen S. Boyle and Margaret M. Andrews

Appendix B   Transcultural Nursing Assessment Guide for Families, Groups, and Communities 435
Joyceen S. Boyle and Margaret M. Andrews

Appendix C   Transcultural Nursing Assessment Guide for Health Care Organizations and Facilities 438
Joyceen S. Boyle, Margaret M. Andrews, and Patti A. Ludwig-Beymer

Appendix D   Transcultural Nursing Assessment for Refugees 440
Joyceen S. Boyle and Martha B. Baird

Index 445

Foundations
of Transcultural Nursing

PART

ONE

Foundations
of Transcultural Nursing

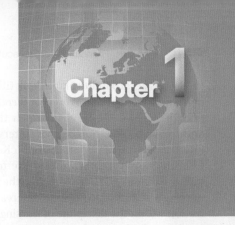

Theoretical Foundations of Transcultural Nursing

- Margaret M. Andrews and Joyceen S. Boyle

Key Terms

Anthropology
Assessment
Assumptions
Chronemics
Communication
Core curriculum
Cross-cultural communication
Cultural competence
Cultural context
Cultural-specific
Cultural universals
Culturally competent care
Culturally congruent nursing
  care

Culture
Culture-specific nursing care
Culture-universal nursing care
Ethnicity
Ethnonursing research
Evaluation
Evidence-based practice
Hijab
Implementation
Interprofessional collaboration
Interprofessional health care
  team
Language
Modesty
Monochronic culture

Mutual goal setting
Nonverbal communication
Paralanguage
Personal space
Polychronic culture
Problem-solving process
Proxemics
Race
Subculture
Transcultural Interprofessional
  Practice (TIP) Model
Transcultural nursing
Transcultural nursing
  certification
Verbal communication

Learning Objectives

1. Explore the historical and theoretical foundations of transcultural nursing.
2. Critically examine the relevance of transcultural nursing in addressing contemporary issues and trends in nursing.
3. Analyze Madeleine Leininger's contributions to the creation and development of transcultural nursing as a theory- and evidence-based formal area of study and practice within the nursing profession.
4. Critically examine the contributions of selected transcultural scholars to the advancement of transcultural nursing theory and practice.
5. Discuss key components of the Andrews/Boyle Transcultural Interprofessional Practice (TIP) Model.

In her classic, groundbreaking book titled *Nursing and Anthropology: Two Worlds to Blend*, Leininger (1970) analyzed the ways in which the fields of anthropology and nursing are interwoven and interconnected (c.f., Brink, 1976; McKenna, 1985; Osborne, 1969). Leininger used the term **transcultural nursing (TCN)** to describe the blending of nursing and anthropology into an area of specialization within the discipline of nursing. Using the concepts of culture and care, Leininger established TCN as a theory- and evidence-based formal area of study and practice within nursing that focuses on people's culturally based beliefs, attitudes, values, behaviors, and practices related to health, illness, healing, and human caring (Leininger, 1991, 1995; Leininger & McFarland, 2002, 2006; McFarland & Wehbe-Alamah, 2016, 2018).

TCN is sometimes used interchangeably with cross-cultural, intercultural and multicultural nursing. The *goal* of TCN is to develop a scientific and humanistic body of knowledge in order to provide **culture-specific** and **culture-universal nursing care** practices for individuals, families, groups, communities, and institutions of similar and diverse cultures. *Culture-specific* refers to particular values, beliefs, and patterns of behavior that tend to be special or unique to a group and that do not tend to be shared with members of other cultures. *Culture-universal* refers to the commonly shared values, norms of behavior, and life patterns that are similarly held among cultures about human behavior and lifestyles (Leininger, 1978, 1991, 1995; Leininger & McFarland, 2002, 2006; McFarland & Wehbe-Alamah, 2016, 2018). For example, although the need for food is a culture-universal, there are culture-specifics that determine what items are considered to be edible; methods used to prepare and eat meals; rules concerning who eats with whom, the frequency of meals, and gender- and age-related rules governing who eats first and last at mealtime; and the amount of food that individuals are expected to consume.

Given that culture is the central focus of anthropology and TCN, we begin this chapter by introducing, defining, and describing the concept of culture. We'll then discuss the historical and theoretical foundations of TCN, including its relevance in contemporary nursing practice and the significant contributions of Leininger and other TCN scholars, leaders, and clinicians to the global advancement of TCN research, theory, education, and clinical practice. In the remainder of the chapter, we examine the Andrews/Boyle **Transcultural Interprofessional Practice (TIP) Model** as a framework for delivering client-centered, high-quality nursing and health care that are culturally congruent and competent, safe, affordable, and accessible to people from diverse backgrounds across the lifespan. The term client is used throughout the book because nursing concerns not only the care of people who are ill but also those who strive for optimum health and wellness in their lives.

Anthropology and Culture

To understand the history and foundations of TCN, we begin by providing a brief overview of **anthropology**, an academic discipline that is concerned with the scientific study of humans, past and present. Anthropology builds on knowledge from the physical, biological, and social sciences as well as the humanities. A central concern of anthropologists is the application of knowledge to the solution of human problems. Historically, anthropologists have focused their education on one of four areas: sociocultural anthropology, biological/physical anthropology, archaeology, and linguistics. Anthropologists often integrate the perspectives of several of these areas into their research, teaching, and professional lives (American Anthropological Association, 2018; Council on Nursing and Anthropology, 2018). One of the central concepts that anthropologists study is **culture**. A complicated, multifaceted concept, culture has literally hundreds of definitions. The earliest recorded definition comes from a 19th-century British pioneer in the field of anthropology named Edward Tylor, who defined culture as the complex whole that includes knowledge, beliefs, art, morals, law, customs, and any other capabilities and habits acquired by members of a society (Tylor, 1871). Influenced by her formal academic preparation in anthropology (Mead, 1937), Leininger defines culture as the "learned, shared, and transmitted values, beliefs, norms, and lifeways of a particular group of people that guide thinking, decisions, and actions in a patterned way.... Culture is the blueprint that provides the broadest and most comprehensive means to know, explain, and predict people's lifeways over time and in different geographic locations" (McFarland & Wehbe-Alamah, 2015a, p. 10).

Culture influences a person's definition of health and illness, including when it is appropriate to self-treat and when the illness is sufficiently serious to seek assistance from one or more healers outside of the immediate family. The choice of healer and length of time a person is allowed to recover, after the birth of a baby or following the onset of an illness, are culturally determined. How a person behaves during an illness and the help rendered by others in facilitating healing also are culturally determined. Culture determines who

is permitted, or expected, to care for someone who is ill. Similarly, culture determines when a person is declared well and when they are healthy enough to resume activities of daily living and/or return to work. When someone is dying, culture often determines where, how, and with whom the person will spend his or her final hours, days, or weeks. Although the term culture sometimes connotes a person's racial or ethnic background, there are also many other examples of *nonethnic cultures*, such as those based on *socioeconomic status*, for example, the culture of poverty or affluence and the culture of the homeless; *ability or disability*, such as the culture of the deaf or hearing impaired and the culture of the blind or visually impaired; *sexual orientation*, such as the lesbian, gay, bisexual, and transgender (LGBT) cultures; *age*, such as the culture of adolescence and the culture of the elderly; and *occupational* or *professional* cultures, such as nursing (see Figure 1-1), medicine, and other professions in health care, the military, business, education, and related fields.

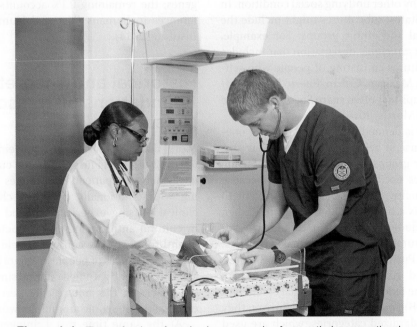

Figure 1-1. The profession of nursing is an example of a nonethnic occupational culture. The faculty member on the left is transmitting the requisite knowledge and skills from one generation to the next by mentoring the nursing student on the right.

In a classic study of culture by the anthropologist Edward Hall (1984), three levels of culture are identified: primary, secondary, and tertiary. The *primary level* of culture refers to the implicit rules known and followed by members of the group, but seldom stated or made explicit, to outsiders. The *secondary level* refers to underlying rules and **assumptions** that are known to members of the group but rarely shared with outsiders. The primary and secondary levels are the most deeply rooted and most difficult to change. The *tertiary level* refers to the explicit or public face that is visible to outsiders, including dress, rituals, cuisine, and festivals.

The term **subculture** refers to groups that have values and norms that are distinct from those held by the majority within a wider society. Members of subcultures have their own unique shared set of customs, attitudes, and values, often accompanied by group-specific language, jargon, and/or slang that sets them apart from others. A subculture can be organized around a common activity, occupation, age, ethnic background, race, religion, or any other unifying social condition. In the United States, subcultures might include the various racial and ethnic groups. For example, Hispanic is a *panethnic* designation that includes many subcultures consisting of people who self-identify with Mexican, Cuban, Puerto Rican, and/or other groups that often share Spanish language and culture (Morris, 2015).

Ethnicity is defined as the perception of oneself and a sense of belonging to a particular ethnic group or groups. It can also mean a feeling that one does not belong to any group because of multiethnicity. Ethnicity is not equivalent to race, which is a biological identification. Rather, ethnicity includes commitment to and involvement in cultural customs and rituals (Douglas, Pacquiao, & Purnell, 2018). In the United States, ethnicity and race are defined and numbers tracked by the federal Office of Management and Budget (OMB) and the U.S. Census Bureau; they provide standardized categories, which are used in the collection of census information on racial and ethnic populations and are also often used by biomedical researchers. The following ethnic and racial categories were used to collect data in the most recent U.S. census: White American, Native American, and Alaska Native; Asian American, Black, or African American; Native Hawaiian and other Pacific Islander; and people of two or more races; a race called "some other race" is also used in the census and other surveys but is not official. The Census Bureau also classifies Americans as "Hispanic or Latino" and "not Hispanic or Latino," which identifies Hispanic and Latino Americans as a racially diverse *ethnicity*.

In the traditional anthropological and biological systems of classification, **race** refers to a group of people who share genetically transmitted traits such as skin color, hair texture, and eye shape or color. Races are arbitrary classifications that lack definitional clarity because all cultures have their own ways of categorizing or classifying their members. (Some define race as a geographically and genetically distinct population, whereas others suggest that racial categories are socially constructed.) The most current scientific data indicate that all humans share the same 99.1% of genes; the remaining 0.1% accounts for the differences in humans (National Human Genome Institute, 2014).

Historical and Theoretical Foundations of Transcultural Nursing

More than 70 years ago, Madeleine Leininger (1925–2012; see Figure 1-2) noted cultural differences between patients and nurses while working with emotionally disturbed children. This clinical nursing experience piqued her interest in cultural anthropology. As a doctoral student in anthropology, she conducted field research on the care practices of people in Papua New Guinea and subsequently studied cultural similarities and differences in the culture care perceptions and expressions of people around the world.

At the same time that Leininger (Leininger, 1978, 1991, 1995, 1997, 1998, 1999; Leininger & McFarland, 2002, 2006; Leininger & Wehbe-Alamah, 2016, 2018) was establishing TCN, other

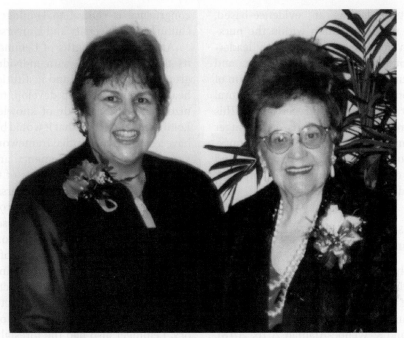

Figure 1-2. Author, Dr. Margaret Andrews (*left*), and Transcultural Nursing Foundress, Dr. Madeleine Leininger (*right*), at a meeting of the American Academy of Nursing.

anthropologists, nurse–anthropologists, and nurses who were studying, teaching, and writing about ethnicity, race, diversity, and/or culture in nursing used terms such as cross-cultural nursing, *ethnic nursing care* (Orque, Bloch, & Monrroy, 1983), or referred to *caring for people of color* (Branch & Paxton, 1976). The term *transcultural nursing* is used in this book, in recognition of the historical, research, and theoretical contributions of Leininger (1978), who used this term in her research and other scholarly works.

Leininger cites eight factors that influenced her to establish TCN as a framework for addressing 20th-century societal and health care challenges and issues, all of which remain relevant today:

1. A marked increase in the migration of people within and between countries worldwide
2. A rise in multicultural identities, with people expecting their cultural beliefs, values, and ways of life to be understood and respected by nurses and other health care providers

3. An increase in health care providers' and patients' use of technologies that connect people globally and simultaneously may become the source of conflict with the cultural values, beliefs, and practices of some of the people receiving care
4. Global cultural conflicts, clashes, and violence that impact health care as more cultures interact with one another
5. An increase in the number of people traveling and working in different parts of the world
6. An increase in legal actions resulting from cultural conflict, negligence, ignorance, and the imposition of health care practices
7. A rise in awareness of gender issues, with growing demands on health care systems to meet the gender- and age-specific needs of men, women, and children
8. An increased demand for community- and culturally based health care services in diverse environmental contexts (Leininger, 1995; McFarland & Wehbe-Alamah, 2018)

TCN exists today as an evidence-based, dynamic area of specialization within the nursing profession because of the visionary leadership of its founder, Madeleine Leininger, and many other nurses committed to the provision of care that is consistent with and "fits" the cultural beliefs and practices of those receiving it. This section explores the contributions of Leininger and then examines the ways in which other nursing scholars contributed to the development and advancement of TCN theory, research, practice, education, and administration globally.

Leininger's Contributions to Transcultural Nursing

Leininger's Theory of Culture Care Diversity and Universality describes, explains, and predicts nursing similarities and differences in care and caring in human cultures (Leininger, 1991; McFarland & Wehbe-Alamah 2016, 2018). Leininger uses concepts such as worldview, social and cultural structure, language, ethnohistory, environmental context, and folk and professional healing systems to provide a comprehensive and holistic view of factors that influence culture care. Culturally based care factors are recognized as major influences on human experiences related to well-being, health, illness, disability, and death. After conducting a comprehensive cultural assessment based on the preceding factors, the three modes of nursing decisions and actions—culture care preservation and/or maintenance, culture care accommodation and/or negotiation, and culture care repatterning and/or restructuring—are used to provide **culturally congruent nursing care** (Leininger, 1991, 1995; Leininger & McFarland, 2002, 2006; McFarland & Wehbe-Alamah, 2018). Culturally congruent nursing care "refers to those cognitively based assistive, supportive, facilitative, or enabling acts or decisions that are mostly tailor-made to fit with an individual's, group's or institution's cultural values, beliefs, and lifeways in order to provide meaningful, beneficial, satisfying care that leads to health and well-being" (Leininger, 1991, p. 47). Cultural congruence is central to Leininger's Theory of Culture Care Diversity and Universality.

Among the strengths of Leininger's theory is its flexibility for use with individuals, families, groups, communities, and institutions in diverse health systems. To help develop, test, and organize the emerging body of knowledge in TCN, Leininger recognized that it would be necessary to have a specific conceptual framework from which various theoretical statements are developed. Figure 1-3 depicts components of the Theory of Culture Care Diversity and Universality, provides a visual representation of the components of Leininger's Sunrise Enabler to Discover Culture Care, and illustrates the interrelationships among the components. As the world of nursing and health care has become increasingly multicultural, the theory's relevance has increased as well.

While creating TCN as a respected and recognized nursing specialty and developing her theory, Leininger also had the foresight to establish the Transcultural Nursing Society (TCNS), generate the *TCNS Newsletter*, and create the *Journal of Transcultural Nursing* (JTN), for which she served as the founding editor. The TCNS holds regional and annual conferences, disseminates the newsletter, and collaborates with a publishing company to produce a quarterly journal, all of which provide forums for the exchange of TCN knowledge, research, and evidence-based best practices relative to the provision of culturally congruent and culturally competent nursing and health care. To integrate TCN into the curricula of schools of nursing, Leininger established the first master's and doctoral programs in nursing with a theoretical and research focus in TCN and provided exemplars for TCN courses and curricula suitable for all levels of nursing education (undergraduate and graduate) through her lectures, publications, and consultations. Leininger also created a new qualitative research method called **ethnonursing research** to investigate phenomena of interest in TCN (Leininger, 1995; Leininger & McFarland, 2002, 2006; McFarland, Mixer, Wehbe-Alamah, & Burk, 2012; McFarland & Wehbe-Alamah, 2016, 2018). Hundreds of

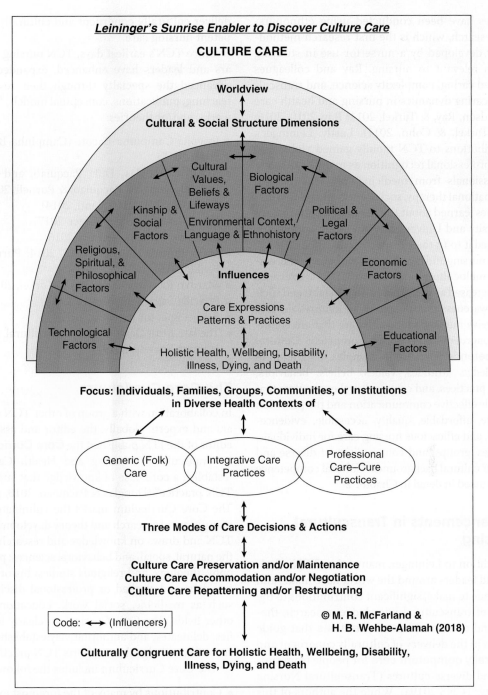

Figure 1-3. Leininger's Sunrise Enabler to Discover Culture Care. Used with permission.
McFarland, M. R., & Wehbe-Alamah, H. B. (2018). Source: McFarland, M. & Wehbe-Alamah, H.
(2018). Transcultural nursing concepts, theories, research, & practice. (4th edition). New York, NY:
McGraw-Hill Education. ISBN: 978-0-07-184113-9.

studies have been conducted using ethnonursing research, which is the first research methodology developed by a nurse for use in studying topics relevant to nursing. Ray and colleagues studied caring, complexity science, and transcultural caring dynamics in nursing and health care (Davidson, Ray, & Turkel, 2011; Ray, 2010, 2016; Ray, Turkel, & Cohn, 2011). Lastly, Leininger's contributions to TCN rapidly gained global and interprofessional recognition as many health care professionals from medicine, physical therapy, occupational therapy, social work, and related disciplines learned about the Theory of Culture Care Diversity and Universality and either adopted or adapted it to fit their respective disciplines.

As nursing and health care have become increasingly multicultural and diverse, TCN's relevance has increased as well. There also is heightened societal awareness that people of all cultures deserve to receive nursing and health care that are culturally congruent and culturally competent. **Cultural competence** refers to the complex integration of knowledge, attitudes, values, beliefs, behaviors, skills, practices, and cross-cultural encounters that include effective communication and the provision of safe, affordable, quality, accessible, evidence-based, and efficacious nursing care for individuals, families, groups, and communities of diverse and similar cultural backgrounds. Cultural competence is discussed in detail in Chapter 2.

Advancements in Transcultural Nursing

In addition to Leininger, many other TCN scholars and leaders around the world have made, and continue to make, significant contributions to the body of transcultural knowledge, research, theory, and **evidence-based practices** that guide nurses in the delivery of culturally congruent and **culturally competent care** for people from similar and diverse cultures (Transcultural Nursing Society, TCNS 2019a). While the authors of this textbook have chosen to emphasize the research and theory generated by Leininger, there are many different ways to conceptualize TCN and

deliver culturally congruent and culturally competent nursing care.

Since TCN's earliest days, TCN nursing scholars and leaders have enhanced, expanded, and advanced the specialty through their research, teaching, publications, conceptual models, frameworks, and/or theories:

- Josepha Campinha-Bacote (Campinha-Bacote, 2011, 2015)
- Marilyn Douglas, Dula Pacquiao, and Larry Purnell (Douglas, Pacquiao, & Purnell, 2018)
- Geri-Ann Galanti (Galanti, 2014)
- Joyce Newman Giger (Giger, 2017)
- Marianne Jeffreys (Jeffreys 2016)
- Larry Purnell (Purnell, 2013, 2014; Purnell & Fenkl, 2018)
- Marilyn Ray (Ray, 2016; Ray & Turkel, 2014)
- Priscilla Sagar (Sagar, 2012, 2014)
- Rachel Spector (Spector, 2017)
- The late Ruth Davidhizar (Transcultural Nursing Society, 2019)

The Core Curriculum

In collaboration with a group of other TCN scholars and experts globally, the editor and associate editor of the JTN published the **Core Curriculum** in Transcultural Nursing and Health Care to "establish a core base of knowledge that supports TCN practice" (Douglas & Pacquiao, 2010, p. S5). The Core Curriculum marks the culmination of many years of research and theory development in TCN and draws on knowledge and research from the natural, social, and behavioral sciences; philosophy, theology, and religious studies; history; the fine arts; and applied or professional disciplines such as medicine, social work, education, and other fields. The Core Curriculum clearly identifies, delineates, and authoritatively establishes the core of knowledge that supports TCN practice.

The Core Curriculum includes the following:

- Contributions by many of the foremost experts in TCN from around the world who provide concrete and specific curricular outline for TCN

- A comprehensive compendium that contains an overview of the key knowledge, research, evidence, and general content areas that collectively form the foundation for TCN practice
- Content on subjects such as global health; comparative systems of health care delivery; cross-cultural communication; culturally based health and illness beliefs and practices across the lifespan; culturally based healing and care modalities; cultural health assessment; educational issues for students, organizational staff, patients, and communities; organizational cultural competency; research methodologies for investigating cultural phenomena and evaluating interventions; and professional roles and attributes of the transcultural nurse
- Content that will prepare nurses to take one or both of the examinations leading to **TCN certification**
- Basic certification in transcultural nursing (CTN-B) and advanced certification in transcultural nursing (CTN-A). Both exams are offered by the TCNS's Certification Commission (Transcultural Nursing Society, 2019) and appear on the list of Magnet national certifications for inclusion on the Demographic Data Collection Tool. See Sagar (2015) for additional information about certification in TCN and/or or visit the Transcultural Nursing Society website for an application (TCNS, 2019b)

The Core Curriculum also is used in schools of nursing, hospitals, health departments, and other health care organizations to determine the key content to be included in seminars, workshops, conferences, and credit-bearing and continuing professional development courses on TCN and cultural competency. Those interested in cultural competence, multiculturalism, diversity, and related topics from multiple disciplines will also find valuable information in the Core Curriculum. As scientific, technological, and discipline-specific advances are made in TCN, the Core Curriculum will be updated and refined.

The coauthors of this book contributed to the Core Curriculum, as did many of the chapter contributors; therefore, the key concepts contained in the Core Curriculum also are found in this book.

Andrews/Boyle Transcultural Interprofessional Practice Model

Conceptual frameworks, theoretical models, and theories in nursing are structured ideas about human beings and their health. Models enable nurses and other health care team members to organize and understand what happens in practice, critically analyze situations for clinical decision-making, develop a plan of care, propose appropriate nursing interventions, predict the outcomes from the care, and evaluate the effectiveness of the care provided (Alligood, 2014).

Goals, Assumptions, and Components of the Model

The goals of the Andrews/Boyle TIP Model are to:

- Provide a systematic, logical, orderly, scientific process for delivering culturally congruent, culturally competent, safe, affordable, accessible, and quality care to people from diverse backgrounds across the lifespan.
- Facilitate the delivery of nursing and health care that is beneficial, meaningful, relevant, culturally congruent, culturally competent, and consistent with the cultural beliefs and practices of clients from diverse backgrounds.
- Provide a conceptual framework to guide nurses in the delivery of culturally congruent and competent care that is theoretically sound and evidence based and utilizes best professional practices.

Fundamental assumptions underlying the TIP Model include those related to TCN (Box 1-1), humans (Box 1-2), and **cross-cultural communication** between and among team members (Box 1-3). These assumptions are ideas that are formed or taken for granted as having veracity without proof or evidence. Assumptions are useful in providing a basis for action and in creating "what-if..." scenarios to simulate possible situations until such time as there is proof or

BOX 1-1 | Assumptions About Transcultural Nursing

- Transcultural nursing is a theoretical and evidence-based formal area of study and practice within professional nursing that focuses on people's culturally based beliefs, attitudes, values, behaviors, and practices related to wellness, health, birth, illness, healing, dying, and death.
- Transcultural nursing requires that nurses engage in an ongoing process of constructively critical, reflective self-assessment that enables them to identify their own culturally based values, attitudes, beliefs, behaviors, biases, stereotypes, prejudices, and practices.
- Transcultural nursing knowledge is interconnected with the knowledge, research, and scholarship of other disciplines in the natural sciences (e.g., biology, chemistry, physics), social and behavioral sciences (e.g., anthropology, sociology, psychology, economics, political science), professional disciplines (e.g., medicine, pharmacy, social work, education), and the humanities (e.g., music, art, history, languages, philosophy, theater).
- Transcultural nursing practice encompasses autonomous and collaborative care of individuals of all ages across the lifespan whether they are sick or well, able or disabled.
- Transcultural nursing engages nurses the care of families, groups, populations, and communities globally.
- Transcultural nursing includes the promotion of health, the prevention of disease, and the care of sick, ill, disabled, and dying people from diverse cultures across the lifespan from birth to old age.
- Transcultural nursing roles include advocacy, research, health policy development, health systems leadership, management, education, clinical practice, and consultation.

- Transcultural nursing practice requires that nurses establish and maintain a caring, empathetic, therapeutic relationship with clients and a collaborative, collegial relationship with other members of the interprofessional health care team.
- Transcultural nursing assessment is facilitated when the nurse's communications are client-centered and focused on establishing and maintaining a therapeutic nurse–client relationship.
- Transcultural nursing practice requires that nurses be aware of changes in the world that influence and challenge their knowledge of the unfolding meaning of diversity and the need for the delivery of nursing and health care that is respectful and responsive to individual needs and differences of the people and communities served.
- Transcultural nursing practice encompasses autonomous and collaborative care of individuals of all ages, families, groups, and communities, sick or well and in all settings.
- Transcultural nursing practice requires that nurses establish and maintain a caring, empathetic, therapeutic relationship with clients; formally educated and/or licensed credentialed healers, such as registered nurses, licensed physicians, and other health professionals; and folk, traditional, religious, spiritual, and other healers are identified by clients as significant to their health and well-being.
- In transcultural nursing practice, the nurse's communications are oriented and focused on what is best for the client's health, well-being, recovery, or peaceful death.
- Transcultural nursing practice requires that nurses be respectful and responsive to individual needs and differences of the people and communities served.

BOX 1-2 | Assumptions About Humans

- Humans are complex biological, cultural, psychosocial, spiritual beings who experience health and illness along a continuum throughout the span of their lives from birth to death.
- All humans have the right to safe, accessible, and affordable nursing and health care, regardless of national origin, race, ethnicity, gender, age, socioeconomic background, religion, sexual orientation, size, and related characteristics.
- Whether rich or poor; educated or illiterate; religious or nonbelieving; male or female; black, white, yellow, red, or brown, each person deserves to be respected by nurses and other members of the health care team.
- As people from different racial, ethnic, and cultural backgrounds travel and comingle with those having backgrounds that differ from their own, the likelihood of intermarriage and offspring of mixed racial and ethnic heritage increases.
- Regardless of their national origin or current citizenship, humans around the world share culture-universal needs for food, shelter, safety, and love; seek well-being and health; and endeavor to avoid, alleviate, or eliminate the pain and suffering associated with disease, illness, dying, and death.
- Although humans have common culture-universal needs, they also have culture-specific needs that are interconnected with their health-related values, attitudes, beliefs, and practices.
- In times of health and illness, humans seek the therapeutic (beneficial) assistance of various types of healers to promote health and well-being, prevent disease, and recover from illness or injury.
- Humans seek therapeutic interventions from family and significant others; credentialed or licensed health care providers; folk, traditional, indigenous, religious, and/or spiritual healers; and companion or therapy animals and pets as they perceive appropriate for their condition, situation, or problem.
- Interventions are judged to have a therapeutic effect when they result in a desirable and beneficial outcome, whether the outcome was expected, unexpected, or even an unintended consequence of the intervention.

BOX 1-3 | Assumptions About Effective Communication

- Effective communication begins with an assessment of the client's ability to read, write, speak, and comprehend messages.
- Effective communication in contemporary society sometimes requires literacy in the use of computers, smartphones, and numerous technology-assisted medical or health devices.
- Effective communication includes the ability to convey sincere interest in others, patience, and willingness to intervene or begin again when misunderstandings occur.
- To provide safe, quality, affordable, accessible, efficacious, culturally congruent, and culturally competent nursing and health care, members of the interprofessional health care team must communicate effectively.
- Communication occurs verbally, nonverbally, in writing, and in combination with technology.
- Communication should be appropriate for the client's age, gender, health status, health literacy, and related factors.
- When nurses communicate with others from cultural and linguistic backgrounds different from their own, the probability of miscommunication increases significantly.
- In promoting effective cross-cultural communication with clients from diverse backgrounds, nurses should avoid technical jargon, slang, colloquial expressions, abbreviations, and excessive use of medical terminology.

evidence available to corroborate or refute the assumption.

The TIP Model consists of the following interconnected and interrelated components:

1. The **context** from which people's health-related values, attitudes, beliefs, and practices emerge
2. The **interprofessional health care team**
3. **Communication**
4. The **problem-solving process**

Cultural Context

Derived from the Latin word *contexere* (*con-* meaning together and *texere* meaning to weave or braid), the term context refers to the conditions, circumstances, and/or situations that exist when and where something happens, thereby providing meaning to what transpired. In the TIP Model, the following factors contribute to the **cultural context** of human experiences and need to be assessed, interpreted, examined, and evaluated when clients interact with nurses and other members of the interprofessional health care team: environmental, social, economic, religious, philosophical, moral, legal, political, educational, biological (genetic/inherited factors), and technological. In TCN, culture is the lens through which nurses see the world, their clients, and other members of the team. When culture is interwoven with the other factors (see Figure 1-4), it forms the health-related cultural values, attitudes, beliefs, and practices of humans worldwide, including clients and other members of the team.

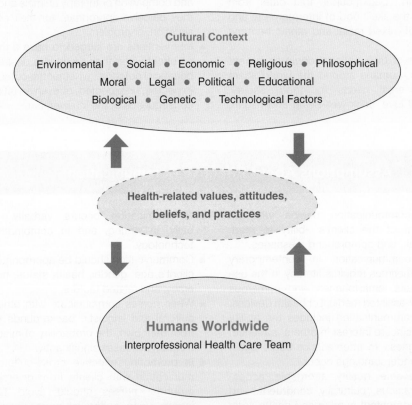

Figure 1-4. Influence of cultural context on health values, beliefs, and practices of the interprofessional health care team. (© Margaret M. Andrews.)

Interprofessional Health Care Team

The transcultural interprofessional health care team has at its core the *client*, who is the team's raison d'être (reason for being). In addition to the client, the team may have one or more of the following members:

- The *client's family* and *others significant in his or her life*, including a legally appointed *guardian* who might not be genetically related
- *Credentialed health professionals* such as nurses; physicians; physical, occupational, respiratory, music, art, dance, recreational, and other therapists; social workers; health navigators; public and community health workers; and related professionals with formal academic preparation, licensure, and/or certification
- *Folk, indigenous, or traditional healers*—unlicensed individuals who learn healing arts and practices through study, observation, apprenticeship, and imitation and sometimes by inheriting healing powers, for example, herbalists, curanderos, medicine men/women, Amish brauchers, bonesetters, lay midwives, sabadors, and healers with related names
- *Religious or spiritual healers*—clergy or lay members of religious groups who heal through prayer, religious or spiritual rituals, faith healing practices, and related actions or interventions, for example, priests, priestesses, elders, rabbis, imams, monks, Christian Science practitioners, and others believed to have healing powers derived from faith, spiritual powers, or religion
- *Others* identified by the client as significant to his or her health, well-being, or healing such as companion animals or pets as culturally appropriate

The World Health Organization defines **interprofessional collaboration** as multiple health workers from different professional backgrounds working together with patients, families, caregivers, and communities to deliver the highest quality of care (World Health Organization, 2013). In collaboration with leaders in nursing, dentistry, and other health care fields, the Institute of Medicine (2011) advocates that interprofessional collaboration be integrated into the curricula of health professions programs, building on recommendations from its earlier report, *To Err is Human*, which focuses on the threat to patient safety caused by human error and ineffective interprofessional communication (Institute of Medicine, 1999).

To be successful in interprofessional collaboration, the following core competencies are required: values and ethics related to interprofessional practice, knowledge of the roles of team members, and a team approach to health care (Fulmer & Gaines, 2014; Institute of Medicine, 1999, 2011; Interprofessional Education Collaborative Expert Panel, 2011; O'Brien, 2013). Interprofessional collaboration is a partnership that starts with the client and includes all involved health care providers working together to deliver client- and family-centered care. Trust must be established and an appreciation of each other's roles must be gained in order for effective collaboration to take place (Interprofessional Education Collaborative Expert Panel). Health professionals must recognize their own individual scope of practice and skill set and have an awareness of and appreciation for other health professionals' capacity to contribute to the delivery of care to clients in order to achieve optimal health outcomes. Working as a member of an interprofessional team requires communication, cooperation, and collaboration (Fulmer & Gaines, 2014; Institute of Medicine, 2011; Interprofessional Education Collaborative Expert Panel, 2011; Interprofessional Education Collaborative, 2016).

Communication

Derived from the Latin verb *communicare*, meaning to share, **communication** refers to the meaningful exchange of information between one or more participants. The information exchanged may be conveyed through ideas, feelings, intentions, attitudes, expectations, perceptions, instructions, or commands. Communication is an organized, patterned system of behavior that makes all nurse–client interactions possible. It is the exchange of messages and the creation of meaning (Munoz & Luckman, 2008). Because communication and culture are acquired simultaneously, they are integrally linked. Figure 1-5 illustrates the ways in which communication, cultural context, and health-related values, attitudes, beliefs, and practices of members of the interprofessional health care team are interconnected and interrelated. In effective communication, there is mutual understanding of the meaning attached to the messages.

Being respectful and polite, using language that is understood by the other(s), and speaking clearly will facilitate **verbal** (or spoken) **communication**. Barriers to effective verbal communication occur when participants are using different languages; when technical terms, abbreviations, idioms, colloquialisms, or regional expressions are used; or when the tone of voice conveys a message that is inconsistent with the words spoken, for example, a client in the postanesthesia care

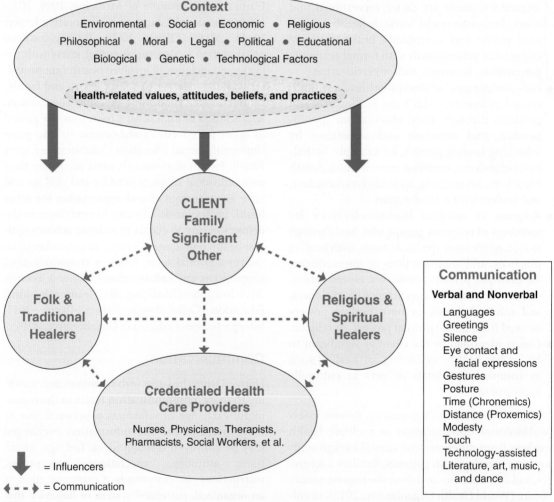

Figure 1-5. Cross-cultural communication among members of the interprofessional health care team—clients, family, significant others, credentialed health professionals, and folk, traditional, religious, and spiritual healers. (© Margaret M. Andrews.)

unit following major surgery verbally denies having pain, but the nurse observes that the client has clenched teeth, taught muscles, pursed lips, and a wrinkled brow, all of which are nonverbal indicators of pain. Whereas **language** refers to what is said, **paralanguage** refers to *how* it is said and relates to all aspects of the voice that are not part of the verbal message. Paralanguage may modify or nuance meaning or convey emotion through rhythm, pitch, stress, volume, speed, hesitations, or intonation. For example, consider the sentence, "I would like to help you." By placing the emphasis on the words I, like, help, and you in four different sentences, the meaning of the sentence changes significantly. **Nonverbal communication** refers to how people convey meaning without words through the use of facial expressions, gestures, posture (body language), and the physical distance between the communicators (proxemics).

The many nuances of verbal and nonverbal communication are interconnected, interwoven, interrelated, and often embedded in one another. Aspects of communication that are of particular importance for the transcultural nurse include language, the use of interpreters, greetings, silence, eye contact and facial expressions, gestures, posture, chronemics (time), proxemics, modesty, touch, technology-assisted communication, and literature, art, music, and dance.

Language

More than 7,000 languages are spoken throughout the world. Three hundred and eighty-two individual languages and language groups are spoken in the United States alone, where nearly 62 million people, aged 5 years or older, speak a language other than English at home (Center for Immigration Studies, 2017). Fifty-six percent of the people who speak a language other than English at home report they speak English "very well" (U.S. Census Bureau, 2018). Spanish is the second most commonly spoken language in the United States, spoken by 37 million people aged 5 and older; 9% of those individuals indicated that they did not speak English at all (U.S. Census Bureau, 2018). After English (230.9 million speakers) and Spanish

(37.5 million), Chinese (2.8 million) was the language most commonly spoken at home. More than 350 languages are spoken in U.S. homes including North American languages such as Pennsylvania Dutch and > 150 different ones spoken by Native Americans (U.S. Census Bureau, 2015). Language is one of the primary ways that culture is transmitted from one generation to the next.

Interpreters

One of the greatest challenges in cross-cultural communication for nurses occurs when the nurse and client speak different languages. After assessing the language skills of the client who speaks a different language from the nurse, the nurse may be in one of two situations: either struggling to communicate effectively through an interpreter or communicating effectively when there is no interpreter. Box 1-4 provides recommendations for overcoming language barriers.

Even a person from another culture or country who has a basic command of the language spoken by the majority of nurses and other health professionals may need an interpreter when faced with the anxiety-provoking situation of entering a hospital, encountering an unfamiliar symptom, or discussing a sensitive topic such as birth control or gynecologic or urologic concerns. A trained medical interpreter knows interpreting techniques, has knowledge of medical terminology, and understands patients' rights. The trained interpreter is also knowledgeable about cultural beliefs and health practices. This person can help bridge the cultural gap and can give advice concerning the cultural appropriateness of nursing and medical recommendations.

Although the nurse is in charge of the focus and flow of the interview, the interpreter should be viewed as an important member of the health care team. It can be tempting to ask a relative, a friend, or even another client to interpret because this person is readily available and likely is willing to help. However, this violates confidentiality for the client, who may not want personal information shared. Furthermore, the friend or relative, though fluent in ordinary language usage, is likely to be unfamiliar with medical terminology,

BOX 1-4 | Overcoming Language Barriers

Using an Interpreter

- Before locating an interpreter, determine the language the client speaks at home; it may be different from the language spoken publicly (e.g., French is sometimes spoken by well-educated and upper-class members of certain Asian or Middle Eastern cultures).
- After assessing client's health literacy, use electronic devices such as cell phones, tablets, and laptop computers to connect client with Web-based translation programs.
- Avoid interpreters from a rival tribe, state, region, or nation (e.g., a Palestinian who knows Hebrew may not be the best interpreter for a Jewish client).
- Be aware of gender differences between interpreter and client. In general, the same gender is preferred.
- Be aware of age differences between interpreter and client. In general, an older, more mature interpreter is preferred to a younger, less experienced one.
- Be aware of socioeconomic differences between interpreter and client.
- Ask the interpreter to translate as closely to verbatim as possible.
- Expect an interpreter who is not a relative to seek compensation for services rendered.

Recommendations for Institutions

- Keep pace with assistive equipment and technology for people who are deaf, hard of hearing, blind, visually impaired, and/or disabled.
- Maintain a computerized list of interpreters, including those certified in sign language, who may be contacted as needed.
- Network with area hospitals, colleges, universities, and other organizations that may serve as resources.

What to Do When There Is No Interpreter

- Be polite and formal.
- Greet the person using the last or complete name. Gesture to yourself and say your name. Offer a handshake or nod. Smile.
- Proceed in an unhurried manner. Pay attention to any effort by the patient or family to communicate.
- Speak in a low, moderate voice. Avoid talking loudly. There is often a tendency to raise the volume and pitch of your voice when the listener appears not to understand, but this may lead the listener to perceive that the nurse is shouting and/or angry.
- Use any words known in the patient's language.
- Use simple words, such as *pain* instead of *discomfort*. Avoid medical jargon, idioms, and slang. Avoid using contractions. Use nouns repeatedly instead of pronouns. For example, do *not* say, "He has been taking his medicine, hasn't he?" Do say, "Does Juan take medicine?"
- Pantomime words and simple actions while verbalizing them.
- Give instructions in the proper sequence. For example, do *not* say, "Before you rinse the bottle, sterilize it." Do say, "First, wash the bottle. Second, rinse the bottle."
- Discuss one topic at a time. Avoid using conjunctions. For example, do *not* say, "Are you cold and in pain?" Do say, "Are you cold [while pantomiming]?" "Are you in pain?"
- Validate whether the client understands by having him or her repeat instructions, demonstrate the procedure, or act out the meaning.
- Write out several short sentences in English, and determine the person's ability to read them.
- Try a third language. Many Southeast Asians speak French. Europeans often know three or four languages.
- Ask if a family member or friend of the same gender could serve as an interpreter.
- Use online translation program for the appropriate languages, contact hospitals for a list of interpreters, and use both formal and informal networking to locate a suitable interpreter.

Adapted from Andrews, M. (2000). Transcultural considerations in health assessment. In C. Jarvis (Ed.), *Physical examination and health assessment* (p. 69). Philadelphia, PA: W.B. Saunders.

hospital or clinic procedures, and health care ethics. In ideal circumstances, ask the interpreter to meet the client beforehand to establish rapport and obtain basic descriptive information about the client such as age, occupation, educational level, and attitude toward health care. This eases the interpreter and client into the relationship and allows the client to talk about aspects of his or her life that are relatively nonthreatening.

When using an interpreter, expect that the interaction with the client will require more time than is needed if the nurse and client speak the same language. It will be necessary to organize nursing care so that the most important interactions or procedures are accomplished first, before the client becomes fatigued. In the absence of an interpreter, try using electronic devices with translation software and other applications that may be helpful in effectively communicating and delivering care for people who speak a language different from the nurse.

Greetings

Some cultures value formal greetings at the start of the day or whenever the first encounter of the day occurs—a practice found even among close family members. When communicating with people from cultures that tend to be more formal, it is important to call a person by his or her title, such as Mr., Mrs., Ms., Dr., Reverend, and related greeting as a sign of respect, and until such time as the individual gives permission to address them less formally. The recommended best practice at the time the nurse initially meets a client or new member of the health care team is to state his or her name and then ask the client or team member by what name he or she prefers to be called.

Silence

Wide cultural variations exist in the interpretation of silence. Some individuals find silence extremely uncomfortable and make every effort to fill conversational lags with words. By contrast, many Native Americans consider silence essential to understanding and respecting the other person. A pause following a question signifies that what has been asked is important enough to be given thoughtful consideration. In traditional Chinese and Japanese cultures, silence may mean that the speaker wishes the listener to consider the content of what has been said before continuing. Other cultural meanings of silence may be found. Arabs may use silence out of respect for another's privacy, whereas people of French, Spanish, and Russian descent may interpret it as a sign of agreement. Asian cultures often use silence to demonstrate respect for elders. Among some African Americans, silence is used in response to a question perceived as inappropriate.

Eye Contact and Facial Expressions

Eye contact and facial expressions are the most prominent forms of nonverbal communication. Eye contact is a key factor in setting the tone of the communication between two people and differs greatly between cultures and countries. In the United States, Canada, Western Europe, and most parts of Australia, eye contact is interpreted similarly: conveying interest, active engagement with the other person, forthrightness, and honesty. People who avoid eye contact when speaking are viewed negatively and may be perceived as withholding information and/or lacking in confidence. In some parts of Asia, Africa, and the Middle East and certain Native American nations, however, direct eye contact may be seen as disrespectful, a sign of aggression, or a sign that the other person's authority is being challenged. In some cultures, staring at someone for a prolonged period of time communicates that the person doing the staring has a sexual interest in the other person. People who make eye contact, but only briefly, are viewed as respectful and courteous. In some Native American cultures, the person might look at the floor while someone in a position of authority is speaking as a sign of respect and interest. Among some African American and White cultures, *occulistics* (eye rolling) takes place when someone speaks or behaves in a manner that is regarded as inappropriate.

Strongly influenced by a person's cultural background, facial expressions include *affective displays* that reveal emotions, such as happiness through a smile or sadness through crying, and various other nonverbal gestures that may be perceived as appropriate or inappropriate according to the person's age and gender. These nonverbal expressions are often unintentional and can conflict with what is being said verbally.

Gestures

Gestures that serve the same function as words are referred to as *emblems*. Examples of emblems include signals that mean okay, the "thumbs-up" gesture, the "come here" hand movement, or the hand gesture used when hitchhiking. Gestures that accompany words to illustrate a verbal message are known as *illustrators*. Illustrators mimic the spoken word, such as pointing to the right or left while verbally saying the words right or left. *Regulators* convey meaning through gestures such as raising one's hand before verbally asking a question. Regulators also include head nodding and short sounds such as "uh huh" or "Hmmmm" and other expressions of interest or boredom. Without feedback, some people find it difficult to carry on a conversation. *Adaptors* are nonverbal behavior that either satisfy some physical need such as scratching or adjusting eyeglasses or represent a psychological need such as biting fingernails when nervous, yawning when bored, or clenching a fist when angry. Although normally subconscious, adaptors are more likely to be restrained in public places than in private gatherings of people. Adaptive behaviors often accompany feelings of anxiety or hostility (Galvin, Prescott, & Huseman, 1988). All of the nonverbal communication previously described varies widely cross-culturally and cross-nationally.

Posture

Posture reflects people's emotions, attitudes, and intentions. Posture may be open or closed and is believed to convey an individual's degree of confidence, status, or receptivity to another person. An open posture is characterized by hands apart or comfortably placed on the arms of a chair while directly facing the person speaking. The person often leans forward, toward the speaker. Open posture communicates interest in someone and a readiness to listen. Someone seated in a closed posture might have his or her arms folded and legs crossed or be positioned at a slight angle from the person with whom they are interacting. The person may also allow his or her eyes to dart quickly from one spot to another in an unfocused, distracted manner. Closed posture usually conveys disinterest or discomfort.

Chronemics

There are cultural variations in how people understand and use time. **Chronemics** is the study of the use of time in nonverbal communication. The manner in which a person perceives and values time, structures time, and reacts to time contributes to the context of communication. Social scientists have discovered that individuals are divided in two major groups in the ways they approach time: **monochronic** or **polychronic**. In monochronic cultures, such as many groups in the United States, Northern Europe, Israel, and much of Australia, time is seen as a commodity, and people tend to use expressions such as "waste time" or "lose time" or "time is money." Given that time is so highly valued, showing up late, especially for a meeting or a dinner, is usually perceived as very disrespectful to the individuals who are made to "waste their time" waiting (Lombardo, n.d.). A monochronic culture functions on clock time. People tend to focus on one thing at a time and usually prefer to complete objectives in a systematic way. In a meeting, for example, it's considered culturally appropriate to follow the predetermined agenda and avoid straying from the agenda by talking about unrelated topics (Rutledge, 2013).

People in **polychronic cultures**, such as some groups in Southern Europe, Latin America, Africa, and the Middle East, take a very different view of time. People from these cultures often believe that time cannot be controlled, and it is flexible. Days are planned based on events rather than the clock. For many people in these cultures, when one event is finished, it is time to start the next, regardless of what time it is. In a polychronic culture, following an agenda might not be very important. Instead, many tasks, such as building relationships, negotiating, and/or problem-solving, can be accomplished at the same time. In many Asian cultures, such as Japanese, Chinese, and Taiwanese groups, people tend to arrive a little early. In many parts of Europe, the United States, Canada, Israel, and Australia, people tend to arrive precisely on time and may perceive it as an inconvenience to others if they arrive too early. In many parts of Latin America, Arab areas in the Middle East, and Africa, people tend to be more flexible in their notion of arrival times and may show up significantly later than the mutually agreed-upon time. Among certain Native American groups, an appointment or event begins "when everyone arrives," and there is considerable tolerance for those who show up after the appointed time. These examples are stereotypes, and not all of members of a culture or subculture will perceive time in the same manner.

Proxemics

Another form of nonverbal communication is manifested in closeness and **personal space**. The study of space and how differences in that space can make people feel more relaxed or more anxious is referred to as **proxemics**, a term that was coined in the 1950s by the anthropologist and cross-cultural researcher Edward T. Hall. Distances have been identified based on the relationship between or among the people involved (Hall, 1984, 1990):

1. *Intimate space* (touching to 1 foot) is typically reserved for whispering and embracing; however, nurses and other health care providers sometimes need to enter this intimate space when providing care for clients.

2. *Personal space* (ranges from 2 to 4 feet) is used among family and friends or to separate people waiting in line at the drug store or ATM.
3. *Social space* (4 to 10 feet) is used for communication among business or work associates and to separate strangers, such as those taking a course on natural child birth.
4. *Public space* (12 to 25 feet) is the distance maintained between a speaker and the audience.

Cultural and ethnic variations occur in proxemics. For example, when having a conversation, people from Arab parts of the Middle East, France, and Latin America generally prefer to stand closer to one another than those from Canadian, American, and British cultures, who also tend to feel more uncomfortable when they have to sit close to one another (Munoz & Luckman, 2008). There are also important gender and age factors to consider in cross-cultural communication. In general, clients are likely to prefer a nurse or other health care provider of the *same gender*, particularly when care requires entering his or her personal space and/or touching the client. Similarly, the same gender may be preferred when the health history and/or physical examination includes the reproductive organs. In some ethnic and religious groups, it may be inappropriate or forbidden for health care providers of the opposite gender to shake hands, provide care, or otherwise touch the client. For example, observant Muslim women are not permitted to shake hands with male physicians, nurses, or other health professionals. As a sign of respect to the man, some Muslim women will place one or both arms over their chest and slightly bow their head. Whenever an observant Muslim is having a conversation with a person of the opposite gender, a third person needs to be present to avoid the appearance of impropriety. Among some people from Chinese, Japanese, or other Asian cultures, there may be both gender and age factors to be considered in cross-cultural communication.

Modesty

Modesty is a form of mixed nonverbal and verbal communication that refers to reserve or propriety in speech, dress, or behavior. It conveys a message that is intended to avoid encouraging sexual attention or attraction in others (aside from a person's spouse). In cultures that have been studied by anthropologists or transcultural nurses, men and women have cultural beliefs about modesty and rules concerning which behavior and dress are appropriate in various situations and circumstances. The following are examples of groups that have required rules or optional guidelines pertaining to modesty.

Traditional Muslim women beyond the age of puberty wear a headscarf to cover their head and hair as a sign of modesty and religious faith. The word **hijab** describes the act of covering up generally but is sometimes used to describe the headscarves worn by Muslim women (Figure 1-6). These scarves come in many styles and colors and have different names around the world, such as *niqab, al-mira, shayla, khimar, chador,* and *burka.*

The type of hijab most commonly worn in the United States, Canada, Australia, and Western Europe covers the head and neck but leaves the face clear. In various parts of the Arab world, cultural expectations for women may include covering the head, face, neck, or entire body in order to conform to certain standards of modesty established by various Islamic denominations and groups. The *burka* is the most concealing of all Islamic coverings. It is a one-piece veil that conceals the face and body, often leaving just a mesh screen to see through. There are differences between modesty at home and modesty in public. At home, Muslim women typically do not wear veils, scarves, or other coverings in the presence of male family members such as their fathers, husbands, sons, and other male or female relatives.

Women from observant Orthodox and Hasidic Judaism, Amish, Mennonite, and some conservative Catholics cover their heads, arms, and/or legs as a cultural and/or religious expression of modesty and often as a sign of their affiliation with a particular religious order within Catholicism.

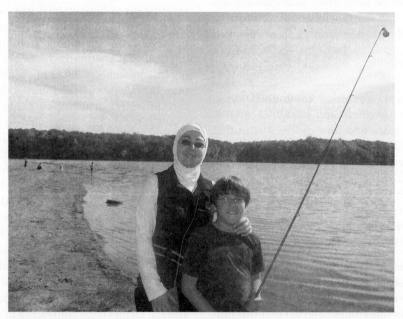

Figure 1-6. When in public places, some Muslim women wear a headscarf (hijab) to cover their hair, head, and neck, as a sign of modesty and religious faith.

The Hebrew word *tznius* or *tzniut* means modesty. It is generally used in reference to women and also relates to humility and general conduct, especially between men and women. Hasidic, Sikh, and Amish men often cover their heads and/or wear clothing that conveys modesty. For Buddhists, modesty is the quality of being unpretentious about one's virtues or achievements. The most important thing is not what type of clothes an individual wears or their color but the quality of his or her heart. Buddhist monks have modesty guidelines pertaining to the manner in which they wear their robes, never allowing skin to show on both sides of the body.

The Church of Jesus Christ of Latter-day Saints (LDS), also known as the Mormon Church, has issued official statements on modesty and dress for its members. Modesty is an attitude of propriety and decency in dress, grooming, language, and behavior. Clothing such as "short shorts" and short skirts, shirts that do not cover the stomach, and clothing that does not cover the shoulders or is low cut in the front or the back are discouraged. Men and women are also encouraged to avoid extremes in clothing or hairstyles. Most LDS members do not wear sleeveless shirts or blouses or shorts that fail to reach the knee. Women do not wear pants or slacks to religious services, and members of both genders attend services well-groomed and well-dressed (Church of Jesus Christ of Latter Day Saints, 2019).

All cultures have rules, often unwritten, concerning who may touch whom, where, when, how, for what reason, and for how long. In general, it is best for nurses to refrain from touching clients or coworkers of either gender unless necessary for the accomplishment of a job-related task, such as the provision of safe client care. Typically, people from Asian cultures are not as overtly demonstrative of affection or as tactile as Whites, Hispanics, or African Americans. Generally, they refrain from public embraces, kissing, loud talking, laughter, and boisterous behavior in public. Affection is expressed in a more reserved manner, usually in private rather than public places. In some instances, nurses and other members of the health care team from cultures that differ from the client's may send unintended messages through their use of touch. Special attention to male–female relationships and to the age of the client is warranted in nurse–client interactions and especially when it is necessary to touch members of the opposite gender.

Technology-Assisted Communication

Communication sometimes uses a combination of verbal, nonverbal, and written signals. With innovations in health care devices and software, technological advances are changing how care is delivered and the nature of the nursing profession. One of the major challenges of technology from a transcultural perspective is the gap between the regions and nations that have greater resources than others. While some strides are being made, it will still be many years before technological capabilities are mobilized in ways that benefit people globally by enhancing safe, quality, accessible, affordable, evidence-based, culturally congruent, and culturally competent nursing and health care. This is a matter of social justice that needs to be addressed as an integral component of TCN.

Although linguists have known that language changes over time, the digital language is changing faster than any other language in recorded history. For example, the first chat room was invented at the University of Illinois in 1973. In 1992, the first mobile text message was sent.

By 2018, people in the world were sending 180 billion texts per month. Ninety-five percent of all adults in the United States own a cell phone—94% of Whites, 98% of African Americans, and 97% of Hispanics (Pew Internet Research Center, 2018). In many health care agencies, nurses are given smartphones, pagers, tablets, and other technology-assisted devices for job-related activities to improve patient outcomes.

While the Internet, social media, and texting enable people to communicate more often, use of technology is primarily about saving time or taking digital shortcuts. It has become easy for nurses to use technology instead of interacting more directly with clients or other members of the health care team. While the digital shortcuts may be expedient and time-saving, the quality of the communication for this generation and the next is currently being studied to determine the ways in which technology is rewriting the neuropathways in children's brains (Brackett et al., 2013).

The average adult in the United States spends more than 10 hours per day using a tablet, smartphone, personal computer, multimedia device, video game, radio, DVD, DVR, and/or television (Nielson, 2017). When people spend so much time communicating through technology, they're not developing their verbal or emotional skills; screen time needs to be balanced with face time. An emoji cannot truly convey emotion— ☺ is not the same as a human smile—nor can a text message replace a warm embrace or hug when a client needs emotional support from family and friends during times of injury or illness. Nurses and other members of the health care team need to communicate in multiple ways, balancing face-to-face and digital interactions. It is important for the nurse to identify the client's preferred mode for communication as an integral component of the overall assessment of communication used by the client, his or her family, and significant others.

Literature, Art, Music, and Dance

The literature, art, music, and dance of various cultural groups communicate to the world the cherished values, beliefs, history, traditions, and contributions of people from nations, tribes, and population groups. The creative products, in the form of books, poems, artwork, music, and dance, describe the social climate of the day; portray religious, racial, gender, political, class, and other perspectives; and serve as unique historical documents and artifacts to help people better see, hear, know, understand, and appreciate the richness of the world's diverse cultures as they are communicated through the literary works, artistic and musical creations, and dance of people from cultures around the world.

Problem-Solving Process

The TIP Model is intended to guide members of the interprofessional health care team in determining what decisions, actions, and interventions the client needs to achieve an optimal state of well-being and health. As indicated in Figure 1-7, the model helps nurses to conceptualize the care of people from diverse backgrounds in a logical, orderly, systematic, scientific five-step process:

1. A comprehensive cultural **assessment**. The cultural assessment includes a self-assessment and a holistic assessment of the client that includes a health history and physical examination (Chapter 3 provides an in-depth discussion of these topics).
2. **Mutual goal setting** that takes into account the perspectives of each member of the health care team—the client, the client's family and significant others, and all those who are coparticipants with the client in the decision-making and goal-setting processes including credentialed health professionals and folk, traditional, indigenous, religious, and/or spiritual healers
3. **Planning** care that includes input from and dialogue with members of the interprofessional health care team
4. **Implementation** of the care plan through a wide range of actions and interventions
5. **Evaluation** of the care plan from multiple, diverse perspectives to determine the degree to which the plan:
   a. Is effective in achieving the intended goal(s)
   b. Provides care that is *culturally congruent* with and fits the client's culturally based beliefs and practices related to wellness, health, illness, disease, healing, dying, and death
   c. Reflects the delivery of *culturally competent* care by nurses and other members of the interprofessional team
   d. Provides *quality* care that is *safe, affordable*, and *accessible*
   e. Integrates *research, evidence-based, and best practices* (Melnyk, 2015) into the care

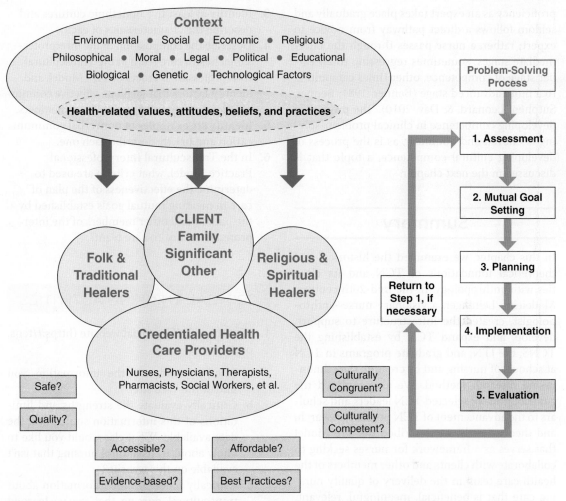

Figure 1-7. The five-step problem-solving process is a key part of the Transcultural Interprofessional Practice (TIP) Model. This client-centered model also includes the context from which people's health-related values, attitudes, beliefs, and practices emerge, the interprofessional health care team; and communication. (© Margaret M. Andrews.)

Data from the formal evaluation of the plan guide the nurses and other team members in determining if modifications or changes to the plan are necessary to accomplish the mutual goal(s) in step 2 or if new goals need to be discussed, proposed, planned, and established. If changes are needed, return to assessment, the first step in the problem-solving process, and repeat the other steps as appropriate until each of the mutual goals is met.

As indicated in Benner's classic work titled *From Novice to Expert*, a nurse passes through levels of proficiency in the acquisition and development of problem-solving skills: novice, advanced beginner, competent, proficient, and expert (Benner, 1984). The development of proficiency in using the previously described problem-solving process requires time and repeated simulated and/or in situ clinical experiences. As Benner aptly observes, the process leading to proficiency as an expert takes place gradually and seldom follows a direct pathway from novice to expert; rather, a nurse passes through the intermediate stages, sometimes regressing to an earlier stage of competence, other times catapulting to a more advanced stage (Benner, 1984; Benner, Sutphen, Leonard, & Day, 2010). The process of developing competence in clinical problem-solving is uneven and nonlinear, as is the process of developing cultural competence, a topic that is discussed in the next chapter.

Summary

In this chapter, we examined the historical and theoretical foundations of TCN and its close ties with anthropology. In the mid-20th century, Madeleine Leininger, a visionary nurse–anthropologist, created the infrastructure to support, develop, and expand TCN by establishing the TCNS, the JTN, and graduate programs in TCN at schools of nursing and by creating the ethnonursing research method. We also explored the contributions of selected TCN leaders and scholars to the advancement of TCN practice, research, and theory. Lastly, we described the TIP Model that serves as a framework for nurses seeking to collaborate with clients and other members of the health care team in the delivery of quality nursing care that is beneficial, meaningful, relevant, culturally congruent, culturally competent, and consistent with the cultural beliefs and practices of clients from diverse backgrounds.

REVIEW QUESTIONS

1. When Dr. Madeleine Leininger established transcultural nursing in the middle of the 20th century, she identified eight reasons why this specialty was needed. Review the reasons and discuss the relevance of these reasons in contemporary nursing and health care.
2. In your own words, describe the meaning of culture and its relationship to nursing.

3. Identify at least five nonethnic cultures and describe the characteristics of each.
4. Describe the composition of the interprofessional health care team in the Transcultural Interprofessional Practice (TIP) Model, and identify factors that facilitate effective communication between and among team members.
5. Identify six examples of nonverbal communication and briefly describe each one.
6. In the Transcultural Interprofessional Practice Model, what criteria are used to determine the effectiveness of the plan of care in meeting mutual goals established by the patient and other members of the interprofessional health care team?

CRITICAL THINKING ACTIVITIES

1. Visit the TCNS's official website (https://tcns.org):
   a. Briefly summarize the information you find at the Web site.
   b. Critically evaluate the strengths and limitations of this information source and the data available. What else would you like to know about transcultural nursing that isn't available on this website?
   c. Critically reflect on the information about transcultural nursing that you've learned and indicate how it will help you to provide nursing care for people from cultures that differ from your own.
   d. Search for other websites on transcultural nursing. What are the similarities and differences in the perspectives on transcultural nursing presented by the TCNS and other websites? How is it helpful or unhelpful to review different viewpoints on the same subject?

2. Read the following article: Andrews, M., & Friesen, L. (2011). Finding electronically available information on cultural competence in health care. *Online Journal of Cultural*

Competence in Nursing and Healthcare, 1(4), 27–47 (available on the OJCCNH website). Using the key word *transcultural nursing*, search for online resources that were posted during the past year. How many references did you find? If you want information about a specific cultural, ethnic, or minority group, what key words will help you to narrow the search? Consult a reference librarian for assistance if you need help.

3. Conduct an electronic search for websites about modesty among observant Muslims and Orthodox and Hasidic Jews:

   a. Evaluate the credibility, accuracy, veracity, and currency of each website and the information available on the topic.
   b. Compare and contrast the beliefs and practices of each group for men and women.
   c. What are the clinical implications of this information?

4. Maria Rodriguez is a 61-year-old female who self-identifies as being Mexican American.

She reads, writes, and speaks Spanish; it is her primary language. Although she speaks English well enough to manage activities of daily living, she has difficulty reading and comprehending medical documents in English. Maria is scheduled to be discharged from the hospital on her 3rd day postoperatively following a below-the-knee amputation of her right leg. She is diagnosed with peripheral vascular disease, diabetes mellitus, obesity, and hypertension. Maria lives alone in a two-story single dwelling. Her son, age 30, is on active duty in Iraq. Her 21-year-old daughter is 8 months pregnant and lives out-of-state. Unable to manage her care at home, Maria is unhappy that she will need to be discharged to a rehabilitation center for the next several weeks. She tells the nurse manager that she is severely depressed and threatens to commit suicide. Using the Transcultural Interprofessional Practice (TIP) Model as a guiding framework, analyze the case and develop a plan of care for Maria.

REFERENCES

Alligood, M. R. (2014). *Nursing theory: Utilization and application.* Maryland Heights, MO: Mosby-Elsevier.

American Anthropological Association. (2018). What is anthropology? Retrieved from https://www.americananthro.org/AdvanceYourCareer/Content.aspx?ItemNumber=2150&navItemNumber=740

American Nurses Association. (2013). What is nursing? Retrieved from http://www.nursingworld.org/especiallyforyou/what-is-nursing

Benner, P. (1984). *From novice to expert: Excellence and power in clinical nursing practice.* Menlo Park, CA: Addison-Wesley.

Benner, P., Sutphen, M., Leonard, V., & Day, L. (2010). *Educating nurses: A call for a radical transformation.* San Francisco, CA: Jossey-Bass.

Blue Cross/Blue Shield. (2014). Limit screen time for a happier family. *Living Healthy, Fall, 2014,* 16.

Brackett, M. A., Bertoli, M., Elbertson, N., Bausseron, E., Castillo, R., & Salovey, P. (2013). Emotional intelligence: Reconceptualizing the cognition-emotion link. In M. D. Robinson, E. Watkins, & E. Harmon-Jones (Eds.), *Handbook of cognition and emotion* (pp. 365–379). New York, NY: Guilford Press.

Branch, M. F., & Paxton, P. P. (Eds.). (1976). *Providing safe nursing care for ethnic people of color.* New York, NY: Appleton-Century-Crofts.

Brink, P. J. (1976). *Transcultural nursing care.* Englewood Cliffs, NJ: Prentice-Hall, Inc.

Campinha-Bacote, J. (2011). Delivering patient-centered care in the midst of cultural conflict: The role of cultural competence. *Online Journal of Issues in Nursing, 16*(2), 5. doi: 10.3912/OJIN.Vol16No02Man05

Campinha-Bacote, J. (2015). *A biblically based model of cultural competence in the delivery of healthcare services.* Cincinnati, OH: Transcultural C.A.R.E. Associates. Retrieved from http://transculturalcare.net/a-biblically-based-model-of-cultural-competence/

Center for Immigration Studies. (2017). Almost half speak a foreign language in America's biggest cities. Retrieved from https://cis.org/Report/Almost-Half-Speak-Foreign-Language-Americas-Largest-Cities

Church of Jesus Christ of Latter Day Saints. (2019). Modesty. Retrieved from https://www.lds.org/topics/modesty?lang=eng

Council on Nursing and Anthropology. (2018). Retrieved from https://www.conaa.org/index.php/about-us/what-is-conaa

Courtney, R., & Wolgamott, S. (2015). Using Leininger's theory as the building block for cultural competence and cultural assessment for a collaborative care team in a primary care setting. In M. R. McFarland & H. B. Wehbe-Alamah (Eds.), *Leininger's culture care diversity and universality: A worldwide nursing theory* (pp. 345–368). Burlington, MA: Jones and Bartlett Learning.

Davidson, A., Ray, M., & Turkel, M. (Eds.). (2011). *Nursing, caring, and complexity science: For human-environment well-being.* New York, NY: Springer Publishing Company.

deRuyter, L. M. (2015). Culture care education and experience of African American students in predominantly EuroAmerican associate degree nursing programs. In M. R. McFarland & H. B. Wehbe-Alamah (Eds.), *Leininger's culture care diversity and universality: A worldwide nursing theory* (pp. 389–442). Burlington, MA: Jones and Bartlett Learning.

Douglas, M. K., & Pacquiao, D. F. (Eds.). (2010). Core curriculum in transcultural nursing and health care. *Journal of Transcultural Nursing, 21*(Suppl. 1), 53S–136S.

Douglas, M., Pacquiao, D., & Purnell, L. (Eds.). (2018). *Global applications of culturally competent health care: Guidelines for practice.* Cham, Switzerland: Springer International Publishing AG part of Springer Nature.

Eipperle, M. (2015). Application of the three modes of culture care decisions and actions in advanced practice primary care. In M. R. McFarland & H. B. Wehbe-Alamah (Eds.), *Leininger's culture care diversity and universality: A worldwide nursing theory* (pp. 317–344). Burlington, MA: Jones and Bartlett Learning.

Fleming, R., & Willgerodt, M. A. (2017). Interprofessional collaborative practice and school nursing: A model for improved health outcomes. *The Online Journal of Issues in Nursing, 22*(3). doi: 10.3912/OJIN.Vol22No03Man02

Fulmer, T., & Gaines, M. (Eds.). (2014). Conference conclusions and recommendations. In G. E. Thibault, T. Fulmer, & M. Gaines. *2014 Conference conclusions and recommendations. Partnering with patients, families, and communities to link interprofessional practice and education.* Proceedings of a conference sponsored by the Josiah Macy Foundation, Arlington, VA, 3–6 April (pp. 27–45). New York, NY: Josiah Macy Foundation.

Galanti, G. A. (2014). *Cultural sensitivity: A pocket guide for health care professionals.* Philadelphia, PA: University of Pennsylvania Press.

Galvin, M., Prescott, D., & Huseman, R. C. (1988). *Business communication: Strategies and skills.* New York, NY: Holt, Rinehart, & Winston.

Giger, J. N. (2017). *Transcultural nursing: Assessment and intervention* (7th ed.), Saint Louis, MO: Mosby/Elsevier.

Hall, E. T. (1984). *The dance of life: The other dimension of time.* New York, NY: Anchor Press Double Press/Doubleday.

Hall, E. T. (1990). *Distance: The hidden dimension.* New York, NY: Anchor Press/Doubleday.

Hesmondhalgh, D., & Saha, A. (2013). Race, ethnicity, and cultural production. *Popular Communication, 11*(3), 179–193.

Hunt, L. M., Truesdell, N. D., & Kreiner, M. J. (2013). Genes, race, and culture in clinical care. *Medical Anthropology Quarterly, 27*(2), 253–271.

Institute of Medicine. (1999). *To err is human.* Washington, DC: The National Academies Press.

Institute of Medicine. (2011). *The future of nursing: Leading change, advancing health.* Washington, DC: The National Academies Press.

International Council of Nurses. (2014). Definition of nursing. Retrieved from http://www.icn.ch/about-icn/icn-definition-of-nursing/

Interprofessional collaborative practice in primary health care: Nursing and midwifery perspectives. Human Resources for Health Observer, No. 13. Retrieved from http://www.who.int/hrh/resources/observer13/en/

Interprofessional Education Collaborative Expert Panel. (2011). *Core competencies for interprofessional collaborative practice: Report of an expert panel.* Washington, DC: Interprofessional Education Collaborative.

Interprofessional Education Collaborative (2016). *Core competencies for interprofessional collaborative practice: 2016 update.* Retrieved from https://nebula.wsimg.com/

Jeffreys, M. R. (2016). *Teaching cultural competence in nursing and health care: Inquiry,* action and innovation (3rd ed.), New York: Springer Publishing.

Larson, M. (2015). The Greek connection: Discovering the cultural and social care dimensions of the Greek culture using Leininger's Theory of Culture Care: A model for a baccalaureate study-abroad experience. In M. R. McFarland & H. B. Wehbe-Alamah (Eds.), *Leininger's culture care diversity and universality: A worldwide nursing theory* (pp. 503–520). Burlington, MA: Jones and Bartlett Learning.

Leininger, M. M. (1970). *Nursing and anthropology: Two worlds to blend.* New York, NY: John Wiley & Sons.

Leininger, M. M. (1978). *Transcultural nursing: Concepts, theories and practices.* New York, NY: John Wiley & Sons.

Leininger, M. M. (1991). *Culture care diversity and universality: A theory of nursing.* New York, NY: National League for Nursing.

Leininger, M. M. (1995). *Transcultural nursing: Concepts, theories, research and practices.* New York, NY: McGraw-Hill.

Leininger, M. M. (1997). Future directions in transcultural nursing in the 21st century. *International Nursing Review, 44*(1), 19–23.

Leininger, M. M. (1998). Twenty five years of knowledge and practice development transcultural nursing society annual research conferences. *Journal of Transcultural Nursing, 9*(2), 72–74.

Leininger, M. M. (1999). What is transcultural nursing and culturally competent care? *Journal of Transcultural Nursing, 10*(1), 9.

Leininger, M. M., & McFarland, M. R. (2002). *Transcultural nursing: Concepts, theories and practices.* New York, NY: McGraw-Hill.

Leininger, M. M., & McFarland, M. R. (2006). *Culture care diversity and universality: A worldwide theory for nursing* (2nd ed.). Sudbury, MA: Jones & Bartlett, Publishers.

Lombardo, J. (n.d.). Monochronic and polychronic cultures: Definitions and communication styles. Retrieved from http://education-portal.com/academy/lesson/mono-chronic-vs-polychronic-cultures-definitions-communication-styles.html

McFarland, M. R., Mixer, S. J., Webhe-Alamah, H., & Burk, R. (2012). Ethnonursing: A qualitative research method for all disciplines. *International Journal of Qualitative Methods, 11*(3), 259–279.

McFarland, M. R., & Wehbe-Alamah, H. B. (2016a). *Leininger's culture care diversity and universality: A worldwide theory of nursing* (3rd ed.). Burlington, MA: Jones & Bartlett Learning.

McFarland, M. R., & Wehbe-Alamah, H. B. (2016b). The theory of culture care diversity and universality. In M. R. McFarland & H. B. Wehbe-Alamah (Eds.), *Leininger's culture care diversity and universality: A worldwide nursing theory* (pp. 1–34). Burlington, MA: Jones and Bartlett Learning.

McFarland, M. R., & Wehbe-Alamah, H. B. (2018). *Transcultural nursing: Concepts, theories, research, and practices* (4th ed.). New York, NY: McGraw-Hill, Medical Publishing Division.

McFarland, M. R., Wehbe-Alamah, H. B., Vossos, H., & Wilson, M. (2015). Synopsis of findings discovered within a descriptive metasynthesis of doctoral dissertations guided by the culture care theory with use of the eth-nonursing research method. In M. R. McFarland & H. B. Wehbe-Alamah (Eds.), *Leininger's culture care diversity and universality: A worldwide nursing theory* (pp. 287–315). Burlington, MA: Jones and Bartlett Learning.

McFarland, M. R., Wehbe-Alamah, H., Wilson, M., & Vossos, H. (2011). Synopsis of findings discovered within a descriptive meta-synthesis of doctoral dissertations guided by the Culture Care Theory with use of the eth-nonursing research method. *Online Journal of Cultural Competence in Nursing and Health Care, 1*(2), 24–39.

McKenna, M. (1985). Anthropology and nursing: The inter-action between two fields of inquiry. *Western Journal of Nursing Research, 6*(4), 423–431.

Mead, M. (1937). *Cooperation and collaboration among primitive peoples*. New York, NY: McGraw-Hill.

Melnyk, B. (2015). *Evidence-based practice in nursing and healthcare* (3rd ed.). Philadelphia, PA: Wolters Kluwer Health.

Mixer, S. J. (2015). Application of culture care theory in teaching cultural competence and culturally congruent care. In M. R. McFarland & H. B. Wehbe-Alamah (Eds.), *Leininger's culture care diversity and universality: A worldwide nursing theory* (pp. 369–388). Burlington, MA: Jones and Bartlett Learning.

Morris, E. (2015). An examination of subculture as a theoretical social construct through an ethnonursing study of urban African American adolescent gang members. In M. R. McFarland & H. B. Wehbe-Alamah (Eds.), *Leininger's culture care diversity and universality: A worldwide nursing theory* (pp. 255–286). Burlington, MA: Jones and Bartlett Learning.

Munoz, C., & Luckman, J. (2008). *Transcultural communication in nursing* (2nd ed.). Clifton Park, NJ: Delmar Learning.

National Human Genome Institute. (2014). *Fact sheet on science, research, ethics, and the institute*. National Institutes of Health, last updated August 7, 2014. Retrieved from https://www.genome.gov/10000202/

Nielson Report. (2017). The Total Audience Report: 2016. Retrieved from https://www.nielsen.com/us/en/insights/reports/2016/the-total-audience-report-q1-2016.html

Olukotun, O., Mkandawire, L., Kreuziger, S., Dressel, A., Wesp, L., Sima, C., ... Stevens, P. (2018). Preparing culturally safe student nurses: An analysis of undergraduate cultural diversity course reflections. *Journal of Professional Nursing, 34*(4), 245–252.

Omeri, A. (2015). Culture care diversity and universality: A pathway to culturally congruent practices in transcultural nursing education, research, and practice in Australia. In M. R. McFarland & H. B. Wehbe-Alamah (Eds.), *Leininger's culture care diversity and universality: A worldwide nursing theory* (pp. 443–474). Burlington, MA: Jones and Bartlett Learning.

Orque, M. S., Bloch, B., & Monrroy, L. S. (1983). *Ethnic nursing care*. St. Louis, MO: C.V. Mosby.

Osborne, O. (1969). Anthropology and nursing: Some common traditions and interests. *Nursing Research, 18*(3), 251–255.

Pacquiao, D. (2018). Conceptual framework for culturally competent care. In M. Douglas, D. Pacquiao, & L. Purnell (Eds.), *Global applications of culturally competent health care: Guidelines for practice* (pp. 1–27). Cham, Switzerland: Springer International Publishing AG part of Springer Nature.

Pew Internet Research Center. (2018). Mobile technology fact sheet. Retrieved from http://www.pewinternet.org/fact-sheet/mobile

Purnell, L. (2013). *Transcultural health care: A culturally competent approach* (4th ed.), Philadelphia: F. A. Davis.

Purnell. L. (2014). *Guide to culturally competent health care*. Philadelphia: F.A. Davis Co.

Purnell, L., & Fenkl, E. (2018). *Guide to culturally competent health care*. Philadelphia, PA: F.A. Davis Company.

Ray, M. (2016). *Transcultural caring dynamics in nursing and health care*. Philadelphia, PA: F.A. Davis.

Ray, M., & Turkel, M. (2014). Caring as emancipatory nursing praxis: The theory of Relational Caring Complexity. *Advances in Nursing Science, 37*(2), 132–146.

Raymond, L. M., & Omeri, A. (2015). Transcultural midwifery: Culture care for Mauritian immigrant childbearing families living in New South Wales, Australia. In M. R. McFarland &

H. B. Wehbe-Alamah (Eds.), *Leininger's culture care diversity and universality: A worldwide nursing theory* (pp. 183–254). Burlington, MA: Jones and Bartlett Learning.

Rutledge, B. (2013). Cultural differences—Monochronic vs polychronic. The Articulate CEO, February 2013. Retrieved from http://hearticulateceo.typepad.com/my-blog/2011/08/cultural-differences-monochronic-versus-polychronic.html

Sagar, P. L. (2012). *Transcultural nursing theory and models: Application in nursing education, practice, and administration.* New York, NY: Springer Publishing Company.

Sagar, P. L. (2014). *Transcultural nursing education strategies.* New York, NY: Springer Publishing Company.

Sagar, P. L. (2015). Transcultural nursing certification: Its role in nursing education, practice, and administration. In M. R. McFarland & H. B. Wehbe-Alamah (Eds.), *Leininger's culture care diversity and universality: A worldwide theory of nursing* (3rd ed., pp. 579–592). Burlington, MA: Jones & Bartlett Learning.

Spector, R. E. (2017). *Cultural diversity in health and illness* (9th ed.). Upper Saddle River, NJ: Pearson.

Stanford Center on Poverty and Inequality. (2014). *State of the union: Poverty and inequality report 2014.* Palo Alto, CA: Author.

Transcultural Nursing Society, TCNS. (2019a). Transcultural nursing certification. Retrieved from https://tcns.org/tcncertification/

Transcultural Nursing Society, TCNS. (2019b). Transcultural nursing theories and models. Retrieved from https://tcns.org/theoriesandmodels/

Tylor, E. B. (1871). *Primitive culture, Vols. 1 and 2.* London: Murray.

U.S. Census Bureau (2015). *Census Bureau reports at least 350 languages spoken in U.S. homes.* Retrieved from https://www.census.gov/newsroom/press-releases/2015/cb15-185.html

U.S. Census Bureau (2018). *American community survey 5-year estimates.* Retrieved from https://www.census.gov/programs-surveys/acs/news/updates/2018.html

Wehbe-Alamah, H. B. (2015). Folk care beliefs and practices of traditional Lebanese and Syrian Muslims in the Midwestern United States. In M. R. McFarland & H. B. Wehbe-Alamah (Eds.), *Leininger's culture care diversity and universality: A worldwide nursing theory* (pp. 137–181). Burlington, MA: Jones and Bartlett Learning.

Wehbe-Alamah, H. B., & McFarland, M. R. (2015). Leininger's enablers for use with the ethnonursing research method. In M. R. McFarland & H. B. Wehbe-Alamah (Eds.), *Leininger's culture care diversity and universality: A worldwide nursing theory* (pp. 73–100). Burlington, MA: Jones and Bartlett Learning.

Wehbe-Alamah, H. B., & McFarland, M. R. (2016). The ethnonursing research method. In M. R. McFarland & H. B. Wehbe-Alamah (Eds.), *Leininger's culture care diversity and universality: A worldwide nursing theory* (pp. 35–71). Burlington, MA: Jones and Bartlett Learning.

World Health Organization (WHO). (2010). *Framework for action on interprofessional education and collaborative practice.* Geneva, Switzerland: World Health Organization.

World Health Organization (WHO). (2018). *Nursing and midwifery.* Retrieved from http://www.who.int/news-room/fact-sheets/detail/nursing-and-midwifery

Zimitri, E. (2013). Throwing the genes: A renewed biological imaginary of "race", place and identification. *Theoria: A Journal of Social and Political Theory, 60*(136), 38–53.

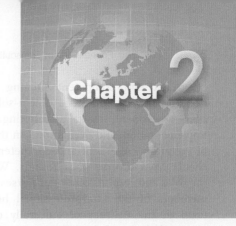

Chapter 2

Culturally Competent Nursing Care

• Margaret M. Andrews

Key Terms

Bias
Cross-cultural communication
Cultural assessment
Cultural baggage
Cultural competence (individual and organizational)
Cultural imposition
Cultural self-assessment
Cultural stereotype
Culture of the deaf

Disabling hearing loss
Discrimination
Diversity
Emic
Emigrate
Ethnocentrism
Etic
Folk healer
Hard of hearing
Health tourism
Immigrant

Immigrate
Interprofessional
    collaborative practice
Language access services (LAS)
Prejudice
Racism
Refugee
Self-location
Social determinants of health
Traditional healer
Vulnerable populations

Learning Objectives

1. Critically analyze the complex integration of knowledge, attitudes, and skills needed for the delivery of culturally competent nursing care.
2. Compare and contrast individual cultural competence and organizational cultural competence.
3. Evaluate guidelines for the practice of culturally competent nursing care.
4. Use a transcultural interprofessional framework for the delivery of culturally congruent and culturally competent nursing care for clients with special needs.

In this chapter, we provide an overview of the rationale for cultural competence in the delivery of nursing care and describe individual and organizational cultural competence, topics that will be discussed throughout the remainder of the book. We analyze cultural self-assessment, a valuable exercise that enables nurses to gain insights into their own unconscious cultural attitudes (biases, cultural stereotypes, prejudice, and tendencies to discriminate against people who are different from themselves). We discuss the need for cultural knowledge about other ethnic and nonethnic groups and psychomotor skills that are required for the delivery of culturally

31

congruent and competent nursing care. We examine the use of the problem-solving process—assessment, mutual goal setting, planning, implementation, and evaluation—in the delivery of culturally congruent and competent care for clients from diverse backgrounds. We explore the roles and responsibilities of nurses and other members of the interprofessional health care team in the delivery of culturally competent care and the need for effective **cross-cultural communication**. We analyze the importance of assessing the cultural context and social determinants of health (Office of Disease Prevention and Health Promotion, 2018) that influence the delivery of culturally competent care for clients from diverse cultures, for example, environmental, social, economic, religious, philosophical, moral, legal, political, educational, biological, and technological factors. By introducing national and global guidelines for the delivery of culturally competent nursing care and identifying cultural assessment instruments, we provide nurses with tools to guide them in the delivery of care that is culturally acceptable and congruent with the client's beliefs and practices; culturally competent, affordable, and accessible; and rooted in state of the science research, evidence-based, and best practices. Lastly, we examine clients with special needs including those at high risk for health disparities, those who are deaf, and those with communication and language needs.

Rationale for Culturally Competent Care

Multiple factors are converging at this time in history to heighten societal awareness of cultural similarities and differences among people. In many parts of the world, there is growing awareness of social injustice for people from diverse backgrounds and the moral imperative to safeguard the civil and health care rights of vulnerable populations. **Vulnerable populations** are groups that have experienced social or economic obstacles in accessing the health care system because of ethnic, cultural, geographic (rural and urban settings), or health characteristics, such as disabilities or multiple chronic conditions (Douglas, Pacquiao, & Purnell, 2018; Pacquiao & Douglas, 2019).

Immigration and migration result in growing numbers of **immigrants**, people who move from one country or region to another for economic, political, religious, social, and personal reasons. The verb **emigrate** means to leave one country or region to settle in another; **immigrate** means to enter another country or region for the purpose of living there. People *emigrate from* one country or region and *immigrate to* a different nation or region.

In the United States, for example, 42 million people (13.2% of the population) are foreign born, a term used by the Census Bureau in reference to anyone who is not a US citizen at birth, including those who eventually become citizens through naturalization (U.S. Census Bureau, 2016). Additionally, an estimated 8 to 10 million people from other countries are living in the United States without documentation. In many countries, national borders have become increasingly porous and fluid, enabling people to move more freely from one country or region to another.

Nurses respond to global health care needs such as infectious disease epidemics and the growing trends in **health tourism**, in which patients travel to other countries for medical and surgical health care needs. By traveling to another nation, clients often obtain more affordable care services or receive specialized care that is unavailable in their own country. Nurses also respond to natural and human-made disasters around the world and provide care for **refugees** (people who flee their country of origin for fear of persecution based on ethnicity, race, religion, political opinion, or related reasons) and other casualties of civil unrest or war in politically unstable parts of the world. In all of these situations, nurses are expected to demonstrate effective cross-cultural communication and deliver culturally congruent and culturally competent nursing care to people from diverse countries and cultures.

Technological advances in science, engineering, transportation, communication, information and computer sciences, health care, and health profession education result in increased electronic and face-to-face communications between nurses and people from diverse backgrounds. Population demographics, health care standards, laws, and regulations make cultural competence integral to nursing practice, education, research, administration, and interprofessional collaborations.

Interprofessional collaborative practice refers to multiple health providers from different professional backgrounds working together with patients, families, caregivers, and communities to deliver the highest quality care (Moss, Seifert, & O'Sullivan, 2016). Interprofessional teams have a collective identity and shared responsibility for a client or group of clients. Culturally competent care is an extension of interprofessional collaborative practice (Institute of Medicine, 2011; Interprofessional Education Collaborative Expert Panel, 2011; Moss et al., 2016), involving clients and their families; credentialed or licensed health professionals; folk or traditional healers from various philosophical perspectives, such as herbalists, medicine men or women, and others; and religious and spiritual leaders, such as rabbis, imams, priests, elders, monks, and other religious representatives or clergy, all of whom are integral members of the interprofessional team. The religious and spiritual healers are especially helpful when the client is discerning which decision or action in health-related matters is best, especially when there are moral, ethical, or spiritual considerations involved (see Chapter 12, Religion, Culture, and Nursing, and Chapter 13, Cultural Competence in Ethical Decision-Making).

Guidelines for the Practice of Culturally Competent Nursing Care

A set of guidelines for implementing culturally competent nursing care was recently developed by a task force consisting of members of the American Academy of Nursing (AAN) Expert Panel on Global Nursing and Health and the Transcultural Nursing Society (TCNS). In addition to endorsement by the membership of the AAN and TCNS, these guidelines have been endorsed by the International Council of Nurses. Intended to present universally accepted guidelines that can be embraced by nurses around the world, the ten items listed in Table 2-1 provide a useful framework for implementing culturally competent care. The guidelines include knowledge of culture, education, and training in culturally competent care, critical reflection, cross-cultural communication, culturally competent practice, cultural competence in systems and organizations, patient advocacy and empowerment, multicultural workforce, cross-cultural leadership, and evidence-based practice and research. The guidelines have their foundation in principles of social justice, such as the belief that everyone is entitled to fair and equal opportunities for health care and to have their dignity protected. The guidelines and accompanying descriptions are intended to serve as a resource for nurses in clinical practice, administration, research, and education (Douglas et al., (Douglas, et al., 2018).

Definitions and Categories of Cultural Competence

There is no universally accepted definition of **cultural competence**. Rather, there are hundreds of definitions that have "evolved from diverse perspectives, interests, and needs and are incorporated in state legislation, Federal statutes and programs, private sector organizations, and academic settings" (National Center for Cultural Competence, n.d.a, n.d.b, n.d.c, n.d.d). Although definitions vary, there is general consensus that cultural competence conceptually can be divided into two major categories: (1) **individual cultural competence**, which refers to the care provided for an individual client by one or more nurses, physicians, social workers, and/or other health care, education, or social service professionals, and (2) **organizational cultural competence**, which focuses on the organizational leadership (Douglas, 2018; Marrone, 2014),

Table 2-1	Guidelines for the Practice of Culturally Competent Nursing Care
Guideline	**Description**
1. Knowledge of cultures	Nurses shall gain an understanding of the perspectives, traditions, values, practices, and family systems of culturally diverse individuals, families, communities, and populations they care for, as well as knowledge of the complex variables that affect the achievement of health and well-being.
2. Education and training in culturally competent care	Nurses shall be educationally prepared to provide culturally congruent health care. Knowledge and skills necessary for assuring that nursing care is culturally congruent shall be included in global health care agendas that mandate formal education and clinical training as well as required ongoing, continuing education for all practicing nurses.
3. Critical reflection	Nurses shall engage in critical reflection of their own values, beliefs, and cultural heritage in order to have an awareness of how these qualities and issues can impact culturally congruent nursing care.
4. Cross-cultural communication	Nurses shall use culturally competent verbal and nonverbal communication skills to identify client's values, beliefs, practices, perceptions, and unique health care needs.
5. Culturally competent practice	Nurses shall utilize cross-cultural knowledge and culturally sensitive skills in implementing culturally congruent nursing care.
6. Cultural competence in health care systems and organizations	Health care organizations should provide the structure and resources necessary to evaluate and meet the cultural and language needs of their diverse clients.
7. Patient advocacy and empowerment	Nurses shall recognize the effect of health care policies, delivery systems, and resources on their patient populations and shall empower and advocate for their patients as indicated. Nurses shall advocate for the inclusion of their patient's cultural beliefs and practices in all dimensions of their health care.
8. Multicultural workforce	Nurses shall actively engage in the effort to ensure a multicultural workforce in health care settings. One measure to achieve a multicultural workforce is through strengthening of recruitment and retention efforts in the hospitals, clinics, and academic settings.
9. Cross-cultural leadership	Nurses shall have the ability to influence individuals, groups, and systems to achieve outcomes of culturally competent care for diverse populations. Nurses shall have the knowledge and skills to work with public and private organizations, professional associations, and communities to establish policies and guidelines for comprehensive implementation and evaluation of culturally competent care.
10. Evidence-based practice and research	Nurses shall base their practice on interventions that have been systematically tested and shown to be the most effective for the culturally diverse populations that they serve. In areas where there is a lack of evidence of efficacy, nurse researchers shall investigate and test interventions that may be the most effective in reducing the disparities in health outcomes.

Source: Douglas, M. K., Rosenkoetter, M., Pacquiao, D. F., Callister, L. C., Hattar-Pollara, M., Lauderdale, J., ... Purnell, L. (2014). Guidelines for implementing culturally competent nursing care. *Journal of Transcultural Nursing, 25*(2), 110–129. Reprinted with permission from Sage Publications, Inc.

collective competencies of the members of an organization, and their effectiveness in meeting the diverse needs of their clients, patients, staff, and community (see Chapter 9, Creating Culturally Competent Health Care Organizations).

Before nurses can provide culturally competent care for individual clients or contribute to organizational cultural competence, they need to engage in a cultural self-assessment to identify their cultural baggage. **Cultural baggage** refers to the tendency for a person's own culture to be foremost in his/her assumptions, thoughts, words, and behavior. People are seldom consciously aware that culture influences their worldview and interactions with others.

Cultural Self-Assessment

The purpose of the **cultural self-assessment** is for nurses to critically reflect on their own culturally based attitudes, values, beliefs, and practices and gain insight into, and awareness of, the ways in which their background and lived experiences have shaped and informed the person the nurse has become today. Cultural critical self-reflection is an ongoing process whereby nurses continuously review their thoughts, feelings, and beliefs about others with backgrounds different from their own and their professional, moral, and ethical obligation to care for all without bias or prejudice (Purnell & Fenkl, 2018).

The nurse's cultural self-assessment is a personal and professional journey that emphasizes strengths as well as areas for continued growth, thereby enabling nurses to set goals for overcoming barriers to the delivery of culturally congruent and competent nursing care (National Center for Cultural Competence, n.d.a, n.d.b, n.d.c, n.d.d).

Part of the cultural self-assessment process includes nurses' awareness of their human tendencies toward bias, ethnocentrism, cultural imposition, cultural stereotyping, prejudice, and discrimination. **Bias** refers to the tendency, outlook, or inclination that results in an unreasoned judgment, positive or negative, about a person, place, or object.

> *If anyone, no matter who, were given the opportunity of choosing from amongst all the nations in the world the set of beliefs which he thought best, he would inevitably—after careful considerations of their relative merits—choose that of his own country.*
>
> Herodotus, ancient Greek historian,
> *Histories*, circum. *450 to 420* BC

The term **ethnocentrism** refers to the human tendency to view one's own group as the center of and superior to all other groups. People born into a particular culture grow up absorbing and learning the values and behaviors of the culture, and they develop a worldview that considers their culture to be the norm. Other cultures that differ from that norm are viewed as inferior. Ethnocentrism may lead to pride, vanity, belief in the superiority of one's own group over all others, contempt for outsiders, and cultural imposition. Box 2-1 identifies other examples of—"-isms"—preconceived, unfavorable judgments about people based on personal characteristics of another. "-Isms" are derived from cultural baggage, biases, stereotypes, prejudice, and/or discrimination related to someone with a background that differs from one's own. As indicated in Evidence-Based Practice 2-1, **racism**, the belief that one's own race is superior and has the right to dominate others, has a profound impact on the body's stress management system. Exposure to racism over prolonged periods of time may result in severe cardiovascular disease.

Cultural imposition is the tendency of a person or group to impose their values, beliefs, and practices onto others. **Cultural stereotype** refers to a preconceived, fixed perception or impression of someone from a particular cultural group without meeting the person. The perception generally has little or no basis in fact but nonetheless is perpetuated by individuals who are unwilling to re-examine or change their perceptions even when faced with new evidence that disproves the incorrect perception. Cultural stereotypes fail to recognize individual differences, group changes that occur over time, and personal preferences. Ethnocentrism, cultural imposition, and cultural stereotypes are barriers to effective cross-cultural communication and the provision of culturally competent care, as are prejudice and discrimination.

Prejudice refers to inaccurate perceptions of others or preconceived judgments about people based on ethnicity, race, national origin, gender, sexual orientation, social class, size, disability,

BOX 2-1	Selected Examples of "-Isms" Based on Preconceptions About Others

Characteristic	Type of -Ism
Race	Racism
Ethnicity	Ethnocentrism
National origin	Nationalism
Socioeconomic class	Classism
Gender	Sexism, feminism
Sexual orientation	Homophobism*
Disability	Ableism*
Religion	Islamism* (political ideology associated with some denominations of Islam)
	Anti-Semitism (anti-Jewish)
	Anti-(name of religion), e.g., anti-Mormonism
Political opinion	Anti-(name of ideology), e.g., anticapitalism, anticommunism
Size	Sizeism*

*Neologism—a newly coined term or phrase that is in the process of entering common or mainstream use but isn't yet found in dictionaries.

religion, language, political opinion, or related personal characteristics (Dunagan, Kimble, Gunby, & Andrews, 2016). Whereas prejudice concerns perceptions and attitudes, **discrimination** refers to the *act* or behavior of setting one individual or group apart from another, thereby treating one person or group differently from other people or groups. In the context of civil rights law, *unlawful* discrimination refers to unfair or unequal treatment of an individual or group based on age, disability, ethnicity, gender, marital status, national origin, race, religion, and sexual orientation (Titles I and V of the Americans with Disabilities Act of 1990; Title VII of the Civil Rights Act of 1964 [Public Law 88–352]; U.S. Equal Employment Opportunity Commission, 2016).

By engaging in cultural self-assessments and demonstrating genuine interest in and curiosity about the client's cultural beliefs and practices, nurses learn to develop their cultural competency and learn to put aside their own ethnocentric tendencies. Box 2-2 contains a cultural self-assessment tool that enables nurses to gain insights into how they relate to people from five different categories: racial/ethnic groups, social issues/problems, religious differences, physical and emotional handicaps, and different political perspectives. After completing and scoring the cultural self-assessment contained in Box 2-2, continue to the next section, which focuses on the cultural assessment of clients.

Cultural Assessment of Clients

The foundation for culturally competent and culturally congruent nursing care is the **cultural assessment**, a term that refers to the collection of data about the client's health state. There are two major categories of data: *subjective data* (i.e., what clients say about themselves during the admission or intake interview) and *objective data* (i.e., what health professionals observe about clients during the physical examination through observation, percussion, palpation, and auscultation). See Chapter 3, Cultural Competence in the

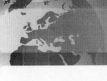

Effects of Racism on the Health and Well-Being of African Americans

With the growing frequency of the complex interrelationship among genetics, the **social determinants of health** (environment, neighborhood, lifestyle, stress, unemployment), and various forms of racism, are being studied by multidisciplinary teams comprised of biologists, geneticists, physicians, nurses, ethicists, and social and behavioral scientists (Pacquiao & Douglas, 2019; World Health Organization, n.d.).

Racism triggers stress-related biological mechanisms in African Americans that, in turn, stimulate a series of processes originating as perceived social exclusion. Exposure to racism increases sympathetic nervous system activation and affects the *HPA (hypothalamus, pituitary, and adrenal) axis*, a neuroendocrine system that controls reactions to stress. The HPS axis regulates many body processes, including digestion, the immune system, mood and emotions, sexuality, and energy storage and expenditure. Consequently, racism is associated with morbidities including low birth weight, hypertension, abdominal obesity, and cardiovascular disease even when there is no socioeconomic hardship among affected African Americans.

Racism impacts the ability of individuals, families, and communities to access health care and often results in the following:

- Fewer diagnostic and treatment options (e.g., cardiac catheterizations)
- Less follow-up or referral appointments for postoperative community services after discharge
- Increased presence of epinephrine, resulting in increased heart rate and blood pressure
- Higher mortality rates for African American men with cardiovascular disease:

Due to the presence of epinephrine, both blood pressure and heart rate are raised significantly; therefore, racism influences the prevalence of hypertension through stress exposure, prolonged elevation of blood pressure, strain on the myocardium and left ventricle, and hypertrophy as a compensatory mechanism to offset the increased vascular resistance produced by hypertension. The process of sustained sympathetic activation eventually causes heart failure. Renal failure may result when the kidneys respond to hypertension. When a person experiences racism on a daily basis, the stress response becomes overwhelmed, and the adrenal system is no longer able to maintain homeostasis. Chronic adrenal fatigue often leads to depression, obesity, hypertension, diabetes, cancer, ulcers, allergies, eczema, autoimmune diseases, headaches, and liver disease.

Clinical Implications

Nurses need to position themselves strategically to bring about change in the health care system by acting as patient advocates, addressing racism for individual clients, and acting collectively as members of the nursing profession to rid the system of racism through systemic changes. Strategies for action include the following:

- Acknowledging the ways in which nurses' own race, culture, class, gender, socioeconomic background, and other social identities influence their beliefs, attitudes, and the care provided to patients from similar and different racial and ethnic backgrounds
- Addressing how inequities intersect and overlap to deepen disadvantage and how advocacy by nurses can bring about change
- Providing leadership in analyzing organizational approaches to racial diversity and workplace policies to foster inclusiveness, equity, and justice in health systems

(*continued*)

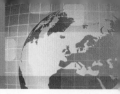

Effects of Racism on the Health and Well-Being of African Americans (continued)

- Conducting research on populations experiencing racism in their daily lives and within the health care system
- Ensuring that people from a variety of racial backgrounds are represented in investigations and on research councils that review proposals and allocate funds for nursing and health care research

References: Goosby, B. J., Cheadle, J. E., & Colter, M. (2018). Stress-related biosocial mechanisms of discrimination and African American Health Inequities. *Annual Review of Sociology, 44*(1), 319–340.

Hill, L. K., Hoggard, L. S., Richmond, A. S., Gray, D. L., Williams, D. P., & Thayer, J. F. (2017). Examining the association between perceived discrimination and heart rate variability in African Americans. *Cultural Diversity and Ethnic Minority Psychology, 23*(1), 5–14.

World Health Organization. (2018). Fact sheet. Deafness and hearing loss. Retrieved from http://www.who.int/en/news-room/fact-sheets/detail/deafness-and-hearing-loss

World Health Organization. (n.d.). What are the social determinants of health? Retrieved from http://www.int/social_determinants/en/

BOX 2-2 | How Do You Relate to Various Groups of People in the Society?

Described below are different levels of response you might have toward a person.

Levels of Response

1. *Greet*: I feel I can *greet* this person warmly and welcome him or her sincerely.
2. *Accept*: I feel I can honestly *accept* this person as he or she is and be comfortable enough to listen to his or her problems.
3. *Help*: I feel I would genuinely try to *help* this person with his or her problems as they might relate to or arise from the label–stereotype given to him or her.
4. *Background*: I feel I have the *background* of knowledge and/or experience to be able to help this person.
5. *Advocate*: I feel I could honestly be an *advocate* for this person.

The following is a list of individuals. Read down the list and place a check mark next to anyone you would *not* "greet" or would hesitate to "greet." Then, move to response level 2, "accept," and follow the same procedure. Try to respond honestly, not as you think that might be socially or professionally desirable. Your answers are only for your personal use in understanding your initial reactions to different people. Your answers will be used in the second part of the survey.

Level of Response	1	2	3	4	5
Individual	Greet	Accept	Help	Background	Advocate
1. Haitian or Haitian American	☐	☐	☐	☐	☐
2. Reformed criminal	☐	☐	☐	☐	☐
3. Observant Jewish person	☐	☐	☐	☐	☐
4. Obese person	☐	☐	☐	☐	☐

BOX 2-2	How Do You Relate to Various Groups of People in the Society? (continued)

5. Neo-Nazi activist ☐ ☐ ☐ ☐ ☐

6. Mexican or Mexican American ☐ ☐ ☐ ☐ ☐

7. Cigarette smoker ☐ ☐ ☐ ☐ ☐

8. Practicing Roman Catholic ☐ ☐ ☐ ☐ ☐

9. Older adult with Alzheimer's disease ☐ ☐ ☐ ☐ ☐

10. Member of a worker's union ☐ ☐ ☐ ☐ ☐

11. Navajo ☐ ☐ ☐ ☐ ☐

12. Sex worker ☐ ☐ ☐ ☐ ☐

13. Practicing Muslim ☐ ☐ ☐ ☐ ☐

14. Person in a wheelchair ☐ ☐ ☐ ☐ ☐

15. Feminist ☐ ☐ ☐ ☐ ☐

16. Iraqi or Iraqi American ☐ ☐ ☐ ☐ ☐

17. Transgender person ☐ ☐ ☐ ☐ ☐

18. Atheist ☐ ☐ ☐ ☐ ☐

19. Person who is HIV positive ☐ ☐ ☐ ☐ ☐

20. Vegan/vegetarian ☐ ☐ ☐ ☐ ☐

21. Chinese exchange student ☐ ☐ ☐ ☐ ☐

22. Unmarried pregnant teenager ☐ ☐ ☐ ☐ ☐

23. Member of Jehovah's Witnesses ☐ ☐ ☐ ☐ ☐

24. Person with cancer ☐ ☐ ☐ ☐ ☐

25. Ku Klux Klansman ☐ ☐ ☐ ☐ ☐

26. Irish or Irish American ☐ ☐ ☐ ☐ ☐

27. Opioid-dependent person ☐ ☐ ☐ ☐ ☐

28. Amish person ☐ ☐ ☐ ☐ ☐

29. Person with anorexia or bulimia ☐ ☐ ☐ ☐ ☐

30. Proponent of socialized health care ☐ ☐ ☐ ☐ ☐

31. Computer hacker or pirate ☐ ☐ ☐ ☐ ☐

32. Shoplifter ☐ ☐ ☐ ☐ ☐

Scoring Guide: The above activity may help you anticipate the various levels of clients that you will encounter as a nurse. The 32 types of individuals can be grouped into five categories: ethnicity and/or race, social/moral/legal, spiritual and/or lifestyle choice, current physical and/or mental health status, and political viewpoint. Transfer your check marks to the following form. If you have a concentration of checks within a specific category of individuals or at specific levels, this may indicate a conflict that could hinder you from rendering effective professional help.

(continued)

BOX 2-2	How Do You Relate to Various Groups of People in the Society? (continued)

Level of Response	1	2	3	4	5
Individual	Greet	Accept	Help	Background	Advocate
Ethnicity and/or race					
1. Haitian or Haitian American	☐	☐	☐	☐	☐
6. Mexican or Mexican American	☐	☐	☐	☐	☐
11. Navajo	☐	☐	☐	☐	☐
16. Iraqi or Iraqi American	☐	☐	☐	☐	☐
21. Chinese exchange student	☐	☐	☐	☐	☐
26. Irish or Irish American	☐	☐	☐	☐	☐
Social/moral/legal					
2. Reformed criminal	☐	☐	☐	☐	☐
12. Sex worker	☐	☐	☐	☐	☐
22. Unmarried pregnant teenager	☐	☐	☐	☐	☐
31. Computer hacker or pirate	☐	☐	☐	☐	☐
32. Shoplifter	☐	☐	☐	☐	☐
Spiritual and/or lifestyle choice					
3. Observant Jewish person	☐	☐	☐	☐	☐
8. Practicing Roman Catholic	☐	☐	☐	☐	☐
17. Transgender person	☐	☐	☐	☐	☐
13. Practicing Muslim	☐	☐	☐	☐	☐
18. Atheist	☐	☐	☐	☐	☐
20. Vegan/vegetarian	☐	☐	☐	☐	☐
23. Member of Jehovah's Witnesses	☐	☐	☐	☐	☐
28. Amish person	☐	☐	☐	☐	☐
Current physical and/or mental health status					
4. Obese person	☐	☐	☐	☐	☐
9. Older adult with Alzheimer's disease	☐	☐	☐	☐	☐
14. Person in a wheelchair	☐	☐	☐	☐	☐
19. Person who is HIV positive	☐	☐	☐	☐	☐
24. Person with cancer	☐	☐	☐	☐	☐
29. Person with anorexia or bulimia	☐	☐	☐	☐	☐

BOX 2-2	How Do You Relate to Various Groups of People in the Society? (continued)				
7. Cigarette smoker	☐	☐	☐	☐	☐
27. Opioid-dependent person	☐	☐	☐	☐	☐
Political viewpoint					
5. Neo-Nazi activist	☐	☐	☐	☐	☐
10. Member of a worker's union	☐	☐	☐	☐	☐
15. Feminist	☐	☐	☐	☐	☐
30. Socialized health care proponent	☐	☐	☐	☐	☐
25. Ku Klux Klansman	☐	☐	☐	☐	☐

Adapted from Randall-David, E. (1989). Assessing your own cultural heritage. In *Strategies for working with culturally diverse communities and clients* (1st ed., pp. 7–9). Bethesda, MD: Association for the Care of Children's Health. Retrieved from https://archive.org/details/strategiesforwor00rand

Health History and Physical Examination, for an in-depth discussion of cultural competence in the health history and physical examination (Jarvis, 2016).

When conducting a comprehensive cultural assessment of clients, nurses need to be able to successfully form, foster, and sustain relationships with people who may frequently come from a cultural background that is different from the nurse's, thus making it necessary to quickly establish rapport with the client. The ability to see the situation from the client's point of view is known as an **emic** or insider's perspective; looking at the situation from an outsider's vantage point is known as an **etic** perspective. The ability to successfully form, foster, and sustain relationships with members of a culture that differs from one's own requires effective cross-cultural communication. Social/moral/legal is based on knowledge of many factors, such as the other person's values, perceptions, attitudes, manners, social structure, decision-making practices, and an understanding of how members of groups communicate both verbally and nonverbally.

Knowledge about a client's family and kinship structure helps nurses to ascertain the values, decision-making patterns, and overall communication within the household. It is necessary to identify the significant others whom clients perceive to be important in their care and who may be responsible for decision-making that affects their health care. For example, for many clients, familism—which emphasizes interdependence over independence, affiliation over confrontation, and cooperation over competition—may dictate that important decisions affecting the client be made by the family, not the individual alone. When working with clients from cultural groups that value cohesion, interdependence, and collectivism, nurses may perceive the family as being overly involved and usurping the autonomy of both the client and the nurse. At the same time, clients are likely to perceive the involvement with family as a source of mutual support, security, comfort, and fulfillment.

The family is the basic social unit in which children are raised and where they learn culturally based values, beliefs, and practices about health and illnesses. The essence of family consists of living together as a unit. Relationships that may seem obvious sometimes warrant further exploration when the nurse interacts with clients from culturally diverse backgrounds. For example, most European Americans define siblings as two persons with the same mother, the same father, the same mother and father, or the same adoptive parents. In some Asian cultures, a sibling relationship is defined as any infant breast-fed by the same woman. In other cultures, certain kinship patterns, such as maternal first cousins, are defined as sibling relationships. In some African cultures, anyone from the same village or town may be called brother or sister.

Among some Hispanic groups, for example, female members of the nuclear or extended family such as sisters and aunts are primary providers of care for infants and children. In some African American families, the grandmother may be the decision-maker and primary caretaker of children. To provide culturally congruent and competent care, nurses must effectively communicate with the appropriate decision-maker(s).

When making health-related decisions, some clients may seek assistance from other members of the family. It is sometimes culturally expected that a relative (e.g., parent, grandparent, eldest son, or eldest brother) will make decisions about important health-related matters. For example, in Japan, it is the obligation and duty of the eldest son and his spouse to assume primary responsibility for aging parents and to make health care decisions for them. Among the Amish, the entire community is affected by the illness of a member and pays for health care from a common fund. The Amish join together to meet the needs of both the sick person and his or her family throughout the illness, and the roles of dozens of people in the community are likely to be affected by the illness of a single member. The individual value orientation concerning relationships is predominant among the dominant cultural majority in North America. Although members of the nuclear family may participate to varying degrees, decision-making about health and illness is often an individual matter. Nurses should ascertain the identity of all key participants in the decision-making process; sometimes, decisions are made after consultation with family members, but the individual is the primary decision-maker.

Individual Cultural Competence

Individual cultural competence is a complex integration of knowledge, attitudes, values, beliefs, behaviors, skills, practices, and cross-cultural nurse–client interactions that include effective communication and the provision of safe, affordable, accessible, research-based, evidence-based, and best practices and acceptable, quality, and efficacious nursing care for clients from diverse backgrounds. The term diverse or **diversity** refers to the client's uniqueness in the dimensions of race; ethnicity; national origin; socioeconomic background; age; gender; sexual orientation; philosophical and religious ideology; lifestyle; level of education; literacy; marital status; physical, emotional, and psychological ability; political ideology; size; and other characteristics used to compare or categorize people (Kroeber, 2018).

Although the connotation of diversity is generally positive, it is sometimes argued that the term diversity is itself an ethnocentric term because it focuses on how different the other person is from *me*, rather than how different I am from *the other person*. In using the term *cultural diversity*, the White panethnic group frequently is viewed as the norm against which the differences in everyone else (ethnocentrically referred to as non-Whites) are measured or compared.

Cultural competence is not an end point but a dynamic, ongoing, lifelong, developmental process that requires self-reflection, intrinsic motivation, and commitment by the nurse to value, respect, and refrain from judging the beliefs, language, interpersonal styles, behaviors, and culturally based, health-related practices of individuals and families receiving services as well as the professional and auxiliary staff who are providing such services (Kroeber, 2018). Culturally competent nursing and health care require an effective cross-cultural communication and a diverse workforce and are provided in a variety of social, cultural, economic, environmental, and other contexts across the life span. Scholars from nursing, medicine, psychology, social work, physical therapy, education, anthropology, and many other disciplines have written about cultural competence (American Medical Association, 2013; Andrews, et al., 2011; Andrews & Collins, 2015; McFarland & Wehbe-Alamah, 2018; Montgomery, 2019; Purnell & Fenkl, 2018; Spector, 2017).

Given the large number of cultures and sub-cultures in the world, it's impossible for nurses to know everything about them all; however, it is possible for nurses to develop excellent cultural assessment and cross-cultural communication skills and to follow a systematic, orderly process for the delivery of culturally competent care. Nurses are encouraged to study in depth the top two or three cultural groups that they encounter most frequently in their clinical practice and develop the affective (feelings or emotions), cognitive (conscious mental activities such as thinking), and psychomotor (combined thinking and motor) skills necessary to deliver culturally competent nursing care. As new groups move into a geographic area, nurses need to update their knowledge and skills in order to be responsive to the changing demographics. For nurses in large multicultural urban centers, the challenge of keeping pace with client diversity is complex and needs to become an integral component of the nurse's continuing professional development. Professional organizations, employer-sponsored in-service programs, and Web-based resources provide nurses with valuable sources of information on culturally based health beliefs and practices of clients from diverse backgrounds.

Figure 2-1 provides a more detailed view of the five-step problem-solving process for delivering culturally congruent and competent nursing care for individual clients introduced in Chapter 1. Clients (the individual, their family, and significant others) are at the center and are the focus of the interprofessional health care team (which includes credentialed and/or licensed health professionals and folk, traditional, religious, and spiritual healers).

Step 2 of the process is assessment—of both the nurse and the client. This begins with nurses' *self-assessment* of their attitudes, values, and beliefs about people from backgrounds that differ

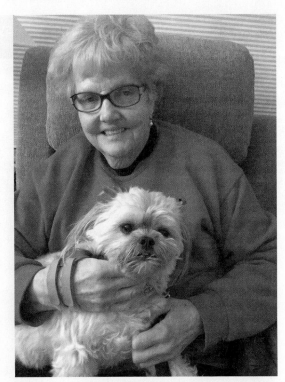

Figure 2-1. During visiting hours, this pet is a frequent companion to a patient recovering from knee replacement surgery in a rehabilitation facility with a pet-friendly policy.

from their own; their *knowledge* of their own **self-location** (cultural, gender, class, and other social self-identities) compared to those of clients and other team members; and the *psychomotor skills* needed for the delivery of culturally congruent and competent care (see Box 2-3). The self-assessment includes self-reflection and reflexivity (analysis of cause–effect relationships) for the purpose of uncovering the nurse's unconscious biases, cultural stereotypes, prejudices, and discriminatory behaviors. Nurses then have the opportunity to change, or rectify, affective, cognitive, or psychomotor deficits by reframing their attitude toward certain individuals and groups from diverse backgrounds, learning more about the cultures and subcultures most frequently encountered in their clinical practice, and developing psychomotor skills that enhance their

BOX 2-3	Selected Examples of Psychomotor Skills Useful in Transcultural Nursing

Assessment

- Techniques for assessing biocultural variations in health and illness, for example, assessing cyanosis, jaundice, anemia, and related clinical manifestations of disease in darkly pigmented clients, differentiating between Mongolian spots and ecchymoses (bruises)
- Measurement of head circumference and fontanelles in infants using techniques not in violation of taboos for selected cultural groups
- Growth and development monitoring for children of Asian heritage using culturally appropriate growth grids
- Cultural modification of the Denver II and other developmental tests used for children
- Conducting culturally appropriate obstetric and gynecologic examinations of women from various cultural backgrounds

Communication

- Speaking and writing the language(s) used by clients
- Using alternative methods of communicating with non–English-speaking clients and families when no interpreter is available (e.g., pantomime, e-translators for smartphones, tablets, and other devices)

Hygiene

- Skin care for people of various racial/ethnic backgrounds
- Hair care for people of various ethnic/racial backgrounds, for example, care of African American clients' hair

Activities of Daily Living

- Assisting Chinese American clients to regain the use of chopsticks as part of rehabilitation regimen after a stroke
- Assisting paralyzed Amish client with dressing when buttons and pins are used
- Assisting West African client who uses "chewing stick" for oral hygiene

Religion

- Emergency baptism and anointing of the sick for Roman Catholics
- Care before and after ritual circumcision by *mohel* (performed 8 days after the birth of a male Jewish infant)

ability to use and their clinical skills to deliver culturally congruent and competent nursing care.

The comprehensive cultural assessment of the client and his/her family and significant others (people, companion animals, and pets) (Figure 2-1) requires nurses to gather subjective and objective data through the health history and the physical examination (see Chapter 3). The nurse should consider the influence of the following factors: environmental, social, economic, religious, philosophical, moral, legal, political, educational, biological (genetic and acquired diseases, conditions, disorders, injuries, and illnesses), and technological. In addition, the nurse may have professional and organizational cultures that influence the nurse–patient interaction, such as hospital or agency policies that determine visiting hours or laws governing the nurse's scope of practice and professional responsibilities within a particular jurisdiction or setting. The influence of cultural and health belief systems (on the nurse and the client) must also be considered in relation to disease causation, healing modalities, and choice of healer(s). See Chapter 4, The Influence of Cultural Belief Systems on Health Care Practices, for detailed information.

In steps 2 to 4, the nurse collaborates with the client, the client's family and significant others, and members of the health care team (credentialed, folk, traditional, religious, and spiritual healers). The terms **folk healer** and **traditional healer** sometimes are used interchangeably. Folk healers typically learn healing practices through an apprenticeship with someone experienced in folk healing. Folk healers primarily use herbal remedies, foods, and inanimate objects in a therapeutic manner. Traditional or indigenous healers often are divinely chosen and/or learn the art of healing by applying knowledge, skills, and practices based on experiences indigenous to their culture, for example, Native American medicine men/women and shamans. The focus of most traditional and indigenous healers is on establishing and restoring balance and harmony in the body–mind–spirit through the use of spiritual healing interventions, such as praying, chanting, drumming, dancing, participating in sweat lodge rituals, and storytelling. The definition and scope of practice of religious and spiritual healers vary widely, but these healers often help clients analyze complex health-related decisions involving moral and/or ethical issues (see Chapter 12, Religion, Culture, and Nursing, and Chapter 13, Cultural Competence in Ethical Decision-Making). All healers whom the client wants to be involved in care should be included in steps 2 to 5 to the extent feasible.

In *step 2*, mutual goals are set, and objectives are established to meet the goals and desired health outcomes.

In *step 3*, the plan of care is developed using approaches that are client centered and culturally congruent with the client's socioeconomic, philosophical, and religious beliefs, resources, and practices. Members of the health care team assume roles and responsibilities according to their educational background, clinical knowledge, and skills. For credentialed or licensed members of the team such as nurses; physicians; physical, occupational, and respiratory therapists; social workers; and similar health professions, roles, responsibilities, and scope of practice are delineated by ministries of health, provincial or state health professions licensing, and/or registration boards. In most instances, the credentialed or licensed healer has formal academic

preparation and has passed an examination that tested knowledge and skills deemed necessary for clinical practice.

In *step 4*, decisions, actions, treatments, and interventions that are congruent with the patient's health-related cultural beliefs and practices are implemented by those team members who are best prepared to assist the client. In some instances, there is overlapping of scope of practice, roles, and responsibilities between and among team members (Figure 2-2). Client-centered interprofessional team conferences are usually helpful in sorting out roles and responsibilities of

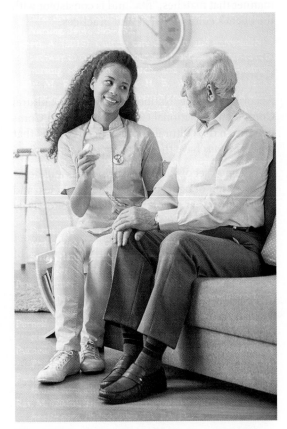

Figure 2-2. Effective cross-cultural communication is vital to the establishment of a strong nurse–client relationship. It is important to understand both verbal and nonverbal cues when communicating with people from different cultural backgrounds (Photographee.eu\ Shutterstock.com).

team members when there is lack of clarity about who will deliver a particular service.

Lastly, in *step 5*, the client and members of the health care team collaboratively evaluate the care plan and its objectives to determine if the care is safe; culturally acceptable, congruent, and competent; affordable; accessible; of high quality; and based on research, scientific evidence, and/ or best practices. If modifications or changes are needed, the nurse should return to previous steps and repeat the process. Throughout the five steps of the process for the delivery of culturally congruent and competent nursing care, the nurse behaves in an empathetic, compassionate, caring manner that matches, "fits," and is consistent with the client's cultural beliefs and practices.

Organizational Cultural Competence

According to the National Center for Cultural Competence (National Center for Cultural Competence, n.d.), cultural competence requires that *organizations* have the following characteristics:

- A defined set of values and principles and demonstration of behaviors, attitudes, policies, and structures that enable them to work effectively cross-culturally
- The capacity to (1) value diversity, (2) conduct self-assessments, (3) manage the dynamics of difference, (4) acquire and institutionalize cultural knowledge, and (5) adapt to diversity and the cultural contexts of the communities they serve
- Incorporation of the previously mentioned items in all aspects of policy making, administration, practice, and service delivery and systematic involvement of consumers, key stakeholders, and communities (National Center for Cultural Competence, n.d.c; Marrone, 2014)

Organizational cultural competence is discussed in detail in Chapter 9, Creating Culturally Competent Organizations. Appendix C contains the Andrews/Boyle Transcultural Nursing Assessment Guide for Health Care Organizations and Facilities.

Clients with Special Needs

In the remainder of this chapter, we discuss the delivery of culturally competent nursing care for three groups of clients with special needs: those at high risk for health inequities and health disparities, those who are deaf, and those with communication and special language needs.

Health Disparities

The Health Resources and Services Administration defines health disparities as population-specific differences in the presence of disease, health outcomes, or access to health care. These differences can affect how frequently a disease affects a group, how many people get sick, or how often the disease causes death (U.S. Department of Health and Human Services, 2015). Many different populations are affected by disparities. These include the following:

- Racial and ethnic minorities
- Residents of rural areas
- Women, children, and older adults
- Persons with disabilities
- Other special populations such as the deaf and hearing impaired or blind and visually impaired

In the United States, health disparities are a well-known problem among panethnic minority groups, particularly African Americans, Asian Americans, Native Americans, and Latinos. When examining health disparities within countries and globally, the World Health Organization uses the term health inequities (World Health Organization, 2018a).

Recent studies indicate that despite the steady improvements in the overall health of the United States, clients from racial and ethnic minority backgrounds experience a lower quality of health services, are less likely to receive routine medical procedures, and have higher rates of morbidity and mortality than nonminorities. Disparities in health care exist even when controlling for gender, condition, age, and socioeconomic status (Frieden, 2013; Mandal, 2018; Narayan & Scafide, 2017; Office of Minority Health, n.d.; Purnell & Fenkl, 2018). The

U.S. Department of Health, Health Resources and Services Administration identifies culturally competent nursing care as an effective approach in reducing and eliminating health disparities and inequities in high-risk populations such as Blacks, Latinos, and American Indians. Studies demonstrate that these groups have a higher prevalence of chronic conditions, along with higher rates of mortality and poorer health outcomes, when compared with counterparts in the general population. For example, African Americans have the highest overall cancer incidence and death rates compared to other major racial/ethnic groups, 10% and 23% higher, respectively, than non-Hispanic White males and Hispanic males (American Cancer Society, 2018). African Americans and Latinos are also approximately twice as likely to develop diabetes as counterparts in the general population. Throughout the remaining chapters of the book, we will discuss interventions and strategies for reducing health disparities and inequities through the delivery of culturally congruent and culturally competent nursing and health care for people from diverse backgrounds across the life span.

Culture of the Deaf

Although nurses tend to think about clients from racially and ethnically diverse backgrounds, when discussing culturally competent nursing care, there are many people who self-identify with *nonethnic cultures,* such as the **cultural of the deaf**, and/or with more than one culture or subculture. For example, more than 5% of the world's population (466 million adults and 34 million children) experience disabling hearing loss (World Health Organization, 2018). Additionally, nurses will encounter clients who are of "double minority," both Black and deaf, gay and deaf, Native American and deaf, and many other combinations of two or more cultures (Nelson Schmitt & Leigh, 2015). **Disabling hearing loss** is defined as the loss of greater than 40 decibels in the better ear in adults and the loss of greater than 30 decibels in the better ear in children. Disabling hearing loss means that a client has very little or no hearing, which has consequences for interpersonal communication, psychosocial well-being, quality of life, and economic independence. Hearing loss may affect one or both ears, can be congenital or acquired, and occurs on a continuum from mild to severe. Hearing loss leads to difficulty in hearing conversational speech or loud sounds. Clients who are **hard of hearing** usually communicate through spoken language and can benefit from hearing aids, captioning, and assistive listening devices (National Institute on Deafness and Other Communication Disorders, 2018; World Health Organization, 2018b).

If hearing loss develops in childhood, it impedes speech and language development and, in severe cases, requires special education. In adulthood, disabling hearing loss can lead to embarrassment, loneliness, social isolation, stigmatization, prejudice, abuse, mental health problems such as depression, difficulties in interpersonal relationships with partners and children, restricted career choices, occupational stress, and lower earnings when compared with counterparts who do not have disabling hearing loss. Approximately one-third of people over 65 years of age are affected by disabling hearing loss. The prevalence in this age group is greatest in South Asia, Asia Pacific, and sub-Saharan Africa (World Health Organization, 2018).

Some clients with congenital deafness or others with significant hearing losses may benefit from cochlear implants, but the decision to have a cochlear implant is interconnected with an animated debate within and between members of the deaf culture and members of the culture of medicine concerning the appropriateness of cochlear implants. The fundamental issues underlying the debate concern the philosophical belief about deafness and the concept of deaf culture.

From an **emic** perspective, many deaf people see their bodies as well, whole, and non-impaired, and they self-identify as members of a linguistic minority, not with the culture of disability (Carter & Mireles, 2016; Harrington, 2016; Harris, 2014; Holcomb, 2013; Humphries, 2014; Leigh & Andrews, 2017; Mandal, 2018). As members of a cultural minority, some deaf people perceive themselves as being on a journey of cultural awareness, one of several stages on the way to achieving a positive sense of self- and deaf identity. On the other hand, others who are deaf advocate reframing the concept of a deaf culture and conceptualizing it as the deaf experience based on values stemming from a visual orientation. Recognizing that the literature and the arts provide forums for cultural awareness, appreciation, and expression of ideas and feelings, there are a growing number of deaf people using these media to communicate their experiences with one another and with hearing members of society.

From an **etic** (outsider's) perspective, some physicians and other members of the hearing society embrace concepts about deaf peoples' bodies that emphasize their differences from the bodies of people in the hearing society, thereby placing unwanted, unwarranted, and unnecessary limitations on deaf people's lives and capabilities. In the biological sciences, for example, the bodies of hearing people historically have been constructed with a normative bias. In other words, the body that hears is the normative prototype. Some physicians engage in the cultural imposition of medical and surgical interventions on members of the deaf culture through eugenics (a science that tries to improve the human race by controlling which people become parents), genetic engineering, and insistence that deaf people should use hearing aids, agree to cochlear implant surgery, and embrace other technologies that profoundly change their lives and their culture.

Box 2-4 uses the framework of the five-step process for delivering culturally congruent and competent nursing care for people who self-identify as members of the deaf culture, beginning with a cultural assessment of self and the client, mutual goal setting, planning, implementation, and evaluation. Box 2-5 identifies measures that nurses can take to prevent deafness.

There are hundreds of sign language dialects in use around the world. Each culture has developed its own form of sign language to be compatible with the language spoken in that country. In the United States, an estimated 500,000 people communicate by using American Sign Language (ASL), including many who are deaf and hearing impaired and family members, friends, or teachers of people with hearing impairments (Harrington, 2016). An ASL interpreter is often helpful in avoiding communication difficulty when caring for someone who is deaf or hearing impaired. Signaling and assistive listening devices, alerting devices, telecommunication devices for the deaf (TDD), and telephone amplifiers might also help promote effective communication and facilitate the provision of culturally competent care in home, community, hospital, and other settings.

Communication and Language Assistance

With growing concerns about racial, ethnic, and language disparities in health and health care and the need for health care systems to accommodate increasingly diverse patient populations, **language access services (LAS)** have become a matter of increasing national importance. Currently, about 20% of the US population speaks a language other than English at home, and 9% has limited English proficiency. By 2050, more than half of the population will come from racial or ethnic minority backgrounds. Diversity is even greater when dimensions such as geography, socioeconomic status, disability status, sexual orientation, and gender identity are considered. Attention to these trends is critical for ensuring that health disparities narrow, rather than widen, in the future. The Office of Minority Health's National Standards for Culturally and Linguistically Appropriate Services in Health and Health Care (the National CLAS Standards) are in Box 2-6.

Standards under the theme "Communication and Language Assistance" include the recommendation that language assistance should be provided as needed, in a manner appropriate to the organization's size, scope, and mission (Larson, 2017). Clients are informed about the availability of assistance in their preferred language after being

BOX 2-4 | Culturally Congruent and Competent Care for Deaf Clients

1. **Cultural Assessment**
   - **Self-Assessment**
     - What is your attitude toward people who are deaf?
     - Do you think of people who are deaf as able-bodied or disabled?
     - How do you feel about those who use hearing aids and other assistive devices for hearing?
     - How do you assess your self-location with regard to culture, gender, class, age, and other self-identities compared to the client's background?
     - What do you know about deafness, for example, causes, categories or types, and assistive devices?
     - Do you know anyone who is deaf?
       - If so, how do you feel about the interactions you had with this person(s)?
   - **Client Assessment**
     Health History (Subjective Data)—*See Appendix A, Transcultural Nursing Assessment Guide for Individuals and Families, for questions you might want to pose in the following categories:*
     - Cultural affiliations or self-identities associated with deafness?
     - Client's preferred method for communication?
       - Sign language?
       - Written communication?
       - Verbal communication?

   - Are any assistive devices needed for effective communication?
   - Has exclusion from communication significantly impacted everyday life?
   - Is there any evidence of feelings of loneliness, isolation, and frustration, particularly for older adults with hearing loss?
   - Cultural sanctions and restrictions?
   - Economic or financial concerns?
   - Adults with hearing loss have a much higher unemployment rate and earn less than counterparts who have hearing. Is the client employed?
   - Education and health literacy levels?
   - In developing countries, children with hearing loss and deafness rarely receive any schooling. What is the educational and health literacy level of the client? Improving access to education and vocational rehabilitation services and raising awareness, especially among employers, would decrease unemployment rates among adults with hearing loss.
   - Health-related beliefs and practices?
   - Kinship and social support network?
   - Nutrition and diet?
   - Religion and spirituality?
   - Value orientation of the client, including his/her perspective on culturally acceptable interventions to improve hearing?
   Physical Examination (Objective Data): *See Chapter 3, Cultural Competence in the Health History and Physical Examination.*

2. **Mutual Goal Setting**
3. **Care Planning**
4. **Implementation of Care Plan**
5. **Evaluation of Care**

> In collaboration with client's family; significant others; credentialed, licensed members of the health care team (e.g., audiologist, speech–language pathologist); and folk, traditional, religious, and/or spiritual healers

- Culturally acceptable, congruent, and competent?
- Affordable?
- Accessible?
- Quality?
- Evidence based?
- Best practices?

BOX 2-5 | Prevention of Deafness

Fifty percent of all cases of hearing loss can be prevented through primary prevention. Strategies for prevention include:

- Immunizing children against childhood diseases, including measles, meningitis, rubella, and mumps
- Immunizing adolescent girls and women of reproductive age against rubella before pregnancy
- Screening for and treating syphilis and other infections in pregnant women
- Improving antenatal and perinatal care, including promotion of safe childbirth
- Avoiding the use of ototoxic drugs, unless prescribed and monitored by a qualified physician, nurse practitioner, or other health care providers
- Referring infants with high-risk factors (such as those with a family history of deafness and those born with low birth weight, birth asphyxia, jaundice, or meningitis) for early assessment of hearing, prompt diagnosis, and appropriate management, as required
- Reducing exposure (both occupational and recreational) to loud noises by creating awareness, using personal protective devices, and developing and implementing suitable legislation

Data from World Health Organization (2018). Deafness prevention. Retrieved from https://www.who.int/deafness/en/

BOX 2-6 | National Standards for Culturally and Linguistically Appropriate Services in Health and Health Care

The National Standards for Culturally and Linguistically Appropriate Services in Health and Health Care (the National CLAS Standards) aim to improve health care quality and advance health equity by establishing a framework for organizations to serve the nation's increasingly diverse communities.

Principal Standard

1. Provide effective, equitable, understandable, and respectful quality care and services that are responsive to diverse cultural health beliefs and practices, preferred languages, health literacy, and other communication needs.

Governance, Leadership, and Workforce

2. Advance and sustain organizational governance and leadership that promotes CLAS and health equity through policy, practices, and allocated resources.

3. Recruit, promote, and support a culturally and linguistically diverse governance, leadership, and workforce that are responsive to the population in the service area.
4. Educate and train governance, leadership, and workforce in culturally and linguistically appropriate policies and practices on an ongoing basis.

Communication and Language Assistance

5. Offer language assistance to individuals who have limited English proficiency and/or other communication needs, at no cost to them, to facilitate timely access to all health care and services.
6. Inform all individuals of the availability of language assistance services clearly and in their preferred language, verbally and in writing.

| BOX 2-6 | National Standards for Culturally and Linguistically Appropriate Services in Health and Health Care (continued) |

7. Ensure the competence of individuals providing language assistance, recognizing that the use of untrained individuals and/or minors as interpreters should be avoided.

8. Provide easy-to-understand print and multimedia materials and signage in the languages commonly used by the populations in the service area.

Engagement, Continuous Improvement, and Accountability

9. Establish culturally and linguistically appropriate goals, policies, and management accountability, and infuse them throughout the organizations' planning and operations.

10. Conduct ongoing assessments of the organization's CLAS-related activities and integrate CLAS-related measures into assessment measurement and continuous quality improvement activities.

11. Collect and maintain accurate and reliable demographic data to monitor and evaluate the impact of CLAS on health equity and outcomes and to inform service delivery.

12. Conduct regular assessments of community health assets and needs and use the results to plan and implement services that respond to the cultural and linguistic diversity of populations in the service area.

13. Partner with the community to design, implement, and evaluate policies, practices, and services to ensure cultural and linguistic appropriateness.

14. Create conflict and grievance resolution processes that are culturally and linguistically appropriate to identify, prevent, and resolve conflicts or complaints.

15. Communicate the organization's progress in implementing and sustaining CLAS to all stakeholders, constituents, and the general public.

Source: Office of Minority Health. (2018). The national CLAS standards. Retrieved from https://www.minorityhealth.hhs.gov/omh/browse.aspx?lvl=2&lvlid=53

asked to indicate their language needs (Burkle et al., 2017; U.S. Department of Health & Human Services, n.d.). Health care organizations and providers that receive federal financial assistance without providing free language assistance services could be in violation of Title VI of the Civil Rights Act of 1964 and its implementation regulations. The director of the U.S. Department of Health and Human Services Office for Civil Rights encourages requests for information and technical assistance concerning the law (Hoh, Garcia, & Alvarez, 2014).

Summary

In this chapter, the reader was introduced to individual and organizational cultural competence and provided with the knowledge and skills needed to deliver culturally congruent and competent nursing care to individual clients from diverse cultures. Nurses are encouraged to think about the delivery of care as a five-step process consisting of:

1. A constructively critical self-assessment of the nurse's own attitudes, knowledge, and skills and a cultural assessment of clients from diverse backgrounds by gathering subjective and objective data using the health history and physical examination

2. Mutual goal setting in collaboration with the client and other members of the interprofessional health care team (family, significant others, credentialed, licensed, folk, traditional, religious, and/or spiritual healers)

3. Development of the plan of care

4. Implementation of the care plan

5. Evaluation of the plan for client acceptance, cultural congruence, cultural competence, affordability, accessibility, and use of research, evidence, and best practices

If necessary, the steps in the process may be repeated. Interprofessional collaboration with the client and members of the health care team is integral to the provision of culturally congruent and competent nursing care. Lastly, we examined clients with special needs including those at high risk for health disparities, those who are deaf, and those with communication and language needs.

REVIEW QUESTIONS

1. Compare and contrast individual and organizational cultural competence.
2. Describe the five steps in the process for delivering culturally congruent and competent care for clients from diverse backgrounds.
3. In your own words, define the following terms: cultural baggage, ethnocentrism, cultural imposition, prejudice, and discrimination.
4. Identify key strategies to assist clients with communication and language needs.

CRITICAL THINKING ACTIVITIES

1. After critically analyzing the definitions of cultural competence presented in the chapter, craft a definition of the term in your own words.

2. In discussions of culturally competent nursing care, the culture of the deaf and hearing impaired is sometimes overlooked because it is categorized as a nonethnic culture. Search the Internet for information on the culture of the deaf. What cultural characteristics do deaf people have in common with members of other cultural groups? If a client is both deaf and self-identifies as a member of another ethnic or nonethnic culture, how does this influence your ability to deliver culturally congruent and culturally competent nursing care?

3. To provide culturally competent nursing care, you should engage in a cultural self-assessment. Answer the questions in Box 2-2, How Do You Relate to Various Groups of People in the Society? Score your answers using the guide provided. What did you learn about yourself? How would you approach learning more about the health-related beliefs and practices of groups for which you need more background knowledge? What resources might you use in your search for information?

4. At the request of the Bureau of Primary Health Care, Health Resources and Services Administration, U.S. Department of Health and Human Services, staff at the National Center for Cultural Competence (NCCC) developed the *Cultural Competence Health Practitioner Assessment*, which is available online. Visit the NCCC website and complete this assessment.

5. Mary Johnson is an African American nurse working in the postanesthesia care unit (PACU). When Mrs. Li, a recent immigrant from China, arrives in the PACU following a major bowel resection for cancer, Mary assesses Mrs. Li for pain. Mary notes that Mrs. Li is not complaining about pain, is lying quietly in her bed, and has a stoic facial expression. Mary comments to another nurse that "all Chinese patients seem to do just fine without postoperative pain medications. I'm not going to administer any analgesics unless she asks me for something." Do you agree with Nurse Johnson's assessment of Mrs. Li's pain? What nonverbal manifestations of pain would you assess? How would you reply to Nurse Johnson's statement that she doesn't intend to administer any pain medication?

REFERENCES

American Cancer Society. (2018). Cancer facts and figures 2018. Retrieved from https://www.cancer.org/content/dam/cancer-org/research/cancer-facts-and-statistics/annual-cancer-facts-and-figures/2018/cancer-facts-and-figures 2018.pdf

American Medical Association. (2013). *Health literacy and patient safety: Helping patients understand.* Chicago, MA: Author.

Andrews, J. D. (2013). *Cultural, ethnic, and religious reference manual for healthcare providers* (4th ed.). Kernersville, NC: JAMARDA Resources.

Andrews, M. M., & Collins, J. W. (2015). Using Leininger's theory as the organizing framework for a federal project on cultural competence. In M. R. McFarland & H. B. Wehbe-Alamah (Eds.), *Leininger's culture care diversity and universality: A worldwide nursing theory* (pp. 537–582). Burlington, MA: Jones and Bartlett Learning.

Andrews, M., Thompson, T., Wehbe-Alamah, H., McFarland, M. R., Hasenau, S., Horn, B., ... Vint, P. (2011). Developing a culturally competent workforce through collaborative partnerships. *Journal of Transcultural Nursing, 22*(3), 300–306.

Burkle, C. M., Anderson, K. A., Xiong, Y., Guerra, A. E., Tschida-Reuter, D. A., & Xiong, Y. (2017). Assessment of the efficiency of language interpreter services in a busy surgical and procedural practice. *BMC Health Services Research, 17*, 1–6. Retrieved from https://doi-org.libproxy.umflint.edu/10.1186/s12913-017-2425-7

Carter, M. J., & Mireles, D. C. (2016). Exploring the relationship between deaf identity verification processes and self-esteem. *Identity, 16*(2), 102–114. doi: 10.1080/15283488.2016.1159963

Clark, L. (2014). A humanizing gaze for transcultural nursing research will tell the story of health disparities. *Journal of Transcultural Nursing, 25*(2), 122–128.

Douglas, M. K. (2018). Building an organizational environment of cultural competence. In M. K. Douglas, D. F. Pacquiao, & L. Prunell (Eds.), *Global applications of culturally competent health care: Guidelines for practice* (pp. 203–313). Cham, Switzerland: Springer International Publishing.

Douglas, M. K., Pacquiao, D. F., & Purnell, L. (2018). *Global applications of culturally competent health care: Guidelines for practice.* Cham, Switzerland: Springer International Publishing.

Douglas, M. K., Rosenkoetter, M., Pacquaio, D. F., Callister, L. C., Hattar-Pollara, M., Lauderdale, J., ... Purnell, L. (2014). Guidelines for implementing culturally competent nursing care. *Journal of Transcultural Nursing,* 25(2), 110–129.

Dunagan, P. B., Kimble, L. P., Gunby, S. S., & Andrews, M. M. (2016). Baccalaureate nursing students' attitudes of prejudice: A qualitative inquiry. *Journal of Nursing Education, 55*(6), 345–348. doi: 10.3928/01484834-20160516-0

Frieden, T. R. (2013). CDC Health disparities and inequalities report—United States, 2013. *Morbidity and Mortality Weekly Report.* Surveillance summaries (Washington, DC: 2002), *62*(Suppl 3), 1–2.

Harrington, T. (2016). Sign language: Ranking and number of users. Retrieved from http://libguides.gallaudet.edu/content.php?pid=114804&sid=991835

Harris, R. (2014). Introduction to American deaf culture. *Sign Language Studies, 14*(3), 406–410.

Hoh, H. K., Garcia, J. N., & Alvarez, M. H. (2014). Culturally and linguistically appropriate services—Advancing health with CLAS. *New England Journal of Medicine, 371*, 198–201.

Holcomb, T. K. (2013). *Introduction to American deaf culture.* New York, NY: Oxford University Press.

Humphries, T. (2014). Our time: The legacy of the twentieth century. *Sign Language Studies, 15*(1), 57–73.

Institute of Medicine. (2011). *Future of nursing: Leading change, advancing health.* Washington, DC: National Academies Press.

Interprofessional Education Collaborative Expert Panel. (2011). *Core competencies for interprofessional collaborative practice: Report of an expert panel.* Washington, DC: Interprofessional Education Collaborative.

Kroeber, A. L. (2018). *Culture: A critical review of concepts and definitions.* London: Forgotten Books. Retrieved from http://www.forgottenbooks.com

Leigh, I. W. & Andrews, J. F. (2017). *Deaf people and society: Psychological, sociological and educational perspectives* (2nd ed.). New York, NY: Routledge.

Mandal, A. (2018). What are health disparities? Retrieved from https://www.news-medical.net/health/What-are-Health-Disparities.aspx

Marrone, S. (2014). Organizational cultural competence. Transcultural Nursing Society Annual Conference, October 2014, Charleston, SC.

McFarland, M. R., & Wehbe-Alamah, H. B. (2018). *Transcultural nursing: Concepts, theories, research, and practices* (4th ed). New York: McGraw-Hill, Medical Publishing Division.

Montgomery, M. (2019). *Language, media, and culture: The key concepts.* New York, NY: Routledge.

Moss, E., Seifert, C. P., & O'Sullivan, A. (2016). Registered nurses as interprofessional collaborative partners: Creating value-based outcomes. *The Online Journal of Issues in Nursing, 21*(3), 4. doi: 10.3912/OJIN.Vol21No03Man04

Narayan, M. C., & Scafide, K. N. (2017). Systematic review of racial/ethnic outcome disparities in home health care. *Journal of Transcultural Nursing, 28*(6), 598–607. doi: 10.1177/1043659617700710

National Center for Cultural Competence. (n.d.a). Definitions of cultural competence. (Georgetown University Center for Child and Human Development). Retrieved from Curricula Enhancement Module Series: http://www.nccccurricula.info/culturalcompetence.html

National Center for Cultural Competence. (n.d.b). Foundations of cultural and linguistic competence. Retrieved from http://nccc.georgetown.edu/foundations/index.html

National Center for Cultural Competence. (n.d.c). Organizational cultural competence. Retrieved from https://nccc.georgetown.edu/foundations/framework.php

National Center for Cultural Competence. (n.d.d). Guiding principles of self-assessment. Retrieved September 28, 2018 from https://nccc.georgetown.edu/assessments/principles.php

National Institute on Deafness and Other Communication Disorders. (2018). Age-related hearing loss. Retrieved from https://www.nidcd.nih.gov/health/age-related-hearing-loss

Nelson Schmitt, S., & Leigh, I. (2015). Examining a sample of black deaf individuals on the deaf acculturation scale. *The Journal of Deaf Studies and Deaf Education, 20*(3), 283–295. doi: https://doi.org/10.1093/deafed/env017

Office of Disease Prevention and Health Promotion. (2018). Social determinants of health. Retrieved from https://www.healthypeople.gov/2020/topics-objectives/topic/social-determinants-of-health

Office of Minority Health. (2018). The national CLAS standards. Retrieved from https://www.minorityhealth.hhs.gov/omh/browse.aspx?lvl=2&lvlid=53

Office of Minority Health. (n.d.). National standards for culturally and linguistically appropriate services in health and health care. Retrieved from https://minorityhealth.hhs.gov/omh/browse.aspx?lvl=2&lvlid=34

Pacquiao, D. F., & Douglas, M. (2019). *Social pathways to health vulnerability: Implications for health professionals.* Cham, Switzerland: Springer International Publishing AG, part of Springer Nature.

Purnell, L., & Fenkl, E. (2018). *Guide to culturally competent health care.* Philadelphia, PA: F.A.Davis.

Ray, M. (2010a). Creating caring organizations and cultures through communitarian ethics. *Journal of the World Universities Forum, 3*(5), 41–52.

Spector, R. E. (2017). *Cultural diversity in health and illness* (9th ed.). Upper Saddle River, NJ: Pearson.

Title VII of the Civil Rights Act of 1964 (Public Law 88–352). Retrieved from http://www.eeoc.gov/laws/statutes/ada.cfmwww.eeoc.gov/laws/statutes/titlevii.cfm

Titles I and V of the Americans with Disabilities Act of 1990 (Pub. L. 101–336) (ADA). Retrieved from http://www.eeoc.gov/laws/statutes/ada.cfm

U.S. Census Bureau. (2016). Selected social characteristics in the United States. Retrieved from https://factfinder.census.gov/faces/tableservices/jsf/pages/productview.xhtml?pid=ACS_16_5YR_DP02&src=pt

U.S. Department of Health and Human Services. (2015). HHS Action Plan to Reduce Racial and Ethnic Health Disparities Implementation Progress Report. Retrieved from https://minorityhealth.hhs.gov/assets/pdf/FINAL_HHS_Action_Plan_Progress_Report_11_2_2015.pdf

U.S. Department of Health and Human Services. (n.d.). National Standards for Culturally and Linguistically Appropriate Services (CLAS) in Health and Health Care. Retrieved from https://www.thinkculturalhealth.hhs.gov/clas

U.S. Equal Employment Opportunity Commission. (2016). EEOC Enforcement Guidance on National Origin Discrimination. Retrieved from https://www.eeoc.gov/laws/guidance/national-origin-guidance.cfm#_ftn1

World Health Organization. (2010). *Framework for action on interprofessional education and collaborative practice.* Geneva, Switzerland: Author.

World Health Organization. (2018a). Social determinants of health: key concepts. Retrieved from http://www.who.int/social_determinants/thecommission/finalreport/key_concepts/en/

World Health Organization. (2018b). Deafness and hearing loss. Retrieved from http://www.who.int/news-room/fact-sheets/detail/deafness-and-hearing-loss

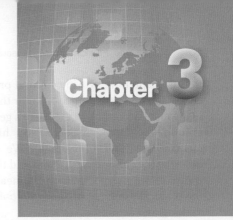

Chapter 3

Cultural Competence in the History and Physical Examination

• Margaret M. Andrews

Key Terms

Addison's disease
Albinism
Biocultural variations
Café au lait spots
Clinical decision-making
Copy-number variants
Cultural assessment
Cultural care accommodation
  or negotiation
Cultural care preservation or
  maintenance
Cultural care repatterning or
  restructuring

Cultural norms
Culture-bound syndromes
Cyanosis
Ecchymoses
Epigenetics
Erythema
Ethnohistory
Evaluation
Genetics
Genome
Genomics
Genotyping
Jaundice
Lactose intolerance

Leukoedema
Mongolian spots
Oral hyperpigmentation
Pain
Pallor
Petechiae
Pharmacogenomics
Presbycusis
Single-nucleotide
  polymorphisms
Steatorrhea
Uremia
Vitiligo

Learning Objectives

1. Explore the process and content needed for a comprehensive cultural assessment of clients from diverse cultures.
2. Identify biocultural variations in health and illness for individuals from diverse cultures.
3. Integrate concepts from the fields of genetics and genomics into the cultural assessment of clients from diverse cultural backgrounds.
4. Discuss biocultural variations in common laboratory tests.
5. Critically review transcultural perspectives in the health history and physical examination.

In this chapter, we provide cultural prompts that enable nurses to customize or tailor their cultural assessment according to the client's genetic background, biographic makeup, and his/her self-identified cultural affiliation(s). We define and describe the cultural assessment and then discuss transcultural perspectives on the health history, the physical examination, and **clinical decision-making** and actions.

In many instances, the health history and physical examination are interconnected and interrelated. For example, the client might complain about shortness of breath during the history, and the nurse might hear the client wheezing during the interview. After the interview is finished, the nurse gathers additional data during the physical examination by observing the client for clinical manifestations of cyanosis, nasal flaring, and intercostal retraction and by auscultating the lungs. Based on the findings in the physical examination, the nurse might ask additional questions, such as the length of time the client has experienced the symptoms, check for family history of respiratory disease, and pursue additional assessment related to the respiratory and cardiovascular systems.

The health history includes cultural perspectives on biographic and genetic data, medications, reasons for seeking care, present health and history of the present illness, past health, family and social history, and the review of systems. In the physical examination, the nurse compares and contrasts normal and abnormal cultural variations in measurements, general appearance, skin, sweat glands, head (hair, eyes, ears, mouth), mammary plexus, and the musculoskeletal system. We also discuss biocultural variations in pain and illness and cultural considerations in selected laboratory tests for which there is evidence of racial and/or ethnic differences. Lastly, we explore transcultural perspectives in clinical decision-making and actions. After completing a comprehensive cultural assessment through the health history, physical examination, and analysis of laboratory test results, the next steps are to analyze the subjective and objective data,

set mutual goals with the client, develop a plan of care, confer with and make referrals to other members of the interprofessional health care team as needed, and implement a plan of care, either alone or with others.

Cultural Assessment

With more than 328 million people, the United States is the third most populous nation in the world, behind China and India (U.S. Census Bureau, 2018). By the year 2050, it is estimated that nearly 50% of the US population will be composed of people from diverse racial and ethnic backgrounds, that is, non-White groups. Hispanic and Asian populations are expected to double between now and 2050 and are followed in growth by Blacks, Native Americans, Native Hawaiians, and other Pacific Islanders (U.S. Census Bureau, 2017). With this growing diversity comes the need for nurses to develop their knowledge and skills in cultural assessment. In the course of their professional careers, nurses will need to assess people from many different racial and ethnic groups and from numerous nonethnic cultures.

Cultural assessment, or *culturologic assessment*, refers to a systematic, comprehensive examination of individuals, families, groups, and communities regarding their health-related cultural beliefs, values, and practices. Although the focus in this chapter is on the individual client, there are some instances in which clients' families and others in close contact might need to be involved, for example, when the cultural assessment reveals the presence of a genetic, infectious, or communicable disorder. Cultural assessments form the foundation for the clients' plan of care, providing valuable data for setting mutual goals, planning care, intervening, and evaluating the care. The goal of the cultural assessment is to determine the nursing and health care needs of people from diverse cultures and intervene in ways that are culturally acceptable, congruent, competent, safe, affordable, accessible, high quality, and based on current research, evidence, and best practices (McFarland & Wehbe-Alamah, 2018).

Given that they deal with cultural values, belief systems, and lifeways, cultural assessments tend to be broad and comprehensive. It is sometimes necessary to conduct an abbreviated assessment when time is limited, the client's reason for seeking care is urgent or time sensitive, the client is unable to provide all of the necessary data, or other circumstances require a shorter, more focused assessment. The cultural assessment consists of both *process* and *content*. *Process* refers to how to approach to the client, consideration of verbal and nonverbal communication, and the sequence and order in which data are gathered. The *content* of the cultural assessment consists of the actual data categories in which information about clients is gathered. Nurses are required to complete assessments before and/or at the time of admission to health care facilities, when opening home health care cases, and prior to many types of medical and surgical procedures. Depending on the circumstances, assessments may be very brief, or they may be detailed and in-depth. Ideally, the cultural assessment is integrated into the overall assessment of the client, family, and significant others. It is usually impractical to expect that nurses will have the time to conduct a separate cultural assessment, so questions aimed at gathering cultural data should be integrated into the overall assessment using the format provided by health care facilities, agencies, or organization for their admissions or intake assessment.

Appendix A is the Andrews and Boyle Transcultural Nursing Assessment Guide for Individuals and Families for use when initially assessing clients from diverse backgrounds, for example, when conducting an admission assessment or opening a case in home health care or ambulatory settings. The major categories in this guide include cultural affiliations, values orientation, communication, health-related beliefs and practices, nutrition, socioeconomic considerations, organizations providing cultural support, education, religion, cultural aspects of disease incidence, bicultural variations, and developmental considerations across the lifespan. Appendix B is the Andrews and Boyle Transcultural Nursing

Assessment Guide for Groups and Communities. The major categories in this guide include family and kinship systems, social life and networks, political or government systems, language and traditions, worldview, values, norms, religious beliefs and practices, health beliefs and practices, and health care systems.

Transcultural Perspectives on the Health History

The purpose of the health history is to gather *subjective data*—a term that refers to things that people say or relate about themselves. The health history provides a comprehensive overview of a client's past and present health, and it examines the manner in which the person interacts with the environment. The health history enables the nurse to assess health strengths, including cultural beliefs and practices that might influence the nurse's ability to provide culturally competent nursing care. The history is combined with the *objective data* from the physical examination and the laboratory results to form a diagnosis about the health status of a person.

For the well client, the history is used to assess lifestyle, which includes activity, exercise, diet, and related personal behaviors and choices that nurses may gather to identify potential risk factors for disease. For the ill client, the health history includes a chronologic record of the health problem(s). For both well and ill clients, the health history is a screening tool for abnormal symptoms, health problems, and concerns. The health history also provides valuable information about the coping strategies and health-related behaviors and responses used previously by clients and family members.

In many health care settings, the client is expected to fill out a printed history form or checklist. From a transcultural perspective, this approach has both positive and negative aspects. On the positive side, this approach provides the client with ample time to recall details such as relevant family history and the dates of health-related events such as surgical procedures and illnesses. It is expedient for nurses because it takes less time to review a form or a checklist than to elicit the information in a face-to-face or telephone interview.

However, this approach has limitations. First, the form is likely to be in English. Those whose primary language is not English might find the form difficult or impossible to complete accurately. Although some health care facilities provide forms translated into Spanish, French, or other languages, translating forms can be costly and is not always effective. In some instances, the literal translation of medical terms is not possible. In other instances, the symptom or disease is not recognized in the culture with which the client identifies. For example, in asking about symptoms of depression, there might be many cultural factors that influence the client's interpretation of the question. In Chinese languages, there is no literal translation for the word *depression*. In Chinese culture, it is more acceptable to somaticize emotional pain with expressions of physical discomfort such as chest pain or "heaviness of the heart" (Zhu, 2018). In rural Guatemala, Mayans might refer to *dolor de corazón* or pain in the heart. *Nervios* may be cited by Guatemalan Mayan women as the cause of somatic disorders such as ulcers, diabetes, and dizziness (Nogueira, Mari, & Razzouk, 2015). If health care providers fail to understand the cultural meaning of the symptom "heaviness of the heart" or "pain in the heart," unnecessary, invasive, and costly tests might be performed to rule out cardiovascular disease. Nearly 9% of the US population has limited English proficiency (LES) and can be described as speaking English "less than very well" (U.S. Census Bureau, 2017). In some instances, clients might be unable to read or write in any language; thus, an assessment of the client's literacy level should precede the use of printed history forms or checklists.

Although there is wide variation in health history formats, most contain the following categories: *biographic data, reason for seeking care, review of medications and allergies, present health or history of present illness, past history, family and social history*, and *review of systems. Genetic data* are also an important area for the transcultural nurse to consider as part of the health history. This chapter will not provide a comprehensive overview of these categories but will present them as they relate to providing culturally congruent and culturally competent nursing care.

Biographic Data

Although the biographic information (name, address, phone, age, gender, preferred language, and so forth) might seem straightforward, several cultural variations in recording age are important to note. In some Asian cultures, an infant is considered 1 year old at birth. Having an accurate age has many clinical implications, including assessing developmental milestones and determining appropriate medication dosages, and certain legal implications as well. For many reasons, age may not be reported correctly. Some clients may not wish to report their correct age; other clients may not know or be able to provide a specific age in the way health care providers may expect it.

One of the first areas that nurses should assess is the client's self-reported cultural affiliation. With what cultural group(s) does the client report affiliation? Where was the client born? What is the ancestry or **ethnohistory** of the client? When the client self-identifies with multiple races or ethnicities, it is often useful to determine with which group the client *primarily* identifies. Knowledge of the client's ethnohistory is important in determining risk factors for genetic and acquired diseases and in understanding the client's cultural heritage. In addition to the standard descriptive information about clients, it is necessary to record who has furnished the data. Whereas this is usually the client, the source might be a relative, guardian, or friend. Note whether an interpreter is used and indicate the relationship to the client.

Genetic Data

Genetics is a branch of biology that studies heredity and the variations of inherited characteristics. This area continues to be a rapidly evolving science; genetics exerts a significant influence on the health of people from cultures around the world. Whereas genetics scrutinizes the functioning and composition of a specific gene, genomics addresses all genes and their interrelationship to identify their combined influence on the growth and development of the organism. The Human Genome Project, which concluded in 2003, revealed there are around 20,500 human genes, which is a surprising revelation as it was once estimated there were more than 50,000 human genes. It is an error in one of these genes that can potentially lead to a recognizable genetic disease in a human (McCance & Huether, 2019; National Institute of Health, 2016). A genome is an organism's complete set of DNA, including all of its genes. Each genome contains all of the information needed to build and maintain that organism. In humans, a copy of the entire genome—more than three billion DNA base pairs—is contained in all cells that have a nucleus. Genetic mapping is continuing at a rapid rate, and these numbers and discoveries are constantly being updated. Epigenetics is the study of how genes are influenced by forces such as the environment, obesity, or medication. Although the children in Figure 3-1 are twins, epigenetic modifications can cause individuals with the same DNA sequences to have different disease profiles (McCance & Huether, 2019). As a result of epigenetic research, the critical role played by external forces is better understood and can now be integrated into client assessment and care.

While each person has approximately 20,500 genes, any two individuals share 99.9% of their DNA sequence, reflecting that the diversity among individuals accounts for approximately 0.1% of the DNA (National Institute of Health, 2016; Porth, 2015). Although humans are more alike than different, the growing inventory of human genetic variation facilitates an understanding of why susceptibility to common diseases differs among individual clients and populations. It is the combinations of multiple genetic variants that influence not only susceptibility to disease but also the disease course, as well as response to therapy and the

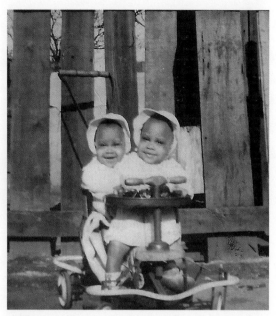

Figure 3-1. Due to diet, environment, and lifestyle, these identical twins have different disease profiles as they have matured into adulthood; however, both became registered nurses and nursing faculty.

response to certain medications (Eyre, Orozco, & Worthington, 2017). These genetic variations provide the knowledge that health care professionals need to safely administer medications and counsel clients regarding the prevention and risk of disease. This discussion provides a foundation in genetic and genomic science to ensure that the nursing assessment is customized according to each client's unique background and current care needs.

Human genetic variation contributes significantly to the physical variation occurring among individuals. The two most important components of human genetic variation are single-nucleotide polymorphisms (SNPs) and copy-number variants. SNPs are single DNA base pairs that differ among individual DNA sequences; copy-number variants are larger blocks of DNA sequence that vary. Most common SNPs are shared among populations from different continents, which reflect continued migration and gene flow among humans through history. Many studies have shown that 85% to 90% of genetic variation can be found within any human population. Samples of persons from Great Britain and Ghana have genetic similarity. Only an additional 10% to 15% of variation is gained when the entire human population is considered. A genetic variation may be relatively common in one population but absent in another due to a recent emergence of a variant that has not yet had time to spread. Hereditary hemochromatosis, a disorder that causes the body to absorb too much iron from food, is common in Europe, but very rare elsewhere. Hereditary lactase, as another example, is prevalent among European and African pastoral populations where milk consumption beyond childhood has had a selective advantage (Du & Gray, 2017).

Genetic research studies are now readily available regarding the safety and efficacy of medications for a variety of conditions. This information extends far beyond traditional inherited disease such as sickle cell anemia or cystic fibrosis. This growing inventory of human variation facilitates an understanding of why susceptibility to common disease varies among individuals and populations. Analyses of two key heart failure (HF) trials comparing African Americans to Whites reveal significant ethnic differences in response to treatment.

The African-American Heart Failure Trial (A-HeFT) demonstrates that therapy with fixed-dose combined isosorbide dinitrate/hydralazine (BiDil) added to customary therapy significantly improved survival in self-identified African American men and women with advanced HF (Ofili et al., 2017).

The American College of Cardiology Foundation/American Heart Association guidelines recommend combined isosorbide dinitrate (ISDN) and hydralazine to reduce mortality and morbidity for African Americans with symptomatic HF as earlier studies reflected a significant reduction in death and improvement in outcomes. Hypertension contributes to HF, especially in African Americans. The A-HeFT and its more recent substudies demonstrate improvements in ventricular performance based on echocardiogram, morbidity, and mortality as well as a decrease in hospitalizations, potentially affecting burgeoning HF health care costs. The importance of genetic characteristics in determining response to ISDN–hydralazine was reinforced a decade after the original study. The Genetic Risk Assessment in Heart Failure substudy confirmed an important hypothesis and generated relevant pharmacogenomic data, and further studies are echoing these findings (Ferdinand et al., 2014; McNamara et al., 2016).

Investigators have focused on genetic variations in populations, which may yield a more complete characterization of risk, and thereby permit more specifically targeted treatment of HF clients. In the future, more precise selection of beta-blocker therapy for HF and hypertension based on genotype may be superior to selecting therapy based on a client's race/ethnicity.

Recent attention has been drawn to the association of chronic traumatic encephalopathy (CTE) with contact sports such as boxing, American football, soccer, hockey, and wrestling. CTE is a progressive neurodegenerative disease that is a long-term consequence of single or repetitive closed head injuries for which there is no treatment and no definitive premortem diagnosis. Researchers from Boston University discovered significant cases of CTE in college and professional football players. Subsequently, it was discovered that a significant number of these athletes had two copies of the ApoE4 gene variant; this version of the ApoE gene has been shown to substantially increase the risk of Alzheimer's disease (National Institute on Aging, 2015). This raises questions about offering genetic screening for the ApoEv4 to linebackers, boxers, and parents whose children play sports that put players at risk for CTE. Sports transcend all cultures, yet may be more prevalent in certain racial and ethnic groups, for example, almost 70% of all NFL football players are African American (Lapchick & Marfatia, 2017). Juvenile traumatic brain injury leaves survivors facing a potential lifetime of cognitive, somatic, and emotional symptoms; therefore, prevention and education are currently the most compelling ways to combat CTE and are emphasized by nurses with parents, athletic trainers, and coaches (Centers for Disease Control and Prevention, 2015).

The apolipoprotein genotype also has a potential role in cognitive function of postmenopausal women with early-stage breast cancer (American Cancer Society, n.d.; Domchek, 2014). Koleck et al. (2014) examine the role of apolipoprotein E (ApoE) in the cognitive function of postmenopausal women with early-stage breast cancer prior to the initiation of adjuvant therapy, that is, assisting in the prevention, amelioration, or cure of the disease. Performance or changes in performance on tasks of executive function, attention, verbal/visual learning, and memory were influenced. ApoE genotype along with other biomarkers may be used in the future to assist nurses in identifying women with breast cancer most at risk for cognitive decline.

Nurses should consider how the client will use genetic and genomic information and potential racial, ethnic, and cultural factors and be prepared to provide support if clients experience moral or ethical issues. Most hospitals have ethics committees, chaplains, pastoral teams, and other resources to assist clients facing religious, moral, and ethical dilemmas.

The addition of genetics and genomics to the traditional nursing assessment will inform and engage clients to make key decisions in their personal health care plan. By virtue of their race or ethnicity, clients are sometimes said to be "at risk" for certain diseases. Examples include diabetes mellitus among Native Americans, breast cancer among Ashkenazi Jews, and prostate cancer among African Americans. Particular forms of treatment are also believed to be more (or less) effective among certain racial/ethnic groups compared with others.

Among African Americans (compared with Whites), angiotensin-converting enzyme (ACE) inhibitors are less effective for essential hypertension, and a therapeutic response to selective serotonin reuptake inhibitor (SSRI) antidepressants occurs at lower doses. Considerations about health by racial and ethnic groups require the context that environmental factors and health disparities as well as genetic factors are operative in determining health risk. The nurse should avoid oversimplifying the relationship between race/ethnicity and genetics when communicating to clients and their families. Knowledge of race or ethnicity might prompt genetic testing or detailed family history taking in particular instances; however, the issues are often too complex for the nurse to make unqualified assertions to clients that they are "at risk" for a particular illness or unlikely to respond to therapies solely on the basis of their racial/ethnic background. In most instances, the full interprofessional health care team will be the best catalyst for client information and interventions. Table 3-1 provides an overview of the distribution of selected genetic traits and disorders by population or ethnic group. Knowledge of the client's race or ethnicity might prompt the nurse to gather a detailed family history and/or collaborate with physicians and nurse practitioners to order genetic testing.

Human genetic information is accumulating at a rapid pace, and almost 7,000 diseases can now be diagnosed by testing for specific mutations (McCance & Huether, 2019; National Center for Biotechnology Information, 2017). The following genetic screenings may be useful to clients, nurses, and other members of the health care team:

- *Drug efficacy or sensitivity*: **Pharmacogenomics**, the study of the role of inherited and acquired genetic variation in drug response, is an evolving field that facilitates the identification of biomarkers that can help health providers optimize drug selection, dose, and treatment duration as well as eliminate adverse drug reactions. For example, researchers have identified an HLA allele that is associated with hypersensitivity reactions to the anticonvulsant and mood-stabilizing drug carbamazepine (Tegretol) in persons of European descent (Yip & Pirmohamed, 2017). For other drugs such as warfarin (Coumadin) and clopidogrel (Plavix), genetic testing for variants in specific genes may be warranted to help guide the drug dosage.
- *Carrier screening*: Genetic tests can identify heterozygous carriers for many recessive diseases such as cystic fibrosis, sickle cell disease,

Table 3-1 | Selected Genetic Diseases and Clinical Implications

Disease or Condition	Group Impacted	Clinical Implications
Alpha-1 antitrypsin deficiency (AAT) Autosomal recessive disorder resulting in early-onset emphysema and liver disease	Northern European, Scandinavian, and Iberian ancestry. Rare in Jewish, Black, and Japanese populations AAT deficiency affects 1%–2% of patients with chronic obstructive pulmonary disease	**Consider diagnosis in** adults with emphysema with onset at ≤40 years of age and without risk factors (no history of smoking or occupational dust exposure) **Diagnosis made by** serum alpha-1 antitrypsin levels and confirmed with genetic testing
Breast cancer **BRCA1 and BRCA2** Autosomal dominant; accounting for ~5% US cases	Ashkenazi Jewish women Estimated that 0.2%–0.33% of general population have gene mutations	**Counseling:** U.S. Preventive Services Task Force recommends genetic counseling and evaluation for BRCA testing for Ashkenazi Jewish women with any first-degree relative with breast or ovarian cancer or second-degree relatives on same side of family with breast or ovarian cancer
G6PD deficiency (Glucose-6-phosphate dehydrogenase deficiency) X-linked genetic defect with clinical manifestations of neonatal jaundice and/or acute or chronic hemolytic anemia triggered by medications, infections, and fava beans	Highest frequency found in Africa, southern Europe (Mediterranean region), the Middle East, Southeast Asia, and central and southern Pacific islands Deficiency is found in 10% of Blacks and can occur in Sephardic Jews, Greeks, Iranians, Chinese, Filipinos, and Indonesians with a frequency ranging from 5% to 40% Kurdish Jews 50% of males reported to be affected Most common human enzyme defect worldwide	**Relevant history:** Ask about family history of G6PD deficiency and hemolytic factors that can be transmitted to infants via mother's milk (such as fava bean ingestion, drugs, or herbal remedies). Hemolytic anemia occurs about 24 hours after ingestion of fava beans **Medication history:** Ask about recent history of medications that may have precipitated hemolytic anemia, such as antimalarials, nitrofurantoin (urinary tract infections), phenazopyridine (for dysuria), and topical application of henna
Leiden V The most common hereditary abnormality of hemostasis predisposing to thrombosis Autosomal dominant inheritance single mutation causes mild hypercoagulable state	Highest in US and European White populations. Prevalence may be higher in some Middle Eastern countries including Jordan (12.3%) and Lebanon (14.4%)	**Relevant assessment** May have no clinical symptoms Mutation is present in about 15%–20% patients with first deep vein thrombosis and up to 50% of patients with recurrent venous thromboembolism **Medication history:** Risk for thromboembolism increased with oral contraceptives, hormone replacement therapy (HRT), and selective estrogen receptor modulators (SERMs)

Table 3-1	Selected Genetic Diseases and Clinical Implications (continued)	
Disease or Condition	**Group Impacted**	**Clinical Implications**
Sickle cell disease Autosomal recessive genetic disorder; patients with same genotype may have highly variable phenotypes, ranging from asymptomatic to life-threatening complications; interaction of environmental factors with genetic polymorphisms may explain disease variation Chronic inflammation, ischemia, and vaso-occlusion contribute to chronic organ damage	African, Mediterranean, Middle Eastern, Indian ancestry, Caribbean, and parts of Central and South America Most prevalent disease detected by neonatal blood screening Alpha-thalassemia and beta-thalassemia may be coinherited 1 out of every 12 African Americans carries the sickle cell trait Sickle cell disease affects ~70,000–100,000 Americans, occurs in 1 out of every 365 Blacks, and occurs in 1 out of every 36,000 Hispanic American births	**Relevant assessment** Affected infants not identified through neonatal screening usually present clinically during infancy/early childhood with painful swelling of the hands and feet (dactylitis), pneumococcal sepsis or meningitis, severe anemia and acute splenic enlargement (splenic sequestration), acute chest syndrome, jaundice, and pallor **Counseling:** Many adolescents and young adults are unaware of their sickle cell trait status—higher risk for rhabdomyolysis during rigorous sports Prenatal diagnosis may be made in first and second trimester PGD is available during in vitro fertilization. Embryos not affected with sickle cell disease may be selected
Tay–Sachs disease Neurodegenerative disorder caused by inborn error of metabolism, deficiency in enzyme, and hexosaminidase A Genetic mutation results in central nervous system degeneration and loss of organ function	Ashkenazi Jews Incidence of 1/3,600 among Ashkenazi Jewish births Carrier rate of 1/30 among Jewish Americans of Ashkenazi descent Additional at-risk groups include French Canadians living in Eastern Quebec or New England, select Cajun communities in Louisiana, and Pennsylvania Dutch semi-isolates	**Relevant assessment** Classic or acute infantile is the most common type Infants appear normal at birth Rapidly progressive neurodegenerative disorder characterized by progressive motor weakness beginning at 3–6 months old, loss of developmental milestones and death within first few years of life
Alpha-thalassemia Hereditary anemia caused by defect during hemoglobin production and various clinical phenotypes—from silent carrier to more severe	Inhabitants or descendants of Southeast Asia, the Middle East, and Mediterranean countries 80%–90% may be carriers of alpha-thalassemia in tropical and subtropical regions Some studies have estimated that as much as 5% of the world's population carries an alpha-thalassemia variant	**Relevant assessment** Patients can be asymptomatic or have mild symptoms of anemia including fatigue and dyspnea, poor growth in children, and jaundice Abnormal physical findings occur with more severe phenotypes
Beta-thalassemia An autosomal recessive inherited anemia caused by absent or decreased beta–globin chain synthesis during hemoglobin production. Also referred to as Cooley's or Mediterranean anemia	Inhabitants or descendants of Mediterranean countries, the Middle East, Central Asia, India, Southern China, the Far East, South America, and north coast of Africa Estimated annual incidence of symptomatic individuals: 1 in 100,000 people globally and 1 in 10,000 people in European community	**Relevant assessment** Symptoms emerge at 6–12 months—failure to thrive, feeding problems, diarrhea, fever, and progressive enlargement of the abdomen due to hepatosplenomegaly Symptoms in patients who have not been treated or who have received inadequate transfusion treatments may include growth retardation, jaundice, and craniofacial changes

(continued)

Table 3-1	Selected Genetic Diseases and Clinical Implications (continued)	
Disease or Condition	**Group Impacted**	**Clinical Implications**
von Willebrand disease Bleeding disorder resulting in platelet and clotting defect Varies from mild to more severe forms Three types exist, most commonly autosomal dominant	Found in 1% of the general population Type 3 may be more prevalent in Swedish communities Males and females are both approximately equally affected Racial characteristics of all patients: 75.1% White 10.9% Hispanic 7.5% Black 2.6% Asian/Pacific Islander 0.4% American Indian/Alaska native	**Preoperative assessment** May be asymptomatic All patients having major surgery should be screened Symptoms typical of bleeding disorder, most commonly mucosal bleeding such as nosebleed, gingival bleeding, easy bruising, or menorrhagia (most common bleeding disorder in women who present with menorrhagia, 12%–20%)

Data from Centers for Disease Control and Prevention. (2017). Sickle cell disease: Data and statistics. Retrieved from https://www.cdc.gov/ncbddd/sicklecell/data.html; Centers for Disease Control and Prevention. (n.d.). About BRCA1, BRCA2, and hereditary breast and ovarian cancers. Retrieved from https://www.knowbrca.org/Provider/FNA/about-brca1-brca2-and-hereditary-breast-and-ovarian-cancers; Echahdi, H., El Hasbaoui, B., El Khorassani, M., Agadr, A., & Khattab, M. (2017). Von Willebrand's disease: Case report and review of literature. *The Pan African Medical Journal, 27*, 147. Retrieved from http://doi.org/10.11604/pamj.2017.27.147.12248; Fishbach, F., & Dunning, M. B. (2015). *A manual of laboratory and diagnostic tests* (9th ed.). Philadelphia, PA: Wolters Kluwer; Harteveld, C. L., & Higgs, D. R. (2010). Alpha-thalassaemia. *Orphanet Journal of Rare Diseases, 5*, 13; Kaback, M., & Desnick, R. J. (2011). Hexosaminidase A deficiency. *Gene Reviews, 8*(11); McCance, K. L., & Huether, S. E. (2019). *Pathophysiology: The biologic basis for disease in adults and children* (8th ed.). St. Louis, MO: Elsevier, Inc.; McGrady, T., Mannino, D. M., Malanga, E., Thomashow, B. M., Walsh, J., Sandhaus, R. A., & Stoller, J. K. (2015). Characteristics of chronic obstructive pulmonary disease (COPD) patients reporting alpha-1 antitrypsin deficiency in the WebMD Lung Health Check Database. Retrieved from https://www.ncbi.nlm.nih.gov/pmc/articles/PMC5556968/; Mohr, H. (2006). Acquired von Willebrand syndrome: Features and management. *American Journal of Hematology, 81*(8), 616–623; National Organization for Rare Diseases. (2018). Beta thalassemia. Retrieved from https://rarediseases.org/rare-diseases/thalassemia-major/; National Organization for Rare Diseases. (2017). Alpha thalassemia. Retrieved from https://rarediseases.org/rare-diseases/alpha-thalassemia/; National Organization for Rare Diseases. (2017). Tay Sachs disease. Retrieved from https://rarediseases.org/rare-diseases/tay-sachs-disease/; Porth, C. M. (2015). *Essentials of pathophysiology: Concepts of altered health states* (4th ed.). Philadelphia, PA: Lippincott Williams & Wilkins; Rotimi, C. N., & Jorde, L. B. (2010). Ancestry and disease in the age of genomic medicine. *New England Journal of Medicine, 36*, 1551–1558; Taylor, C., Kavanagh, P., & Zuckerman, B. (2014). Sickle cell train-neglected opportunities in the era of genomic medicine. *JAMA, 311*(15), 1495–1496.

and Tay–Sachs disease. A couple may wish to undergo carrier screening to help make reproductive decisions, especially in populations where specific diseases are relatively common, for example, Tay–Sachs disease in Ashkenazi Jewish populations and beta-thalassemia in Mediterranean populations.

- *Prenatal diagnostic tests*: Several of these tests can tell parents-to-be, with as much certainty as possible, if their fetus has a genetic disorder. Amniocentesis is usually performed at 16 weeks' gestation and chorionic villus sampling (CVS) is carried out at 10 to 12 weeks' gestation. Preimplantation genetic diagnosis

(PGD) is carried out on early embryos (8 to 12 cells) prior to implantation, and fetal DNA analysis in maternal circulation is done at 6 to 8 weeks' gestation (American College of Obstetrics and Gynecology, 2016; Centers for Disease Control and Prevention, 2017; March of Dimes, 2017; National Center for Biotechnology Information, 2017).

Review of Medications and Allergies

The review of medications includes all current prescription, over-the-counter, and home remedies, including herbs that a client might purchase or grow in a home garden. During the health history, note the name, dose, route of administration, schedule, frequency, purpose, and length of time that each medicine has been taken. Because of cultural differences in clients' perceptions of what substances are considered medicines, it is important to ask about specific items by name. Inquire about vitamins, birth control pills, aspirin, antacids, herbs, teas, inhalants, poultices, vaginal and rectal suppositories, ointments, essential oils, and any other items taken by the client for therapeutic purposes. The nurse also gathers data on the client's allergies to medicines and foods.

Table 3-2 provides an overview of commonly used herbs, their sources, uses, dosage, and warnings, such as contraindications (e.g., pregnancy, childhood, people with compromised immune systems) and interactions with prescription drugs. Many of the active ingredients in herbs or plant-derived drugs are unknown. These herbs and plant-derived drugs remain

Table 3-2	Herbal Remedies
Aloe vera	
Source	Leaf of *Aloe barbadensis*
Action	Topical analgesic, anti-inflammatory, antioxidant, and antifungal agent
Traditional uses	Applied as topical ointment for treatment of inflammation, minor burns, sunburn, cuts, bruises, and abrasions; administered orally as a laxative
Current uses	Promotes wound healing in soft tissue injuries and is used as a folk or traditional remedy for diabetes, asthma, epilepsy, and osteoarthritis *Aloe vera* gel, contained in the leaves of the plant, is found in skin products such as lotions and sunblocks Prevents wound pain by inhibiting the action of the pain-producing agent bradykinin
Dosage	Apply topically as needed; the FDA ruled that aloe is not safe as a stimulant laxative
Warnings	Rarely, skin rash follows topical application Can cause diarrhea and abdominal cramps when taken orally and can decrease the absorption of many drugs
Dong quai (Chinese Angelica, Angelica sinensis)	
Source	Dried root of a member of the parsley family
Action	Smooth muscle relaxant; antispasmodic
Traditional uses	A highly regarded herb in Chinese medicine, also used in traditional Korean and Japanese medicine Has been called "female ginseng" because it is used for health conditions in women Used for both men and women to treat heart conditions, high blood pressure, inflammation, headache, infections, and nerve pain Believed to help nourish the blood and balance energy
Current uses	Used for menstrual cramps, anemia during menstruation, pregnancy, premenstrual syndrome (PMS), pelvic pain, recovery from childbirth or illness, muscle spasms, and fatigue or low energy Used in combination with other herbs for liver and spleen problems
Dosage	Varies by condition: Available in capsule, in liquid extract, or in tea form
Warnings	Contraindicated for pregnant and breast-feeding women and persons with abdominal distention or diarrhea Not recommended for use with aspirin, ibuprofen, anticoagulants, antiplatelet drugs, diabetic clients taking insulin, or other herbs, such as *Ginkgo biloba* Large doses may cause contact dermatitis and photosensitivity

(continued)

Table 3-2	Herbal Remedies (continued)

Echinacea (Echinacea angustifolia, E. pallida, E. purpurea)

Source	Member of the daisy family, also known as purple coneflower
Action	Reduces cold symptoms
Traditional uses	Used to treat wounds and skin problems, such as acne or boils
Current uses	Enhances the immune system to fight infection and to treat colds, flu, and other illnesses. The parts of the plant above ground are used to make teas, juice, or extracts
Dosage	Follow directions on label, needed at onset of symptoms, usually taken for no longer than 2 weeks
Warnings	Contraindicated for pregnant or breast-feeding women, children, and those who are allergic to plants in the daisy family, including ragweed, chrysanthemums, marigolds, and daisies. Not recommended for people with severely compromised immune systems such as those with HIV/AIDS, tuberculosis, or multiple sclerosis

Evening primrose oil (Oenothera biennis)

Source	Seeds of the wildflower evening primrose
Action	Antihypertensive, immunostimulant, weight reduction
Traditional uses	Used as a folk remedy to treat eczema since the 1930s
Current uses	Believed to help inflammation, PMS, diabetes mellitus, eczema, fatigue, diabetic neuropathy, and rheumatoid arthritis
Dosage	Follow directions on label; will take at least 1 month to experience benefits
Warnings	Side effects include occasional reports of headache, nausea, and abdominal discomfort; not recommended for children Some capsules may be altered with other types of oil such as soy or safflower

Ginger

Current uses	Currently is used to treat postsurgery nausea; nausea caused by motion, chemotherapy, and pregnancy; rheumatoid arthritis; osteoarthritis; and joint and muscle pain
Dosage	Boil 1-oz dried ginger root in 1 cup water for 15–20 minutes Follow label directions on ginger supplements

Ginkgo (Ginkgo biloba)

Source	Extract from leaves of the ginkgo tree, one of the oldest types of trees in the world; is cultivated worldwide for its medicinal properties
Action	Antioxidant; improves blood circulation
Traditional uses	Used in traditional Chinese medicine for asthma, bronchitis, fatigue, circulatory disorders, sexual dysfunctions, and tinnitus
Current uses	Promotes vasodilation and improves memory, attention span, and mood in early stages of Alzheimer's disease or dementia by improving oxygen metabolism in the brain; used to treat intermittent claudication, sexual dysfunction, multiple sclerosis, tinnitus, and other health conditions
Dosage	Available in tablets, capsules, teas, and occasionally skin products Follow labels on supplements

Table 3-2 | Herbal Remedies (continued)

Warnings	Side effects may include headaches, diarrhea, nausea and vomiting, and dizziness Some people have reported allergic skin reactions Fresh ginkgo seeds can cause serious adverse reactions—including seizures and death Contraindicated for women who are pregnant or breastfeeding Contraindicated for persons with clotting disorders or those who are about to have surgery Not recommended for children

Ginseng (Panax quinquefolius [American], Panax ginseng [Asian])

Source	Dried root of several species of the genus *Panax* of the family Araliaceae
Action	Tonic
Traditional uses	Treatment of anemia, atherosclerosis, edema, ulcers, hypertension, influenza, colds, inflammation, and disorders of the immune system (American) Treatment of shock, diaphoresis, dyspnea, fever, thirst, irritability, diarrhea, vomiting, abdominal distention, anorexia, and impotence; considered a "heat-raising" tonic for the blood and circulatory system (Asian)
Current uses	Used to enhance sexual experience and treat impotence, though there is no current research to support this claim Also used to improve athletic performance, strength, and stamina, as well as to treat diabetes and cancer (American) Used to treat diabetes, cancer, and HIV/AIDS and as an immunostimulant or to improve athletic performance (Asian) Improved sense of well-being (Asian)
Dosage	American: Follow directions on label Asian: 100 mg BID
Warnings	American: May cause headaches, insomnia, anxiety, breast tenderness, rashes, asthma attacks, hypertension, cardiac arrhythmias, and postmenopausal uterine hemorrhage Should be used with caution for the following conditions: pregnancy, insomnia, hay fever, fibrocystic breasts, asthma, emphysema, hypertension, clotting disorders, and diabetes mellitus Asian: Same as American

Gotu kola (Centella asiatica)

Source	Dried and powdered leaves of a member of the parsley family
Action	Improves memory
Traditional uses	In ancient India, considered a rejuvenating herb that increases intelligence, longevity, and memory while slowing the aging process In China, used as a tea for colds and for lung and urinary tract infections; used topically for snakebite, wounds, and shingles
Current uses	Acceleration of wound healing, diuretic, treatment of phlebitis, varicose veins, and scleroderma
Dosage	Follow directions on label; lower dose needed for children and older adults
Warnings	Side effects include headaches and skin rash Contraindicated for pregnant or breast-feeding women and children younger than 18 years Contraindicated for those diagnosed with liver disease

(continued)

Table 3-2	Herbal Remedies (continued)

Saint John's wort (Hypericum perforatum)

Source	Tea made from the leaves and flowering tops of the perennial *H. perforatum*, which is particularly abundant in late June, the feast of St. John the Baptist
Action	Antidepressant
Traditional uses	Used first in ancient Greece and historically to treat mental disorders and nerve pain. Also used to treat malaria, as a sedative, and topically for wounds, burns, and insect bites Also used by Native Americans to treat wounds, snakebites, and diarrhea
Current uses	Treatment of mild to moderate depression, anxiety, seasonal affective disorder, and sleep disorders
Dosage	300 mg daily
Warnings	Fair-skinned people may experience photosensitivity Reduces effectiveness of some anticancer agents Can interact with antidepressants, birth control pills, cyclosporine, heart medications, HIV medications, anticoagulants, and seizure control medications Clinical manifestations of depression should be considered seriously Encourage client to see a mental health care provider

Valerian (Valeriana officinalis)

Source	Dried rhizome and roots of the tall perennial *V. officinalis*
Action	Mild tranquilizer and sedative
Traditional uses	Used as medicinal herb since Ancient Greece and Rome for insomnia
Current uses	Used as a mild tranquilizer and sedative; relieves muscle spasms, anxiety, headaches, depression, irregular heartbeat, and trembling Especially effective for insomniac persons and older adults
Dosage	Available in capsules, tablets, liquid extracts, and teas
Warnings	Reported side effects include headache, gastrointestinal upset, and dizziness Must not be taken in combination with other tranquilizers or sedatives Client should be cautioned against operating a motor vehicle after ingesting Should discontinue use at least 1 week before surgery because it may interact with anesthesia

Table based on data from Mayo Clinic. (2017). Drugs and supplements. Retrieved from http://www.mayoclinic.org; Memorial Sloan-Kettering Cancer Center. (2018). About herbs, botanicals and other products. Retrieved from http://www.mskcc.org/cancer-care/integrative-medicine/about-herbs-botanicals-other-products; National Center for Complementary and Integrative Health. (2015). Herbs at a glance. Retrieved from https://nccih.nih.gov/health/herbsataglance.htm; United States National Library of Medicine. (2018). Herbs and supplements. Retrieved from https://medlineplus.gov/druginfo/herb_All.html; University of Maryland Medical Center. (2018). Retrieved from https://umm.edu/health/medical/altmed/herb.

largely unregulated by government agencies, except for customs officials who make efforts to control the flow of illegal drugs and the Food and Drug Administration (FDA)'s guidance information. FDA's guidance documents do not establish legally enforceable responsibilities related to herbs/botanicals; rather, they are the agencies' view on the topic and provide recommendations (U.S. Department of Health and Human Services,

2016). Fresh or dried herbs are usually brewed into a tea, with the dosage adjusted according to the chronicity or acuteness of the illness, age, and size of the client. Traditional Chinese medicine usually is used only as long as symptoms persist. Some clients may extend this same logic to prescription medicines. For example, they might stop taking an antibiotic as soon as the symptoms subside instead of completing the course of treatment for the prescribed length of time. Be sure to also consider the potential interaction of herbs with prescription medicines. The root of the shrub *ginseng*, for example, is widely used for the treatment of arthritis, back and leg pains, and sores. Because ginseng is known to potentiate the action of some antihypertensive drugs, nurses need to ask clients whether they are experiencing side effects or toxicity and should frequently monitor the client's blood pressure. It might be necessary to withhold doses of the prescribed antihypertensive medicine if the blood pressure is low or to ask the client to discontinue or reduce the strength of the ginseng. When assessing the client's use of traditional Chinese medicine, nurses should be aware that some Chinese Americans who use herbs topically do not consider them drugs; therefore, nurses might not know that the person is taking these medicines. For further information about herbs, ask the client and family, consult an herbalist, search for reputable sources on the Internet, or check reference books on herbal remedies. People sometimes fail to disclose that they are taking herbs and plant-based medicines or using essential oils because they are concerned that their health care provider will disapprove. The National Center for Complementary and Integrative Health (2018) provides fact sheets with basic information about specific herbs or botanicals—common names, what the science says, potential side effects and cautions, and resources for more information.

For many years, people have attempted to identify plants, marine organisms, arthropods, animals, and minerals with healing properties. According to the World Health Organization, the majority of the world depends on traditional medicine for health care needs, with around 80% of people residing in less developed countries using indigenous medicinal plants for many of their primary health care needs (Bukar, Dayom, & Oguru, 2016). The estimated global market for botanical and plant-derived drugs is valued at $29.4 billion as of 2017 and is projected to grow to $39.6 billion by 2022 (BCC Research, 2017). Respiratory problems, such as asthma,

represent one of the largest medical applications of plant-derived drugs. Botanicals, as a subgroup of all plant-derived medications sold as prescription drugs, are expected to grow at higher levels relative to the entire pharmaceutical sector at a rate of 49.5% from 2017 to 2022 (BCC Research, 2017). In particular, nurses should be aware of the widespread use of plant-derived medications among various cultures and utilize this awareness when conducting a thorough health history (see Table 3-2).

The client's genetic makeup results in distinctive patterns of drug absorption, metabolism, excretion, and effectiveness. Knowledge of clients' individual genotypes guides pharmacologic treatment and allows customization of choice of drug and dosage to ensure a therapeutic response and avoid toxicity (Kliegman, Stanton, Saint Geme, Schor, & Behrman, 2016). For example, Evidence-Based Practice 3-1 describes genetically linked racial and ethnic differences in the conversion of codeine to morphine for analgesia. Another example concerns the possibility of reduced effectiveness of the widely prescribed platelet aggregation inhibitor clopidogrel (Plavix), which is used in the prevention of myocardial infarction and stroke. The cause of the reduced effectiveness is related to genetic variations in cytochrome P450 and polypeptide 19 (CYP2C19). A black box warning from the U.S. Food and Drug Administration recommends that all clopidogrel users be tested. It is estimated that between 2% and 14% of the US population are poor metabolizers. While previous studies have explored the impact of this variation in metabolism on heart disease, researchers found that a proportion of the poor/intermediate clopidogrel metabolizers have an increased risk of recurrent cerebrovascular events, including stroke. Around 2% of Caucasians, 4% of African Americans, and 14% of Chinese are CYP2C19 poor metabolizers, and up to 45% of patients are CYP2C19 intermediate metabolizers. This finding is comparable to cardiovascular studies and warrants routine CYP2C19 testing and monitoring of people taking clopidogrel (Dean, 2018). Table 3-3 identifies

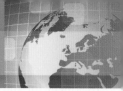

Racial and Ethnic Variations in the Conversion of Codeine to Morphine for Analgesia

CYP2D6 is one of the most important enzymes involved in the metabolism of xenobiotics in the body. In particular, CYP2D6 is responsible for the metabolism and elimination of approximately 25% of clinically used drugs. Xenobiotics are foreign chemical substances found within an organism that are not normally naturally produced by or expected to be present within it. In humans, antibiotics are xenobiotics because the human body does not produce them itself nor are they typically part of normal food.

There is considerable variation in the efficiency and amount of CYP2D6 enzyme produced by individuals from different racial and ethnic backgrounds. For drugs that are metabolized by CYP2D6, certain individuals eliminate the drugs quickly (ultrarapid metabolizers), while others eliminate them slowly (poor metabolizers). If a drug is metabolized too quickly, it may decrease the drug's efficacy. If the drug is metabolized too slowly, toxicity may result. CYP2D6 catalyzes the conversion of codeine to morphine.

In 7% to 10% of US Whites, an active form of the CYP2D6 enzyme, which is necessary to convert codeine into its active metabolite, morphine, is missing. These individuals experience the side effects of morphine without pain relief. Other variations in metabolic efficiency among ethnic groups are apparent. For example, Chinese produce less morphine from codeine than do Whites and also are less sensitive to morphine's effects. The reduced sensitivity to morphine may be due to decreased production of morphine-6-glucuronide.

Clinical Implications

In approximately 10% of US Whites, codeine is ineffective as an analgesic, and 4% to 5% of the US population and 16% to 28% of North Africans, Ethiopians, and Arabs are ultrarapid metabolizers with increased sensitivity to codeine's effects, and therefore, nurses need to observe for the following signs of toxicity:

- Bluish-colored fingernails and lips
- Slow and labored breathing, shallow breathing, and no breathing

- Cold, clammy skin
- Coma (decreased level of consciousness and lack of responsiveness)
- Confusion
- Dizziness
- Drowsiness
- Fatigue
- Light-headedness
- Low blood pressure
- Muscle twitches
- Pinpoint pupils
- Spasms of the stomach and intestines
- Weakness
- Weak pulse

Consider the possibility of metabolic genetic variations in any client who experiences toxicity or does not receive adequate analgesia from codeine or other opioid drugs (e.g., hydrocodone and oxycodone). Red heads also have variations. Dysfunctional melanocortin 1 receptor on certain cells that gives people their red hair also increases production of a hormone that causes heightened pain sensitivity.

References: Binkley, C. J., Beacham, A., Neace, W., Gregg, R. G., Liem, E. B., & Sessler, D. I. (2010). Genetic variations associated with red hair color and fear of dental pain, anxiety regarding dental care and avoidance of dental care. *Journal of the American Dental Association, 140*(7), 896–905.

Liu, F., Struchalin, M. V., van Duijn, K., Hofman, A., Uitterlinden, A. G., van Duijn, C., …, Kayser, M. (2011). Detecting low frequent loss-of-function alleles in genome wide association studies with red hair color as example. *PLoS One, 6*(11), e28145.

Sammer, C. F., Daali, Y., Wagner, M., Hopfgartner, G., Eap, C. B., Rebsamen, M. C., …, Desmueles, J. A. (2010). The effects of CYP2D6 and CYP3A activities on the pharmacokinetics of immediate release oxycodone. *British Journal of Pharmacology, 160*(4), 907–918.

Teh, L. K., & Bertilsson, L. (2012). Pharmacogenomics of CYP2D6: Molecular genetics, interethnic differences and clinical importance. *Drug Metabolism and Pharmacokinetics, 27*(1), 55–67.

Walko, C. M., & McLeod, H. (2012). Use of CYP2D6 genotyping in practice: Tamoxifen dose adjustment. *Pharmacogenomics, 13*(6), 691–707.

Table 3-3 | Cultural Differences in Response to Drugs

Drug Category	Group	Remarks
Analgesics	Blacks	Despite decreased sensitivity to pain-relieving therapeutic action of drugs, there are increased gastrointestinal side effects, especially with acetaminophen
Narcotic analgesics	Chinese	May be less sensitive to the respiratory depressant and hypotensive effects of morphine but more likely to experience nausea; have a significantly higher clearance of morphine
Antiarrhythmics	Arab Americans	Some may need lower dosage
Anticoagulants	Asian	Require lower doses of warfarin (Coumadin) than White counterparts
	Blacks	Require higher doses of warfarin (Coumadin) than White or Asian counterparts
Anticonvulsants	Chinese, Filipinos, Malaysians, Thai, Singaporeans, Taiwanese, East Indians, and Japanese	Higher toxicity observed with the use of carbamazepine (Tegretol) including incidence of drug-induced Stevens–Johnson syndrome
Antihypertensives	Arab Americans	Some may need lower dosage
	Asian/Pacific Islanders	Respond best to calcium antagonists
	Blacks	Respond best to treatment with a single drug (vs. combined antihypertensive therapy) Research suggests favorable response to diuretics, calcium antagonists, and alpha-blockers Less responsive to beta-blockers (e.g., propranolol) and ACE inhibitors (e.g., enalapril, imidapril) Increased side effects such as mood response (e.g., depression) to thiazides (e.g., hydrochlorothiazide), which may explain reluctance to take drug as prescribed
Fat-soluble drugs	Asian Americans	Due to average lower percentage of body fat, dosage adjustments must be made for fat-soluble vitamins and other drugs, for example, vitamin K used to reverse the anticoagulant effect of Coumadin (warfarin); consider dietary intake of vitamins when calculating doses
Immunosuppressants	Blacks	Black clients with kidney failure require higher doses of tacrolimus (Prograf, Advagraf, Protopic) to reach trough concentrations similar to those observed in White counterparts
Muscle relaxants	Native Alaskans	May experience prolonged muscle paralysis and an inability to breathe without mechanical ventilation for several hours postoperatively when succinylcholine has been administered in surgery
Mydriatics	Blacks	Higher dose required; less dilation occurs with dark-colored eyes

(continued)

Table 3-3	Cultural Differences in Response to Drugs (continued)	
Drug Category	**Group**	**Remarks**
Neuroleptics	Arab Americans	Some may need lower dosage
	Asian/Pacific Islanders	Require lower dose than do Whites or Blacks
Oxidizing drugs	Greeks, Italians, and others of Mediterranean descent with G6PD deficiency	The following drugs may precipitate a hemolytic crisis: primaquine, quinidine, thiazolsulfone, furazolidone, haloperidol, nitrofural, naphthalene, toluidine blue, phenylhydrazine, chloramphenicol, and aspirin
Psychotropics	Asian/Pacific Islanders	Require lower dose, sometimes as little as half the normal dose for lithium and tricyclic antidepressants (TCAs) such as desipramine and trimipramine
	Blacks	Increased extrapyramidal side effects with TCAs such as haloperidol, relatively prolonged clearance and half-life of carbamazepine
	Hispanics	May require lower dosage and experience higher incidence of side effects with TCAs
	Jewish North Americans (Ashkenazi)	Agranulocytosis develops in 20% when clozapine (Clozaril or ODT) is used to treat schizophrenia; thus, the granulocyte count should be checked before the drug is administered
Steroids	Blacks	When methylprednisolone is used for immunosuppression in renal transplant clients, there is increased toxicity such as steroid-associated diabetes; although Blacks are four times as likely to develop end-stage renal disease as Whites, they have the poorest long-term graft survival of any ethnic group
Tranquilizers	Blacks	15%–20% are poor metabolizers of Valium (diazepam)

Table based partially on data from Bress, A., Han, J., Patel, S. R., Desai, A. A., Mansour, I., Groo, V., ..., Cavallari, R. L. (2013). Association of aldosterone synthase polymorphism (*CYP11B2* -344T>C) and genetic ancestry with atrial fibrillation and serum aldosterone in African Americans with heart failure. *PLoS One, 8*(7), e71268; Buttaro, T. M., Trybulski, J., Polgar Bailey, P., & Sandberg-Cook, J. (2016). *Primary care: A collaborative practice*. St. Louis, MO: Elsevier; Casorbi, I., Bruhn, O., & Werk, A. N. (2013). Challenges in pharmacogenetics. *European Journal of Pharmacology, 69*(Suppl. 1), S17–S23; Center for Disease Control and Prevention. (2017). Genetic testing. Retrieved from http://www.cdc.gov/genomics/gtesting/index.htm; Marino, S. E., Birnbaum, A. K., Leppik, I. E., Conway, J. M., Musib, L. C., Brundage, R. C., ..., Cloyd, J. C. (2012). Steady-state carbamazepine pharmacokinetics following oral and stable-labeled intravenous administration in epilepsy clients: Effects of race and sex. *Clinical Pharmacology and Therapeutics, 91*(3), 483–488.

drug categories for which clients from certain racial or ethnic backgrounds respond differently from the general population.

Reason for Seeking Care

The *reason* or *reasons for seeking care* refers to a brief statement in the client's own words

describing why he/she is visiting a health care provider. This part of the health history previously was called the *chief complaint*, a term that is now avoided because it focuses on illness rather than wellness and tends to label the person as a complainer. Not only does this terminology reflect a negative implication, it also misdirects the focus of a clinical visit by suggesting to clinicians that patients typically arrive at a health care visit with a single issue they want to address. In reality, literature shows that patients typically have multiple reasons for seeking care (Krupat, 2017).

Symptoms are defined as phenomena experienced by an individual or a patient that signify a departure from normal function, sensation, or appearance and that might include physical aberrations. By comparison, *signs* are objective abnormalities that the examiner can detect on physical examination or through laboratory testing. As individuals experience symptoms, they interpret them and react in ways that are congruent with their **cultural norms**, unconscious behavior patterns that are typical of specific groups. Such behaviors are learned from parents, teachers, peers, and others whose values, attitudes, beliefs, and behaviors take place in the context of their own culture. Some cultural norms are healthy; others are not.

Symptoms cannot be attributed to another person; rather, individual clients experience symptoms from their knowledge of bodily function and sociocultural interactions. Symptoms are perceived, recognized, labeled, reacted to, ritualized, and articulated in ways that make sense within the cultural worldview of the person experiencing them. Symptoms are defined according to the client's perception of the meaning attributed to the event. This perception must be considered in relation to other sociocultural factors and biologic knowledge. People develop culturally based explanatory models to explain how their illnesses work and what their symptoms mean. The search for cultural meaning in understanding symptoms involves a translation process that includes both the nurse's worldview and the client's. Assess the symptoms within the client's sociocultural and ethnohistorical context. It is important to use the same terms for symptoms that the client uses. For example, if the client refers to "swelling" of the leg, nurses should refrain from medicalizing that to "edema." Knowledge of the cultural expression of symptoms influences the decisions nurses make and will facilitate their ability to provide culturally congruent and culturally competent nursing care

(Leininger & McFarland, 2002, 2006; McFarland & Wehbe-Alamah, 2015).

Present Health and History of Present Illness

Although all illnesses are defined and conceptualized through the lens of culture, the term **culture-bound syndromes** refers to disorders or patterns of behavior created by personal, social, and cultural reactions to malfunctioning biological or psychological processes and can be understood only within defined contexts of meaning and social relationships. Culture-bound syndromes have been described all over the world, and they often encompass various symptoms ranging from anxiety to psychotic symptoms (Kleinman, 1980; Prakash, Sharan, & Sood, 2016; Simons & Hughes, 1985). When assessing clients with a culture-bound syndrome, it is important for the nurse to find out what the client, family, and other concerned individuals believe is happening, what prior efforts for help or cure have been tried, and what the results or outcomes from the treatment were.

Past Health

Past illnesses are important for multiple reasons. First, past illnesses may have residual effects on the current state of health or have sequelae that appear many months or years later. For example, the varicella–zoster virus responsible for chicken pox may remain latent until a person notices the characteristic rash or blisters of shingles; chicken pox and shingles are caused by the same herpes zoster virus. Although there has been a varicella vaccine available in the United States since 1995, protection from one dose is not lifelong, and a second dose is necessary 5 years after the initial immunization. Further, those born prior to 1995 and those born outside the United States may not be immunized. Second, the assessment of past illnesses includes other childhood conditions with known sequelae such as rheumatic fever, scarlet fever, and poliomyelitis. The nurse also gathers information about the date and nature of accidents, serious and chronic illnesses, hospitalizations, surgeries, obstetric history, and the last examination (Jarvis, 2016).

Family and Social History

In this era of genetics and genomics, a comprehensive and accurate family history highlights those diseases and disorders for which a client may be at increased risk. Table 3-4 provides an alphabetical listing of common diseases and identifies racial and ethnic groups for which the conditions are more prevalent. When conducting the family history, the nurse can refer to the table for conditions that tend to be more prevalent among certain groups. If clients are aware that they are at increased risk for a certain condition, they may arrange with

Table 3-4	Biocultural Aspects of Disease
Disease	**Remarks**
Alcoholism	American Indians have double the rate of Whites and 12% of all Native American deaths linked to alcohol; lower tolerance to alcohol among Chinese and Japanese Americans
Anemia	High incidence among Vietnamese because of the presence of infestations among immigrants and low-iron diets; low hemoglobin and malnutrition found among 18.2% of Native Americans, 32.7% of Blacks, 14.6% of Hispanics, and 10.4% of White children under 5 years of age
Arthritis	*Increased incidence among Native Americans*
	Blackfoot 1.4%
	Pima 1.8%
	Chippewa 6.8%
Asthma	Six times greater for Native American infants <1 year, same as the general population for Native Americans aged 1–44 years
Bronchitis	Six times greater for Native American infants <1 year, same as the general population for Native Americans aged 1–44 years. Main cause of death for Aboriginal Canadian infants in the postnatal period
Cancer	*Nasopharyngeal*: High among Chinese Americans and Native Americans
	Breast: Overall, White women are more likely to develop breast cancer than Black women. But under the age of 45, Black women are more likely than White to develop breast cancer (American Cancer Society, 2018)
	Higher prevalence of BRCA1 and BRCA2 mutations (linked to breast and ovarian cancers) in Ashkenazi Jews, Norwegians, Dutch, and Icelandic peoples; also higher in African Americans, Hispanics, Asian Americans, and non-Hispanic Whites (National Cancer Institute, 2018)
	Colorectal: Blacks 40% higher than Whites in the United States
	Ashkenazi Jews have one of the highest colorectal cancer risks of any ethnic group in the world
	Esophageal: No. 2 cause of death for Black men aged 35–54 years
	Incidence
	White men 3/100,000
	Black men 16.8/100,000
	Liver: Highest among all ethnic groups are Filipino Hawaiians; Latinos have twice the rate of Whites

Table 3-4	Biocultural Aspects of Disease (continued)
Disease	**Remarks**
	Stomach: Black men twice as likely as White men, low among Filipinos
	Cervical: 120% higher in Black women than in White women
	Mexican American and Puerto Rican women 2–3 times higher than Whites
	Uterine: 53% lower in Black women than White women
	Prostate: Black men have highest incidence of all groups
	Most prevalent cancer among Native Americans: biliary, nasopharyngeal, testicular, cervical, renal, and thyroid (females) cancer
	Lung cancer among Navajo uranium miners 85 times higher than among White miners
	Most prevalent cancer among Japanese Americans: esophageal, stomach, liver, and biliary cancer
	Among Chinese Americans, there is a higher incidence of nasopharyngeal and liver cancer than among the general population
Cholecystitis	*Incidence*
	Whites 0.3%
	Puerto Ricans 2.1%
	Native Americans 2.2%
	Chinese 2.6%
Colitis	High incidence among Japanese Americans
Diabetes mellitus	Three times as prevalent among Filipino Americans as Whites, higher among Hispanics than Blacks or Whites
	Death rate is 3–4 times as high among Native Americans aged 25–34 years, especially those in the West such as Utes and Tohono O'odham (Pimas and Papagos)
	Complications
	Amputations: Twice as high among Native Americans vs. the general US population
	Renal failure: 20 times as high as the general US population, with tribal variation, for example, Utes have 43 times higher incidence
G6PD deficiency	Present among 30% of Black males
Influenza	Increased death rate among Native Americans aged 45+
Ischemic heart disease	Responsible for 32% of heart-related causes of death among Native Americans; Blacks have higher mortality rates than all other groups
Lactose intolerance	Present among 66% of Hispanic women; increased incidence among Blacks and Chinese
Myocardial infarction	Leading cause of heart disease in Native Americans, accounting for 43% of death resulting from heart disease; low incidence among Japanese Americans
Otitis media	7.9% incidence among school-aged Navajo children vs. 0.5% in Whites
	Up to 1/3 of Eskimo children <2 years have chronic otitis media
	Increased incidence among bottle-fed Native Americans and Eskimo infants

(continued)

Table 3-4	Biocultural Aspects of Disease (continued)	
Disease	**Remarks**	
Pneumonia	Increased death rate among Native North Americans aged 45+	
Psoriasis	Affects 2%–5% of Whites but <1% of Blacks; high among Japanese Americans	
Renal disease	Lower incidence among Japanese Americans	
Sickle cell anemia	Increased incidence among Blacks; 1 in 12 African Americans carries the sickle cell trait	
Trachoma	Increased incidence among Native Americans and Eskimo children (3–8 times greater than the general population)	
Tuberculosis	Highest among Asian Americans, Pacific Islanders, and non-Hispanic Blacks	
	Increased incidence among Native Americans	
	Apache	2.0%
	Sioux	3.2%
	Navajo	4.6%
	Aboriginals living on Canadian reserves are 10 times more likely to have TB than non-Aboriginal Canadians	
	US-born persons, 37.1% of TB cases were reported among Blacks, followed by 29.5% non-Hispanic Whites	
Ulcers	Decreased incidence among Japanese Americans	

Table based on data accessed on October 8, 2018 at American Cancer Society (http://www.cancer.org); American Diabetes Association (http://www.diabetes.org); American Heart Association (http://www.americanheart.org); Centers for Disease Control and Prevention (http://www.cdc.gov/DiseasesConditions/); Fishbach, F., & Dunning, M. B. (2015). *A manual of laboratory and diagnostic tests* (9th ed.). Philadelphia, PA: Wolters Kluwer; Kim, A., Ashman, P., Ward-Peterson, M., Lozano, J. M., & Barengo, N. C. (2017). Racial disparities in cancer-related survival in patients with squamous cell carcinoma of the esophagus in the US between 1973 and 2013. *PLoS One, 12*(8). Retrieved from http://dx.doi.org.libproxy.umflint.edu/10.1371/journal.pone.0183782; Office of Minority Health (http://www.omhrc.gov/omh/whatsnew/2pgwhatsnew/special128a.htm); National Center for Health Statistics (http://www.cdc.gov/nchs); National Center on Minority Health & Health Disparities, National Institutes of Health (ncmhd.nih.gov); National Institute on Alcohol Abuse and Alcoholism (2014) Spotlight on Minority Health (http://www.cdc.gov/omh/populations/populations.htm); National Cancer Institute (2018). *Cancer disparities*. Retrieved from https://www.cancer.gov/about-cancer/understanding/disparities.

their health care provider to seek early screening and periodic surveillance and may choose to adopt a healthier lifestyle, for example, stop smoking, exercise regularly, and/or lose weight.

In addition to diagramming a family tree to identify familial relationships and the presence of disease conditions among those related to the client, the nurse should assess the broader socioeconomic factors influencing the client. The health history should include in-depth data pertaining to the client's family and/or close social friends, including identification of *key decision-makers*. Although personal financial information is often

a sensitive topic, it is important to determine the overall economic factors that influence a client. For example, regardless of race or ethnicity, people from lower socioeconomic categories have poorer health and shorter lives. There is a disproportionately high level of poverty among Blacks, Latinos/Latinas, American Indians/Alaska Natives (U.S. Census Bureau, 2017), and First Nation People of Canada (Wien, 2017). Economic factors have been identified as causes of less favorable outcomes among clients with cancer (Centers for Disease Control and Prevention, 2018). Research suggests that this is caused by a lack of health insurance and/or diminished access to health care services, both of which contribute to a situation in which less affluent clients receive diagnosis and treatment later in the course of the disease (Becares et al., 2012; Centers for Disease Control and Prevention, 2018; Dubay & Lebrun, 2012; Haeok, Fitzpatrick, & Baik, 2013; Kaiser Family Foundation, 2014; Obeig-Odoom, 2012; Pardasani & Bandyopadhyay, 2014).

See Appendix A for suggested interview topics aimed at eliciting information about family and social history.

Review of Systems

The purpose of the review of systems is threefold: (1) to evaluate the past and present health state of each body system, (2) to provide an opportunity for the client to report symptoms not previously stated, and (3) to evaluate health promotion practices. For example, when reviewing the gastrointestinal system with clients from Native American, Asian, African, and South American descent, the nurse should inquire about symptoms of lactose intolerance, such as diarrhea, nausea, vomiting, abdominal cramps, bloating, and flatus, usually beginning 30 minutes to 2 hours after eating or drinking foods that contain lactose (e.g., milk, cheese, and ice cream). **Lactose intolerance** means that the body cannot easily digest lactose, a type of natural sugar found in milk and dairy products. Some people who have lactose intolerance cannot digest any milk products. Others can eat or drink small amounts of milk products or certain types of milk products without problems (Mayo Clinic, 2018).

Knowledge of current research on diseases prevalent in specific ethnic and racial groups might be useful in asking appropriate questions in the review of systems. For example, if the nurse is gathering review of systems information from a middle-aged African American man, it is useful to know that there is a statistically higher incidence of hypertension, sickle cell anemia, and type 2 diabetes in this group than in counterparts from other racial and ethnic groups. This will assist in customizing the review of systems questions and ensuring that symptoms of disease specific to the client's ethnic or racial heritage are included.

Transcultural Perspectives on the Physical Examination

There are a number of **biocultural variations** that nurses may encounter when conducting the physical examination of clients from different cultural backgrounds. Accurate assessment and **evaluation** of clients require knowledge of normal biocultural variations among healthy members of selected populations, as well as variations that occur in illness. The data about biocultural variations presented here are evidence based and reflect the findings of classic studies that have been conducted over a period of years. The work of Dr. Theresa Overfield, a renowned nurse–anthropologist who published extensively on biological variations in health and illness, is cited frequently in the discussion that follows. The original work of Dr. Overfield was first published in 1995 and has recently been reissued as of 2017. As more research on biocultural variations is conducted, there will be additions and modifications to the current body of knowledge. The information provided here is intended to be helpful and illustrative, not exhaustive.

Biocultural Variations in Measurements

Racial and ethnic differences are found in measurements such as height (or length in infants and young children), body proportions, weight, and vital signs.

Height

Average heights for men and women from selected cultural groups are summarized in Table 3-5. In all groups, height increases up to 1.5 inches as socioeconomic status improves. First-generation immigrants might be up to 1.5 inches taller than their counterparts in the country of origin, due

Table 3-5	Biocultural Variations in Height for Selected Groups			
Average Height (in Inches)				
	White American	**African American**	**Mexican American**	**Asian**
All groups of men (*n*)				
69.2	69.7	69.5	67.3	67.0
All groups of women (*n*)				
63.7	64.1	64.2	61.9	61.8

Table developed using data from Centers for Disease Control and Prevention. (2017). Body measurements. Retrieved from https://www.cdc.gov/nchs/fastats/body-measurements.htm.

to better nutrition and decreased interference with growth by infectious diseases. There was a trend of height increase in this country, with the height of men from the United States increasing by 0.7 inches in a 10-year span; women from the United States grew an average of 0.5 inches taller in the same time period. In more recent years, the Centers for Disease Control and Prevention (CDC) reports that the height of men in the United States has leveled off. In 2008, American men were a mean height of 69.4 inches according to CDC data, while in 2014, the mean height was 69.2 inches (Centers for Disease Control and Prevention, 2008, 2017). On average, Black men and White men have similar mean heights (69.5 inches vs. 69.7 inches), as do Black and White women (64.2 inches vs. 64.1 inches) (Centers for Disease Control and Prevention, 2017; Overfield, 2017).

Body Proportions

Biocultural variations are found in the body proportions of individuals, largely because of differences in bone length. In comparing sitting/standing height ratios, Blacks of both genders have longer arms and legs and shorter trunks than Whites, Native Americans, or Asians. Because proportionately most of the body's weight is in the trunk, White men appear more obese than do their Black counterparts. The reverse is true of women. Clients of Asian heritage are markedly shorter, weigh less, and have smaller body frames

than their White counterparts and/or the overall population (Jarvis, 2016; Overfield, 2017).

Weight

Biocultural differences exist in the amount of body fat and the distribution of fat throughout the body. Generally, people from the lower socioeconomic class are more obese than those from the middle class, who are more obese than members of the upper class. On average, Black men weigh less than their White counterparts throughout adulthood (166.1 pounds vs. 170.6 pounds). The opposite is true of women. Black women are consistently heavier than White women of every age (149.6 pounds vs. 137 pounds) (Overfield, 2017). Between the ages of 35 and 64 years, Black women weigh on average 20 pounds more than White women. Mexican Americans weigh more in relation to height than non-Hispanic Whites because of differences in truncal fat patterns (Howell et al., 2018).

Some differences in the amount of body fat are related to socioeconomic factors, which in turn influence nutrition and exposure to communicable diseases. In a study of college-age women in Hawaii, researchers found that current weight (body mass index [BMI]) appears to play a larger role in the desire for a lower body weight than does race/ethnicity, suggesting a desired BMI may be more personal than cultural. All of the young women were found to desire a body weight consistent with a normal BMI, including the Hawaiians/Pacific Islanders, who traditionally have been reported to value a larger body size. This possible shift in preference could potentially lead to an increase in the prevalence of eating disorders in this population, as studies have shown that stronger identification with one's cultural group attenuates the link between perceived discrimination and eating and body image disturbance (Masuda, Latnera, Barliea, & Sargent, 2018).

Around the world, people in cold climates tend to have more body fat, whereas those residing in warmer areas have less. Blacks have smaller skinfold thicknesses on their trunks and arms than do their White counterparts (Overfield, 2017). Bottle-fed infants are heavier on average than those who are breast-fed, although their lengths are similar (Kliegman et al., 2016; Overfield, 2017).

Vital Signs

Although the average pulse rate is comparable across cultures, there are racial and gender differences in *blood pressure*. Black men have lower systolic blood pressures than their White counterparts from ages 18 to 34, but between the ages of 35 and 64, it reverses: Blacks have an average systolic blood pressure 5 mm Hg higher between 35 and 64 years of age. After age 65, there is no difference between the two races. Black women have a higher average systolic blood pressure than their White counterparts at every age. After age 45,

the average blood pressure of Black women might be as much as 16 mm Hg higher than that of White women in the same age group.

Hypertension develops earlier in life for African Americans and the incidence is twice as high in African Americans as it is in Whites. In addition, African Americans have the highest incidence of hypertension of anywhere in the world (American Heart Association, 2015). Studies have consistently reported a higher prevalence of hypertension in Blacks than in Whites, with hypertension being a main reason for the higher incidence of cardiovascular disease in Blacks. The long list of causes for this higher prevalence suggests that the real reasons are still unknown. Biological differences in the mechanisms of blood pressure control or in the differences in the environment and habits of Whites and Blacks are among the potential causes. The higher prevalence of hypertension in Blacks living in the United States as compared to those living in Africa demonstrates that environmental and behavioral characteristics are the more likely reasons for the higher prevalence in Blacks living in the United States. These factors could act directly or by triggering mechanisms of blood pressure increase that are dormant in Blacks living in Africa (American Heart Association, 2015; Jarvis, 2016; Musemwa & Gadegbeku, 2017). In Figure 3-2, a nurse practitioner checks the blood pressure of a client who is being seen for primary care services at an urban multicultural nurse-managed clinic.

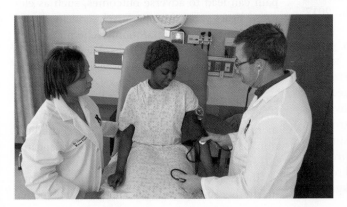

Figure 3-2. A nurse practitioner gathers subjective data during the health history and objective data (such as the blood pressure measurement) during the physical exam as part of the cultural assessment of a client being seen at an urban nurse–managed primary health care clinic.

Biocultural Variations in the Assessment of Pain

Pain is the most frequent and compelling reason that people seek health care and is sometimes referred to as the fifth vital sign. A universally recognized phenomenon, the term **pain** is defined as an unpleasant sensory and emotional experience conveyed by the brain through sensory neurons arising from actual or potential tissue damage to the body. Derived from the Greek word for penalty, pain is often associated with punishment in Judeo–Christian thought. Pain is a culture universal that is experienced by people in all parts of the world. Pain and ethnicity are multidimensional, subjective, and shaped by culture. The American Academy of Pain Medicine classifies pain as **acute** or **chronic**. In *acute pain*, a direct, one-to-one relationship exists between an injury and pain, and the pain is frequently short-lived and self-limiting. Acute pain, however, can become persistent and intractable if the underlying cause continues for a prolonged period. *Chronic pain* is described as pain that persists greater than 3 months. Chronic pain is now considered the most frequent cause of disability in industrialized nations globally. As a multi–billion-dollar public health concern and major cause of disability, careful attention needs to be given to provision of culturally and linguistically appropriate care. Data show that in the United States, an estimated 100 million people experience chronic pain, at a cost of $560 to $635 billion in health care treatment and lost productivity (National Center for Complimentary and Integrative Health, 2017; Robinson-Lane & Booker, 2017).

In terms of pain measurement, it is generally believed that humans experience similar sensation thresholds. However, pain perception thresholds, pain tolerance, and encouraged pain threshold vary considerably among individuals from different racial and ethnic backgrounds. *Sensation threshold* refers to the lowest stimulus that results in tingling or warmth. *Pain threshold* refers to the point at which the individual reports that a stimulus is painful. Cultural background has an effect on this measure of pain as well as on pain threshold, the point at which the individual reports that a stimulus is painful, and pain tolerance, the point at which the individual withdraws or asks to have the stimulus stopped.

In a meta-analysis of 26 studies on racial and ethnic pain threshold and tolerance, Rahim-Williams, Riley, Williams, and Fillingim (2012) found that African Americans and non-Hispanic Whites are the most frequently studied groups. Both groups have the same pain threshold, but African Americans have lower pain tolerance. In a study of pain among African Americans and Whites, it was reported similar finding with African Americans having lower pain thresholds than Whites for cold, heat, pressure, and ischemia. In addition, a more recent meta-analysis by Kim et al. (2017) looked at 44 studies of racial and ethnic differences in pain sensitivity. These studies echoed previous research and found that racial and ethnic minorities not only had lower pain tolerance but higher pain ratings across all pain modalities. Research on racial and ethnic group differences has translational merit for culturally competent clinical care and addressing and reducing pain treatment disparities among racially and ethnically diverse groups.

Research reveals that chronic disease, psychological distress, Medicaid insurance, lower education levels, and other social determinants of health are associated with higher incidences of severe pain (Meghani et al., 2012; Turk & Gatchel, 2018; Wyatt, 2013). Failure to adequately treat pain can lead to adverse outcomes, such as elevated heart rates postoperatively and increased risk of myocardial infarction, ischemic stroke, and hemorrhage resulting from elevated systemic vascular resistance and elevated levels of catecholamines. Other consequences of uncontrolled pain include reduced mobility, loss of strength, sleep disturbances, immune system impairment, increased susceptibility to disease, and medication dependence (Wang, Kennedy, & Caggana, 2013; Wyatt, 2013).

The assessment of pain is complicated primarily because pain is an inherently subjective experience that necessitates the reliance on self-reporting, rather than objective measurements. Rating scales do not resolve uncertainties inherent in self-reporting methods. For example, self-report measures can be difficult to understand for people with limited English proficiency as well as for children and people with cognitive impairments. Pain assessment is influenced by three factors: (1) characteristics of the client, such as race and ethnicity, (2) the environmental context, and (3) the nurse's background and experience. Nurses and other health care providers sometimes project their own attitudes, beliefs, and opinions about pain onto their clients, a situation that encourages cultural stereotyping when assessing the client's self-reported level of pain (Henschke et al., 2016; Tait & Chibnall, 2014).

Nurses and other health care providers are challenged to avoid bias when assessing pain and to take appropriate action commensurate with the level of self-reported pain. Research indicates that minority clients are likely to be more active in their communications when the clinical encounter is race concordant, that is, when the health care provider is from the same racial group, and to be less active in their communications when the encounter is race discordant, that is, the health care provider is from a different racial group than the client (Poma, 2017). Studies of primary care physicians reveal that provider race bias exists, especially between White providers and Black or Hispanic clients (FitzGerald & Hurst, 2017).

Negative stereotypes have been documented for members of racial and ethnic groups who experience pain. For example, some primary care physicians underestimate pain intensity in Black clients compared to other sociodemographic groups, and African Americans and Hispanics are sometimes perceived as requiring more scrutiny for potential drug abuse and misuse, despite evidence to the contrary (Becker et al., 2011; Centers for Disease Control and Prevention, 2018; Henschke et al., 2016; Kwok & Bhuvanakrishna, 2014; Tait & Chibnall, 2014). Blacks are more likely than non-Hispanic Whites to underreport pain unpleasantness in the clinical setting, especially in the presence of physicians who are perceived as having higher social status or are from a different racial background (Mack, Hunnicutt, Jesdale, & Lapane, 2018). Blacks demonstrate higher levels of posttreatment disability than do Whites for conditions such as low back pain, osteoarthritis, and other chronic pain conditions. Blacks also demonstrate more affective distress in response to chronic pain, with the distress contributing to levels of pain-related disability (Allen et al., 2018). Compared to non-Hispanic Whites, Native Americans have higher ischemic pain tolerance, higher electric pain threshold tolerance, lower ratings of electrical stimuli, and delay in withdrawing the hand from a noxious stimulus (nociceptive flexion reflex) (Kim et al., 2017). There is extensive evidence that Blacks and other minorities lack trust in the health care system and in their physicians, nurse practitioners, and other health professionals with different cultural backgrounds from their own (Cuevas & O'Brien, 2017); therefore, the client may fail to accurately report symptoms of pain, withhold information about the type and amount of medications he/she is using to control pain, and seek treatment for folk, traditional, religious, and/or spiritual healers when credentialed or licensed healers are unsuccessful in providing treatments that control pain to the client's satisfaction.

Factors contributing to racial and ethnic disparities in pain assessment include stereotypes and biases of nurses conducting the client assessment, nurse–client communication, the nurse's ability to empathize with clients from racial/ethnic groups different from his/her own, the client's educational and socioeconomic background, and the client's pain reporting skills, pain-coping ability, and level of trust of health care providers. The client's perception of the seriousness of the cause of pain (e.g., pain caused by cancer) may also influence the client's experience of pain (Booker, 2016; Henschke et al., 2016).

Evidence-Based Practice 3-2 summarizes the results of a study of African American, Latino/Latina, and White clients with chronic pain who

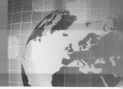

Interdisciplinary Team Approach to Chronic Pain Management

The purpose of this study was to identify ethnic differences in interdisciplinary pain treatment outcome for clients from diverse ethnic backgrounds experiencing chronic pain. The study was a retrospective chart review of prospective data. Participant data were obtained from medical record of clients who had been assessed, evaluated, and subsequently treated using an interdisciplinary pain management program in the Chicago area. Clients participated in either full- or half-day programs that included individual pain psychology, physical therapy, occupational therapy, biofeedback, relaxation training, vocational counseling, and medical management. In addition to the individual sessions, all clients participated in the following groups: psychology (e.g., pain cycles and cognitive restructuring), relaxation training, physical therapy (e.g., conditioning and core strengthening exercises), Feldenkrais (a movement-based therapy), occupational therapy (e.g., body mechanics and community outing), pool therapy, vocational counseling, and nursing lectures (e.g., sleep hygiene and use of laughter). The investigators assessed a sample of 116 White, African American, and Latino/Latina clients with chronic pain who participated in a 4-week interdisciplinary pain treatment program. The outcome measure consisted of pre- and posttreatment and change scores on the Multidimensional Pain Inventory, Pain Anxiety Symptoms Scale, Chronic Pain Acceptance Questionnaire, Coping Strategies Questionnaire-Revised, and Center for Epidemiologic Studies Depression Scale—short form.

Ethnic minorities differed from Whites on a number of treatment outcome measures at pre- and posttreatment. At pretreatment, Latinos/Latinas reported greater levels of pain-related anxiety, pain severity, and pain catastrophizing than White counterparts experiencing chronic pain. Both Latinos/Latinas and African Americans reported greater use of prayer at pre- and posttreatment, with Whites showing the greatest decrease in the use of prayer in response to treatment. At posttreatment, African American clients had a slightly greater level of anxiety than Whites. There was a significant difference in levels of depression at posttreatment with African Americans having higher levels of depression than Whites or Latinos/Latinas. There was a significant ethnic difference in the use of pain catastrophizing at pretreatment with Latinos/Latinas compared to Whites. There were also significant ethnic differences pre- and posttreatment with both Latinos/Latinas and African Americans using prayer as a coping strategy more than Whites. There was significant ethnicity effect for pain severity at pretreatment with both African Americans and Latinos/Latinas reporting a significantly greater level of pain severity than Whites. There was also significant posttreatment ethnicity effect for general activity level with Whites having a significantly higher level of activity than African Americans.

Clinical Implications

Although the researchers reported that ethnic minority groups have a greater level of distress when experiencing chronic pain when compared to Whites, African American, Latino/Latina, and White clients with chronic pain who participated in the study all demonstrated a significant reduction in emotional distress, pain-related anxiety, use of maladaptive coping strategies such as catastrophizing, and perception of pain severity when they participated in a 4-week interdisciplinary team intervention to manage their pain. As an integral part of the interdisciplinary team, nurses have a key role to play in assisting clients from diverse ethnic backgrounds to effectively manage chronic pain. Nurses should seek opportunities to collaborate with health professionals from other disciplines to plan, implement, and evaluate interdisciplinary interventions such as the one described in this study in order to help clients manage their chronic pain.

Reference: Gagon, C. M., Matsura, J. T., Smith, C. C., & Stanos, S. P. (2013). Ethnicity and interdisciplinary pain treatment. *Pain and Practice, 14*(6), 532–540.

participated in a 4-week interdisciplinary team intervention that supported the notion that ethnic differences in pain assessment, perception, and treatment can be effectively managed using an interdisciplinary team approach, with nurses either leading or being key members of the team.

Biocultural Variations in General Appearance

In assessing general appearance, survey the person's entire body. Note the general health state and any obvious physical characteristics and readily apparent biologic features unique to the individual. In assessing the client's general appearance, consider four areas: physical appearance, body structure, mobility, and behavior.

1. *Physical appearance* includes age, gender, level of consciousness, facial features, and skin color (evenness of color tone, pigmentation, intactness, and presence of lesions or other abnormalities).
2. *Body structure* includes stature, nutrition, symmetry, posture, position, and overall body build or contour.
3. *Mobility* includes gait and range of motion.
4. *Behavior* includes such variables as facial expression, mood and affect, fluency of speech, ability to communicate ideas, appropriateness of word choice, grooming, and attire or dress. For example, observant members of the following groups often wear culture-specific attire: Amish, Mennonites, Hasidic and Orthodox Jewish, and Muslims. Members of the Church of Jesus Christ of Latter-day Saints (LDS) (also known as Mormons) wear undergarments that symbolize their temple covenants. Many clients will want to leave the garments on during physical examinations. Nurses should respect the attire or clothing of people from diverse cultures and religions and those who ask to leave their garments on during the physical examination. In some instances, the client will not want nurses to handle their clothing.

In assessing a client's hygiene, it is useful to ask about typical bathing habits and customary use of various hygiene-related products. The level of self-care may suggest poor hygiene if unkempt and dirty. Recent immigrants from some arid nations where water is scarce might bathe less frequently than those from countries where water is more abundant.

People in most cultures in the United States and Canada make a great effort to disguise their natural body odors by bathing frequently, using douches, or applying antiperspirants, colognes, and/or perfumes with scents that are deemed to be desirable. These practices may mask the symptoms of some diseases and infections. There are dozens of diseases associated with odors of the breath, skin, urine, stool, penis, and vagina (National Geographic, 2018).

During the assessment, the nurse should:

- Note the nature of breath odor—sweet may suggest diabetic ketoacidosis (sickly sweet smell), alcoholism (distinctive), liver failure (a sweet smell), or maple syrup urine disease; unpleasant or foul may suggest renal failure (urine or fishlike breath due to ammonia) and infections of the mouth, nose, pharynx, or chest (putrid odor).
- Examine state of teeth and teeth hygiene and note whether the teeth are real or false—loose-fitting teeth may be responsible for mouth ulcers or decayed teeth, which may cause halitosis (bad breath odor).
- Check the following test results for indications of abnormalities:
  - *Blood tests* such as full blood count and the erythrocyte sedimentation rate will be helpful in determining the presence of infection.
  - *Renal function tests* may suggest renal failure as cause of breath odor.
  - *Liver function tests* may suggest hepatic coma as cause of breath odor.
  - *Blood sugar* may suggest diabetic ketoacidosis as a cause of breath odor.
  - *Blood alcohol level* to establish if alcoholism may be the cause of the breath odor.

- Urine analysis:
  - Glucose and ketones present may suggest diabetic ketoacidosis as cause of breath odor.
  - Urine microscopy and culture may detect urinary tract infection.
- Culture of the mouth, gums, and nasopharynx may be necessary to diagnose anaerobic infections that may be the cause of breath odor.
- Sputum microscopy and culture.
- Vaginal or penile discharge swab for culture, if appropriate.
- Stool tests:
  - Stool microscopy for ova, parasites, and culture for bacteria
  - *Giardia* antigen
  - Twenty-four-hour stool analysis of fecal fat—if **steatorrhea** is present (i.e., fatty, pale-colored, extremely smelly stools that float in the toilet and are difficult to flush away due to excess fat in the stool)
- Radiological investigations:
  - X-ray or CT scan of the chest or sinuses—if suspect respiratory infection as a cause of breath odor.
  - Esophagogram will help detect a diverticulum (a pouch opening from the esophagus) that may cause bad breath odor (Mayo Clinic, 2019).

Biocultural Variations in Skin

An accurate and comprehensive examination of the skin of clients from culturally diverse backgrounds requires knowledge of biocultural variations and skill in recognizing color changes, some of which might be subtle. Awareness of normal biocultural differences and the ability to recognize the unique clinical manifestations of disease are developed over time as the nurse gains experience with clients with various skin colors.

The assessment of a client's skin is subjective and is highly dependent on observational skill, the ability to recognize subtle color changes, and repeated exposure to individuals having various gradations of skin color. *Melanin* is responsible for the various colors and tones of skin observed in different people. Melanin protects the skin against harmful ultraviolet rays—a genetic advantage accounting for the lower incidence of skin cancer among darkly pigmented Black and Native American clients (Jarvis, 2016).

Normal skin color ranges widely. Some health care practitioners have attempted to describe the variations by labeling their observations with some of the following adjectives: *copper*, *olive*, *tan*, and various shades of *brown* (*light, medium, and dark*). In observing pallor in clients, the term *ashen* is sometimes used. Skin color is one of the most important biological variations to assess in nursing care and of great clinical significance. The nurse's ability to establish a reliable description of baseline skin color and subsequently recognize when variations occur in an individual is of great importance, especially for clients whose health condition may be linked to changes in skin color (Giger, 2017).

Mongolian Spots

Mongolian spots are irregular areas of deep blue pigmentation usually located in the sacral and gluteal areas but sometimes occurring on the abdomen, thighs, shoulders, or arms. During embryonic development, the melanocytes originate near the embryonic nervous system in the neural crest. They then migrate into the fetal epidermis. Mongolian spots are embryonic pigment that has been left behind in the epidermal layer during fetal development. The result looks like a bluish discoloration of the skin.

Mongolian spots are a normal variation in children of African, Asian, or Latin descent. By adulthood, these spots become lighter but usually remain visible. Mongolian spots are present in 90% of Blacks, 80% of Asians and Native Americans, and 9% of Whites (Jarvis, 2016; Overfield, 2017). To the unfamiliar eye, mongolian spots sometimes can be confused with bruises. Recognition of this normal variation is particularly important when dealing with children who might be erroneously identified as victims of child abuse, causing much anguish to the parents or guardians.

Vitiligo

Vitiligo, a condition in which the melanocytes become nonfunctional in some areas of the skin, is characterized by unpigmented, patchy, milky white skin patches that are often symmetric bilaterally. Vitiligo affects an estimated two to five million Americans. There is no greater prevalence among dark-skinned individuals, although the disorder may cause greater psychosocial stress in some groups because it is more visible (Buttaro, Trybulski, Polgar Bailey, & Sandberg-Cook, 2016). Although it is more visible, several studies have shown that even though the burden on daily life was greater for darker-skinned individuals with vitiligo, self-perceived stress was similar regardless of skin color (Grimes & Miller, 2018). People with vitiligo also have a statistically higher-than-normal risk for pernicious anemia, diabetes mellitus, and hyperthyroidism. These factors are believed to reflect an underlying genetic abnormality.

Hyperpigmentation

Other areas of the skin affected by hormones and, in some cases, differing for people from certain ethnic backgrounds are the sexual skin areas, such as the nipples, areola, scrotum, and labia majora. In general, these areas are darker than other parts of the skin in both adults and children, especially among African American and Asian clients. When assessing these skin surfaces on dark-skinned clients, observe carefully for erythema, rashes, and other abnormalities because the darker color might mask their presence.

Cyanosis

A severe condition indicating a lack of oxygen in the blood, **cyanosis,** is the most difficult clinical sign to observe in darkly pigmented persons. Because peripheral vasoconstriction can prevent cyanosis, be attentive to environmental conditions such as air conditioning, mist tents, and other factors that might lower the room temperature and thus cause vasoconstriction. For the client to manifest clinical evidence of cyanosis, the level of deoxygenated hemoglobin in the arteries is usually below 5 g/dL with an oxygen saturation below 85% (Adeyinka & Kondamudi, 2017; Overfield, 2017). Only severe cyanosis is apparent in skin. It is best to check the conjunctivae, oral mucosa, and nail beds rather than to rely on the assessment of the skin, which will appear dull and lifeless in darkly pigmented people.

Given that most conditions causing cyanosis also cause decreased oxygenation of the brain, other clinical symptoms, such as changes in the level of consciousness, will be evident. Cyanosis usually is accompanied by increased respiratory rate, use of accessory muscles of respiration, nasal flaring, and other manifestations of respiratory distress. Exercise caution when assessing persons of Mediterranean descent for cyanosis because their circumoral region is normally dark blue.

Jaundice

In both light- and dark-skinned clients, **jaundice** is best observed in the sclera. When examining culturally diverse individuals, exercise caution to avoid confusing other forms of pigmentation with jaundice. Many darkly pigmented people, for example, African Americans, Filipinos, and others, have heavy deposits of subconjunctival fat that contain high levels of carotene in sufficient quantities to mimic jaundice. The fatty deposits become denser as the distance from the cornea increases. The portion of the sclera that is revealed naturally by the palpebral fissure is the best place to accurately assess color. If the palate does not have heavy melanin pigmentation, jaundice can be detected there in the early stages (i.e., when the serum bilirubin level is 2 to 4 mg/100 mL). The absence of a yellowish tint of the palate when the sclerae are yellow indicates carotene pigmentation of the sclerae rather than jaundice. Light- or clay-colored stools and dark golden urine often accompany jaundice in both light- and dark-skinned clients. To distinguish between carotenemia and jaundice, it is necessary to inspect the posterior portion of the hard palate using bright daylight or good artificial lighting. Also, check the palms and soles for a yellow-orange color (Jarvis, 2016; Overfield, 2017). The ingestion of large amounts of carotene-rich foods may mimic jaundice; therefore, ask if the person recently ingested significant amounts of sweet potatoes, carrots, dark green leafy vegetables, butternut squash, or romaine lettuce.

Pallor

Assessing for **pallor** in darkly pigmented clients can be difficult because the underlying red tones are absent. This is significant because these red tones are responsible for giving brown or black skin its luster. The brown-skinned individual will manifest pallor with a more yellowish brown color, and the black-skinned person will appear ashen or gray. Generalized pallor can be observed in the mucous membranes, lips, and nail beds. The palpebrae, conjunctivae, and nail beds are preferred sites for assessing the pallor of anemia. When inspecting the conjunctiva, lower the lid sufficiently to see the conjunctiva near the inner and outer canthi. The coloration is often lighter near the inner canthus.

In addition to changes seen on skin assessment, the pallor of impending shock is accompanied by other clinical manifestations, such as increasing pulse rate, oliguria, apprehension, and restlessness. Anemia, particularly chronic iron deficiency anemia, might be manifested by the characteristic "spoon" nails, which have a concave shape. A lemon-yellow tint of the face and slightly yellow sclerae accompany pernicious anemia, which is also manifested by neurologic deficits and a red, painful tongue. Also, fatigue, exertional dyspnea, rapid pulse, dizziness, and impaired mental function accompany the most severe anemia (Jarvis, 2016; Overfield, 2017).

Erythema, Petechiae, and Ecchymoses

Erythema (redness) can also be difficult to assess in darkly pigmented clients because the contrast between white and red is more pronounced than it is when the skin color is darker. Erythema is frequently associated with localized inflammation and is characterized by increased skin temperature. The degree of redness is determined by the quantity of blood in the subpapillary plexus, whereas the warmth of the skin is related to the rate of blood flow through the blood vessels. In the assessment of inflammation in dark-skinned clients, it is often necessary to palpate the skin for increased warmth, tautness, or tightly pulled surfaces that might indicate edema and hardening of deep tissues or blood vessels. The dorsal surfaces of the fingers are the most sensitive to temperature sensations and should be used to assess for erythema.

The erythema associated with rashes is not always accompanied by noticeable increases in skin temperature. Macular, papular, and vesicular skin lesions are identified by a combination of palpation and inspection. In addition, it is important to listen to the client's description of symptoms. For example, persons with macular rashes will usually complain of itching, and evidence of scratching will be apparent. When the skin is only moderately pigmented, a macular rash might become recognizable when the skin is gently stretched. Stretching the skin decreases the normal red tone, thus providing more contrast and making the macules appear brighter. In some skin disorders with a generalized rash, the rash is most readily visible on the hard and soft palates.

Petechiae are best visualized in the areas of lighter melanization, such as the abdomen, buttocks, and volar surface of the forearm. Usually, the petechiae are found in clusters and consist of small, pinpoint spots that vary in color from red, brown, or purple (Mayo Clinic, 2018). When the skin is black or very dark brown, petechiae cannot be seen in the skin. Most of the diseases that cause bleeding and the formation of microscopic emboli, such as thrombocytopenia, subacute bacterial endocarditis, and other septicemias, are characterized by petechiae in the mucous membranes and skin. Petechiae are most easily seen in the mouth, particularly the buccal mucosa, and in the conjunctiva of the eye (Jarvis, 2016).

Ecchymoses caused by systemic disorders are found in the same locations as petechiae, although their larger size makes them more apparent on dark-skinned individuals. When differentiating petechiae and ecchymoses from erythema in the mucous membrane, pressure on the tissue will momentarily blanch erythema but not petechiae or ecchymoses.

Addison's Disease

The cortisol deficiency characteristic of **Addison's disease** causes an increase in melanin production, which turns the skin a bronze color that resembles suntan. The nipples, areola, genitalia, perineum, and pressure points such as the axillae, elbow, inner thighs, and buttocks look bronze. Addison's disease is very difficult to recognize in people with darkly pigmented skin; therefore, laboratory tests and other clinical manifestations of the disease should be used to corroborate the skin changes (Jarvis, 2016; Vashi & Maibach, 2017).

Uremia

Uremia is the illness accompanying kidney failure characterized by unexplained changes in extracellular volume, inorganic ion concentrations, or lack of known renal synthetic products. Uremic illness is due largely to the accumulation of organic waste products, not all identified, that are normally cleared by the kidneys. Renal failure causes retained urochrome pigments in the blood to turn the skin of a person with uremia gray or orange-green. In people with darkly pigmented skin, it may be difficult to visualize these skin color changes; therefore, skin manifestations of uremia are often masked. Laboratory tests and other clinical findings are needed to corroborate the observation of skin color change when assessing a person with suspected uremia.

Albinism

The term **albinism** refers to a group of inherited conditions. People with albinism have little or no pigment in their eyes, skin, or hair. They have inherited altered genes that do not make the usual amounts of the pigment melanin. One person in 18,000 to 20,000 in the United States has some type of albinism. In other parts of the world, the occurrence of albinism could be as high as 1 in 3,000 (National Organization for Albinism and Hypopigmentation, 2018). Albinism affects people from all races. Most children with albinism are born to parents who have normal hair and eye color for their ethnic backgrounds. Sometimes, people do not recognize that they have albinism. There are different types of albinism, and the amount of pigment in the eyes varies. Although some individuals with albinism have reddish or violet eyes, most have blue eyes, whereas others have hazel or brown eyes.

Vision problems are associated with all forms of albinism. People with albinism always have impaired vision (not correctable with eyeglasses) and many have low vision. Low vision refers to impaired vision in which there is a significant reduction in visual function that cannot be corrected by conventional glasses. With low vision, it may become hard or seem impossible to do normal tasks, yet this may be improved with special aids or devices to make the most out of the vision that is available (American Academy of Ophthalmology, 2018a). The degree of vision impairment varies with the type of albinism. Many people with albinism are legally blind due to abnormal development of the retina and abnormal patterns of nerve connections between the eye and the brain. The presence of these eye problems defines the diagnosis of albinism. Therefore, the main test for albinism is an eye examination. People with albinism also need to take precautions to avoid damage to the skin caused by the sun, such as wearing sunscreen lotions, hats, and sun-protective clothing (American Academy of Ophthalmology, 2018b; National Organization for Albinism and Hypopigmentation, 2018).

Normal Age-Related Skin Changes

Although aging is accompanied by the growing presence of wrinkles in all cultures, Blacks, Asian Americans, American Indians, and Eskimos wrinkle later in life than their Anglo American counterparts (Vashi & Maibach, 2017). Light skin shows the effects of sun damage more than dark skin, regardless of race or ethnicity, and the area of the skin that is exposed to the sun shows the effects of aging more than protected skin, such as those parts covered by clothing. **Café au lait spots**, tan to light brown irregularly shaped oval patches with well-defined borders, are caused by increased melanin pigment in the basal cell layer of the skin (Vashi & Maibach, 2017).

Regardless of climate, dry skin is inevitable in individuals older than 70 years of age. Transepidermal water loss will result in a dry, tight, and often inflamed-looking appearance. It gives an impaired acid mantle and impaired immune response, impacting and compromising the skin's structural integrity. Examples of severe transepidermal water loss are eczema or psoriasis. These conditions occur when vital fluids evaporate and the skin becomes very dry and inflamed. Restoring free water levels and thickening the matrix of the skin are an integral part of returning the skin back to a healthy functional state. African Americans have a slightly higher transepidermal water loss than Whites, which correlates with the water content of the stratum corneum layer of the skin (Vashi & Maibach, 2017).

Moles occur when cells in the skin grow in a cluster instead of being spread throughout the skin. These cells are called melanocytes, and they make the pigment that gives skin its natural color. Moles may darken after exposure to the sun, during the teen years, and during pregnancy. Because the number of moles increases with age, they are thought to be the result of long-term exposure to the sun. People with lighter skin have more moles than those with darkly pigmented skin. Whites have more moles than Asian Americans or African Americans (Overfield, 2017). Most moles are benign; however, moles that are more likely to be cancer are those that look different than other existing moles or those that first appear after age 30. If nurses notice changes in a mole's color, height, size, or shape, they should consult with a dermatologist. Any client who has a mole that bleeds, oozes, itches, or becomes tender or painful should be referred immediately to a dermatologist (American Cancer Society, 2016; Jarvis, 2016).

Nurses and other health care providers often overestimate or underestimate age when dealing with clients whose cultural heritage is different from their own. Whites tend to underestimate the age of Africans, Asians, and American Indians, whereas African Americans, Asians, and American Indians tend to overestimate the age of White clients (Gunn et al., 2013). Yet, it must be noted that as the intermixing of races, cultures, and ethnicities occurs, over time we will start to see more heterogenous groups rather than homogenous groups in relation to the skin and the age-related skin changes (Vashi, De Castro Maymone, & Kundu, 2016).

Biocultural Variations in Sweat Glands

The *apocrine* and *eccrine sweat glands* are important for fluid balance and thermoregulation. Approximately two to three million glands open onto the skin surface through pores and are responsible for the presence of sweat. When glands are contaminated by normal skin flora, odor results. Most Asians and Native Americans have a mild to absent body odor, whereas Whites and African Americans tend to have strong body odor.

Eskimos have made an environmental adaptation whereby they sweat less than Whites on their trunks and extremities but more on their faces (Overfield, 2017). This adaptation allows for temperature regulation without causing perspiration and dampness of their clothes, which would decrease their ability to insulate against severe weather and would pose a serious threat to their survival.

The amount of chloride excreted by sweat glands varies widely, and African Americans have lower salt concentrations in their sweat than Whites do. A study of Ashkenazi Jews (of European descent) and Sephardic Jews (of North

African and Middle Eastern descent) revealed that those of European origin had a lower percentage of sweat chlorides (Levin, 1966; Overfield, 2017). This variation might be significant in the care of clients with renal or cardiac conditions or of children with cystic fibrosis (Gunn et al., 2013; Taylor & Machado-Moreira, 2013).

Biocultural Variation in the Head

Nurses will notice marked, biocultural variations when examining the hair, eyes, ears, and mouths of clients from diverse racial and ethnic backgrounds. The ability to distinguish normal variations from abnormal ones could have serious implications as some variations are associated with systemic sometimes life-threatening conditions.

Hair

Perhaps one of the most obvious and widely variable cultural differences occurs with assessment of the hair. African American hair varies widely in texture. It is very fragile and ranges from long and straight to short, spiraled, thick, and kinky. The hair and scalp have a natural tendency to be dry and require daily combing, gentle brushing, and the application of oil. By comparison, clients of Asian backgrounds generally have straight, silky hair.

Obtaining a baseline hair assessment is significant in the diagnosis and treatment of certain disease states. For example, hair texture is known to become dry, brittle, and lusterless with inadequate nutrition. The hair of Black children with severe malnutrition, as in the case of marasmus, frequently changes not only in texture but also in color. The child's hair often becomes straighter and turns a reddish copper color. Certain endocrine and genetic disorders are also known to affect the amount, thickness, and texture of the client's hair (Vashi & Maibach, 2017).

Although gray hair correlates with age for both men and women, there are cultural differences in the rate of hair graying. In general, Whites gray faster than other ethnic groups, with Whites starting to gray in their mid-30s and African Americans in their mid-40s (Park, Khan, & Rawnsley, 2018). Among some Asian Americans, graying might be delayed significantly, with some in their eighth or ninth decade of life showing little or no graying.

Eyes

Biocultural differences in both the structure and the color of the eyes are readily apparent among clients from various cultural backgrounds. Racial differences are evident in the palpebral fissures. Persons of Asian background are often identified by their characteristic epicanthal eye folds, whereas the presence of narrowed palpebral fissures in non-Asian individuals might be diagnostic of a serious congenital anomaly known as Down's syndrome or trisomy 21.

There is culturally based variability in the color of the iris and in retinal pigmentation: darker irises are correlated with darker retinas. Clients with light retinas generally have better night vision but can experience pain in an environment that is too light. The majority of African Americans and Asians have brown eyes, whereas many individuals of Scandinavian or Northern European descent have blue eyes (Overfield, 2017).

It is clinically relevant that differences in visual acuity (clearness of vision) occur among people from different cultures. When eyeglasses are prescribed to improve visual clarity, Blacks have poorer corrected visual acuity than do Whites. The visual acuity of Hispanic Americans is between that of Blacks and Whites (Qiu, Wang, Singh, & Lin, 2014). American Indians are comparable to Whites in visual acuity; Japanese and Chinese Americans have the poorest corrected visual acuity because of a high incidence of myopia (Overfield, 2017; Qiu et al., 2014). Dutch German Mennonites have an X chromosome disorder that causes night blindness (and low phosphate levels) (National Institute of Health, 2018).

Ears

Ears come in a variety of sizes and shapes. Earlobes can be freestanding or attached to the face. Ceruminous glands are located in the external ear canal and are functional at birth. Cerumen (earwax) is genetically determined and comes in two major types, dry cerumen, which is gray and flaky and frequently forms a thin mass in the ear canal, and wet cerumen, which is dark brown and moist. Asians and Native Americans (including Eskimos) have an 84% frequency of dry cerumen. Wet cerumen is found in 99% of African Americans and 97% of Whites (Overfield, 2017). The clinical significance of this occurs when examining or irrigating the ears; the presence and composition of cerumen are not related to poor hygiene, and flaky, dry cerumen should not be mistaken for the dry lesions of eczema.

Hearing loss may be genetic, congenital, or acquired through aging, injury, infection, or accident. On rare occasions, hearing loss is caused by surgery when the excision of a brain tumor is necessary. Age-related hearing loss, or **presbycusis**, is the slow loss of hearing that occurs as people get older and the cilia (tiny hair cells) in the inner ear become damaged or die. The following factors that contribute to age-related hearing loss should be considered in the health history and physical examination: family history (age-related hearing loss tends to run in families), repeated exposure to loud noises, smoking (smokers are more likely to have hearing loss than nonsmokers), certain medical conditions such as diabetes, and some prescription medicines (e.g., the antibiotic gentamicin). Although hearing loss caused by noise and aging previously has been considered permanent, there is animal research using vitamin B_3 that offers promise for restoring hearing loss (Gladstone Institute, 2014). After age 40, men have poorer hearing than women. Blacks have better hearing at high and low frequencies; Whites have better hearing at middle frequencies. Melanin pigmentation is significantly more abundant in the cochlea of African Americans than Whites. Research detailing pigmentation in the cochlea helps to explain the observed racial differences in hearing thresholds between African Americans and Whites and may be the reason that African Americans are less susceptible to noise-induced hearing loss such as that caused by loud music or occupational exposure to noise (Healthy Hearing Foundation, 2016).

Mouth

Oral hyperpigmentation also shows variation by race. Usually absent at birth, hyperpigmentation increases with age. By age 50, 10% of Whites and 50% to 90% of African Americans will show oral hyperpigmentation, a condition believed to be caused by a lifetime of accumulation of postinflammatory oral changes (Kliegman et al., 2016; Overfield, 2017).

Cleft uvula, a condition in which the uvula is split either completely or partially, occurs in up to 10% of some Native American groups and up to 10% of Asians, as well (Jarvis, 2016; Kliegman et al., 2016). Ethnic differences exist in the incidence of cleft lip and palate with American Indians having the highest incidence (3.6 per 1,000), followed by Asians (2.1 per 1,000) and Whites (1 per 1,000). Blacks have the lowest incidence (0.41 per 1,000) (Noorollahian et al., 2015). The incidence of cleft lip and palate rises with increased parental age; older mothers with additional parity have an increased incidence of having children with cleft palate (Berg, Lie, Siversten, & Haaland, 2015).

Leukoedema, a grayish-white benign lesion occurring on the buccal mucosa, is present in 68% to 90% of Blacks and 43% of Whites. Care should be taken to avoid mistaking leukoedema for oral thrush or related infections that require treatment with medication (Overfield, 2017).

Teeth

Teeth are often used as indicators of developmental, hygienic, and nutritional adequacy, and there are important biocultural differences. It is rare for a White baby to be born with teeth (1 in 3,000), but the incidence was quite high among

Alaskan Tlingit Indian infants (9%) with 62% of those newborns' relatives also affected by these teeth. Although congenital teeth are usually not problematic, extraction is necessary for some breast-fed infants (Kliegman et al., 2016; Malki, Al-Badawi, & Dahlan, 2015; Overfield, 2017).

The size of teeth varies widely, with the teeth of Whites being the smallest, followed by Blacks and then Asians and Native Americans. The largest teeth are found among Native Alaskans and Australian Aborigines. Larger teeth cause some groups to have prognathic (protruding) jaws, a condition that is seen more frequently in African and Asian Americans. The condition is normal and does not reflect a serious orthodontic problem.

Agenesis (absence of teeth) varies by race, with missing third molars occurring in 18% to 35% of Asians, 9% to 25% of Whites, and 1% to 11% of Blacks. Throughout life, Whites have more tooth decay than do Blacks, which might be related to a combination of socioeconomic factors and biocultural variation. Current data show that dental caries continue to be high in non-Hispanic White adults (94%), as compared with non-Hispanic Black (86%). Statistics have shifted in relation to loss of teeth and race. Previously, it was reported that complete loss of teeth was highest among Whites (Overfield, 2017), yet more recent data from the CDC are challenging this. The CDC is reporting that tooth retention is currently lowest among non-Hispanic Black adults (38%) compared with non-Hispanic White (51%), non-Hispanic Asian (49%), and Hispanic (45%) adults (Centers for Disease Control and Prevention, 2015). Further, data are showing that complete tooth loss is highest in non-Hispanic Black adults, with a 29% complete tooth loss, as compared with the non-Hispanic White population at 16.9% complete tooth loss (Centers for Disease Control and Prevention, 2015).

Dental caries or tooth decay is significant because there are known correlations between dental caries and other conditions such as cleft lip and palate, renal failure, cystic fibrosis, immunosuppression, heart defects, low birth weight, seizures, maternal illness, and rickets (Kliegman et al., 2016). The differences in tooth decay between African Americans and Whites can be explained by the fact that African Americans have harder and denser tooth enamel, which makes their teeth less susceptible to the organisms that cause caries. The increase in periodontal disease among African Americans is believed to be caused by poor oral hygiene. When obvious signs of periodontal disease are present, such as bleeding and edematous gums, a dental referral should be initiated.

Biocultural Variations in the Mammary Venous Plexus

Regardless of gender, the superficial veins of the chest form a network over the entire chest that flows in either a transverse or a longitudinal pattern. In the transverse pattern, the veins radiate laterally and toward the axillae. In the longitudinal pattern, the veins radiate downward and laterally like a fan. These two patterns occur with different frequencies in the two populations that have been studied, Whites and Navajos. The recessive longitudinal pattern occurs in 6% to 10% of White women and in 30% of Navajos. The only known alteration of either pattern is produced by breast tumor. Although this variation has no clinical significance, it is mentioned so that if nurses note its presence during physical assessment, they will recognize it as a normal variation (Overfield, 2017; Yang et al., 2012).

Biocultural Variations in the Musculoskeletal System

Many normal biocultural variations are found in clients' musculoskeletal systems. The long bones of Blacks are significantly longer, narrower, and denser than those of Whites. Bone density measured by race and gender shows that Black males have the densest bones, accounting for the relatively lower incidence of osteoporosis and hip fractures in this population. Similarly, Black women have lower incidence of these two conditions when compared with Hispanic and White women (Jarvis, 2016; Zengin et al., 2016). Bone density in Chinese, Japanese, and Native Alaskans is below that of Whites (Overfield, 2017). Low bone mineral density is just one of the factors associated with higher prevalence of bone fracture in all ethnic groups. In addition to bone density, other risk factors such as genetics, bone size, bone geometry, physical activity, smoking history, and alcohol consumption must be looked at (International Osteoporosis Foundation, 2017).

Curvature of the body's long bones varies widely among culturally diverse groups. Native Americans and First Nation People of Canada have anteriorly convex femurs, whereas Blacks have markedly straight femurs, and Whites have intermediate femurs. This characteristic is related to both genetics and body weight. The femurs of thin Blacks and Whites have less curvature than average, whereas those of obese Blacks and Whites display increased curvatures. It is possible that the heavier density of the bones of Blacks helps to protect them from increased curvature caused by obesity. Blacks tend to be wide shouldered and narrow hipped; Asians tend to be wider in the hips and narrower in the shoulders. The clavicle is a long bone that is responsible for shoulder width; therefore, taller people generally have wider shoulders than shorter people (Overfield, 2017; Silva et al., 2011).

As the largest component of adipose tissue–free body mass in humans, skeletal muscle is central to the body's nutritional, physiologic, and metabolic processes. Blacks tend to have more lean body mass than Whites, with this greater muscle mass correlating with the greater bone mass in Blacks. Between the ages of 18 and 80 years, Blacks have more skeletal muscle than White, Hispanic, and Asian counterparts across the entire age range, even when adjusting for weight and height. Body composition should be interpreted according to ethnicity and gender. Different standards for skeletal muscle should be applicable for multiethnic populations (Overfield, 2017; Silva et al., 2011).

Table 3-6 summarizes biocultural variations occurring in the musculoskeletal system that have been identified through observation and study of people from various cultures and subcultures.

Biocultural Variations in Illness

Researchers have abundant evidence that there is a relationship between ethnicity and the incidence of certain diseases across the lifespan, from infancy to old age. Knowledge of normal biocultural variations and those occurring during illness helps nurses to conduct more accurate, comprehensive, and thorough physical examinations of clients from diverse cultures.

Biocultural Variations in Laboratory Tests

As summarized in Table 3-7, biocultural variations occur with some laboratory tests, such as measurement of hemoglobin, hematocrit, cholesterol, serum transferrin, blood glucose, creatinine, and estimated glomerular filtration rate. There are also biocultural differences in the results of tests conducted during pregnancy. For example, the multiple marker screening test and two tests of amniotic fluid constituents are routinely used to screen pregnant women for potential fetal problems.

Caution should be used in interpreting genetic data as population categories are not discrete and separate entities. African Americans and Latinos have complex recent ancestral histories. African Americans on average are estimated to have approximately 20% European ancestry, and this proportion varies substantially among different African American populations within North America. Genetic analysis of individual ancestry indicates that some self-identified European Americans have substantial recent African genetic ancestry. Population categories including race and ethnic groups are inadequate and misleading to fully describe the pattern and range of variation among individual clients. The more

Table 3-6 | Biocultural Variations in the Musculoskeletal System

Bone/Muscle	Remarks
Bone	
Frontal	Thicker in Black males than in White males
Parietal occiput	Thicker in White males than in Black males
Palate	Tori (protuberances) along the suture line of the hard palate
	Problematic for denture wearers
	Incidence
	Blacks 20%
	Whites 24%
	Asians Up to 50%
	Native Americans Up to 50%
Mandible	Tori (protuberances) on the lingual surface of the mandible near the canine and premolar teeth
	Problematic for denture wearers
	Most common in Asians and Native Americans, exceeds 50% in some Eskimo groups
Humerus	Torsion or rotation of the proximal end with muscle pull
	Greater degree of torsion observed in Whites than Blacks
	Torsion in Blacks is symmetric; torsion in Whites tends to be greater on the right side than the left side
Radius	Length at the wrist variable
Ulna	The ulna and radius are not always of equal length, useful for assessing radial and ulnar fractures and postop recovery of bone healing
	Equal length
	Swedes 61%
	Chinese 16%
	Ulna longer than radius
	Swedes 16%
	Chinese 48%
	Radius longer than ulna
	Swedes 23%
	Chinese 10%
Vertebrae	Twenty-four vertebrae are found in 85%–93% of all people; racial and sex differences reveal 23 or 25 vertebrae in select groups
	Vertebrae Population
	23 11% of Black females
	25 12% of Native Alaskan and Native American
	Related to lower back pain and lordosis

(continued)

Table 3-6 | Biocultural Variations in the Musculoskeletal System (continued)

Bone/Muscle	Remarks	
Pelvis	Hip width is 1.6 cm (0.6 in.) less in Black women than in White women; Asian women have significantly smaller pelvises	
Femur	Convex anterior	Native American
	Straight	Black
	Intermediate	White
Second tarsal	The second toe longer than the great toe	
	Incidence	
	Whites	8%–34%
	Blacks	8%–12%
	Vietnamese	31%
	Melanesians	21%–57%
	Clinical significance for joggers and athletes	
Height	White males are 1.27 cm (0.5 in.) taller than Black males and 7.6 cm (2.9 in.) taller than Asian males	
	White females = Black females	
Composition of long bones	Longer, narrower, and denser in Blacks than in Whites; bone density in Whites > Chinese, Japanese, and Native Alaskan	
	Osteoporosis is lowest in Black males and highest in White females	
Muscle		
Peroneus tertius	Responsible for dorsiflexion of the foot	
	Muscle absent	
	Asians, Native Americans, and Whites	3%–10%
	Blacks	10%–15%
	Berbers (Sahara desert)	24%
	No clinical significance because the tibialis anterior also dorsiflexes the foot	
Palmaris longus	Responsible for wrist flexion	
	Muscle absent	
	Whites	12%–20%
	Native Americans	2%–12%
	Blacks	5%
	Asians	3%
	No clinical significance because three other muscles are also responsible for flexion	

Based on data reported by Overfield, T. (2017). *Biologic variation in health and illness: Race, age, and sex differences.* New York, NY: CRC Press; Shin, M., Zmuda, J., Barrett-Connor, E., Sheu, Y., Patrick, A., Leung, P., …, Cauley, J. (2014). Race/ethnic differences in associations between bone mineral density and fracture history in older men. *Osteoporosis International, 25*(3), 387–845.

Table 3-7	Biocultural Variations and Clinical Significance for Selected Laboratory Tests

Test	Remarks
Hemoglobin/hematocrit	1 g lower for Blacks than other groups; Blacks < counterparts in other groups
Serum transferrin	Biocultural variation in children aged 1–3½ years Mean for Blacks 22 mg/100 mL > Whites *Note*: May be due to lowered hemoglobin and hematocrit levels found in Blacks *Clinical significance*: Transferrin levels increase in the presence of anemia, thus influencing the diagnosis, treatment, and nursing care of children with anemia
Serum cholesterol	Biocultural variation across the lifespan Birth　　　　　　　　Blacks = Whites Childhood　　　　　　Blacks 5 mg/100 mL > Whites Tohono O'odham (Pima) Indians 20–30 mg/100 mL >Whites Adulthood　　　　　　Blacks < Whites Tohono O'odham (Pima) Indians 50–60 mL/100 mL < Whites *Clinical significance*: Prevention, treatment, and nursing care of clients with cardiovascular disease
High-density lipoproteins (HDLs)	Biocultural variation in adults Blacks > Whites Asians ≥ Whites Mexican Americans < Whites
Ratio of HDL to total cholesterol	Blacks < Whites
Low-density lipoproteins (LDLs)	Biocultural variation in adults Blacks < Whites *Clinical significance*: Prevention, treatment, and nursing care of clients with cardiovascular disease
Blood glucose	Biocultural variation in adults North American Indians, Hispanics, Japanese > Whites Blacks = Whites (for equivalent socioeconomic groups) *Clinical significance*: Diagnosis, treatment, and nursing care of adults and children with hypoglycemia and diabetes mellitus
Creatinine	For patients >49 years of age, the average creatinine level is 0.6–1.2 mg/dL in adult males and 0.5–1.1 mg/dL in adult females (In the metric system, a milligram is a unit of weight equal to one-thousandth of a gram, and a deciliter is a unit of volume equal to one-tenth of a liter.) A person with only one kidney may have a normal level of about 1.8 or 1.9 Creatinine levels that reach 10.0 or more in adults indicate severe kidney impairment and the need for dialysis to remove wastes from the blood For Blacks, the normal average is 13% higher than counterparts in the general population *Clinical significance*: Interpretation of test results for Blacks with suspected or diagnosed renal disease needs to take racial difference into account

(continued)

Table 3-7	Biocultural Variations and Clinical Significance for Selected Laboratory Tests (continued)
Test	**Remarks**
Estimated glomerular filtration rate (eGFR)	Blacks have more extreme rate of eGFR, followed by Hispanics, Whites, and Asians
Clinical significance: eGFR predicts onset of end-stage renal disease (ESRD) and need for dialysis and renal transplantation. Projected kidney failure during chronic kidney disease stages 3 and 4 was high in Blacks, Hispanics, and Asians relative to Whites. Mortality for those with projected kidney failure is highest in Whites. Differences in eGFR decline and mortality contribute to racial disparities in ESRD incidence
Multiple marker screening	Biocultural variations in blood levels for protein and hormones in pregnant women
Alpha-fetoprotein (AFP), hCG, and estriol levels in Black and Asian women > Whites
Clinical significance: High AFP levels signal that the woman is at increased risk for being delivered of an infant with spina bifida and neural tube defects, whereas low levels may signal Down syndrome; Down syndrome also is associated with low levels of estriol and high levels of hCG
Black and Asian American women have higher average levels of AFP, hCG, and estriol than White counterparts
Using a single median for women of all cultures:
• Causes Black and Asian women to be falsely identified as being *at risk* for having infants with spina bifida and neural tube defects; by being classified as *high risk*, women are more likely to be subjected to invasive and expensive procedures such as amniocentesis; some may elect to abort the pregnancy based on screening test results
• Inappropriately lowers the identified Down syndrome risk for Black and Asian women
Lecithin/sphin-gomyelin ratio	Biocultural variations in amniotic fluid measures of fetal pulmonary maturity
Blacks have higher ratios than Whites from 23 to 42 weeks' gestation
Clinical significance: The ratio is used to calculate the risk of respiratory distress in premature infants; lung maturity in Blacks is reached 1 week earlier than in Whites (34 weeks vs. 35 weeks); racial differences should be considered in making decisions about inducing labor or delivering by cesarean section

Table based on data from Adigun, O., & Bhimji, S. S. (2016). Alpha fetoprotein. Retrieved from https://www.ncbi.nlm.nih.gov/books/NBK430750/; Allanson, A., Michie, S., & Matreau, T. M. (1997). Presentation of screen negative results on serum screening for Down's syndrome. *Journal of Medical Screening, 4*(1), 21–22; Chapman, S. J., Brumfield, C. G., Wenstrom, K. D., & DuBard, M. B. (1997). Pregnancy outcomes following false-positive multiple marker screening test. *American Journal of Perinatology, 14*(8), 475–478; Chan, R. L. (2014). Biochemical markers of spontaneous preterm birth in asymptomatic women. *Biomedical Research, 2014*, 164081. doi: 10.1155/2014/164081; Derose, S. F., Rutkowski, M. P., Crooks, P. W., Shi, J. M., Wang, J. Q., Kalantar-Zadeh, K., …, Jacobsen, S. J. (2013). Racial differences in estimated glomerular filtration decline, ESDR, and mortality in an integrated health system. *American Journal of Kidney Disease, 62*(2), 236–244; Fishbach, F., & Dunning, M. B. (2015). *A manual of laboratory and diagnostic tests* (9th ed.). Philadelphia, PA: Wolters Kluwer; O'Brien, J. E., Dvorin, E., Drugan, A., Johnson, M. P., Yaron, Y., & Evans, M. I. (1997). Race-ethnicity-specific variation in multiple-marker biochemical screening: Alpha-fetoprotein, hCG, and estriol. *Obstetrics and Gynecology, 89*(3), 355–358; National Down Syndrome Society (2014); Overfield, T. (2017). *Biologic variation in health and illness: Race, age, and sex differences*. New York, NY: CRC Press.

accurate assessment of disease risk is obtained by genotyping. **Genotyping** refers to the process of identifying differences in genetic makeup using biological testing rather than assuming their population affiliation as a surrogate.

Although the reasons for differences are not always known, genetics, environment, diet, socioeconomic background, race, ethnicity, and lifestyle factors contribute to the differences in test results.

Transcultural Perspectives in Clinical Decision-Making and Actions

After completing a comprehensive cultural assessment through the health history and physical examination, analyze the subjective and objective data. Leininger suggests three major modalities to guide nursing decisions and actions for the purpose of providing culturally congruent care that is beneficial, satisfying, and meaningful to clients—*cultural care preservation or maintenance, cultural care accommodation or negotiation,* and *cultural care repatterning or restructuring* (Leininger, 1991; Leininger & McFarland, 2002; McFarland & Wehbe-Alamah, 2015):

- **Cultural care preservation or maintenance** refers to those professional actions and decisions that help people of a particular culture to retain and/or preserve relevant care values so that they can maintain their well-being, recover from illness, or face handicaps and/or death (Leininger, 1991; Leininger & McFarland, 2002; McFarland & Wehbe-Alamah, 2015).
- **Cultural care accommodation or negotiation** refers to professional actions and decisions that help people of a designated culture to adapt to or to negotiate with others for beneficial or satisfying health outcomes with professional care providers (Leininger, 1991; Leininger & McFarland, 2002; McFarland & Wehbe-Alamah, 2015).
- **Cultural care repatterning or restructuring** refers to professional actions and decisions that help clients reorder, change, or greatly modify their lifeways for new, different, and beneficial health care patterns while respecting the clients' cultural values and beliefs and yet providing more beneficial or healthier lifeways than before the changes were coestablished with the clients (Leininger, 1991; Leininger & McFarland, 2002, 2006; McFarland & Wehbe-Alamah, 2015).

Whether the nurse uses Leininger's three modes for decisions and actions or engages in other analytic processes, the next step in the process leading to culturally competent decision-making and actions is to set mutual goals with the client, develop a plan of care, confer with and make referrals to other members of the interprofessional health care team (when needed), and implement a plan of care, either alone or with others. This process, presented primarily from the nurse's vantage point, is based on the health histories and physical examinations by the nurse and other team members and focuses on the nurse–client interaction and those aspects of the care plan that fall within the scope of practice and responsibilities of professional nurses.

Credentialed or licensed health professionals (e.g., physicians, pharmacists, social workers, dieticians, and physical, occupational, respiratory, and other therapists) have been educated to follow a similar process. Although some folk, traditional, religious, and spiritual healers may follow a comparable process, others might rely on a different approach, for example, reliance on subjective data from the client that are based on a spiritual assessment. They may prefer to practice their healing interventions with the client in private and may or may not want to collaborate with other members of the team. Be mindful that the federal Health Insurance Portability and Accountability Act (HIPAA) regulations may prohibit the sharing of some information, especially when the client is too ill to provide informed consent to release medical information with family, friends, and healers without authorization.

Once the plan has been implemented, it should be evaluated in collaboration with the client, with the client's family and significant others, and with other credentialed, licensed, folk, traditional, religious, and spiritual healers who are members of the team. The evaluation includes a comprehensive analysis of the plan's effectiveness in meeting mutually established goals and desired outcomes. As indicated in Figure 3-3, nurses collaborate with clients, physicians, and other members of the health care team to determine if the care delivered was culturally acceptable, congruent and competent, safe, affordable, accessible,

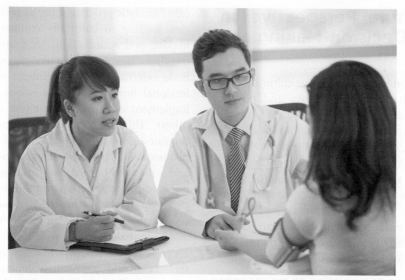

Figure 3-3. When conducting a comprehensive cultural assessment, the nurse collaborates with the client and physician as members of an interprofessional health care team (Dragon Images/Shutterstock.com).

high quality, and based on research, scientific evidence, and best professional practices. Gather additional subjective and objective data to determine the effectiveness of the intervention(s) and the client's overall satisfaction with care delivery and outcomes. Health care facilities, home and community health agencies, and related health care organizations usually have comprehensive evaluation processes and instruments that they administer to clients or patients and then subsequently review individually and in the aggregate for the purpose of improving the quality of care.

Summary

Many biocultural variations in health and illness are apparent in the health assessment and physical examination. For example, nurses will note differences based on the client's gender, age, race, ethnicity, and/or genetic makeup. In gathering subjective and objective assessment data, note biocultural differences in body measurements, pain perception, general appearance, and

symptom manifestation. For example, in assessing the skin of lightly and darkly pigmented clients, there are notable differences in the manifestations of cyanosis, jaundice, pallor, erythema, petechiae, and ecchymoses. From the head to the toes, systematically use multiple techniques to gather data through observation, inspection, auscultation, palpation, and smell to conduct a comprehensive physical examination of the client. Upon completion of the health assessment and physical examination, analyze and synthesize subjective and objective findings from the assessment, review the results of laboratory tests, and collaborate with the client and other members of the health care team to develop mutual goals, make clinical decisions, plan care, implement the plan, and evaluate the care. After evaluating the care, it may be necessary to ask the client additional questions, conduct a more focused physical examination on a particular body system, and/or revise the plan of care to ensure that it provides safe, culturally acceptable, congruent, competent, affordable, accessible, high-quality care that is evidence based and reflects best professional practices.

REVIEW QUESTIONS

1. In your own words, describe the key components of a comprehensive cultural assessment.
2. Compare and contrast your approach to the assessment of light- and dark-skinned clients for cyanosis, jaundice, pallor, erythema, and petechiae.
3. Review the biocultural variations in laboratory tests for hemoglobin, hematocrit, serum cholesterol, serum transferrin, creatinine, eGFR, multiple marker screening, and amniotic fluid constituents.
4. Critically analyze the reasons for the current interest in herbal medicines by nurses, physicians, pharmacists, and other health care providers. How does knowledge of these medicines facilitate the nurse's ability to provide culturally competent and congruent nursing care?
5. If you are a student or nurse who is in a clinical practice setting with patients from diverse racial, ethnic, or cultural backgrounds, how will you use the information in this chapter to facilitate the collection of objective and subjective data in the health assessment and physical examination?

CRITICAL THINKING ACTIVITIES

1. Critically analyze the instrument, tool, or form used by nurses when conducting an initial client or resident admission assessment at a hospital, extended care facility, or other health care agency in terms of its relevance to the health and nursing needs of persons from diverse cultures. From a transcultural nursing perspective, identify the strengths and limitations of the admission assessment instrument. What suggestions would you make to enhance the effectiveness of the instrument in assessing the cultural needs of newly admitted clients or residents? Be sure to consider the practical constraints that nurses face in the current health care environment, such as time limitations, external forces that require nurses to care for increasingly large numbers of clients, and other constraints, before you suggest modifications to the existing instrument.

2. Using the Andrews and Boyle Transcultural Nursing Assessment Guide for Individuals and Families (Appendix A), interview someone from a cultural background different from your own to assess his or her health-related cultural values, attitudes, beliefs, and practices. After you have completed the interview, compare and contrast those responses with your own responses in Question 2. Identify the ways in which you are *alike*. Critically analyze the *differences* as potential sources of cross-cultural conflict, and explore ways in which they might influence the nurse–client interaction.

3. Conduct a head-to-toe physical examination of a person from a racial background different from your own. Summarize your findings in writing. In a constructively self-critical manner, reflect on what aspects of the exam were (1) easiest and (2) most difficult for you. Try to determine the reason(s) why some aspects were relatively easy or difficult for you. What further information or skill development would assist you in gaining confidence in your ability to conduct physical examinations on people from diverse racial backgrounds?

4. If you are in a clinical setting with refugees, use the Boyle/Baird Transcultural Nursing Assessment Guide for Refugees instrument found in Appendix D. How did this assessment guide assist you in assessing the unique needs of refugees? What other data might have been gathered to develop a plan of care that is culturally congruent with the cultural beliefs and practices of this refugee population?

REFERENCES

Adeyinka, A., & Kondamudi, N. P. (2017). NCBI Resources. Bookshelf. Cyanosis. Retrieved October 22, 2018 from https://www.ncbi.nlm.nih.gov/books/NBK482247/

Allen, K. D., Arbeeva, L., Cené, C. W., Coffman, C. J., Grimm, K. F., Haley, E., ..., Campbell, L. C. (2018). Pain coping skills training for African Americans with osteoarthritis study: Baseline participant characteristics and comparison to prior studies. *BMC Musculoskeletal Disorders, 19*(1), 337. Retrieved from https://doi.org/10.1186/s12891-018-2249-6

American Academy of Ophthalmology. (2018a). What is low vision? Retrieved October 23, 2018 from https://www.aao.org/eye-health/diseases/low-vision

American Academy of Ophthalmology. (2018b). What is albinism? Retrieved October 23, 2018 from https://www.aao.org/eye-health/diseases/albinism-diagnosis

American Cancer Society. (n.d.). Genetics and breast cancer. Retrieved from http://www.cancer.org/cancer/breastcancer/index

American Cancer Society. (2016). Signs and symptoms of basal and squamous cell skin cancers. Retrieved October 26, 2018 from https://www.cancer.org/cancer/basal-and-squamous-cell-skin-cancer/detection-diagnosis-staging/signs-and-symptoms.html

American College of Obstetrics and Gynecology. (2016). Prenatal genetic diagnostic tests. Retrieved October 15, 2018 from https://www.acog.org/Patients/FAQs/Prenatal-Genetic-Diagnostic-Tests

American Heart Association. (2015). African Americans and heart disease, stroke. Retrieved October 9, 2018 at http://www.heart.org/en/health-topics/consumer-healthcare/what-is-cardiovascular-disease/african-americans-and-heart-disease-stroke

BCC Research. (2017). Botanical and plant-derived drugs [Report]. Retrieved October 5, 2018 from https://www.bccresearch.com/market-research/biotechnology/botanical-and-plant-derived-drugs-global-markets-bio022h.html

Becares, L., Shaw, R., Nazroo, S., Stefford, M., Albor, C., & Atkin, K. (2012). Ethnic diversity effects on physical morbidity, mortality, and health behaviors: A systematic review of the literature. *American Journal of Public Health, 102*(12), e33–e66.

Becker, W. C., Starrels, J. L., Heo, M., Li, X., Weiner, M. G., & Turner, B. J. (2011). Racial differences in primary care opioid risk reduction strategies. *Annals of Family Medicine, 9*, 219–225.

Berg, E., Lie, R. T., Siversten, A., & Haaland, O. A. (2015). Parental age and the risk of isolated cleft lip: A registry-based study. *Annals of Epidemiology, 25*(12), 942–947. Retrieved from https://doi.org/10.1016/j.annepidem.2015.05.003

Booker, S. Q. (2016). African Americans' perceptions of pain and pain management: A systematic review. *Journal of Transcultural Nursing, 27*(1), 73–80. doi:10.1177/1043659614526250.

Bukar, B. B., Dayom, D. W., & Uguru, M. O. (2016). The growing economic importance of medicinal plants and the need for developing countries to harness from it: A mini review. *IOSR Journal of Pharmacy, 6*(5), 42–52. Retrieved from http://iosrphr.org/papers/v6i5/G0654252.pdf

Buttaro, T. M., Trybulski, J., Polgar Bailey, P., & Sandberg-Cook, J. (2016). *Primary care: A collaborative practice* (5th ed.). St. Louis, MO: Elsevier.

Centers for Disease Control and Prevention. (2008). Anthropometric reference data for children and adults: United States, 2003–2006. Retrieved October 19, 2018 from https://www.cdc.gov/nchs/data/nhsr/nhsr010.pdf

Centers for Disease Control and Prevention. (2015a). Concussion at play: Opportunities to reshape the culture around concussion. Retrieved from https://www.cdc.gov/headsup/pdfs/resources/concussion_at_play_playbook-a.pdf

Centers for Disease Control and Prevention. (2015b). Dental caries and tooth loss in adults in the United States, 2011–2012. Retrieved October 26, 2018 from https://www.cdc.gov/nchs/products/databriefs/db197.htm

Centers for Disease Control and Prevention. (2017a). Genetic testing. Retrieved from http://www.cdc.gov/genomics/gtesting/index.htm

Centers for Disease Control and Prevention. (2017b). Body measurements. Retrieved from https://www.cdc.gov/nchs/fastats/body-measurements.htm

Centers for Disease Control and Prevention. (2018a). Cigarette smoking and tobacco use among people of low socioeconomic status. Retrieved from https://www.cdc.gov/tobacco/disparities/low-ses/index.htm

Centers for Disease Control and Prevention. (2018b). Drug poisoning mortality in the United States, 1999–2016. Retrieved from https://www.cdc.gov/nchs/data-visualization/drug-poisoning-mortality/index.htm

Cuevas, A. G., & O'Brien, K. (2017). Racial centrality may be linked to mistrust in healthcare institutions for African Americans. *Journal of Health Psychology*, 1–9. Retrieved from https://doi.org/10.1177/1359105317715092

Dean, L. (2018). Clopidogrel therapy and CYP2C19 genotype. Retrieved from https://www.ncbi.nlm.nih.gov/books/NBK84114/

Domchek, S. M. (2014). Evolution of genetic testing for inherited susceptibility to breast cancer. *Journal of Clinical Oncology, 33*(4), 295. doi: 10.1200/JCO.2014.59.3178

Du, X., & Gray, P. M. (2017). Evolution of lactase persistence. *Western Undergraduate Research Journal: Health and Natural Sciences, 8*(1), 1–3. doi: 10.5206/wurjhns.2017-18.28. Retrieved October 19, 2018 from https://ir.lib.uwo.ca/cgi/viewcontent.cgi?article=1158&context=wurjhns

Dubay, L., & Lebrun, A. (2012). Health, behavior, and health care disparities: Disentangling the effects of income and race in the United States. *International Journal of Health Services, 42*(4), 607–625.

Eyre, S., Orozco, G., & Worthington, J. (2017). The genetics revolution in rheumatology: Large scale genomic arrays and genetic mapping. *Nature Reviews Rheumatology, 13*(6), 421–432. Retrieved from https://doi-org.libproxy.umflint.edu/10.1038/nrrheum.2017.80

Ferdinand, K. C., Elkayam, U., Mancini, D., Ofili, E., Pina, I., Anand, I., & Leggett, C. (2014). Use of isosorbide, dinitrate and hydralazine in African-Americans with heart failure 9 years after the African-American Heart Failure Trial. *American Journal of Cardiology, 114*(1), 151–159.

FitzGerald, C., & Hurst, S. (2017). Implicit bias in healthcare professionals: A systematic review. *BMC Medical Ethics, 18*, 19. Retrieved from http://doi.org/10.1186/s12910-017-0179-8

Gagon, C. M., Matsura, J. T., Smith, C. C., & Stanos, S. P. (2013). Ethnicity and interdisciplinary pain treatment. *Pain and Practice, 14*(6), 532–540.

Giger, J. N. (2017). *Transcultural nursing: Assessment and intervention* (7th ed.). St. Louis, MO: Elsevier.

Gladstone Institute. (2014). Vitamin supplement successfully prevents noise-related hearing loss. *Science Daily*. Retrieved from http://www.sciencedaily.com/releases/2014/12/141202123840.htm

Grimes, P. E., & Miller, M. M. (2018). Vitiligo: Patient stories, self-esteem, and the psychological burden of disease. *International Journal of Women's Dermatology, 4*(1), 32–37. Retrieved from https://www.ncbi.nlm.nih.gov/pmc/articles/PMC5986114/

Gunn, D. A., de Craen, A. J. M., Dick, J. L., Tomlin, C. C., van Heemest, D., Catt, S., ..., Westendorp, R. G. J. (2013). Facial appearance reflects human familial longevity and cardiovascular disease risk in healthy individuals. *Journals of Gerontology Series A: Biological Medical Sciences, 68*(2), 145–152.

Haeok, B., Fitzpatrick, J., & Baik, S. (2013). Why isn't evidence-based practice improving health care for minorities in the United States? *Applied Nursing Research, 26*(2013), 263–268.

Healthy Hearing Foundation. (2016). Examining the relationship between race and hearing loss. Retrieved October 26, 2018 from https://hearinghealthfoundation.org/blogs/examining-the-relationship-between-race-and-hearing-loss

Henschke, N., Lorenz, E., Pokora, R., Michaleff, Z. A., Quartey, J., & Oliveira, V. C. (2016). Understanding cultural influences on back pain and back pain research. *Best Practice and Research Clinical Rheumatology, 30*(6), 1037–1049. doi: 10.1016/j.berh.2017.08.004

Howell, C. R., Mehta, T., Ejima, K., Ness, K. K., Cherrington, A., & Fontaine, K. (2018). Body composition and mortality in Mexican American adults: Results from the National Health and Nutrition Examination Survey. *Obesity, 26*(8), 1372–1380. Retrieved from https://doi-org.libproxy.umflint.edu/10.1002/oby.22251

International Osteoporosis Foundation. (2017). Facts and statistics. Retrieved October 29, 2018 from https://www.iofbonehealth.org/facts-statistics

Jarvis, C. (2016). *Physical examination and health assessment* (7th ed.). St. Louis, MO: Elsevier/Saunders.

Kaiser Family Foundation. (2014). Poverty rate by race and ethnicity. Retrieved from https://www.kff.org/other/state-indicator/poverty-rate-by-raceethnicity/

Kim, H. J., Yang, G. S., Greenspan, J. D., Downton, K. D., Griffith, K. A., Renn, C. L., ..., Dorsey, S. G. (2017). Racial and ethnic differences in experimental pain sensitivity: Systematic review and meta-analysis. *Pain, 158*(2), 194–211. doi: 10.1097/j.pain.0000000000000731

Kleinman, A. (1980). *Patients and healers in the context of culture*. Berkeley, CA: University of California Press.

Kliegman, R. M., Stanton, B. F., Saint Geme, J. W., Schor, N. F., & Behrman, R. E. (2016). *Nelson's textbook of pediatrics* (20th ed.). Philadelphia, PA: Elsevier/Saunders.

Koleck, T. A., Bender, C. M., Sereika, S. M., Ahrendendt, G., Jankowitz, R. C., McGuire, K. P., ..., Conley, Y. P. (2014). Apolipoprotein E genotype and cognitive function in postmenopausal women with early-stage breast cancer. *Oncology Nursing Forum, 41*(6), E313–E325.

Krupat, E. (2017). When I say ... chief complaint. *Medical Education, 51*(2), 134–135. Retrieved from https://doi-org.libproxy.umflint.edu/10.1111/medu.13146

Kwok, W., & Bhuvanakrishna, T. (2014). The relationship between ethnicity and the pain experience of cancer patients: A systematic review. *Indian Journal of Palliative Care, 20*(3), 194–200.

Lapchick, R., & Marfatia, S. (2017). The 2017 Racial and Gender Report Card: National Football League. Retrieved from http://nebula.wsimg.com/1a7f83c14af6a516176740244d8afc46?AccessKeyId=DAC3A56D8FB782449D2A&disposition=0&alloworigin=1

Leininger, M. M. (1991). *Culture care diversity and universality: A theory of nursing*. New York, NY: NLN Press.

Leininger, M. M., & McFarland, M. R. (2002). *Transcultural nursing: Concepts, theories, research and practices*. New York, NY: McGraw-Hill.

Leininger, M. M., & McFarland, M. R. (2006). *Culture care diversity and universality: A worldwide nursing theory*. Sudbury, MA: Jones & Bartlett.

Levin, S. (1966). Effect of age, ethnic background and disease on sweat chloride. *Israeli Journal of Medical Science, 2*(3), 333–337.

Mack, D. S., Hunnicutt, J. N., Jesdale, B. M., & Lapane, K. L. (2018). Non-Hispanic Black-White disparities in pain and pain management among newly admitted nursing home residents with cancer. *Journal of Pain Research, 11*, 753–761. doi: 10.2147/JPR.S158128

Malki, G. A., Al-Badawi, E. A., & Dahlan, M. A. (2015). Natal teeth: A case report and reappraisal. *Case Reports in Dentistry, 2015*. http://dx.doi.org/10.1155/2015/147580. Retrieved October 29, 2018 from https://www.hindawi.com/journals/crid/2015/147580/

March of Dimes. (2017). Prenatal tests. Retrieved October 5, 2018 from https://www.marchofdimes.org/pregnancy/prenatal-tests.aspx

Masuda, A., Latnera, J. D., Barliea, J. P., & Sargent, K. (2018). Understanding self-concealment within a framework of eating disorder cognitions and body image flexibility: Conceptual and applied implications. *Eating Behaviors, 30*(1), 49–54. Retrieved from https://doi.org/10.1016/j.eatbeh.2018.05.005

Mayo Clinic. (2018a). Petechiae. Retrieved October 26, 2018 from https://www.mayoclinic.org/symptoms/petechiae/basics/definition/sym-20050724

Mayo Clinic. (2018b). Lactose intolerance: Symptoms. Retrieved from https://www.mayoclinic.org/diseases-conditions/lactose-intolerance/symptoms-causes/syc-20374232

Mayo Clinic. (2019). *Sweating and body odor.* Retrieved from https://www.mayoclinic.org/diseases-conditions/sweating-and-body-odor/symptoms-causes/syc-20353895

McCance, K. L., & Huether, S. E. (2019). *Pathophysiology: The biologic basis for disease in adults and children* (8th ed.). St. Louis, MO: C.V. Mosby.

McFarland, M. R., & Wehbe-Alamah, H. B. (2015). *Leininger's culture care diversity and universality: A worldwide theory of nursing* (3rd ed.). Burlington, MA: Jones & Bartlett Learning.

McFarland, M. R., & Wehbe-Alamah, H. B. (2018). *Transcultural nursing: Concepts, theories, research, and practices* (4th ed.). New York: McGraw-Hill, Medical Publishing Division.

McNamara, D. M., Feldman, A., Yancy, C., Taylor, A., Dries, D., Hanley-Yanez, K., & Halder, I. (2016). Genomic score to target therapy with a fixed dose combination of hydralazine and isosorbide dinitrate. *Journal of the American College of Cardiology, 67*(13S), 1353. Retrieved from https://doi-org.libproxy.umflint.edu/10.1016/S0735-1097(16)31354-7

Meghani, S., Polomano, R. C., Tait, R. C., Vallerand, A. H., Anderson, K. O., & Gallagher, R. M. (2012). Advancing a national agenda to eliminate disparity in pain care: Directions for health policy, education, practice and research. *Pain and Medicine, 13*(1), 5–28.

Musemwa, N., & Gadegbeku, C. A. (2017). Hypertension in African Americans. *Current Cardiology Reports, 19*(129). Retrieved from https://doi-org.libproxy.umflint.edu/10.1007/s11886-017-0933-z

National Cancer Institute. (2018). *Cancer disparities.* Retrieved from https://www.cancer.gov/about-cancer/understanding/disparities

National Cancer Institute. (2019). Cancer fact sheets. *Cancer types.* Bethesda, MD: National Institutes of Health. Retrieved from https://www.cancer.gov/publications/patient-education

National Center for Biotechnology Information. (2017). Genetic testing registry. Retrieved from https://www.ncbi.nlm.nih.gov/gtr/

National Center for Complementary and Integrative Health. (2018). Herbs at a glance. Retrieved from https://nccih.nih.gov/health/herbsataglance.htm

National Center for Complimentary and Integrative Health. (2017). The Institute of Medicine says chronic pain in the U.S.... Retrieved October 9, 2018 from https://nccih.nih.gov/news/multimedia/infographics/chronic-pain-panel1

National Down Syndrome Society. (2014). Prenatal testing. Retrieved from http://www.ndss.org/About-NDSS/Media-Kit/Position-Papers/CDC-Study-on-Prevalence-of-Down-Syndrome-/

National Geographic. (2018). You can smell when someone's sick—Here's how. Retrieved October 22, 2018 from https://news.nationalgeographic.com/2018/01/smell-sickness-parkinsons-disease-health-science/?user.testname=none

National Institute on Aging. (2015). Alzheimer's disease genetics fact sheet. Retrieved October 4, 2018 from https://www.nia.nih.gov/health/alzheimers-disease-genetics-fact-sheet

National Institute on Alcohol Abuse and Alcoholism. (2014). *Minority health and health disparities.* Rockville, MD: National Institutes of Health, Alcohol Research Centers. Retrieved from http://www.niaaa.nih.gov/alcohol-health/special-populations-co-occurring-disorders/diversity-health-disparities

National Institute of Health. (2016). An overview of the human genome project. Retrieved October 15, 2018 from https://www.genome.gov/12011238/an-overview-of-the-human-genome-project/

National Institute of Health. (2018). X-linked congenital stationary night blindness. Retrieved October 26, 2018 from https://ghr.nlm.nih.gov/condition/x-linked-congenital-stationary-night-blindness#statistics

National Institutes of Health. (2013). Cleft lip and cleft palate. Retrieved from http://www.ncbi.nlm.nih.gov/pubmedhealth/PMH0002046/?report=printable

National Organization for Albinism and Hypopigmentation (2018). *Information for medical professionals.* Retrieved from https://www.albinism.org/medical/

Nogueira, B. L., Mari, J., & Razzouk, D. (2015). Culture-bound syndromes in Spanish speaking Latin America: The case of Nervios, Susto and Ataques de Nervios. *Archives of Clinical Psychiatry (São Paulo), 42*(6), 171–178. Retrieved from https://dx.doi.org/10.1590/0101-60830000000070

Noorollahian, M., Nematy, M., Dolatian, A., Ghesmati, H., Akhlaghi, S., & Khademi, G. R. (2015). Cleft lip and palate and related factors: A 10 years study in university hospitalised patients at Mashhad—Iran. *African Journal of Pediatric Surgery, 12*(4), 286–290.

Obeig-Odoom, F. (2012). Health, wealth, and poverty in developing countries: Beyond the state, market, and civil society. *Health Sociology Review, 21*(2), 156–162.

O'Brien, J. E., Dvorin, E., Drugan, A., Johnson, M. P., Yaron, Y., & Evans, M. I. (1997). Race-ethnicity-specific variation in multiple-marker biochemical screening:

Alpha-fetoprotein, hCG, and estriol. *Obstetrics and Gynecology, 89*(3), 355–358.

Ofili, E., Anand, I., Williams, R. A., Akinboboye, O., Xu, L., & Puckrein, G. (2017). Fixed-dose versus off-label combination of isosorbide dinitrate plus hydralazine hydrochloride: Retrospective propensity-matched analysis in black medicare patients with heart failure. *Advances in Therapy 34*(8), 1976–1988. Retrieved from https://doi-org.libproxy.umflint.edu/10.1007/s12325-017-0584-x

Overfield, T. (2017). *CRC revivals: Biologic variation in health and illness: Race, age and sex differences* (2nd ed.). New York, NY: CRC Press.

Pardasani, M., & Bandyopadhyay, S. (2014). Ethnicity matters: Experiences of minority groups in public health. *Journal of Cultural Diversity, 21*(3), 90–98.

Park, A. M., Khan, S., & Rawnsley, J. (2018). Hair biology: Growth and pigmentation. *Facial Plastic Surgery Clinics of North America, 26*(4), 415–424. doi: 10.1016/j.fsc.2018.06.003

Poma, P. A. (2017). Race/Ethnicity concordance between patients and physicians. *Journal of the National Medical Association, 109*(1), 6–8. Retrieved from http://dx.doi.org.libproxy.umflint.edu/10.1016/j.jnma.2016.12.002

Porth, C. M. (2015). *Essentials of pathophysiology: Concepts of altered health states* (4th ed.). Philadelphia, PA: Lippincott.

Prakash, S., Sharan, P., & Sood, M. (2016). A study on phenomenology of Dhat syndrome in men in a general medical setting. *Indian Journal of Psychiatry, 58*(2), 129–141. Retrieved from https://doi-org.libproxy.umflint.edu/10.4103/0019-5545.183776

Qiu, M., Wang, S. Y., Singh, K., & Lin, S. (2014). Racial disparities in uncorrected and undercorrected refraction errors in the United States. *Investigative Ophthalmological and Visual Sciences, 55*(10), 6996–7005.

Rahim-Williams, B., Riley, J., Williams, A. K., & Fillingim, R. B. (2012). A quantitative review of ethnic group differences in experimental pain response: Do biology, psychology, and culture matter? *Pain Medicine, 13*(4), 522–540.

Robinson-Lane, S., & Booker, S. Q. (2017). Culturally responsive pain management for black older adults. *Journal of Gerontological Nursing, 43*(8), 33–41. Retrieved from http://dx.doi.org.libproxy.umflint.edu/10.3928/00989134-20170224-03

Shin, M. H., Zmuda, J., Barrett-Connor, E., Sheu, Y., Patrick, A., Leung, P., ..., Cauley, J. (2014). Race/ethnic differences in associations between bone mineral density and fracture history in older men. *Osteoporosis International, 25*(3), 837–845.

Silva, A. M., Shen, W., Heo, M., Gallager, D., Wang, Z., & Sardinha, L. B. (2011). Ethnicity-related skeletal muscle differences across the life span. *Human Biology, 22*(1), 76–82.

Simons, R. C., & Hughes, C. C. (1985). *The culture-bound syndromes: Folk illnesses of psychiatric and anthropological interest*. Dordrecht, The Netherlands: D. Reidel/Kluwer Academic.

Tait, R. C., & Chibnall, J. T. (2014). Racial/ethnic disparities in the assessment and treatment of pain. *American Psychologist, 69*(2), 131–141.

Taylor, C., Kavanagh, P., & Zuckerman, B. (2014). Sickle cell train-neglected opportunities in the era of genomic medicine. *JAMA, 311*(15), 1495–1496.

Taylor, N. A., & Machado-Moreira, C. A. (2013). Regional variations in transepidermal water loss, eccrine sweat gland density, sweat excretion rates, and electrolyte composition in resting and exercising humans. *Extreme Physiology and Medicine, 2*(4), 2–4.

Townsend, C., Takishima-Lacasa, J. Y., Latner, J. D., Grandinetti, A., & Keawe'aimoku Kaholokula, J. (2014). Ethnic and gender differences in ideal body size and related attitudes among Asians, Native Hawaiians, and Whites. *Hawaii Journal of Medicine and Public Health, 73*(8), 236–243.

Turk, D. C., & Gatchel, R. J. (2018). *Psychological approaches to pain management: A practitioner's handbook* (3rd ed.). New York, NY: Guilford Publications.

U.S. Census Bureau. (2017a). Selected social characteristics in the United States: 2017 American Community Survey 1-year estimates. Retrieved from https://factfinder.census.gov/faces/tableservices/jsf/pages/productview.xhtml?src=bkmk

U.S. Census Bureau. (2017b). 2017 National Population Projections Tables. Retrieved September 28, 2018 from United States Census Bureau: https://www.census.gov/data/tables/2017/demo/popproj/2017-summary-tables.html

U.S. Census Bureau. (2017c). Income and poverty in the United States: 2016. Retrieved from https://www.census.gov/content/dam/Census/library/publications/2017/demo/P60-259.pdf

U.S. Census Bureau. (2018). U.S. and World Population Clock. Retrieved September 28, 2018 from https://www.census.gov/popclock/

U.S. Department of Health and Human Services. (2016). Botanical drug development guidance for industry. Retrieved October 16, 2018 from https://www.fda.gov/downloads/Drugs/Guidances/UCM458484.pdf

Vashi, N. A., De Castro Maymone, M. B., & Kundu, R. V. (2016). Aging differences in ethnic skin. *Journal of Clinical and Aesthetic Dermatology, 9*(1), 31–38. Retrieved from http://libproxy.umflint.edu/login?url=http://search.ebscohost.com/login.aspx?direct=true&db=a9h&AN=112227388&site=ehost-live&scope=site

Vashi, N. A., & Maibach, H. I. (2017). *Dermatoanthropology of ethnic skin and hair*. Cham, Switzerland: Springer International Publishing.

Wang, Y., Kennedy, J., & Caggana, M. (2013). Sickle cell disease incidence among newborns in New York State by maternal race/ethnicity and nativity. *Genetics in Medicine, 15*(3), 222–228.

Wien, F. (2017). Social determinants of health: Tackling poverty in indigenous communities in Canada. Retrieved October 18, 2018 from https://www.ccnsa-nccah.ca/docs/determinants/FS-TacklingPovertyCanada-SDOH-Wien-EN.pdf

Wyatt, R. (2013). Policy forum: Pain and ethnicity. *American Medical Association Journal of Ethics, 15*(3), 449–454.

Yang, H. J., Gil, Y. C., Jin, J. D., Cho, H., Kim, H., & Lee, H. Y. (2012). Novel findings of the anatomy and variations of the axillary vein and its tributaries. *Clinical Anatomy, 25*(7), 893–902.

Yip, V. L. M., & Pirmohamed, M. (2017). The HLA-A*31:01 allele: Influence on carbamazepine treatment. *Pharmacogenomics and Personalized Medicine, 10,* 29–38. Retrieved from https://www.dovepress.com/the-hla-a3101-allele-influence-on-carbamazepine-treatment-peer-reviewed-fulltext-article-PGPM

Zengin, A., Pye, S. R., Cook, M. J., Adams, J. E., Wu, F. C., O'Neill, T. W., & Ward, K. A. (2016). Ethnic differences in bone geometry between White, Black and South Asian men in the UK. *Bone, 91,* 180–185.

Zhu, L. (2018). Depression symptom patterns and social correlates among Chinese Americans. *Brain Sciences, 8*(1), 16. Retrieved from http://dx.doi.org.libproxy.umflint.edu/10.3390/brainsci8010016

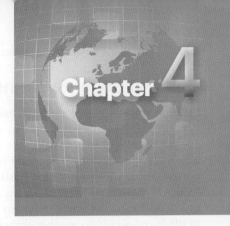

Chapter 4

Influence of Cultural and Health Belief Systems on Health Care Practices

- Marilyn K. Eipperle and Margaret M. Andrews

Key Terms

Allopathic medicine
Alternative health care
Ayurvedic medicine
Complementary and integrative health care
Cultural belief systems
Determinants of illness behavior

Dietary supplements
Folk healers
Folk healing systems
Health behaviors
Health belief systems
Health literacy
Holistic paradigm
Illness behavior
Integrative health care
Magico-religious paradigm

Naturopathy
Osteopathic medicine
Paradigm
Professional care systems
Scientific paradigm
Self-care
Sick role behavior
Traditional Chinese medicine
Values and beliefs
Worldview

Learning Objectives

1. Describe the major belief systems of people from diverse cultures.
2. Compare and contrast professional health care and folk healing systems.
3. Identify the major complementary and alternative health care therapies.
4. Describe cultural influences on illness symptoms and sick role behaviors.
5. Critically appraise the efficacy of selected traditional therapeutic approaches for health problems.

In this chapter, we examine the major **cultural belief systems** embraced by people from diverse cultures and explore the characteristics of three of the most prevalent worldviews (or paradigms) related to health–illness beliefs: magico-religious, scientific/biomedical, and holistic. We explore self-care, integrative professional care, and folk (indigenous, traditional, generic, lay) care approaches

along with their respective systems and healers. After analyzing cultural **values and beliefs** and their influences on symptoms, sick roles, and illness behaviors, we examine selected complementary and alternative therapies used to treat acute and chronic physical and psychological illnesses and diseases.

Cultural Belief Systems

Cultural meanings and cultural belief systems develop from shared social group experiences and are expressed symbolically. The use of symbols to define, describe, and relate to the world around us is a basic characteristic of being human. One of the most common expressions of symbolism is metaphor, wherein one aspect of life is connected to another through a shared symbol. For example, the phrase "what a tangled web we weave" expresses metaphorically the relationship between two normally disparate concepts—human deception and a spider's web. People often use metaphors as a way of thinking about and explaining life events.

All people groups across time have attempted to explain the phenomena of *nature*. From each explanation emerged a common belief system. The explanations usually involved metaphoric imagery of magical, religious, natural/holistic, scientific, or biological forms. The range for these explanations was limited only by the human imagination.

The set of metaphoric explanations used by a group of people to explain life events and offer solutions to life mysteries can be described as its **worldview** or major paradigm. A **paradigm** is a universal interpretation of the world and its phenomena and encompasses the assumptions, premises, and linkages that bind together a prevailing interpretation of reality. Paradigms are slow to change and do so only if and when their explanatory power has been depleted.

Worldview reflects the total configuration of beliefs and practices and permeates every lifeway within a group culture. Members of a culture share a worldview without necessarily recognizing it as such. Group thought is patterned on or derives from this worldview because the culture imparts a particular set of associated relational symbols used in thinking. Because these symbols are taken for granted, people typically do not question the cultural bias of their thoughts. Use of the term *American* by United States (US) citizens as a referent only to themselves collectively reflects such an unconscious cultural bias.

In reality, it is a generic term referring to all people in the Americas, which are the combined continental landmasses of North Central and South America and their islands in the Western Hemisphere from Canada to Peru.

Another example of symbolism and worldview can be seen in the way nurses use terms such as *nursing care, health promotion, illness,* and *disease.* Nurses often take for granted that all their clients define and relate to these concepts in the same way they do. This assumption reflects an unconscious belief that cultural symbols are shared by all and therefore do not require explanation within any given nurse–client context. Such assumptions account for many of the difficulties nurses encounter when communicating with clients and other nonmembers of the health profession culture.

Health Belief Systems

Generally, theories of health and disease or illness causation are based on a group's prevailing worldview. Worldview includes a group's health-related values, beliefs, and practices, sometimes referred to as its *health belief system.* People embrace three major **health belief systems** or worldviews:

1. *Magico-religious*
2. *Scientific/biomedical*
3. *Holistic*

Each has its own corresponding system of health beliefs. In the magico-religious and holistic systems, disease is perceived as an entity separate from the *self,* caused by an agent external to the body but capable of "getting in" and causing damage. The causative agent becomes attributed to a variety of natural and supernatural phenomena. Frequently, people may adhere to or believe in aspects of two or all three of the systems at any given time. For example, a person who is ill may understand the illness has an identified causative agent but at the same time may pray to recover quickly as well as embark on a sacred journey to visit a vortex specialist to realign body, mind, and spirit.

Magico-Religious Health Paradigm

In the **magico-religious paradigm**, the world is an arena dominated by supernatural forces. The fate of the world and those in it, including humans, depends on the actions of God, the gods, or other supernatural forces of good or evil. In some cases, the human individual is at the mercy of such forces regardless of behavior. In other cases, the gods punish humans for their transgressions. Many Latino, African American, native or aboriginal, and Middle Eastern cultures are grounded in the magico-religious paradigm (Quiroz & van Andel, 2018). *Magic* involves the calling forth and control of supernatural forces for and against others. Some African and Caribbean cultures have aspects of magic in their belief system, such as voodoo. In some Western cultures, metaphysical reality intersects within mainstream society. For example, Christian scientists believe that physical healing can be effected through prayer alone.

Writing about the history of medicine, Ackernecht (1946) stated that "...magic or religion seems to satisfy better than any other device a certain eternal psychic or 'metaphysical' need of mankind, sick and healthy, for integration and harmony." Magic and religion are logical in their own way but are not based on empiric premises; they defy the reality of the physical or scientific world known from the use of human senses, particularly observation. In the magico-religious paradigm, disease is viewed as the action and result of supernatural forces that cause intrusion of a disease-producing foreign body or health-damaging spirit.

Throughout the world in the magico-religious paradigm, five categories of events are believed to be responsible for illness: *sorcery, breach of taboo, intrusion of a disease object, intrusion of a disease-causing spirit,* and *loss of soul* (Clements, 1932). One or any combination of these belief categories may be offered to explain the origin of disease. Alaska Natives refer to *soul loss* and *breach of taboo* (i.e., breaking a social norm, such as committing adultery). West Indians and some

Africans and African Americans believe that the malevolence of sorcerers is the cause of many conditions. Belief in *mal ojo* (or the *evil eye*), common in Hispanic and other cultures, is viewed as the projected intrusion of a disease-causing spirit by one person onto another, particularly vulnerable persons such as children (Lloreda-Garcia, 2017).

In the magico-religious paradigm, illness is initiated by a supernatural agent with or without justification, or by another person who practices sorcery or engages the services of sorcerers. The cause-and-effect relationship is not organic; rather, the cause of health or illness is mystical. Health is perceived a reward bestowed as a sign of God's blessing and goodwill. Illness may be seen as a sign of God's possession or punishment; alternatively, it may signify God's special favor permitting the affected person an opportunity to accept *God's will*. Hence, in many Christian religions, the faithful communally gather to pray for God to heal the ill or to practice healing rituals such as *laying on of hands* or *anointing the sick* with oil. Furthermore, health and illness are commonly viewed as belonging first to the community and then to the individual. Thus, one person's actions may directly or indirectly influence the health or illness of another person. This perception of community is virtually absent in the other paradigms.

Scientific/Biomedical Health Paradigm

In the scientific/biomedical paradigm, life is controlled by a series of physical and biochemical processes that humans can study and manipulate. Several specific forms of symbolic thought processes characterize the **scientific paradigm**. The first is *determinism*, which states that a cause-and-effect relationship exists for all natural phenomena. The second, *mechanism*, assumes that it is possible to control life processes through mechanical, genetic, and other engineered interventions. The third form is *reductionism*, in which all life can be reduced or divided into smaller parts; study of the unique characteristics of these isolated parts is thought to reveal aspects or properties of the whole (i.e., the human genome and its component parts). The final thought process is *objective materialism*, wherein reality is only what can be observed and measured. Further distinctions between *subjective* and *objective* realities are made within this paradigm.

When the scientific paradigm is applied to matters of health, it is often referred to as the *biomedical model*. The scientific/biomedical paradigm considers only forces that can be observed and measured. Dominant Western cultural groups in the United States, Canada, Europe, Australia, and New Zealand espouse this paradigm. In the biomedical model (generally practiced as either **allopathic** or **osteopathic** medicine), all aspects of human health are viewed through the natural sciences (biology, chemistry, physics, and mathematics). This mindset fosters the belief that psychological and emotional processes can be reduced to the study of biochemical exchanges. Effective treatments consist of physical and chemical interventions, often with lesser or no regard for human values, beliefs, or relationships.

In this model, disease is viewed metaphorically as the breakdown of the human machine due to wear and tear (stress), external trauma (injury, accident), external invasion (pathogens), or internal damages (fluid and chemical imbalances, genetic or other structural changes). Disease causes illness, generally has a specific cause, follows a predictable time course, and requires a specified set of treatments. The scientific/biomedical paradigm parallels the magico-religious belief in external agents but replaces *supernatural forces* with *infectious and genetic agents*.

With the metaphor of the machine, the computer is analogous for the brain. Biomedicine specialists take care of the "parts" and "fixing" a part restores the machine's function ability; engineering becomes a task for biomedical practitioners. The discovery of DNA and development of the human genome have led to the research field of *genetic engineering*, another eloquent biomedical

metaphor. The symbols used to discuss health and disease reflect the US cultural values of *dominance* and *mastery*. Thus, when microorganisms attack the body, war is waged against the invaders, money is donated for the campaign against cancer, and illness is a struggle in which the patient must put up a good defense. The biomedical model defines *health as the absence of disease or the signs and symptoms of disease*. To be healthy, one must be free of all disease. In comparison, the World Health Organization (WHO) defined health more holistically as "...a state of complete physical, mental, and social well-being and not merely the absence of disease or infirmity" (WHO, 1948, p. 100). This definition is oft-cited, and although it has remained unchanged since 1948, the eight supplemental statements have been updated across time (WHO, 2018).

Holistic Health Paradigm

In the **holistic paradigm**, the *forces of nature* must be kept in natural balance or *harmony*. Human life is but one aspect of nature and the general order of the cosmos. Everything in the universe has its place with a role to perform according to the natural laws that maintain order. Disturbing these laws creates imbalance, chaos, and disease. The holistic paradigm has existed for centuries in many parts of the world, particularly in American Indian and Asian cultures. It has gained wider acceptance in the United States and Canada because it complements the increased sense that the biomedical model fails to account fully for naturally occurring causations and other factors such as cultural values, psychological effects, and **social determinants** of health.

The holistic paradigm seeks to maintain a sense of balance between humans and the larger universe. Explanations for health and disease are based on imbalance or disharmony among the human, geophysical, and metaphysical forces of the universe. For example, in the biomedical model, the cause of tuberculosis is clearly identified as an invasion of mycobacterium. In the holistic paradigm, whereby disease is the result of multiple environment–host interactions, tuberculosis is caused by the interrelationship of poverty, malnutrition, overcrowding, poor sanitation/ventilation/hygiene, and mycobacterium.

The term *holistic*, coined by Smuts (1926), described an attitude or mode of perception wherein the whole person was viewed in the context of the total environment. Its Indo-European root word, *kailo*, means "whole, intact, or uninjured," and from this root have come the words *hale, hail, hallow, holy, whole, heal*, and *health*. Thus, the essence of health and healing became the quality of *wholeness* humans associate with healthy functioning and well-being. In this paradigm, health is viewed as a positive process encompassing more than absent signs and symptoms of disease. Health is not restricted to biologic or somatic wellness but rather involves broader environmental, sociocultural, and behavioral determinants. In this model, diseases of civilization such as unemployment, racism, poverty, urban decay, and pollution are just as much illnesses as are biomedical diseases such as obesity, asthma/allergies, depression, and suicide.

The belief system of Florence Nightingale, who emphasized nursing's control of the environment so that patients could heal naturally, was holistic. Transcultural nursing, founded by Madeleine Leininger, and the Theory of Culture Care Diversity and Universality are also holistic paradigms (McFarland & Wehbe-Alamah, 2015, 2018).

Metaphors used in this paradigm including the *healing power of nature, health foods, mindfulness*, and *Mother Earth* reflect the human connection with the cosmos and nature. A strong metaphor in the holistic paradigm is exemplified by the Chinese concept of yin and yang, in which the forces of nature are balanced to produce harmony (Xiang, Lu, Chen, & Wen, 2017). The *yin* force in the universe represents the female aspect of nature. It is characterized as the negative pole, encompassing darkness, cold, and emptiness. The *yang* or male force, characterized by fullness, light, and warmth, represents the positive pole. An imbalance of these forces creates illness.

Illness is the outward expression of *disharmony*. This disharmony may result from seasonal changes, emotional imbalances, a disrupted pattern, or other chain of events. Illness is not caused by an intruding agent but is perceived as a natural part of life's rhythmic course. Transitioning in and out of balance is accepted as a natural process that happens continually throughout the life span. Health and illness are dimensions of the same process, in which the individual organism responds to the changing environment. In the holistic paradigm, illness is inevitable and thus perfect health is not the goal. Rather, achieving an optimal adaptation to the environment by living according to society's rules and caring appropriately for one's body is the desired outcome. The holistic paradigm places a greater emphasis on preventive care and maintenance measures than typically occurs in biomedicine.

Another common metaphor for health and illness in the holistic paradigm is the hot/cold theory of disease, founded on the ancient Greek concept of the four body humors: yellow bile, black bile, phlegm, and blood. *Humors* are vital components of the blood found in varying amounts throughout the human body. The four humors work together to ensure the optimum nutrition, growth, and metabolism. When the humors are balanced in a healthy individual, the state of *ecrasia* exists. When the humors are in a state of imbalance, this is referred to as *dyscrasia* (Osborn, 2015). The treatment of disease becomes a process of restoring the body's humoral balance through the addition or subtraction of substances that affect each of these four humors. Foods, beverages, herbs, and drugs are all classified as *hot* or *cold* depending on their effect, not their actual physical state. Disease conditions are also classified as either hot or cold. Imbalance or disharmony is believed to cause internal damage and altered physiologic functions. Medicine is directed at correcting this imbalance as well as restoring body functions. Although the concept of hot and cold is found in Asian, Latino, Black, Arab, Muslim, and Caribbean societies, each cultural group defines what it believes to be hot and cold entities, and little agreement exists across cultures.

Health and Illness Behaviors

The series of behaviors typifying the health-seeking process have been labeled *health and illness behaviors.* These behaviors are expressed in the roles people assume after identifying a symptom. Related to these behaviors are the roles individuals assign to others and the status given to the role-players. People assume various types of behaviors once they have recognized a symptom. **Health behavior** is any activity undertaken by a person who believes himself or herself to be healthy to prevent or detect disease at an asymptomatic stage. **Illness behavior** is any activity undertaken by a person who feels ill to define the state of his or her health and discover a suitable remedy. **Sick role behavior** is any activity undertaken by a person who considers himself or herself ill to get well or to deal with the illness.

Three sets of factors influence the course of behaviors and practices carried out to maintain health and prevent disease: (1) one's beliefs about health and illness; (2) personal factors such as age, education, knowledge, or experience with a given disease condition; and (3) cues to action, such as advertisements in the media, the illness of a relative, or the advice of friends. Mechanic (1978) outlined the **determinants of illness** model with 10 facets of illness behavior important to understanding the help-seeking process (see Table 4-1). Awareness of these motivational factors (including cultural influences) provides insights enabling nurses to offer more appropriate assistance to clients transitioning through the illness process.

Types of Healing Systems

The term *healing system* refers to the accumulated sciences, arts, and techniques of restoring and preserving health that are used by any cultural group. In complex societies in which several cultural traditions flourish, healers tend to compete with one another and/or to view their scopes of practice as separate from one another. In some instances, however, practitioners may make referrals to different healing systems.

For example, a nurse may contact a rabbi to assist a Jewish patient with spiritual needs, or a *curandero* may advise a Mexican American patient to visit a professional health care provider for an antibiotic when traditional practices do not heal a wound.

Self-Care

For common minor illnesses and injuries, most people initially try **self-care** with over-the-counter medicines, megavitamins, herbs, exercise, and/or foods that they believe have healing powers. Many self-care practices have been handed down from generation to generation, frequently by oral tradition. Self-care is the largest component of the US health care system with **dietary supplements** accounting for more than $20 billion annually (Faurot et al., 2015). The use of over-the-counter medications, or nonprescription medications, is a common form of self-care. Dietary supplements such as herbs, vitamins, minerals, oils, topical agents, and other substances are very popular and used extensively across all cultures and social strata in the United States. Box 4-1 provides tips for making informed decisions and evaluating information about dietary supplements. When self-care becomes ineffective, people are more likely to seek care from *professional* and/or *folk* (indigenous, generic, traditional, lay) healing systems (see Evidence-Based Practice 4-1).

Professional Care Systems

According to Leininger (1997) and McFarland and Wehbe-Alamah (2015, 2018), **professional care** (also referred to as scientific/biomedical care) is formally taught, learned, and transmitted knowledge and practice skills and approaches for treating acute and chronic illness and maintaining health and wellness that prevails in professional institutions and health care systems with multidisciplinary clinicians and staff. Professional care is characterized by specialized education and knowledge with responsibility for care provision

Table 4-1	Mechanic's Determinants of Illness Behavior
Determinant	**Description**
Quality of symptom	The more frightening or visible the symptom, the greater the likelihood that the individual will intervene.
Seriousness of symptom	The perceived threat of the symptom must be serious for action to be taken. Often, others will step in if the person's behavior is considered dangerous (e.g., suicidal behavior) but will be unaware of potential problems if the person's behavior seems natural ("he always acts that way").
Disruption of daily activities	Behaviors that are very disruptive in work or other social situations are likely to be labeled as illness much sooner than the same behaviors in a family setting. An individual whose activities are disrupted by a symptom is likely to take that symptom seriously even if on another occasion he would consider the same symptom trivial (e.g., acne just before a date).
Rate and persistence of symptom	The frequency of a symptom is directly related to its importance; a symptom that persists is also likely to be taken seriously.
Tolerance of symptom	The extent to which others, especially family, tolerate the symptom before reacting varies; individuals also have different tolerance thresholds.
Sociocognitive status	A person's information about the symptom, knowledge base, and cultural values all influence that person's perception of illness.
Denial of symptom	Often, the individual or family members need to deny a symptom for personal or social reasons. The amount of fear and anxiety present can interfere with perception of a symptom.
Motivation	Competing needs may motivate a person to delay or enhance symptoms. A person who has no time or money to be sick will often not acknowledge the seriousness of symptoms.
Assigning of meaning	Once perceived, the symptom must be interpreted. Often, people explain symptoms within normal parameters ("I'm just tired").
Treatment accessibility	The greater the barriers to treatment—whether psychological, economic, physical, or social—the greater the likelihood that the symptom will not be interpreted as serious or that the person will seek an alternative form of care.

Adapted from Mechanic, D. (1978). *Medical sociology* (2nd ed.). New York, NY: The Free Press. Copyright © 1978 by David Mechanic, with permission.

and outcomes and an expectation of remuneration for services rendered. Nurses, physicians, physical therapists, and other licensed health care clinicians constitute the professional care providers in most health systems in the United States, Canada, Europe, Australia, New Zealand, Japan, and other parts of the world.

Folk Healing System

A **folk healing system** is a set of beliefs that has a shared social dimension and reflects what people typically do when they are ill versus what society says they should do according to a set of social standards (Sandberg et al., 2018). According to McFarland and Wehbe-Alamah (2015, 2018), all cultures of the world have a lay health care system, which is sometimes referred to as indigenous, folk, lay, or generic. The key consideration that defines folk systems is their history of tradition: many folk healing systems have endured over time through oral transmission of beliefs and practices from one generation to the next. A folk healing system uses healing practices that are often divided into secular and sacred components.

BOX 4-1 | Tips for Making Informed Decisions and Evaluating Information About Dietary Supplements

Basic Points to Consider

1. *Do I need to think about my total diet?*

   Yes, dietary supplements are intended to supplement your diet, not to replace the varieties of food that are important for your health

2. *Should I check with my doctor or health care provider before using a supplement?*

   Yes, this is a good idea. Dietary supplements are not always risk-free and may interfere with prescribed medications or therapies.

   Always check with your health care provider if you are pregnant, are breast-feeding, or have a chronic medical condition such as cancer, diabetes, hypertension, kidney disease, or heart disease.

   - Some supplements may interact with prescription and over-the-counter medicines.
   - Some supplements can have unwanted effects during surgery.//Adverse effects from the use of dietary supplements should be reported to the FDA at 1-800-332-1088 or by contacting their state or regional consumer complaint coordinator identifiable at https://www.fda.gov/Safety/ReportaProblem/ConsumerComplaintCoordinators/default.htm.

   Adverse effects from the use of dietary supplements should be reported to the FDA at 1-800-332-1088 or by contacting their state or regional consumer complaint coordinator identifiable at https://www.fda.gov/Safety/ReportaProblem/ConsumerComplaintCoordinators/default.htm.

3. Evaluate product Web sites and labels carefully. By federal law, manufacturers of dietary supplements are responsible for ensuring their products are safe before being marketed:
   - What expert or organization sponsors or validates the Web site?
   - What is the purpose of the Web site?
   - Is the source of the information identified, and does the site contain accessible references?
   - Does the information appear current and accurate?
   - Are the claims significantly different than found elsewhere (i.e., too good to be true)?

4. Think twice about believing what you read. Here are some assumptions that raise safety concerns:

   "Even if a product may not help me, it at least will not hurt me."

   "When I see the term 'natural,' it means that a product is healthful and safe."

   "A product is safe when there is no cautionary information on the product label."

   "A recall of a harmful product guarantees that all such harmful products will be immediately and completely removed from the marketplace."

5. Contact the manufacturer for specific product information before purchasing.

Sources: U.S. Department of Health and Human Services, Food and Drug Administration, Center for Food Safety and Applied Nutrition. (2018, February 23). *Tips for dietary supplement users* [Webpage]. Retrieved from https://www.fda.gov/food/dietary-supplements/usingdietarysupplements/ucm110567.htm#basic

See also U.S. Department of Health and Human Services, Food and Drug Administration, Center for Food Safety and Applied Nutrition. (2017, November 29). *Dietary supplements: What you need to know* [Webpage]. Retrieved from https://www.fda.gov/food/dietarysupplements/usingdietarysupplements/ucm110567.htm

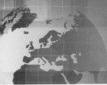

Chronic Disease Self-Management and Health Literacy in Four Ethnic Groups

Health literacy as a social determinant of health has widespread public health implications. It is essential for optimal self-care and is not directly related to intelligence or level of education. Individual health literacy becomes compromised under situations of duress such as illness, pain, stress, high emotion, altered cognitive states, and with aging (Prins & Monnat, 2015).

One interdisciplinary team of investigators studied chronic disease, self-management, and health literacy among four US ethnic groups: Vietnamese, African Americans, Whites, and Latinos. The researchers defined health literacy as the wide range of skills and competencies that people develop to seek out, comprehend, evaluate, and use health information and concepts to make informed choices, reduce health risks, and improve quality of life.

The facilitators of self-management of disease included speaking and listening skills that promote better clinician–patient communication; math (numeracy) skills, such as sliding scales for insulin dosage based on blood glucose levels; reading skills to read educational materials about disease processes and treatment; social support from family members, such as spouse and adult children; and social support from neighbors and friends who have higher levels of literacy than does the patient and, in some instances, more financial resources. For example, a Vietnamese participant with diabetes who lived in a rooming house reported that his landlord's wife buys extra vegetables for him whenever she goes shopping.

Identified barriers to disease self-management included confusion about the name of the diagnosis and the underlying cause of the chronic health problem(s) such as confusing certain aspects of their conditions with other conditions (e.g., misunderstanding the differences among high blood pressure, high blood sugar, and high cholesterol).

One Vietnamese patient stated that he thought his diabetes had been caused by imprisonment during the Vietnam War and the poor diet and forced labor he endured more than 40 years ago. Another patient indicated that hypertension meant that the blood is flowing very fast and stated that a complication of the rapid heartbeat is that the "heart is going to become very agitated," resulting in high cholesterol and obstruction of the veins.

Clinical Implications

- Nurses and other members of the health care team should recognize that patients' cultural health belief systems and explanatory models are interrelated with their health and linguistic literacy, educational background, and socioeconomic status.
- Cultural health beliefs exert important influences on the self-management of chronic diseases such as diabetes and hypertension.
- Cultural health beliefs are part of internally consistent explanatory models constructed by the patient in an effort to make sense of his/her diagnosis and the clinical manifestations of the underlying cause(s) of illness.
- If the patient's cultural health beliefs are not aligned with a biomedical explanation, the patient may decide to adhere to their own beliefs and refrain from following the provided biomedical advice and recommendations by nurses, physicians, and other health professionals.

References: Prins, E., & Monnat, S. (2015). Examining associations between self-rated health and proficiency in literacy and numeracy among immigrants and U.S.-born adults: Evidence from the Program for the International Assessment of Adult Competencies (PIACC). *PLoS ONE, 10*(7), e1–e25. doi: 10.1371/journal.pone.0130257; Shaw, S. J., Armin, J., Torres, C. H., Orzech, K. M., & Vivian, J. (2012). Chronic disease self-management and health literacy in four ethnic groups. *Journal of Health Communication, 17*(S3), 67–81.

Most cultures have **folk healers** (sometimes referred to as traditional, lay, indigenous, or generic healers), sometimes make house calls, usually speak the native tongue of the client, and often charge significantly less than professional/nontraditional health care providers (Leininger, 1997; McFarland & Wehbe-Alamah, 2015, 2018).

In addition, many cultures (and some health care systems) have lay midwives (e.g., *parteras* for Hispanic women), *doulas* (support women for new mothers and babies), or other health care providers available for meeting the needs of clients. Table 4-2 identifies indigenous or folk healers for selected groups.

Table 4-2	Healers and Their Scope of Practice

Cultural/Folk Practitioner	Preparation	Scope of Practice
African American/Black		
"Old lady"	Usually, an older woman who has successfully raised her own family; knowledgeable in child care and folk remedies	Consulted about common ailments and for advice on child care; found in rural and urban communities
Spiritualist	Called by God to help others; no formal training; usually associated with a fundamentalist Christian church	Assists with problems that are financial, personal, spiritual, or physical; predominantly found in urban communities
Voodoo priest and priestess or *Houngan* and *Mambo*	May be trained by other priests/priestesses In the United States, the eldest son of a priest becomes a priest; the daughter of a priest(ess) becomes a priestess if she is born with a veil (amniotic sac) over her face	Knowledgeable about properties of herbs; interpretation of signs and omens; able to cure illness caused by voodoo; uses communication techniques to establish a therapeutic milieu like a psychiatrist; treats Blacks, Mexican Americans, and Native Americans
Amish		
Braucher or *baruch-doktor*	Apprenticeship	Men or women who use a combination of modalities including physical manipulation, massage, herbs, teas, reflexology, and *brauche*, a folk healing art with origins in the 18th- and 19th-century Europe; especially effective in the treatment of bed-wetting, nervousness, and women's health problems; may be generalist or specialist in practice; some set up treatment rooms; some see non-Amish as well as Amish patients
Lay midwives	Apprenticeship	Care for women before, during, and after childbirth
Appalachia		
Granny woman, herb doctor	Lay practitioner familiar with Appalachian culture	Healer usually accessible, familiar with the culture, provides accepted cultural remedies and well known to the family
Chinese		
Herbalist	Knowledgeable in diagnosis of illness and herbal remedies	Both diagnostic and therapeutic; diagnostic techniques include interviewing, inspection, auscultation, and assessment of pulses

Table 4-2 | Healers and Their Scope of Practice (continued)

Cultural/Folk Practitioner	Preparation	Scope of Practice
Acupuncturist	3½–4½ years (1,500–1,800 hours) of courses on acupuncture, Western anatomy and physiology, Chinese herbs; usually requires a period of apprenticeship, learning from someone else who is licensed or certified Licensure required in the United States	Diagnosis and treatment of yin/yang disorders by inserting needles into *meridians*, pathways through which life energy flows; when heat is applied to the acupuncture needle, the term *moxibustion* is used May combine acupuncture with herbal remedies and/or dietary recommendations. Acupuncture is sometimes used as a surgical anesthetic
Greek		
Magissa "magician"	Apprenticeship	Woman who cures *matiasma* or evil eye; may be referred to as doctor
Bonesetter	Apprenticeship	Specialize in treating uncomplicated fractures
Priest (Orthodox)	Ordained clergy Formal theological study	May be called on for advice, blessings, exorcisms, or direct healing
Hispanic		
Family member	Possesses knowledge of folk medicine	Common illnesses of a mild nature that may or may not be recognized by modern medicine
Curandero	May receive training in an apprenticeship; may receive a "gift from God" that enables him or her to cure; knowledgeable in use of herbs, diet, massage, and rituals	Treats most of the traditional illnesses; some may not treat illness caused by witchcraft for fear of being accused of possessing evil powers; usually admired by members of the community
Espiritualista or spiritualist	Born with the special gifts of being able to analyze dreams and foretell future events; may serve apprenticeship with an older practitioner	Emphasis on prevention of illness or bewitchment through the use of medals, prayers, amulets; may also be sought for cure of existing illness
Yerbero	No formal training; knowledgeable in growing and prescribing herbs	Consulted for preventive and curative use of herbs for both traditional and Western illnesses
Sobador	Knowledgeable in massage and manipulation of bones and muscles	Treats many traditional illnesses, particularly those affecting the musculoskeletal system; may also treat nontraditional illnesses
Native American Native Alaskan Native Hawaiian		
Shaman Medicine Man Learned One	Spiritually chosen Apprenticeship	Uses incantations, divination practices, prayers, and herbs to cure a wide range of physical, psychological, and spiritual illnesses
Crystal gazer, hand trembler (Navajo)	Spiritually chosen Apprenticeship	Diviner diagnostician who can identify the cause of a problem, either by using crystals or by placing hand over the sick person; does not implement treatment

Adapted from Hautman, M. A. (1979). Folk health and illness beliefs. *Nurse Practitioner, 4*(4), 23–31; Small, C. C. (2017). Appalachians. In J. N. Giger (Ed.), *Transcultural nursing, assessment, and intervention* (7th ed., pp. 262–280). St. Louis, MO: Elsevier; Specter, R. E. (2013). Health and illness in the American Indian and Alaska Native population. In R. E. Spector (Ed.), *Cultural diversity in health and illness* (8th ed., pp. 210–237). Boston, MA: Pearson, with permission.

When clients use folk healers, these practitioners should be an integral part of the health care team and participate in as many aspects of the client's care as possible. For example, a nurse might include the folk healer in obtaining a health history and in determining what treatments already have been used toward bringing about healing. In discussing traditional remedies, it is important to be respectful and to listen attentively to healers who combine spiritual and herbal remedies for a wide variety of illnesses, both physical and psychological in origin. Chapter 13 provides detailed information about the religious beliefs and spiritual healers in major religious groups.

Complementary, Integrative, and Alternative Health System

Complementary, integrative, and alternative health is an umbrella term for hundreds of therapies used by individuals and cultures worldwide. Some of these therapies have ancient origins in Egyptian, Chinese, Greek, Indian, and American aboriginal (Mayan, Aztecan, Native American, and First Nations) cultures. Other practices such as chiropractic medicine and magnet therapy have evolved more recently. Allopathic or biomedicine and osteopathic medicine are the reference point with all other therapies considered *as complementary* (in addition to), *integrative* (combined selected magico-religious or holistic therapies with scientifically documented efficacy), or *alternative* (instead of).

Integrative health care is defined as a comprehensive, often interdisciplinary, approach to treatment, prevention, and health promotion that brings together complementary and professional care therapies (McFarland & Wehbe-Alamah, 2018). The use of an integrative approach to health and wellness across the United States has grown within care settings including hospitals, hospices, and military health facilities (U.S. Department of Health and Human Services [USDHHS], 2017a). The mission for the National Center for Complementary and Integrative Health is to

discover through rigorous scientific investigation the usefulness and safety of complementary and integrative health approaches and their roles in improving health and health care (USDHHS, 2017a). Their research priorities include the study of approaches such as spinal manipulation, meditation, yoga, and massage to manage pain and other symptoms that may not be well-addressed by conventional biomedical treatments. The center's current research foci encompass chronic pain and integrative approaches including military personnel and veterans, medication compatibilities with natural products, mind–body interactive effects, health promotion/disease prevention, and individual behaviors that support health, wellness, and quality of life (USDHHS, 2017b).

Consider a client who has been diagnosed with breast cancer. Worldwide, increasing numbers of individuals use complementary or integrative therapies to manage symptoms, prevent toxicities, and improve quality of life during chronic illness (Hardorfer & Jentschke, 2017; Jonkman, Schuurmans, Groenworld, Hoes, & Trappenburg, 2016; Richardson et al., 2014). An estimated 75% to 87% of North American cancer survivors self-report using complementary and integrative therapies following diagnosis (John et al., 2016; Judson et al., 2017; Luo & Asher, 2017). In clinical practice guidelines that address the supportive care of patients treated for breast cancer, oncology-recommended complementary or integrative therapies include acupuncture/acupressure, massage therapy, meditation, reflexology, hypnosis, music therapy, yoga, Tai chi, biofeedback, and selected approved supplements for the management of disease-related pain and chemotherapy-associated nausea and other adverse side effects (Greenlee et al., 2017; Solloway et al., 2016; Xiang et al., 2017). In addition, complementary or integrative therapies provide therapeutic supportive care for stress, fatigue, and other disease and treatment symptoms or effects and thereby improve quality of life (Greenlee et al., 2017). Using a special diet in lieu of undergoing specialist-recommended or oncologic treatment is an example of nonrecommended alternative solo therapy.

Complementary Health Approaches

Johns Hopkins Medicine (n.d.) categorizes complementary and integrative health approaches as follows:

1. *Traditional alternative medicine* beliefs are built on complete systems of theory and practice and have evolved earlier and apart from other conventional medical approaches used in the United States or Canada. Traditional health care systems include acupuncture, traditional **Chinese medicine**, **Ayurvedic** medicine, homeopathy, and **naturopathy**.

2. *Body touch* practices include a diverse group of techniques administered by a trained practitioner or teacher that are designed to enhance the mind's capacity to affect bodily functions and symptoms. The most commonly used body touch practices include chiropractic (10.3%; Clarke, Barnes, Black, Stussman, & Nahin, 2018) or osteopathic manipulation, massage, body movement therapies, Tai chi, and yoga. In the United States, adult use of yoga rose from 9.5% to 14.3% from the 2012 prior report (Clarke et al., 2018).

3. *Natural products* include herbs (also known as botanicals or herbal medicine), vitamins, minerals, and probiotics. They are also marketed to the public as *dietary supplements* (Dwyer, Coates, & Smith, 2018). In their study, Mongiovi, Shi, and Greenlee (2016) found 72% of adult participants reported using dietary supplements, most commonly vitamins (74%), minerals (57%), and herbs (43%) (p. 6).

4. *Mind or mind–body* connection practices include deep breathing, meditation, progressive relaxation, and hypnosis. Adult use of meditation in the United States increased

from 4.1% in 2012 to 14.2% in 2017 (Clarke et al., 2018).

5. *Senses* are believed to affect overall health. Practices include guided imagery, visualization, aromatherapy, and art, dance, or music therapy.

6. *External energy therapies* involve the use of energy fields in two ways:
   - *Biofield therapies* are intended to affect energy fields that surround and penetrate the human body. (The existence of such fields has not yet been scientifically proven.) Some forms of energy therapy manipulate biofields by applying pressure and/or manipulating the body by placing the hands in or through these fields. Examples include qigong (Tai chi), Reiki, and therapeutic touch.
   - *Bioelectromagnetic-based therapies* involve the unconventional use of electromagnetic fields, such as pulsed fields, magnetic fields, or alternating-current or direct-current fields.

"Nationally, 22.9% of U.S. adults aged 18–64 met the guidelines for both aerobic and muscle-strengthening activities during leisure-time physical activity in 2010–2015" (Blackwell & Clarke, 2018) with males exceeding females by approximately 10%. For both genders, Southern and Central regions had significantly lower use compared with mountain and coastal regions. Box 4-2 identifies and describes some of the complementary and alternative therapies most commonly used by people in the United States and Canada to promote health and prevent and treat disease. Figure 4-1 shows the age-adjusted percentage of adults who used yoga, meditation, or chiropractic treatments by race and Hispanic origin in the United States during the preceding 12-month period (2017). Other mind–body techniques considered complementary and integrative include meditation, prayer, mental healing, and creative outlet therapies such as art, music, or dance.

BOX 4-2 | Selected Complementary and Alternative Therapies

Acupuncture refers to a family of procedures involving stimulation of anatomical points on the body by a variety of techniques. The acupuncture technique that has been most studied scientifically involves penetrating the skin with thin, solid, metallic needles that are manipulated by the hands or by electrical stimulation. When heat is applied to the needles, it is referred to as moxibustion.

Aromatherapy involves the use of essential oils (extracts or essences) from flowers, herbs, and trees to promote health and well-being.

Ayurvedic medicine includes diet and herbal remedies and emphasizes the use of body, mind, and spirit in disease prevention and treatment.

Chiropractic is a noninvasive system of therapy focused on the relationship between bodily structure (primarily that of the spine) and function and how that relationship affects the preservation and restoration of health. Although chiropractors use a variety of treatment approaches, they primarily perform adjustments (manipulations) to the spine or other parts of the body with the goal of correcting alignment problems, alleviating pain, improving function, and supporting the body's natural ability to heal itself.

Dietary supplements are products (other than tobacco) taken by mouth that contain a *dietary ingredient* intended to supplement the diet. *Dietary ingredients* may include vitamins, minerals, herbs or other botanicals, amino acids, and substances such as enzymes, organ tissues, and metabolites. *Dietary supplements* come in many forms including extracts, concentrates, tablets, capsules, gelcaps, liquids, and powders. The United States and Canada have special requirements for labeling and in both countries these products are regulated as *foods* not drugs.

Guided imagery refers to a wide variety of techniques, including simple visualization and direct suggestion using imagery, metaphor and storytelling, fantasy exploration and game playing, dream interpretation, drawing, and active imagination where elements of the unconscious are invited to appear as images that can communicate with the conscious mind (Academy for Guided Imagery, 2018).

Homeopathic medicine is an alternative medical system. In homeopathic medicine, there is a belief that "like cures like," meaning that small, highly diluted quantities of medicinal substances are given to cure symptoms, even though the same substances given at higher or more concentrated doses would actually cause those symptoms.

Massage therapists manipulate muscle and connective tissue to enhance function of those tissues and promote relaxation and well-being.

Naturopathy is an alternative medical system based on the premise that there is a healing power in the body that establishes, maintains, and restores health. Practitioners work with the patient with a goal of supporting this power through treatments such as nutrition and lifestyle counseling, dietary supplements, medicinal plants, exercise, homeopathy, and traditional Chinese medicine.

Osteopathic medicine is a form of conventional medicine that, in part, emphasizes diseases arising in the musculoskeletal system. There is an underlying belief that all of the body's systems work together, and disturbances in one system may affect function elsewhere in the body. Some osteopathic physicians practice osteopathic manipulation, a full-body system of hands-on techniques to alleviate pain, restore function, and promote health and well-being.

Qigong ("chee-GUNG") or **Tai chi** ("tie Chee") is a component of traditional Chinese medicine that combines movement, meditation, and regulation of breathing to enhance the flow of qi (pronounced "chee" and meaning

BOX 4-2	Selected Complementary and Alternative Therapies (continued)

vital energy) in the body, improve blood circulation, and enhance immune function (Hung, Yeh, & Chen, 2018).

Reiki ("RAY-kee") is a Japanese word representing *universal life energy*. Reiki is based on the belief that when spiritual energy is channeled through a Reiki practitioner, the patient's spirit is healed, which in turn heals the physical body.

Therapeutic touch is based on the premise that the healing force of the therapist affects the patient's recovery; healing is promoted when the body's energies are in balance. By passing their hands over the patient, healers can identify energy imbalances.

Traditional Chinese medicine (TCM) is the current name for an ancient system of health care from China. TCM is based on a concept of

balanced *qi*, or *vital energy*, which is believed to flow throughout the body. Qi regulates a person's spiritual, emotional, mental, and physical balance and is influenced by the opposing forces of yin (negative energy) and yang (positive energy). Disease is proposed to result from the flow of qi being disrupted and yin and yang becoming imbalanced. Among the components of TCM are herbal and nutritional therapy, restorative physical exercises, meditation, acupuncture, and remedial massage.

Yoga is a term derived from a Sanskrit word meaning *yoke* or *union*. Yoga involves a combination of breathing exercises, meditation, and physical postures that are used to achieve a state of relaxation and balance of mind, body, and spirit.

Sources: Academy for Guided Imagery. (2018). *What is guided imagery?* Retrieved from http://acadgi.com/about_sitemap/power_of_guided_imagery/

Hung, H-M., Yeh, S-H., & Chen, C-H. (2018). Effects of Qigong exercise on biomarkers and mental and physical health in adults with at least one risk factor for coronary artery disease. *Biological Research for Nursing, 18*(3), 264–273.

U.S. Department of Health and Human Services, Centers for Disease Control and Prevention. (2014, April 16). *Regional variation in use of complementary health approaches by U.S. adults* [Webpage] (reviewed 2015, November 6). Retrieved from https://www.cdc.gov/nchs/data/databriefs/db146.htm

U.S. Department of Health and Human Services, National Institutes of Health, National Center for Complementary and Alternative Medicine. (2018, October 30). *Use of complementary health approaches in the U.S.* [Webpage]. Retrieved from https://nccih.nih.gov/research/statistics/NHIS/2012

Efficacy of Complementary Health Approaches

Research on complementary health approaches has focused on six main areas: medicinal plants, chiropractic and low back pain, acupuncture and pain, cell processes and diseases (e.g., cancer, asthma), the oxidative degradation of lipids, and diabetes and insulin. Research is also being done on the quality-of-life impact of complementary health approaches, including the influence of exercise and physical therapies on pain

(Feinberg, Jones, Lilly, Umer & Innes, 2018; Nahin, Boineau, Khalsa, Stussman, & Weber, 2016) and end-of-life care (Floriani, 2016; Nyatanga, Cook, & Goddard, 2018). For further evidence-based information related to the efficacy of specific health approaches and the reliability and validity of the studies conducted, visit the Cochrane Library (https://www.cochranelibrary.com/); it serves as the repository for the Cochrane Collaboration, a worldwide organization that prepares systematic reviews of health care research.

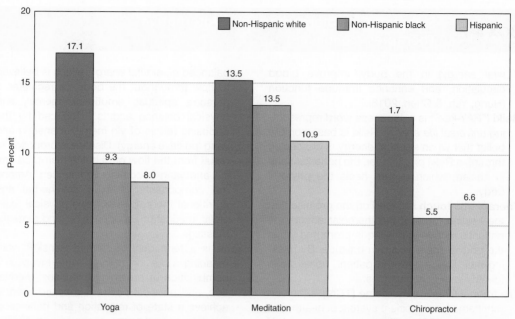

Figure 4-1. Age-adjusted percentage of adults who used yoga, meditation, or a chiropractor during the past 12 months, by race and Hispanic origin: United States, 2017. (From U.S. Department of Health and Human Services, Centers for Disease Control and Prevention, National Center for Health Statistics. (2018, November 15). *Age-adjusted percentage of adults who used yoga, meditation, or a chiropractor during the past 12 months, by race and Hispanic origin: United States, 2017.* Retrieved from https://www.cdc.gov/nchs/products/databriefs/db325.htm)

Summary

Cultural belief systems develop from the shared experiences by members of a social group and are expressed symbolically. The use of symbols to define, describe, and relate to the world around us is one of the basic characteristics of being human. The major cultural belief systems embraced by people worldwide are magico-religious, scientific/biomedical, and holistic health paradigms or worldviews. In the magico-religious cultural belief system, a supernatural agent or agents are believed to bestow health and illness: health may be perceived as a reward given as a sign of blessing and goodwill, while illness may be viewed as a sign of punishment. Most physicians and nurses are formally educated in the scientific or biomedical belief system wherein life is controlled by a series of physical and biochemical processes that can be studied and manipulated by humans through allopathic/osteopathic medicine and other professional care professionals and systems. In holistic cultural belief systems, the forces of nature must be kept in natural balance or harmony. Human life is only one aspect of nature and a part of the general order of the cosmos. Disturbing the laws of nature creates imbalance, chaos, and disease. Order is maintained through balance according to holistic yin/yang and hot/cold theories of health and illnesses.

REVIEW QUESTIONS

1. Describe in your own words the meaning for each of the following terms: (a) cultural belief system, (b) worldview, and (c) paradigm.
2. What are the primary characteristics for each of the three major health belief systems:

magico-religious, scientific/biomedical, and holistic paradigms?

3. What are the main differences between professional care and folk care systems?

4. What is allopathic medicine?

5. What is the primary mission of the U.S. National Center for Complementary and Integrative Health (NCCIH)?

6. Describe the six major categories of complementary or integrative approaches.

CRITICAL THINKING ACTIVITIES

1. Select a complementary health approach that you would like to know more about (such as acupuncture, Ayurveda, chiropractic, yoga, Tai chi, or homeopathy). Search the Internet for information about this practice, and then use a library to locate current research literature. After you have learned more about the practice, contact a healer who uses that health approach and ask the following questions:

   a. How did you prepare to be a practitioner of _____?
   b. What do you believe are the major benefits of _____ to clients or patients?
   c. What health-related conditions do you believe respond best to _____?
   d. Are there any risks to clients resulting from the use of _____?

2. The World Health Organization (2013) estimated that 80% of people worldwide access complementary or integrative health care for acute and chronic illnesses and to maintain health and wellness (pp. 26–28). Select a common illness (such as upper respiratory infection, arthritis, gastrointestinal upset, or a similar condition), and then identify the various complementary and integrative approaches to allopathic medicine that clients might use. What is the efficacy of each modality that you have identified? How effective do you think the complementary and alternative practices are compared with those of allopathic medicine? Compare the cost of each practice as well as its efficacy. What are the risks compared to benefits?

3. Please view the video "Scientific Results of Yoga for Health and Well-being," which can be found on the NCCIH Web site (https://nccih.nih.gov/video/yoga) as part of their Online Continuing Education Series. The presentation will help you to learn more about the use of yoga and Tai chi to improve balance and prevent falls, especially in the elderly. After viewing the video, identify the areas for which you are convinced adequate evidence exists to support integrating yoga as a complementary health approach into your nursing practice.

4. The herb *Echinacea* is frequently used for the prevention and treatment of the common cold. If a patient asked your opinion about the use of *Echinacea*, how would you reply? Would you recommend use of this herb to treat a cold? Explain why or why not.

5. Visit three Web sites from the Internet resources listed on thePoint for further information about specific types of alternative and complementary health care. Select a disease for which you think a complementary or alternative intervention might be helpful (such as breast cancer, hypertension, osteoarthritis, or other chronic condition). Critically appraise the potential benefits and adverse effects of a chosen intervention for clients with this disease. Indicate whether you believe sufficient evidence exists to support recommending the intervention to a client.

REFERENCES

Academy for Guided Imagery. (2018). *What is guided imagery?* Retrieved from http://acadgi.com/about_sitemap/power_of_guided_imagery/

Ackernecht, E. H. (1946). Natural diseases and rational treatment in primitive medicine. *Bulletin of the History of Medicine, XIX*, 467–497. Reprint: (1971). Naturalistic and supernaturalistic diagnosis and treatments. In: *Medicine and ethnology: Selected essays* (pp. 135–161). Baltimore, MD: Johns Hopkins Press.

Blackwell, D. L., & Clarke, T. C. (2018, June 28). *State variation in meeting the 2008 Federal Guidelines for both aerobic and muscle-strengthening activities through leisure time physical activity among adults aged 18–64: United States, 2010–2015. Health Statistics Reports, No. 112.* Hyattsville, MD: U.S. Department of Health and Human Services, Centers for Disease Control and Prevention, National Center for Health Statistics.

Clarke, T. C., Barnes, P. M., Black, L. I., Stussman, B. J., & Nahin, R. L. (2018). *Use of yoga, meditation, and chiropractors among U.S. adults aged 18 and over. NCHS Data Brief, No. 325.* Hyattsville, MD: U.S. Department of Health and Human Services, Centers for Disease Control and Prevention, National Center for Health Statistics.

Clements, F. E. (1932). Primitive concepts of disease. *American Archaeology and Ethnology, 32*(2), 185–252.

Dwyer, J. T., Coates, P. M., & Smith, M. J. (2018). Dietary supplements: Regulatory challenges and research resources. *Nutrients, 10*(1), e1–e24. doi: 10.3390/nu10010041

Faurot, K. R., Siega-Riz, A. M., Gardiner, P., Rivera, J. O., Young, L. A., Poole, C., …, Van Horn, L. (2015). Comparison of a medication inventory and a dietary supplement interview in assessing dietary supplement use in the Hispanic Community Health Study/Study of Latinos. *Integrative Medicine Insights, 2016*(11), e1–e10. doi: 10.4137/IMI.s25587

Feinberg, T., Jones, D. L., Lilly, C., Umer, A., & Innes, K. (2018). The Complementary Health Approaches for Pain Survey (CHAPS): Validity testing and characteristics of a rural population with pain. *PLoS ONE, 13*(5), e1–e20. Retrieved from https://doi.org/10.1371/journal.pone.0196390

Floriani, C. A. (2016). Anthroposophy and integrative care at the end of life. *Alternative and Complementary Therapies, 22*(3), 99–104.

Greenlee, H. G., Dupont-Reyes, M. J., Balneaves, L. G., Carlson, L. E., Cohen, M. R., Deng, G., Johnson, J. A., …, Tripahy, D. (2017). Clinical practice guidelines on the evidence-based use of integrative therapies during and after breast cancer treatment. *Journal of the National Cancer Institute. Monographs, 67*(3), 194–232. doi: 10.3322/caac.21397

Hardorfer, K., & Jentschke, E. (2017). Effect of yoga therapy on symptoms of anxiety in cancer patients. *Oncology Research and Treatment, 41*(9), 526–532. doi: 10.1159/000488989

Hautman, M. A. (1979). Folk health and illness beliefs. *Nurse Practitioner, 4*(4), 23–31.

Hung, H-M., Yeh, S-H., & Chen, C-H. (2018). Effects of Qigong exercise on biomarkers and mental and physical health in adults with at least one risk factor for coronary artery disease. *Biological Research for Nursing, 18*(3), 264–273.

John, G. M., Hershman, D. L., Falci, L., Shi, Z., Tsai, W-Y., & Greenlee, H. (2016). Complementary and alternative medicine use among U.S. cancer survivors. *Journal of Cancer Survivorship: Research and Practice, 10*(5), 850–864. doi: 10.1007/s11764-016-0530-y

Johns Hopkins Medicine. (n. d.). *Types of complementary and alternative medicine* [Webpage]. Retrieved from https://www.hopkinsmedicine.org/healthlibrary/conditions/complementary_and_alternative_medicine/types_of_complementary_and_alternative_medicine_85,P00189

Jonkman, N. H., Schuurmans, M. J., Groenwold, R. H. H., Hoes, A. W., & Trappenburg, J. C. A. (2016). Identifying components of self-management interventions that improve health-related quality of life in chronically ill patients: Systematic review and meta-regression analysis. *Patient Education and Counseling, 99*(7), 1087–1098.

Judson, P. L., Abdallah, R., Xiong, Y., Ebbert, J., & Lancaster, J. M. (2017). *Integrative Cancer Therapies, 16*(1), 96–103.

Leininger, M. M. (1997). Founder's focus alternative to what? Generic vs. professional caring, treatments and healing modes. *Journal of Transcultural Nursing, 91*(1), 37.

Lloreda-Garcia, J. M. (2017). Religion, spirituality, and folk medicine/superstition in a neonatal unit. *Journal of Religion and Health, 56*(6), 2276–2284. doi: 10.1007/s10943-017-0408-y

Luo, Q., & Asher, G. N. (2017). Complementary and alternative medicine use at a comprehensive cancer center. *Integrative Cancer Therapies, 16*(1), 104–109.

McFarland, M. R., & Wehbe-Alamah, H. B. (2015*). Leininger's culture care diversity and universality: A worldwide nursing theory* (3rd ed.). Burlington, MA: Jones & Bartlett Learning.

McFarland, M. R., & Wehbe-Alamah, H. B. (2018). *Transcultural nursing: Concepts, theories, research, and practices* (4th ed.). New York, NY: McGraw-Hill.

Mechanic, D. (1978). *Medical sociology* (2nd ed.). New York, NY: Free Press.

Mongiovi, J., Shi, Z., & Greenlee, H. (2016). Complementary and alternative medicine use and absenteeism among individuals with chronic disease. *Complementary and Alternative Medicine, 16*(248), e1–e12. doi: 10.1186/s12906-016-1195-9

Nahin, R. L., Boineau, R., Khalsa, P. S., Stussman, B. J., & Weber, W. J. (2016). Evidence-based evaluation of complementary health approaches for pain management in the United States. *Mayo Clinic Proceedings, 91*(9), 1292–1306. Retrieved from http://dx.doi.org/10.1016/j.mayocp.2016.06.00

Nyatanga, B., Cook, D., & Goddard, A. (2018). A prospective research study to investigate the impact of complementary therapies in palliative care. *Complementary Therapies in Practice, 31*, 118–125. Retrieved from https://doi.org/10.1016/j.ctcp.2018.02.006

Osborn, D. K. (2015). *Greek medicine: The four humors.* Retrieved from http://www.greekmedicine.net/b_p/Four_Humors.html

Prins, E., & Monnat, S. (2015). Examining associations between self-rated health and proficiency in literacy and numeracy among immigrants and U.S.-born adults: Evidence from the Program for the International Assessment of Adult Competencies (PIACC). *PLoS ONE, 10*(7), e1–e25. doi: 10.1371/journal.pone.0130257

Quiroz, D., & van Andel, T. (2018). The cultural importance of plants in Western African religions. *Economic Botany, 72*(3), 251–262.

Richardson, J., Loyola-Sanchez, A., Sinclair, S., Harris, J., Letts, L., MacIntyre, N. J., & Ginnis, K. M. (2014). Self-management interventions for chronic disease: A systematic scoping review. *Clinical Rehabilitation, 28*(11), 1067–1077.

Sandberg, J. C., Quandt, S. A., Graham, A., Stub, T., Mora, D. C., & Arcury, T. A. (2018). Medical pluralism in the use of *Sobadores* among Mexican immigrants to North Carolina. *Journal of Immigrant and Minority Health, 20*(5), 1197–1205.

Shaw, S. J., Armin, J., Torres, C. H., Orzech, K. M., & Vivian, J. (2012). Chronic disease self-management and health literacy in four ethnic groups. *Journal of Health Communication, 17*(S3), 67–81.

Small, C. C. (2017). Appalachians. In J. N. Giger (Ed.), *Transcultural nursing, assessment, and intervention* (7th ed., pp. 262–280). St. Louis, MO: Elsevier.

Smuts, J. C. (1926). *Holism and evolution.* New York, NY: MacMillan.

Solloway, M. R., Taylor, S. L., Shekelle, P. G., Miake-Lye, I. M., Beroes, J. M., Shanman, R. M., & Hempel, S. (2016). An evidence map of the effect of Tai Chi on health outcomes. *Systematic Reviews, 5*(126), e1–e11. doi: 10.1186/s13643-016-0300-y

Specter, R. E. (2013). Health and illness in the American Indian and Alaska Native population. In R. E. Spector (Ed.), *Cultural diversity in health and illness* (8th ed., pp. 210–237). Boston, MA: Pearson.

U.S. Department of Health and Human Services, Centers for Disease Control and Prevention. (2014). *Regional variation in use of complementary health approaches by U. S. adults* [Webpage]. (2014, April 16; reviewed 2015, November 6). Retrieved from https://www.cdc.gov/nchs/data/databriefs/db146.htm

U.S. Department of Health and Human Services, Food and Drug Administration, Center for Food Safety and Applied Nutrition. (2017, November 29). *Dietary supplements: What you need to know* [Webpage]. Retrieved from https://www.fda.gov/food/dietarysupplements/usingdietarysupplements/ucm110567.htm

U.S. Department of Health and Human Services, Food and Drug Administration, Center for Food Safety and Applied Nutrition. (2018, February 23). *Tips for dietary supplement users* [Webpage]. Retrieved from https://www.fda.gov/food/dietarysupplements/usingdietarysupplements/ucm110567.htm#basic

U.S. Department of Health and Human Services, National Institutes of Health, National Center for Complementary and Alternative Medicine. (2017a, September 24). *About NCCIH* [Web site]. Retrieved from https://nccih.nih.gov/about

U.S. Department of Health and Human Services, National Institutes of Health, National Center for Complementary and Alternative Medicine. (2017b, September 24). *Scientific results of yoga for health and well-being video [Webpage].* Retrieved from https://nccih.nih.gov/video/yoga

U.S. Department of Health and Human Services, National Institutes of Health, National Center for Complementary and Alternative Medicine. (2018, October 30). *Use of complementary health approaches in the U.S.* [Webpage]. Retrieved from https://nccih.nih.gov/research/statistics/NHIS/2012

World Health Organization. (1948). *Preamble to the Constitution of the World Health Organization* as adopted by the International Health Conference, New York, NY, June 19–22, 1946. Geneva, Switzerland: Author.

World Health Organization. (2013). *WHO traditional medicine strategy 2014–2023.* Geneva, Switzerland: Author.

World Health Organization. (2018). *Constitution of WHO: Principles* [Webpage]. Retrieved from https://www.who.int/about/mission/en/

Xiang, Y., Lu, L., Chen, X., & Wen, Z. (2017). Does Tai Chi relieve fatigue? A systematic review and meta-analysis of randomized control trials. *PLoS ONE, 12*(4), e1–e22. Retrieved from doi.org/10.1371/journal.pone.0174872

Lifespan

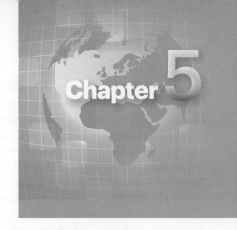

Chapter 5

Transcultural Perspectives in Childbearing

• Melva Craft-Blacksheare

Key Terms

Birth control–related mistrust
Birthing plan
Blended families
Childbearing
De novo

Emergency contraception
Female genital mutilation/
  cutting
Intimate partner violence
Maternal morbidity
Maternal mortality
Participatory women group

Pica
Postpartum depression
Pregnancy
Stereotyping
Taboos
Unintended pregnancy

Learning Objectives

1. Analyze how culture influences the beliefs and behaviors of the childbearing family during pregnancy.
2. Recognize the childbearing beliefs and practices of diverse cultures.
3. Examine the needs of women and childbearing families making alternative lifestyle choices regarding childbirth and childrearing.
4. Explore how cultural ideologies of childbearing populations can affect pregnancy outcomes.

This chapter discusses how culture, family, and social factors influence childbearing. The experiences of women and their support systems during pregnancy, birth, and the postpartum period are examined. Nursing practice recommendations are offered to facilitate the provision of culture-specific care to childbearing women and their families.

Overview of Cultural Belief Systems and Practices Related to Childbearing

Over the past three decades, there has been a dramatic change in contemporary pregnancy and childbirth practices in Western society. Today's global population is increasingly mobile, resulting in new cultural approaches to health and child-birth including a blending of cultural expectations and practices within Western culture. Often, parents from two cultures join together to raise a family, with each parent's cultural norms merging to define the family norms (see **Blended Families**, Figures 5-1 and 5-2). Due to global population shifts, cultural beliefs regarding childbearing must be examined to allow nurses to provide culturally congruent care throughout each patient's pregnancy, birth, and postpartum periods.

Pregnancy and Childbirth Practices in the United States

In their systematic, qualitative review of 35 studies from 19 countries, Downe, Finlayson, Oladapo, Bonet, and Gulmezoglu (2017) explored what mattered to women during childbirth. The authors concluded that women are most valued having a positive birth experience that fulfilled or exceeded their personal and sociocultural beliefs

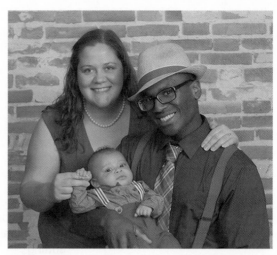
Figure 5-2. African European American family.

and expectations. Due to the mobility of global populations, we are witnessing a dramatic change in contemporary Western culture. To offer culturally congruent care, nurses need to increase their awareness of cultural beliefs regarding childbearing and childrearing. Clearly, offering only Westernized maternity care will not necessarily align with the nursing needs of today's multicultural patients.

Childbearing is a universal phenomenon that crosses all cultures, ethnicities, and socioeconomic levels. Childbirth often is a time of celebration. Indeed, in many cultures, a newborn is not just a new member of the family but also a gift to society. Childbirth is a time of transition and changing needs that are determined by several factors, the cultural norms, values, and socioeconomic influences, that surround the childbearing woman, her family, and her community. Therefore, nurses must know how to assess childbearing patients' cultural needs in order to provide appropriate care.

Historically and in many cultures, birth is considered a wellness event—a time of health and celebration. However, in modern times, it often is considered a hospital event, especially in the United States where more than 98% of infants are born in the hospitals (MacDorman, Matthews,

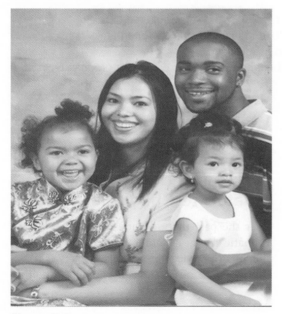
Figure 5-1. African Asian American family.

& Declercq, 2014). Hospital deliveries are routinely followed by trained obstetrical nurses, obstetricians, primatologists, and pediatricians. In most US hospitals, postpartum stays are 36 hours for a typical vaginal delivery and 72 hours for a noncomplicated cesarean delivery. After a 20-year trend of increasing labor induction for singleton births reached a high of 23.8% in 2010, the number began declining slightly in 2011 (23.7%) and 2012 (23.3%) (Osterman & Martin, 2014). Additionally, 85% of women in US hospitals use continuous electronic fetal monitoring, a practice that has increased 45% since 1980 (Berkatsky, 2015). Other routine hospital care includes epidurals for vaginal births and anesthesia for cesarean sections. Hospitals generally have a particular culture of rules and regulations related to OB patient care. However, when a laboring patient presents to the hospital with a **birthing plan** (an individualized list of preferred actions to facilitate a desired childbirth), the optimal outcome will include finding common ground between maternal expectations and the hospital's rules and culture. According to MacDorman and Declercq (2016), out-of-hospital births in the United States increased from 0.87% in 2004 to 1.50% in 2014. Twenty-nine percent of the out-of-hospital births occurred in alternative, freestanding birthing centers where certified nurse midwives (CNM), certified midwives (CM), and obstetricians who promote family-centered care emphasize pregnancy as a normal process requiring minimal technological intervention. During the same period, the remaining percentage of out-of-hospital births took place at home and were attended by lay, professional, or CM (MacDorman & Declercq, 2016).

Compared to other countries, the United States spends more on health care and maternal health than any other type of hospital care (Parente, 2018; Shaw et al., 2016). Despite these expenditures, U.S. mothers have a higher risk of pregnancy-related complications compared to women in 40 other countries. **Maternal morbidity and mortality** are by-products of U.S. health disparities due to the unequal availability of social, economic, and educational opportunities (see Evidence-Based Practice 5-1).

Globalization results in the spread of varied cultural beliefs and practices. In non-Western cultures, the roles of women, men, and social support groups often are different from those of Western society. Many groups have distinct cultural practices including African Americans, Native Americans, Latinos/Hispanics, Middle Eastern groups, Asians, and Orthodox Jewish people. Additionally, subcultures exist related to religious background, regional variations (i.e., urban or rural backgrounds), and sexual preference. It is paramount that those providing care do not assume that a person from a particular racial/ethnic group will act in a certain way. This assumption is the basis for **stereotyping** that likely will be viewed in a negative way by the client. Health care facilities should have cultural information available regarding the clients they serve. Nurses should inquire about patients' cultural practices and preferences and incorporate these in the patient's care plans.

In addition to cultural variations, patients' particular rituals and support systems also may differ from those of Western society. Unfortunately, nurses and health care professionals often expect all clients to act according to dominant Westernized culture. As part of health assessments, nurses should inquire about support systems, cultural practices, taboos, and rituals that are important to patients during childbearing.

Although the US population includes variations in ethnic origin, social class, family structure, and social support, many health care providers erroneously assume that pregnancy and childbirth are experienced the same way by all people. Additionally, nurses may believe that some traditional and cultural maternity practices are old fashioned and therefore do not have a place in modern medicine. It is important to realize that many women strive to maintain their cultural childbearing and childrearing customs. For example, birthing at home with a community midwife may seem unsafe to nurses working in the obstetrical unit of a Westernized hospital.

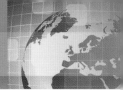

Health Disparities Among the African American Population

Maternal Fetal Medicine Facts

- From 2006 to 2010, African American women in the United States were three times more likely to suffer a pregnancy-related death than were White and Hispanic women. African American women accounted for 14.6% of live births but 35.5% of pregnancy-related deaths.
- Compared to White women, African American women are more likely to experience preventable maternal death.
- African American women experience physical *weathering*, meaning their bodies age faster than White women's due to exposure to chronic stress linked to socioeconomic disadvantages and discrimination. This weathering makes pregnancy riskier for African American women than White women and at an earlier age.
- African American infants die at twice the rate of White infants. Infant mortality is 5.0 deaths per 1,000 live births for White infants and 11.2 per 1,000 live births for African American infants.
- Preterm births occurred at a rate of 9.1% for White women compared to 14% for African American women.
- African American women are significantly less likely than women of other races to express understanding that genetic testing is optional, not required.
- African American women are less likely than women of other races to receive recommended influenza vaccinations during pregnancy.
- African American women have 30% higher odds of having an early cesarean section compared to Whites.
- While low educational attainment can have a negative effect on birth outcomes, for African American women, higher educational attainment does not improve infant survival rates. In other words, African American women with doctorates and professional degrees still have a higher infant mortality rates than do White women who never finished high school.
- A recent analysis of California women enrolled in Medicaid showed that African American women were less likely than White or Latina women to receive postpartum contraception, and when they did receive it, they were less likely to receive a highly effective method.

Clinical Implications

- Social determinants of health must be addressed through polices that raise incomes and provide access to educational attainment; health care; safe, affordable housing; and safe environments.
- It is crucial that nurses assess patients for culture-specific needs and desires and provide culturally sensitive and supportive health care.
- The number of minority health care professionals should be increased to equate with growing ethnic/racial populations.
- Cultural competence education should be required in all professional health curriculums.

References: Eichelberger, K., Doll, K., Edpo, G. E., & Zerden, M. (2016). Black lives matter: Claiming a space for evidence-based outrage in obstetrics and gynecology. *American Journal of Public Health*, *106*(10), 1771–1772. doi: 10.2105/AJPH.2016.303313

National Partnership for Women & Families. (2018). Black women's maternal health: A multifaceted approach to addressing persistent and dire health disparities, Issues brief. Retrieved from http://www.nationalpartnership.org/research-library/maternal-health/black-womens-maternal-health-issue-brief.pdf

Smith, I., Bentley-Edwards, K. L., El-Amin, S., & Darity, W. (2018). Fighting at birth: Eradicating the Black-White infant mortality gap. Retrieved from https://socialequity.duke.edu/sites/socialequity.duke.edu/files/site-images/EradicatingBlackInfantMortality-March2018%20FINAL.pdf

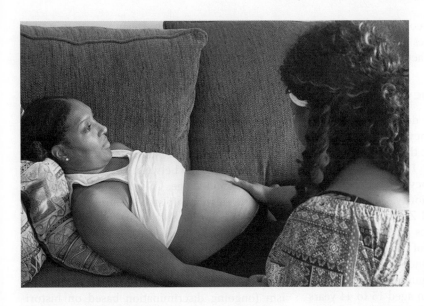

Figure 5-3. Client with home birth midwife.

However, home births are a safe, viable option that allows women to give birth in a familiar, comfortable environment. Figure 5-3 depicts a low-risk mom in her living room with her midwife. For home births, all prenatal appointments take place in the mother's home, where delivery is anticipated with a birthing pool set up in the living room space (see Figure 5-4).

Fertility Control and Culture

A woman's fertility—her ability to conceive a biological child—depends on several factors: nutrition, sexual behavior, endocrinology, timing, emotions, and culture. The significance of culture is paramount because sex and reproduction often are related to the surrounding cultural system. Certainly, cultural practices can influence fertility decisions. Fertility-related cultural practices include the desire to extend the family lineage, early marriages, producing children of a preferable sex, polygamy, and sexual rituals. Gender practices affecting fertility include subordination of women, economic dependence, and multiple home roles. According to Arousell and Carlborm (2016), an increasing number of contemporary research publications acknowledge religion and culture's influence on sexual and reproductive behavior including health care utilization. Gender and culturally sensitive family planning services could provide fertility support, birth interval planning, sexually transmitted infection

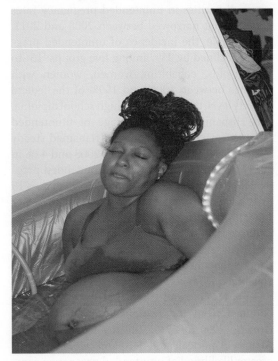

Figure 5-4. Client in home birthing pool.

prevention, and population control maintenance. The following section focuses on the societal elements that influence these factors.

Unintended Pregnancy

The Institute of Medicine defines **unintended pregnancy** as any pregnancy that is mistimed, unplanned, or unwanted at the time of conception (Brown & Eisenberg, 1995). The prevention of unintended pregnancy is a crucial public health and human rights priority.

In their study, Finer and Zolna (2016) calculated US pregnancy statistics for 2008 and 2011. They determined that 45% of pregnancies in the United States were unintended in 2011 compared to 51% in 2008. The unintended pregnancy rate among girls and women aged 15 to 44 years declined by 18% from 2008 (54 per 1,000) to 2011 (45 per 1,000) (Finer & Zolna, 2016). Unintended pregnancy rates for women cohabiting or living below the federal poverty level were two to three times the national average. Population subgroup disparities in unintended pregnancy rates persisted but narrowed between 2008 and 2011. For example, the incidence of unintended pregnancy declined by 25% among five groups: 15- to 17-year-olds, cohabiting women, women with incomes between 100% and 199% of the federal poverty level, those without a high school diploma, and Hispanics. The percentage of unintended pregnancies ending in abortion remained steady during the study period (40% in 2008 and 42% in 2011). Additionally, the rate of unintended pregnancies that ended in birth among women ages 15 to 44 declined from 27 per 1,000 in 2008 to 22 per 1,000 in 2011. The authors concluded that, despite a substantial decline in the unintended pregnancy rate between 2008 and 2011, unintended pregnancies remained most common among poor and cohabiting women (Finer & Zolna, 2016).

Kim, Dagher, and Chen (2016) analyzed data obtained from the *National Survey of Family Growth, 2006 to 2010*. The results showed that African American and Hispanic women had a greater likelihood of unintended pregnancy compared to White women. Decomposition models explained 51% of disparities in unintended pregnancy between African American and White women and 73% of these between Hispanic and White women. Factors contributing to the disparity between African American and White women included age, respondent's mother's age at first birth, federal poverty level, relationship status, and insurance status. Factors contributing to the disparity between Hispanic and White women included age, US-born status, education level, and relationship status (Kim et al., 2016).

After analyzing data from two survey studies, Rosenthal and Lobel (2018) found that, compared to White women, African American and Latina women reported a greater frequency of and concern over stereotype-related gender racism (ongoing discrimination based on historically rooted stereotypes about their sexuality and motherhood) and birth control–related mistrust due to historical abuses. The first study's results ($n = 135$) showed stereotype-related gender racism and **birth control–related mistrust** among African American and Latina women and none among White women. In addition, results of the second study ($n = 343$) showed that general, everyday discrimination and stereotype-related gender racism correlated positively with pregnancy-specific stress for African American and Latina women (Rosenthal & Lobel, 2018). The clinical implications of these findings include the need to educate women's health practitioners about stereotype-related gender racism and birth control–related mistrust to improve the care they provide to these populations. In addition, it would be beneficial to train health practitioners to prevent stereotypes from influencing their perceptions of these women and screen them for gendered racism experiences.

Interventions aimed at reducing the aforementioned disparities in unintended pregnancies should target at-risk groups of women. It is possible that the observed racial and ethnic disparities resulted from psychosocial and economic determinants that must be addressed to improve health outcomes among these women.

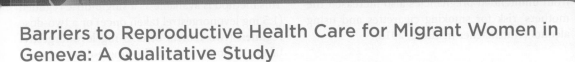

Barriers to Reproductive Health Care for Migrant Women in Geneva: A Qualitative Study

In developed countries, fewer migrant mothers access preventative gynecological services than nonmigrant women, and many experience more complicated pregnancy outcomes. The aim of this study was to explore barriers to reproductive health services experienced by migrant women in Geneva, as their experiences may reflect similar experiences globally. For this qualitative study, the authors conducted 13 focus groups in 7 languages with 78 women aged 18 to 66 years. Barriers were classified as either structural (influencing the accessibility of reproductive health services) or personal (influencing client satisfaction). Five main themes emerged from the data: financial accessibility, language barriers, real or perceived discrimination, lack of information, and embarrassment.

Clinical Implications

- Women should have access to informative material that is easy to understand and available in multiple languages.
- All health professionals should receive mandatory cultural sensitivity training.
- Designated nurses or social assistance staff should be trained to guide migrants through the health system.
- Monitoring and evaluating programs to prevent personal and systemic discrimination should be developed and implemented.

Reference: Schmidt, N. C., Fargnoli, V., Epiney, M., & Irion, O. (2018). Barriers to reproductive health care for migrant women in Geneva: A qualitative study. *Reproductive Health, 15,* 43. doi: 10.1186/s12978-018-0478-7

Preventing unintended pregnancies by addressing the disparities that contribute to them could save money, as well. Expenditures related to unintended pregnancies in the United States totaled to $21 billion in 2010, and the total gross potential savings from averting all unintended pregnancies has exceeded $15 billion (Guttmacher Institute, 2015) (see Evidence-Based Practice 5-2).

Continuation of Unintended Pregnancy

According to Cutler et al. (2018), ambivalence about an unintended pregnancy has been defined as "contradictory or unresolved feelings about whether or not to continue the pregnancy" (p. 75). Pregnancy ambivalence is a risk factor for high-risk sexual behavior and associated with poor pregnancy outcomes. Women with unintended pregnancies report increased levels of anxiety, stress, and depression along with receiving late prenatal care (Cutler et al., 2018). Herd, Higgins, Sicinski, and Merkurieva (2016) examined women's long-term well-being after continuation of an unintended pregnancy by obtaining data from a 60-year longitudinal study of Wisconsin high school graduates from the class of 1957. The aim of the study was to assess later-life depressive symptoms and episodes among women who reported unintended pregnancies before Roe V. Wade. In this cohort of mostly married White women, continuation of unintended pregnancies was strongly associated with poorer mental health outcomes in later life (Herd et al., 2016).

Comparatively, results from the *Turnaway Study* indicated that women were at greater risk for anxiety disorders 3 years after continuing an unintended pregnancy compared to women who terminated an unwanted pregnancy (Biggs, Neuhaus, & Foster, 2015). Additionally, compared to planned births, births from unintended pregnancies were associated with adverse maternal, infant, and child health outcomes such as delayed prenatal care and premature birth. Births from unintended pregnancies also increased the mothers' risk for smoking cigarettes and using alcohol (Guttmacher Institute, 2016).

Contraceptive Methods

According to the Guttmacher Institute (2016), among the 61 million women of childbearing age (15 to 44) in the United States, about 43 million (70%) are at risk for unintended pregnancy. While they are sexually active and do not want to become pregnant, many fail to use a contraceptive method correctly and consistently to prevent pregnancy.

Sixty-seven percent of contraceptive users use nonpermanent methods, primarily hormonal methods (the pill, patch, implant, injectable, and vaginal ring) as well as IUDs and condoms. The remainder rely on female (25%) or male (8%) sterilization.

Women most likely to use the pill are White, in their teens and 20s, college graduates, cohabiting, childless, and never married. Female sterilization is most commonly seen among women who are African American, are Hispanic, are aged 35 or older, are never married, have two or more children, are living 150% of the federal poverty level, have less than a college education, live outside of metropolitan areas, and are publicly insured or uninsured (Guttmacher Institute, 2016).

According to the Guttmacher Institute (2018), 68% of Catholics, 73% of Protestants, and 74% of Evangelicals who are at risk for an unintended pregnancy use a highly effective method (e.g., sterilization, IUD, or the pill or other hormonal methods). Even though Catholicism encourages natural family planning, only about 2% of at-risk Catholics rely on this method, the same percentage as those who attend church once a month or more.

Emergency contraception (EC), available in the United States, is used to prevent pregnancy after unprotected intercourse or contraceptive failure. To be effective, it must be used within 24 and up to 120 hours after unprotected intercourse.

This method is available as a single-dose regimen (1.5 mg levonorgestrel taken once) or a two-dose regimen (two tablets of 0.75-mg levonorgestrel taken 12 hours apart). The single-dose regimen was first made available over the counter in 2013. In addition to hormonal EC, inserting a copper IUD up to 120 hours after unprotected intercourse can be used as an EC method (Holland, Strachan, Pair, Stallworth, & Hodges, 2018).

Global Contraception Concerns

The Global Strategy for Women's Children's and Adolescents' Health (2016–2030) initiative promotes prioritizing ending preventable child and maternal deaths. In their commentary, Fikree, Lane, Simon, Hainsworth, and MacDonald (2017) addressed the Global Consensus Statement (*Expanding Contraceptive Choice for Adolescents and Youth to Include Long Acting and Reversible Contraception* [LARC]) by providing evidence on the safety and effectiveness of LARCs for young people. The authors estimated that more than 12 million married and unmarried adolescents (age 15 to 19) will give birth in 2016 and that pregnancy and childbirth complications are the second leading cause of death in this age group. Evidence supports the fact that early childbearing significantly hinders social and economic prospects for young women. Facilitating the ability of sexually active young people to choose an effective and satisfying contraceptive method will ensure they can exercise their right to prevent, delay, or space pregnancy (Fikree et al., 2017).

Refugees and Reproductive Health

Over the last few years, widely available images have portrayed the intense suffering faced by people in humanitarian crises. Into its 6th year, the largest humanitarian crisis in the world is in Syria, which has displaced 6.3 million people within the country and forced 4.8 million to seek refuge in other countries. Included in the refugee population are 5.3 million women of reproductive age, 440,000 of whom are pregnant (United Nations Population Fund, 2017). Globally in 2015, more than 65 million people—a record high at the time—endured forced displacement due to conflict and persecution. Many of these individuals are women who are pregnant or of childbearing age (Barot, 2017).

Of the 129 million people in need of humanitarian assistance worldwide, approximately one-fourth are women and adolescent girls of reproductive age. Women and girls are at a particular risk for harm when their social and structural support systems collapse. The increased threats to sexual and reproductive health expose women and adolescent girls to unwanted pregnancy, unsafe abortions, STIs (including HIV), maternal illness, and death (Barot, 2017).

Prior to the creation of the Women's Refugee Commission and the Inter-agency Working Group on Reproductive Health in Crisis (IAWG), women living in refugee situations received little assistance when encountering the many barriers to reproductive care. To address this issue, the IAWG has taken a leadership role in research, technical guidance, and guideline development. Because of this work, the IAWG published the *Inter-agency Field Manual on Reproductive Health in Humanitarian Settings*, which was updated in 2010. This manual provides information to help

humanitarian staff provide reproductive health interventions during humanitarian emergencies. The IAWG also created the *Minimum Initial Service Package*, a list of priority activities to be implemented at the onset of every humanitarian emergency (see Box 5-1).

Religion and Fertility Control

Most major religions offer members guidance in sexual and reproductive health matters. Scholars have studied the meaning of sexuality and family planning strategies among the major religious traditions of Judaism, Christianity, Islam, Hinduism, Sikhism, and Buddhism. One commonality among these religions is that each offers a distinct belief system. Depending upon their personal interpretations of their faith, religious followers can be considered devout, conservative, or liberal followers of their religion.

Regarding birth control, the Catholic Church endorses only natural family planning methods (i.e., the rhythm method and cycle beads). Such methods require partner agreement and support to refrain from intercourse during the fertile period. Additionally, the user must understand and become familiar with her menstrual cycle in order to avoid or plan a pregnancy.

BOX 5-1 | Minimum Initial Service Package for Refugee Women and Girls

- Identify an agency to lead the implementation of Minimum Initial Service Package activities.
- Prevent sexual violence, and treat and support survivors through provision of medical and psychosocial services.
- Reduce HIV transmission through infection-control guidelines, freely accessible condoms, and clean blood supply.

- Prevent needless newborn and maternal death and disability.
- Plan for the provision of comprehensive reproductive health services to be integrated into primary health care as soon as possible.

Source: Barot S, *In a state of crisis: meeting the sexual and reproductive health needs of women in humanitarian situations*, Guttmacher Policy Review, Vol. 20, 2017.

Arousell and Carlborm (2016) reported on Moreau and colleagues' findings that regular religious practice among Muslims was associated with a later sexual debut among young people. However, the same study found that sexually active adolescents who regularly practiced their religion were less likely to use contraception. In these situations, controls executed by family and social and religious groups may act as barrier that prevents sexually active adolescents from adopting preventative behaviors. The Muslim value system berates young followers who dishonor their family by deviating from sexual norms or gender roles or become sexually active before marriage (Arousell & Carlborn, 2016) (see Figure 5-5).

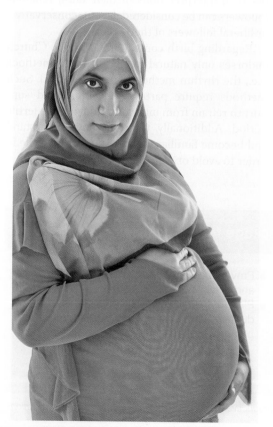

Figure 5-5. Pregnant Muslim woman (ZouZou/Shutterstock.com).

Westoff and Bietsch (2015) analyzed religion influences on reproductive behavior in 29 sub-Saharan African countries. The health surveys conducted over 10 years (2004–2014) categorized the religions as either Muslim or non-Muslim. Results indicated that Muslim fertility rates were higher than were non-Muslim rates. The fertility rate of married Muslim women was higher for those who married at a younger age (17.7 vs. 19.0 years). Polygyny is more common among Muslim women (35%) compared to non-Muslim women (22%). While Islamic law allows a man to have more than one wife, this practice is illegal in Turkey and Tunisia. Higher education levels and urban or rural residence both are associated with marriage and fertility. The percentage of Muslim women with no schooling is higher than for non-Muslim women. The average number of children desired by young Muslim women is 5.1 compared to 4.4 desired by non-Muslim teenagers. Education is inversely related to the number of children desired. Additionally, in most of the 17 countries, the percentage of married Muslim women currently using a contraceptive method is lower than that of non-Muslim women. Finally, in most countries, Muslim women have shorter birth intervals than do non-Muslim women (Westoff & Bietsch, 2015).

Cultural Influences on Fertility Control

Unfortunately, it is common for health professionals to have misconceptions about pregnancy prevention and contraception in cultures different from their own. To ensure that all persons receive optimal care, nurses are challenged to eradicate stigmas, language barriers, stereotyping, discrimination, and patients' lack of information about the health system from care settings (Cesario, 2017).

Salari's (2018) research examined how cultural attitudes affected the fertility decisions of second-generation immigrant women who were born in the United States but kept their heritage language. The results indicated that their original culture had a direct impact on their fertility decisions, with their total fertility rates reflecting the values of the original culture, not their new culture. Additionally, cultural transmission is found to be statically significant among women whose social network is comprised of people of the same culture (Salari, 2018).

According to Wilson and Kuha (2017), cultural entrenchment that predicts immigrants' fertility often resembles their native countries in comparison to their new settlements. A client in the family planning office who has lived in the United States for 10 years may embrace her heritage cultures' value system as it relates to fertility and childbearing rather than the dominate Western culture where she resides. Health providers must be aware of cultural groups existing in the community and have the ability to ask appropriately about their family planning preferences in alignment with their cultural norms.

Between 2008 and 2016, Mutumba, Wekesa, and Stephenson (2018) examined how communities influenced the fertility decisions of 15- to 24-year-old women from 52 countries: 32 in Africa, 6 in Southeast Asia, 5 from the Eastern Mediterranean region, 20 from the Western Pacific region, 5 from the European region, and 8 from the Americas. These researchers concluded that pronatal attitudes—which act as social scripts women are expected to follow—may discourage contraceptive by increasing pressure for young women to prove their fertility or promote prevailing fears and misconceptions that modern contraceptive methods may reduce a woman's fertility. These results also indicated that young women who live in communities with families who have more children than they consider ideal were less likely to report using modern contraceptive methods. However, young women with the following characteristics were more likely to use modern contraceptive measures: higher education, residing in a wealthier household, living in urban areas with greater mass media exposure, and having a higher number of living children (Mutumba et al., 2018).

Nurses providing family planning services should strive to be culturally sensitive to help their patients feel comfortable examining their own attitudes, beliefs, and sense of gynecologic well-being regarding fertility control. Nurses should acquire patients' history of previous contraceptive use including identifying their satisfaction or problems with the methods they used. Providing an explanation of contraceptive benefits, side effects, and risks is crucial. If necessary, an interpreter should be used to address language barriers.

Pregnancy and Culture

All cultures recognize **pregnancy** as a special transition period in a woman's life. Most societies have customs and beliefs that dictate a woman's behavior, activities, and lifestyle during the childbearing period. Due to the US population's varied cultural and ethnic backgrounds, childbirth customs not only reflect the dominant Western society but also allow for the accommodation and blending of other cultural practices to satisfy maternal and family wishes. The following section describes some of the biologic and cultural variations that could influence nursing care during pregnancy.

Biologic Variations

Nurses who provide care to pregnant women need to learn about biologic variations resulting from genetic and environmental backgrounds. In the United States, pregnant African American women are screened for sickle cell disease (SCD), a serious, chronic hemolytic anemia resulting from homozygosity for the mutant allele of the hemoglobin S gene. While SCD prevalence is approximately 1 in 400 African American women, the carrier frequency of the heterozygote sickle cell trait (SST) is 1 in 10. Because pregnant women with SST are at an increased risk for asymptomatic bacterial urinary tract infections, pyelonephritis, and preterm labor, frequent urine cultures are obtained during their antenatal care. If a woman has an SST, a paternal blood test is taken and genetic counseling offered. If the father

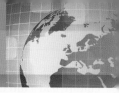

Sickle Cell Disease and Pregnancy Outcomes: A Study of the Community-Based Hospital in a Tribal Block of Gujarat, India

Sickle cell disease (SCD), a hereditary blood disorder, is a serious public health concern that presents mainly in tropical countries, primarily Africa. SCD also is prevalent in Central America, Saudi Arabia, India, and Mediterranean countries. The purpose of this study was to report on the analysis of tribal maternal admissions in the community-based hospital of SEWA Rural (Kasturba Maternity Hospital) in Jhagadia Block, Gujarat, India. Data were collected from March 2011 to September 2015 during which there were 14,640 total tribal maternal admissions and 10,519 deliveries. Overall, 12% (131 out of 10,519) of tribal deliveries were sickle cell admissions and 0.6% (1,645 out of 10,519) of tribal delivery admissions had the sickle cell trait. The percentage of stillborns among SCD deliveries was 9.2%, compared to 4.2% of non–sickle cell patients. Additionally, almost half of sickle cell deliveries required a blood transfusion. Forty-five percent of sickle cell deliveries were preterm births compared to only 17.3% of non-SCD patients. The odds of severe anemia, stillbirth, blood transfusion, cesarean section, and low birth weight was significantly higher for sickle cell admissions compared to non–sickle cell admissions. These findings indicated that there is a high risk of adverse pregnancy outcomes for women with SCD. Identification of tribal women with SCD and SCT is crucial for decreasing morbidity/mortality.

Clinical Implications

- This study highlights the need for sickle cell screening and care for women in remote and tribal rural areas in India.
- Tribal women with SSD need regular third-trimester fetal growth screening.
- Providing blood transfusions for women with SCD (as needed) may help reduce adverse maternal outcomes.
- Health professionals must assess a client's country of ancestral origin to determine if sickle cell blood testing is warranted.

Reference: Desai, G., Anand, A., Shah, P., Shah, S., Dave, K., Bhatt, H., ..., Modi, D. (2017). Sickle cell disease and pregnancy outcomes: A study of the community-based hospital in a tribal block of Gujarat, India. *Journal of Health, Population and Nutrition, 36*(1), 3. doi: 10.1186/s41043-017-0079-z

is heterozygous for the gene, there is a one in four chance that the infant will be born with the disease. Even though SSD and SST predominately occur among people of African descent, SSD also is found among people from the Mediterranean region, South America, and India. A cultural immigration history may be beneficial to determine the necessity of testing for SST (see Evidence-Based Practice 5-3).

Diabetes mellitus is another biologic variation relative to pregnancy. While diabetes has serious implications for the mother and fetus, survival rates have improved over the last few decades. According to Carson et al. (2015), 16.3% of American Indians (AI) and Alaska Natives (AN) have type 2 diabetes, and 30% have prediabetes. This group is 2.2 times more likely to have type 2 diabetes than non-Hispanic Whites and 4 times more likely to experience an amputation as a complication of diabetes than are their White counterparts. In Oklahoma's federally recognized tribes, 24% of AIs with type 2 diabetes experience retinopathy as a complication of their condition (Carson et al., 2015). The rate of gestational diabetes mellitus among the AI/AN exceeds that of the White population and is as high as 15% among some tribes (Carson et al., 2015).

Pregnant women with any form of diabetes are at risk for fetal and neonatal complications. Women with pregestational type 1 diabetes are at an increased risk for pre-eclampsia and adverse neonatal outcomes. Because there is an increased risk of urinary tract infections with every type of diabetes, asymptomatic bacteriuria screening should be performed to help reduce the impact of this problem. In addition, hydramnios (increased amniotic fluid) and fetal macrosomia (baby ≥4,000 g) are more common among pregnant women with diabetes.

Carson et al. (2015) conducted a qualitative research study in which 97 participants from 2 Oklahoma tribes were interviewed to obtain information about variables that could negatively affect diabetes prevention or control. Data analysis revealed the following themes: diabetes self-care adherence as well as fear of neonatal complications, injections, amputation, blindness, and death. Many participants repeated stories about the disease they heard from friends and family members. The researchers concluded that patients might have explanatory models, influenced by their social network members that differ from the practice-based explanatory models health practitioners use. Additionally, effective communication and culturally sensitive care help promote patient compliance with recommended treatments (Carson et al., 2015).

Cultural Variations Influencing Pregnancy

This section discusses Western cultural practices and variations that can influence pregnancy outcomes: alternative lifestyle choices, maternal role attainment, nontraditional support systems, cultural beliefs about parental activity during pregnancy, and food taboos and cravings. Nurses must be able to assess a client's cultural practices related to childbearing to determine if they are harmful or benign. Nurses also must never assume that clients "don't look like" they engage in practices outside those of the mainstream population or "don't look like" they are from a particular ethnic group or culture (stereotyping). It is important to incorporate questions about cultural practices related to pregnancy, childbirth, and newborn care in the initial assessment and throughout the prenatal period.

Female genital mutilation/cutting (FGM/C) is a dangerous ancient cultural practice that can affect pregnancy. FGM/C, also known as female excision, is a violation of girls and women's human rights. According to a recent UNICEF (2016) publication, at least 200 million girls and women have experienced FGM/C in 30 countries across 3 continents. Even though there has been an overall decline in FGM/C over the last three decades, not all countries have made significant progress and the pace of the decline has been uneven. UNICEF's data illustrate that the progress is insufficient to keep up with increasing population growth. In fact, the number of girls and women undergoing FGMC/C will significantly rise over the next 15 years (UNICEF, 2016). The practice of FGM/C, while violent in nature, is perpetrated by family members whose primary intention is not to inflict violence but adhere to cultural norms. Community members practicing this custom believe that FGM/C will ensure a girl's proper upbringing, future marriage, and honor to the family. Others associate this ritual with religious beliefs, although no religious scriptures require it. The fact that parents allow their daughters to undergo this procedure despite being aware of the harm it causes illustrates the power of this cultural practice. Many are afraid that refraining from the practice will risk their daughter's marriage prospects as well as their family status (see Evidence-Based Practice 5-4).

Alternative Lifestyle Choices

Family composition or family structure refers to how family members are related to each other and society. Structure can refer to the form (e.g., single- or two-parent families), partners

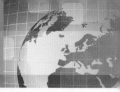

Female Genital Mutilation and Cutting: A Systematic Literature Review of Health Professionals' Knowledge, Attitudes, and Clinical Practice

Due to increased immigration, health professions in high-income countries including the UK, Europe, North America, and Australia care for women and girls with female genital mutilation/cutting (FGM/C). This study reviewed health provider's knowledge, clinical practice, and attitudes regarding FGM/C. Most health professionals were aware of the practice of FGM/C, but few correctly identified the four FGM/C categories defined by WHO. Knowledge about FGM/C legislation varied: 25% of professionals in a Sudanese study, 45% of Belgian labor ward staff, and 94% of health professions from the UK knew that FGM/C was illegal in their country.

Clinical Implications

Female genital mutilation is classified into four major types:

- **Type 1:** Often referred to as clitoridectomy, this is the partial or total removal of the clitoris (a small, sensitive, and erectile part of the female genitals) and, in very rare cases, only the prepuce (the fold of skin surrounding the clitoris).
- **Type 2:** Often referred to as excision, this is the partial or total removal of the clitoris and the labia minora (the inner folds of the vulva), with or without excision of the labia majora (the outer folds of skin of the vulva).
- **Type 3:** Often referred to as infibulation, this is the narrowing of the vaginal opening through the creation of a covering seal. The seal is formed by cutting and repositioning the labia minora, or labia majora, sometimes through stitching, with or without clitoris removal.
- **Type 4:** This includes all other harmful procedures to the female genitalia for nonmedical purposes, for example, pricking, piercing, incising, scraping, and cauterizing the genital area.

Immediate Complications

- Severe pain
- Excessive bleeding

Cultural and Social Factors for Performing FGM

The reasons for performing FGM/C vary from one region to another, as well as over time, and include a mix of sociocultural factors within families and communities. The following are some of the most commonly cited reasons for this practice:

- Where FGM is a social norm, strong motivations to perpetuate the practice include social pressure to conform to what others do and have been doing, the need to be accepted socially, and the fear of community rejection. In some communities, FGM is unquestioned and performed almost universally.
- FGM often is considered a necessary part of raising a girl and a way to prepare her for adulthood and marriage.
- FGM often is motivated by beliefs about what is considered an acceptable sexual behavior. It aims to ensure premarital virginity and marital fidelity. In many communities, FGM is believed to reduce a woman's libido and therefore believed to help her resist extramarital sexual acts. When a vaginal opening is covered or narrowed (type 3), women's fears that opening it will be painful and that doing so will be discovered are expected to discourage extramarital sexual intercourse.
- FGM is more likely to be carried out in communities where it is believed that being cut increases marriageability.
- FGM is associated with cultural ideals of femininity and modesty, which include the notion that girls are clean and beautiful after the removal of body parts considered unclean, unfeminine, or male.
- Though no religious scripts prescribe the practice, practitioners often believe the practice has religious support.
- Religious leaders take varying positions on FGM: some promote it, some consider it irrelevant to religion, and others contribute to its elimination.

Female Genital Mutilation and Cutting: A Systematic Literature Review of Health Professionals' Knowledge, Attitudes, and Clinical Practice (continued)

- Local power and authority structures—such as community leaders, religious leaders, circumcisers, and even some medical personnel—can contribute to upholding the practice.
- In most societies where FGM is practiced, it is considered a cultural tradition, which often is used as an argument for its continuation.
- In some societies, recent adoption of the practice is linked to copying the traditions of neighboring groups. Sometimes, it has started as part of a wider religious or traditional revival movement.

Key Facts About Female Genital Mutilation

- FGM includes procedures that intentionally alter or cause injury to the female genital organs for nonmedical reasons.
- The procedure has no health benefits for girls and women.

- The procedures can cause severe bleeding and problems urinating and later cysts, infections, as well as childbirth complications and increased risk of newborn deaths.
- More than 200 million girls and women alive today have been cut in 30 countries where FGM is concentrated (Africa, the Middle East, and Asia).
- FGM is mostly carried out on young girls between infancy and age 15.
- FGM is a violation of the human rights of girls and women.

References: World Health Organization (WHO). (2018b). Female genital mutilation. Retrieved from http://www.who.int/news-room/fact-sheets/detail/female-genital-mutilation

Zurynski, Y., Sureshkumar, P., Phu, A., & Elliot, E. (2015). Female genital mutilation and cutting: A systematic literature review of health professionals' knowledge, attitudes and clinical practice. *BMC International Health and Human Rights, 15,* 32. doi: 10.1186/s12914-015-0070-y

(e.g., cohabitation, married, or lesbian/gay), or composition (traditional nuclear, extended, or communal family). Regardless of the nurse's perception of what constitutes a family, she must accept whomever clients define as their family members and their relationships with them. In Western culture, the traditional family has changed drastically over the last 30 years. Although the dominate cultural expectations for North American women are for marriage and childbearing to take place within a nuclear family, cultural changes have made it more acceptable for women to delay childbearing in lieu of college education and a formal career. This cultural change has encouraged many couples to have smaller families, women to freeze their embryos (to prevent problems with infertility due to later childbearing), and single women to use donor sperm and raise a child as a single parent.

Lesbian childbearing couples are a distinct subculture with specific needs. More women that are lesbian are choosing to have children in the context of same-sex relationships than ever before (Hayman, Wilkes, Halcomb, & Jackson, 2015). Even though there is a growing number and increasing visibility of families headed by lesbians and gay men throughout Europe and the United States, a study by Costa, Pereira, and Leal (2018) indicated that negative beliefs persist about their competence as parents (see Figure 5-6).

In their qualitative study, Hayman et al. (2015) recruited a convenience sample of 30 self-identified lesbian women (15 couples) to explore how lesbian mothers construct mothering.

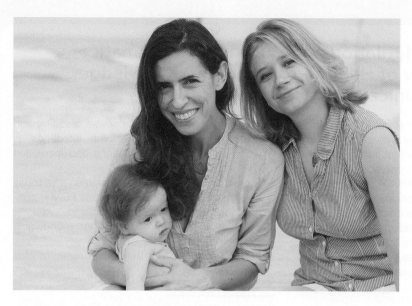

Figure 5-6. Lesbian couple with child (Dubova/ Shutterstock.com).

Participants provided demographic data and participated in semistructured interviews in which they described their journeys into motherhood and parenting. The following four themes emerged from the data analysis: becoming mothers, constructing motherhood, legitimizing our family, and raising our children. Lesbian couples experience several aspects of pregnancy that heterosexual couples do not: discussions about which partner will carry the baby, choosing a sperm donor, and choosing a conception method. Deciding on which partner should be pregnant included several considerations. Some participants selected the younger partner, others selected the healthiest, and one older partner was selected because she did not have much time left to conceive. Partners identifying as "butch" did not recognize childbearing as one of their roles within the relationship, and some outright rejected the idea of conceiving a child even though they had the physical capacity. Choosing a known or unknown donor also was a major decision. Couples had long debates over this decision, reviewing the benefits and limitations of both options. Some couples were artificially inseminated from an unknown donor chosen from a sperm bank, while others chose a relative (e.g., a brother) of the partner that was not carrying the fetus to give that partner a genetic relationship to the child. This choice is seen as a validation of the nonbirth mother's position as a legitimate parent that helped promote social recognition of her maternal identity. Furthermore, choosing a known donor would allow the child to make contact with that relative if they wanted to in the future. Participants who chose an unknown donor ($n = 2$) did so because they felt strongly about not having any donor involvement in childrearing (Hayman et al., 2015).

For young, healthy, heterosexual couples, conception typically takes place via intercourse, and in vitro fertilization (IVF) may be used by those with fertility problems. Because lesbian couples lack access to sperm, they must decide how to impregnate the selected mother. Most couples who used a known sperm donor opted for vaginal insemination. Typically, the nonovulatory partner collected the sperm from the donor's home. Post insemination, many women would elevate legs and buttock for 30 minutes to promote the sperm's movement into the uterus. Often, several trials were necessary for impregnation with this method.

Intrauterine insemination took place at a fertility clinic. As part of this process, health care staff and counselors interviewed the couple to determine their perceived ability to parent. Blood tests and a physical exam were done prior to a 6-month waiting period to determine that the sperm was healthy and disease-free. Generally, only couples who could not get pregnant by other methods used IVF.

In summary, it is obvious that childbearing is a deliberate and conscious decision for lesbian couples. Creating a **de novo** family requires a great deal of planning and preparation. To meet the needs of every childbearing family, health care providers must be mindful of evidence-based research findings and exercise cultural sensitivity when caring for clients who are different from the dominant culture. Simply replacing applications that designate the mother and father with those using the word *parents* shows sensitivity to lesbian couples/families.

Maternal Role Attainment

Based on cross-cultural observations and psychological research, John Bowlby (1999) formulated the theory of attachment as a relationship between a young child and caregiver that is necessary for strong social and emotional development. Klaus and Kennell (1982) further described the importance of maternal and infant interactions, known as bonding behaviors, directly after birth in forming this attachment. Recognizing the importance of maternal–infant bonding for child development, the American Academy of Family Physicians (AAFP) promotes family-centered care, which most hospitals practice today. In the 1980s, bonding rooms—where parents moved to a private room after delivery to hold and marvel at their newborn prior to standard separation—became the norm. Bonding rooms preceded LDRP/LDR (labor, delivery, recovery, postpartum) rooms where bonding takes place today. Not separating the newborn from the family is common practice in many Western hospitals. Obstetrical nurses in LDR settings facilitate maternal role attainment by encouraging evidence-based procedures such as allowing the newborn to rest skin to skin on the mother after delivery, breastfeeding in the first hour, and deferring newborn weighing and other procedures that used to be performed immediately after birth.

An example of successful maternal role attainment is seen in a study conducted with mothers who conceived via IVF. Research indicates that women with infertility issues often experience high levels of stress and anxiety, as well as low self-esteem. Abadi, Zandi, Shiva, Pourshirvani, and Kazemnejad (2018) divided a sample of 60 women who had IVF into control and intervention groups. Each group completed the *Maternal Self-Report Inventory* (MSRI). The intervention group then participated in a four-session maternal preparation program designed to enhance maternal self-esteem. The premise of the program was that higher self-esteem facilitates maternal role fulfillment that promotes mother–infant attachment that, in turn, facilitates positive fetal development. Immediately and 1 month after program completion, both groups took the MSRI again. The intervention group's scores were higher than the control group, indicating program's effectiveness in promoting the maternal role fulfillment. The study findings showed that the program improved the self-esteem of mothers undergoing IVF. The study's clinical implications suggest that nurses working with women conceiving via IVF can help enhance maternal self-esteem and motherhood facilitation by implementing maternal preparation programs as part of their care (Abadi et al., 2018).

Nontraditional Support Systems

In the United States, most pregnant women seek prenatal care from a physician and plan a hospital delivery. According to data collected by the American College of Nurse Midwives (ACNM), CNMs and CMs attended 332,107 of US births in 2014. This number represents 12.1% of all vaginal births or 8.3% of total US births (American College of Nurse Midwives, 2016). The numbers are relatively small compared to the rest of the industrialized world in which more than 70% of pregnant women are cared for by midwives who achieve better birth outcomes compared to the United States (Lake & Epstein, 2008). Because of Western medicine's historically curative focus, many Western medical care providers view pregnancy as a physiologic state that can become pathologic at any movement. With medicine's shift toward disease prevention and health promotion, many nurse practitioners and midwives who view pregnancy as a normal physiologic process do not see pregnant women as sick patients in need of physician-provided curative services unless a medical condition arises. Many cultural groups also perceive pregnancy as a normal physiologic process. Some pregnant women avoid prenatal care classes at medical centers due to their fear of receiving unnecessary medical interventions.

Since the introduction of Lamaze childbirth education classes in the 1970s, pregnant women and their partners have placed an increasing emphasis on the quality of prenatal care and the childbirth experience. While middle-class White women initiated this trend, many traditional cultural groups have continued their indigenous and cultural practices including African Americans, Hispanics, Filipinos, Asians, and Native Americans.

It is essential that nurses conduct a thorough cultural assessment to identify whether the pregnant woman plans to use nontraditional support systems, Western health care, or a blend of both during her pregnancy. Since childbearing is viewed as "women's work" among some cultures, husbands or partners are often not expected to attend prenatal appointments. In contrast, their husbands not only accompany them to prenatal appointments but expect all pregnancy-related questions to be directed to him. Nurses unfamiliar with this custom need to adjust their approach to provide culturally congruent care. Additionally, nurses should discuss patients' use of any herbs or folk medicines. Finally, helping pregnant mothers develop a prenatal care plan can allow nurses to gain an understanding of the cultural traditions that are important to the woman during this period.

A woman's choice about the type of support she wants during labor often is culturally significant and must be explored during the antenatal period. Pregnant women should be encouraged to discuss their needs with the provider and formulate a written birth plan. Research demonstrates that laboring women greatly value and benefit from the presence of someone they trust to provide emotional, psychological, and practical support and advice (Kabakian-Khasholian et al., 2017). Having continuous labor support also has several clinical benefits: a shorter labor, increased rates of spontaneous vaginal birth, decreased use of intrapartum analgesia, fewer cesarean sections, and increased patient satisfaction with the childbirth experience. The World Health Organization's (WHO, 2018a) recommendations encourage all laboring women to have their companion of choice present during labor and childbirth to improve the quality of their care.

Cultural Beliefs Related to Antenatal Care

First-trimester care is encouraged in traditional Western prenatal care. According to *National Vital Statistics Reports*, 77% of women began prenatal care in the first trimester and 4.6% in the third trimester, and 1.6% did received no prenatal care (Osterman & Martin, 2018). The WHO implemented new guidelines and recommendations when they introduced the 2014 WHO Antenatal Care Model (ANC). The four-visit focused ANC (FANC) model recommended that pregnant women have at least four visits with a health care provider. However, this model was replaced in 2016 due to evidence supporting the efficacy of having eight contacts with a health care provider during pregnancy to include screening for anemia, gestational diabetes, and UTIs (WHO, 2016). Box 5-2 compares the WHO's two ANC schedules.

BOX 5-2 | Comparing World Health Organization Antenatal Care Schedules

WHO FANC Model	2016 WHO ANC Model
First trimester	
Visit 1: 8–12 weeks	Contact 1: up to 12 weeks
Second trimester	
Visit 2: 24–26 weeks	Contact 2: 20 weeks
	Contact 3: 26 weeks
Third trimester	
Visit 3: 32 weeks	Contact 4: 30 weeks
Visit 4: 36–38 weeks	Contact 5: 34 weeks
	Contact 6: 36 weeks
	Contact 7: 38 weeks
	Contact 8: 40 weeks
Return for delivery at 41 weeks if not given birth	

Source: World Health Organization (WHO). (2016). WHO recommendations on antenatal care for a positive pregnancy experience. Retrieved from http://www.who.int/reproductivehealth/publications/maternal_perinatal_health/anc-positive-pregnancy-experience/en/

Another way for pregnant women to receive care and support is through **participatory women groups** (PWG). PWG defined by Gram et al. (2018) employs trained facilitators to hold scheduled community meetings where groups of local women are led through a cycle of problem identification, action planning, strategy implementation, and outcome evaluation. Qualitative evidence from providers in high-income countries suggests that such group sessions are enjoyable and informative for clients and an efficient use of provider time (Downe et al., 2017). Pilot studies of PWG have occurred in Ghana, Malawi, and Tanzania. Trials of participatory learning and action groups also were conducted in Bangladesh, India, Malawi, and Nepal. Trained individuals whose aim was to identify, prioritize, and address concerns women faced about pregnancy, childbirth, and postpartum care facilitated these groups. Community women shared information on a monthly basis, and groups participated in activities related to the specific health topic covered that month (WHO, 2016). CenteringPregnancy is a popular PWG model used in the United States. Due to the evidence that PWGs can help reduce maternal and perinatal mortality, the WHO supports this prenatal care approach (WHO, 2016).

Nursing personnel are in an excellent position to teach patients and promote positive prenatal care outcomes. Initially, nurses working in a prenatal setting should examine their own cultural beliefs and practices about pregnancy in order to compare them to and understand other culture's practices. The most important part of reviewing cultural practices is determining if they are safe. Pregnant women who are ingesting culturally accepted foods should be informed if such substances could be harmful to a developing fetus. Immigrant women's country of origin also should be documented, including women who are the second generation in the primary country. Such information is important in discovering potentially harmful cultural and indigenous practices

BOX 5-3 | Risk Factors for Lead Exposure in Pregnant and Lactating Women

- Recent emigration from or residency in areas where ambient lead contamination is high; women from countries where leaded gasoline is still being used (or was recently phased out) or where industrial emissions are not well controlled
- Living near a point source of lead including lead mines, smelters, or battery recycling plants (even if the establishment is closed)
- Working with lead or living with someone who does; women who work in or who have family members who work in an industry that uses lead (e.g., lead production, battery manufacturing, paint manufacturing, shipbuilding, ammunition production, or plastic manufacturing)
- Using lead-glazed ceramic pottery; women who cook, store, or serve food in lead-glazed ceramic pottery made in a traditional process (usually imported by individuals outside the normal commercial channels)
- Eating nonfood substances (pica); women who eat or mouth nonfood items that may be contaminated with lead, such as soil or lead-glazed ceramic pottery
- Using alternative or complementary substances, herbs, or therapies; women that use imported home remedies or certain therapeutic herbs traditionally used by East Indian, Indian,

- Middle Eastern, West Asian, and Hispanic cultures that may be contaminated with lead
- Using imported cosmetics or certain food products; women who use imported cosmetics, such as kohl or surma or certain imported foods or spices that may be contaminated with lead
- Engaging in certain high-risk hobbies or recreational activities; women who engage in high-risk activities (e.g., stained glass production or pottery making with certain leaded glazes and paints) or have family members who do
- Renovating or remodeling older homes without lead-hazard controls in place; women who have been disturbing lead paint, have been creating lead dust, or have been spending time in such a home environment
- Consumption of lead-contaminated drinking water; women whose homes have leaded pipes or source lines with lead
- Having a history of previous lead exposure or evidence of elevated body burden of lead; women who may have high body burdens of lead from past exposure, particularly those who have deficiencies in certain key nutrients (calcium or iron)
- Living with someone identified with an elevated lead level; woman who may have exposure in common with a child, close friend, or other relatives living in the same environment

Source: Centers for Disease Control and Prevention (CDC). (2010). *Guidelines for the identification and management of lead exposure in pregnant and lactating women*. Atlanta, GA: U.S. Department of Health and Human Services. Retrieved from https://www.cdc.gov/nceh/lead/publications/leadandpregnancy2010.pdf

that are uncommon in Western society. For example, performing a lead-exposure assessment is imperative for patients who have emigrated from a country where lead-based cosmetics, pottery, spices, or gas are used (see Box 5-3).

In Western culture, antenatal blood tests, ultrasounds, and pelvic exams are common components of routine care. However, nurses should not expect these practices to be common in other cultures. For example, a nurse should help ease

the anxiety of a Muslim woman receiving a pap smear for the first time at age 30 by explaining the procedure and showing her the instruments to be used. If while doing so the client indicates she does not want to know more but just wants "to get it over with," these feelings should be honored and accepted.

Myunghee, Thongpriwan, Choi, Choi, and Anderson (2018) conducted a qualitative study to understand the prenatal genetic testing decision-making processes among pregnant Korean American women in the United States. Ten Korean American women whose provider recommended they undergo amniocentesis during pregnancy participated in the study. All participants were born in Korea and immigrated to the United States. Four themes emerged from the data analysis: facing the challenges of decision-making, seeking support, determining one's preferred role in the decision-making process, and feeling uncomfortable with the patient's degree of autonomy in the US health care system. Most participants felt it would have been easier to make a decision if they were guided by trustworthy people (mother, sister, God, or fate), while others were unsure if they could make the decision and were afraid that it was even theirs to make. Some participants indicated it was scary that the obstetrician left the decision-making power in their hands. One participant explained that, in Korea, the provider would make the decision and she would honor it. Communication barriers were evident. Nine of the college-educated participants had trouble understanding the genetic counselor and obstetrician even with a translator: "All I could do was listen to [the translator] talk over my head." If the providers involved in this study were more sensitive to Korean culture, they could have allowed more time for test clarification and explained the shared decision-making in the US system. This study supports the practice of health care professionals providing trusting, cultural-sensitive health care that allows pregnant women to ask questions and feel comfortable making autonomous decisions.

Food Taboos and Food Cravings

Due to the body's increasing demand for energy and nutrients during pregnancy, it is important that pregnant women have a nutritious dietary intake. Many cultures have food **taboos** that expand during pregnancy and the postpartum period (Withers, Kharazmi, & Lim, 2018). One cultural practice is that a mother should eat what she craves because "the baby must need this." Unfortunately, food taboos can contribute to unhealthy nutritional practices in pregnancy. For example, in Africa, the giant African snail and grass cutter or cane rat are inexpensive, rich sources of animal protein that can serve as vital nutrition in a balanced diet. However, due to cultural beliefs, they are not readily consumed even though they are available (Ekwochi et al., 2016). **Pica**—eating nonnutritious substances such as clay, red dirt, and starch—is seen often in the Southern United States and among African American populations. Pica has been described for centuries (Hippocrates, 1849) and is found in most cultures. While there can be a relationship between pica and low hemoglobin levels, this is not the case for everyone. Latina American women have been known to have cravings for rocks, sand, ice, chalk, and charcoal during pregnancy (Roy, Furentes-Afflick, Fernald, & Young, 2018). It is extremely important that nurses assess for food taboos and pica during the initial visit as part of the pregnant woman's dietary intake. The nurse should discuss the importance of the nutrients essential to maintaining a healthy pregnancy and the growing fetus' development. In their study, Banu et al. (2016) found that younger women (less than 30) were more likely to eat a balanced diet, take prenatal vitamins with folic acid, take iron and calcium tablets, and attend antenatal care and health education classes. The older women in the study tended to incorporate customary practices and give less credence to eating a balanced diet and receiving antenatal care (Banu et al., 2016). Some food items avoided during pregnancy and the related beliefs are listed in Box 5-4.

It is imperative that nursing professionals determine who the dominate person is in the client's home. In modern Western culture, women often plan and address their own prenatal health needs. In other cultures, however, the pregnant woman's husband/male partner, mother-in-law, mother, or grandmother may handle these issues. If the client lives in a community without blood relatives, her support person could be

BOX 5-4 | Food Taboos During Pregnancy

Food Taboos During Pregnancy: Rural and Urban Tamil Nadu

Food	Beliefs
Ripe papaya	Causes loose stool, abdominal pain
Raw papaya	Causes abortion
Pineapple	Causes cough
Grapes, banana, and custard apple	Causes cold
Grapes (black)	Causes child to be born with a dark complexion
Curd, buttermilk	Causes cough and cold
Maize/corn	Abdominal pain
Yam	Allergy to the child
Hot beverages (especially coffee)	Causes child to be born with a dark complexion
Chicken	Causes loose stools, uterine contractions

Source: Banu, K. K., Prathipa, A., Anandarajan, B., Ismail Sheriff, A. M., Muthukumar, S., & Selvakumar, J. (2016). Food taboos during antenatal and postpartum period among the women of rural and urban areas of Tamilnadu. *International Journal of Biomedical and Advance Research, 7*(8), 393–396. doi: 10.7439/ijbar.v7i8.3539

Food Taboos and Myths for Pregnant Women and Children in Nigeria and Ghana

Food	Beliefs
Snail	Makes baby sluggish in life and spit too much saliva Ghana: do not eat snails out of respect for ancestors
Bush meat like glasscutter (*Thryonomys swinderianus*)	Causes labor to be difficult and prolonged delivery
Starch foods like *garri* (cassava flakes)	Baby will have excess weight making delivery difficult except by surgery
Do not give eggs to children under age 2	It will cause them to start stealing because it is very sweet
Avoid sweet in small children	Children will get worms
Don't allow children to drink garri	Causes eye problems

Source: Ekwochi, U., Osuroah, C. D. I., Ndu, I. K., Ifediora, C., Asinobi, I. N., & Eke, C. B. (2016). Food taboos and myths in South Eastern Nigeria: The belief and practice of mothers in the region. *Journal of Ethnobiology and Ethnomedicine, 12*, 7. doi: 10.1186/s13002-016-0079-x

a community woman elder who attends all her prenatal visits. It is vital that the support person is recognized in accordance with HIPAA laws. While today's nurses are comfortable with the culture of the Westernized health care system, it can be overwhelming to an immigrant from a low- or middle-income country. Nurses should help pregnant women feel comfortable when introducing them to the Westernized health care system. A pregnant client may express a concern about a taboo and its consequences, such as "If you breastfeed the baby before the breast milk is in (colostrum), the baby will become sick." In this case, the nurse—recognizing that she is referring to the vitamin- and nutrient-rich colostrum—can explain the scientific evidence about the benefits of this fluid and encourage the mother to breastfeed. However, the nurse must realize that breastfeeding is the mother's decision, regardless of scientific evidence.

Substance Use

In the United States, a patient's social history is taken as part of prenatal care. This assessment includes asking the patient about cigarette smoking, alcohol consumption, and illicit drug use. In order to complete a thorough assessment, particularly for a client with ties to another culture, nurses must be familiar with substances indigenous to that group. Khat (*Catha edulis*) is a natural stimulant that is widely cultivated and used in East Africa and the Middle East. The most common way to use khat is chewing the raw leaves. Khat enhances mood and alertness as it is consumed but can contribute to depression, anxiety, and insomnia with longer-term usage. In the areas where khat use is common, its use is widely accepted among pregnant women (Nakajima et al., 2017).

According to Sharma, van Teijlingen, Hundley, Angell, and Simkhada (2016), alcohol and pregnancy are culturally linked. In Africa, rum can be given to Akan (a people group in Southern Ghana and adjacent parts of the Ivory Coast) and Igbo (a people group in Southeastern Nigeria) children. Additionally, in Ghana, births are often celebrated with alcohol at naming ceremonies. Greek physicians and Gurung (a people group in Nepal) women may use alcohol to help children go to sleep. Finally, Malaysians may bathe their children in stout (beer) in the belief that it protects babies and cures newborn jaundice.

Cultural Preparation for Childbirth

In the media-filled society, there is plethora of information and education available to support a healthy pregnancy. In the United States as well as many Westernized countries, childbearing women attend childbirth education classes with their birth partner or support person.

Women from culturally diverse backgrounds often want to incorporate culture-specific activities into their care. The fact that pregnancy is viewed in many cultures as a normal event not requiring medical intervention likely contributes to women opting to receive antenatal care and give birth at home using traditional and indigenous birth attendants.

Health professionals must obtain a thorough cultural assessment to determine a pregnant woman's intention to use nontraditional cultural practices during her antenatal care and to assess her birth expectations. A birth plan can incorporate cultural desires along with the beneficial aspects of Westernized hospital culture to ensure a safe, satisfying childbirth. Accommodations should be made to support the childbearing families' cultural desires whenever possible.

Nurses who work in communities that cater to specific cultural groups might consider developing childbirth classes that incorporate specific cultural practices. Facilitating open communication between a hospital's health care providers and cultural group leaders when developing such programs would be beneficial for the hospital and the cultural groups they serve.

Birth and Culture

Childbirth is a biological event where the transition into motherhood happens in one of two ways: vaginal delivery or cesarean section. Culture, religion, family traditions, and values influence birthing plans. A woman's religion could determine what type of provider she uses for childbirth. For example, a Muslim woman may request having only female providers for her delivery. Some cultures believe supernatural forces, either benevolent or malevolent, can affect pregnancy and childbirth. In Bangladesh, people believe in a *jinn* or *bhut* (an evil spirit) that can give the evil eye, a curse, or harm a pregnant woman (Raman, Nicholls, Ritchie, Razee, & Shafiee, 2016). In Western culture, birthing often is a family affair that includes the baby's father, grandparents, siblings, and other family members. The family also plays an active role in the type of birth experience desired. In cultures where birthing is considered "women's work," only the mother-in-law and traditional midwife accompany the laboring woman to the health care clinic or special birthing shed. Cultural practices can dictate the birthplace, position, and members present. Boxes 5-5 and 5-6 describe various cultural practices for birth.

BOX 5-5	Cultural Influences on Antenatal, Intrapartum, and Postpartum Care in Asian Countries

Country	Belief
Antenatal	
Pakistani	Avoid hot foods during pregnancy (sugar, nuts, beans, and maize [hot]) as they are abortifacients. Avoid cold foods (buttermilk, oranges, and curd) because they harm the fetus. Prenatal massages are a common practice to promote maternal and infant health. Use amulets and holy water to solve problems instead of seek help from a health care provider. Lower caste births should take place in a cowshed or specially constructed place.
Indonesia	Eating fish makes breast milk tastes and smells bad. Avoid prenatal vitamins, as they cause excess fetal growth and discourage an easy delivery.
Chinese	Eating shrimp causes the baby to have skin allergies. Eating rabbit meat leads to cleft palate development. Eating meat harms fetal health. Use traditional herbs used for bathing, enemas, ointments, treating nausea and vomiting, and labor stimulation. Use of traditional practitioners, spiritual healers, and religious leaders as to protect a pregnancy. Eating more than half of a banana may cause birth obstruction.
Papua New Guinea	It is the woman's responsibility to dispose of the placenta, as pregnancy and birth is "polluting."
Thailand	Eating shellfish and Northern Thai relishes prevents the perineum from drying out after birth. Thai eggplant will cause anal pain after giving birth.
Labor	
India	Feed women clarified butter, ginger, lentils, milk, or tea to facilitate labor by promoting warmth.
Laotian	Drinks holy water and coconut milk. Places holy water or eggs on the abdomen to ease birth.
Nepal	Drinks cumin seed soup and glucose water to gain strength for birth.
Birthing	
Bangladeshi	Having a hospital delivery is stigmatizing. Pregnancy is normal, so your baby should be delivered at home. "They don't let you bury placenta in hospital." Hospitals and health centers are a place for treating someone with health problems and disease. Giving birth at a hospital lying on your back is not preferred. Sitting, squatting, or kneeling during delivery is desired. "If you go to a hospital, you are forced to have surgery."
Nepal, Bangladesh, India, Papua New guinea	Purifications and rituals protect woman from evil spirits. Malevolent spirits could cause continuous, forceful bleeding and blood clots. Women should seek help from traditional healers. Use mustard oil or turmeric for childbirth; rub it on the newborn and the umbilical cord stump (Nepal).

BOX 5-5	Cultural Influences on Antenatal, Intrapartum, and Postpartum Care in Asian Countries (continued)

Country	Belief
Postpartum	
China, Cambodia, Laos, Nepal, Thailand, Myanmar, Singapore, Vietnam	Restrict mother's movement to help her rest and rebuild strength, as postpartum women are weak, fragile, and vulnerable to illness. Practice sexual abstinence for 30–40 days, and don't bathe, wash hair, or practice dental hygiene (China, "doing the month"). Refrain from reading, eating, or drinking while standing, moving around excessively, experiencing strong emotions, and doing housework. Consume hot foods and avoid cold foods but during the 1st month postpartum. Avoid cold vegetables (e.g., water spinach, spinach, and pumpkins). Hot foods (e.g., beef, mutton, rice with black pepper, anchovies, salted fish, coffee, and milk) are suitable for postpartum mothers.
Cambodia	Spirits (*priey krawlah pleung*) can attack a woman left exposed after birth causing seizures, fainting, and altered consciousness.
Bangladesh, China, Nepal	Women should seek help from trained birthing assistants for any postpartum issues.
China	Cold foods create an imbalance of *qi*, which leads to poor circulation, a weak bladder and uterus, and sore black muscles. Cold foods are fruit and raw or cooked vegetables such as cabbage, bamboo shoots, and turnips. Eating spicy, hot food can cause a baby to be born hairless. Drinking coffee and tea decreases infant intelligence.
Myanmar	Burmese women shave the newborns head at 2 months to remove infants "dirtiness" from coming through the birth canal. Breastfeeding to age 2 is culturally indicated.

Source: Withers, M., Kharazmi, N., & Lim, E. (2018). Traditional beliefs and practices in pregnancy, childbirth and postpartum: A review of the evidence from Asian countries. *Midwifery*, 56, 158–170. doi: 10.1016/j.midw.2017.10.019

The most common health care providers for a childbearing woman throughout the world are midwives, except in the United States where obstetricians and hospitals dominate childbirth. More than 90% of births are under the care of obstetricians in the United States, compared to Europe where midwives are the main providers for 75% of births (Guerra-Reyes & Hamilton, 2017). However, it was not always like this in the United States. During the 1900s, midwives attended 50% of all US births. This number decreased to 12.5% by 1935 despite half of all African American births being attended by midwives. The Sheppard–Towner Act of 1921 resulted in the widespread regulation of African American "granny" midwives. This act was followed by the 1948 push to standardize medicine and eliminate lay healers, which gained a momentum around the time the American Medical Association was formed. As a result, by 1972, midwives attended only 1% of all US births. Today, the trend toward midwife-attended births is highest among non-Hispanic White women (11%) and African American women (8%) (Yoder & Hardy, 2018).

While US birthing typically takes place in a hospital, out-of-hospital births have increased

BOX 5-6 | Childbirth and Postnatal Cultural Practices in Nepal and Other Countries

Cord Cutting Rituals

- Cord is cut with a sickle and then antiseptic, cooking oil, ghee (butter), toothpaste, or ash is applied to the umbilical stump (Nepali).
- Cord is cut with a scythe and stump is cleaned with water (Tamang).
- Placenta is buried at the foot of a tree (Gurung).
- Placenta is buried at a junction or under the road (Newari, Tamang).
- Placenta is buried at a junction in Mexico (old Jewish texts tell pregnant woman not to stand alone at the crossroads, as "they may see the fetus taken away by evil powers").
- Placenta is a dirty object and therefore must be buried and fire burned over it to prevent evil spirits and animals from reaching it. If any part of the woman touches the placenta, the lochia might dry up causing harm to her baby and possibly neonatal death (Lao).
- The placenta must "roast" to provide heat to stimulate the mother's healing (Burmese and Lao).
- Cord cut after the placenta is delivered; the cord cutter remains unholy and cannot go for prayer for 40 days (Bangladesh).
- The child's future health is linked to the placenta.

Rest and Seclusion

- The postnatal mother is not allowed to go into the kitchen until the 9th day; then she is sent to another person's home for about 10 to 15 days and can stay as long as she wishes up to a month (Tamang).
- Mother and new baby are massaged with mustard oil to relax the mother's muscles and help the child grow.
- In the maternal home, the new mother is cared for and fed a diet of lentils and spices (such as cumin) to stimulate breast milk production.
- Isolate women in the stable or shed during menstruation and pregnancy (Tamang and Newari).

Purification, Naming, and Weaning Ceremonies

- The birth of a baby is believed to be unclean.
- A day is set aside to clean the home and bathe the mother and baby.
- At the ceremony, a nwaran name is given to the baby based on the astrological sign.
- The ceremony takes place between the 3rd and 12th day after birth.
- The ritual is celebrated on the 9th day for girl and on the 11th day for boy.
- The new mother cannot go out before the ceremony, she can't go to temple, and no one will touch her or take the child directly from her, as she is considered dirty; fire is used to burn the woven mat women lie on during and after childbirth (Bahun).
- After the ceremony, the mother returns to household activities.
- The sleeping child is placed in sari, as the cloth is believed to offer protection from the evil eye.
- The ceremony timing varies by ethnic groups: Nwaran is on the 3rd day for Tamangs, 7th day among Bahun and Chhetri, and on the 9th or 12th day for Newar communities. The higher the caste of the family, the later the ceremony is held.
- In Greece, birth customs include women and babies resting and being isolated for 40 days after birth (during the "lochia period").
- Women in Zaire and India are secluded in a hut.
- For Muslims, the postnatal seclusion period traditionally lasts 40 days.
- In Burma and Turkey, women are more vulnerable to evil spirits during the postnatal

| BOX 5-6 | Childbirth and Postnatal Cultural Practices in Nepal and Other Countries (continued) |

period: "the grave of a woman who have just gave birth is open for 40 days."

- In Bangladesh, purdah (female seclusion) lasts 5 to 9 days, and dietary restrictions can last up to 6 months.
- For the Negev Bedouin in Israel, the 40-day postnatal period includes seclusion (homestay) followed by congratulatory visits and food.
- Among Mayans, the period lasts 20 days.
- Among Japanese, mothers remain in a birth chamber for 3 weeks.
- The Chinese postnatal period ("sitting month" or "doing the month") lasts 30 or 40 days. Traditional Chinese medicine is given to women who are believed to be in a weak state during the postpartum period.
- In Nepal, new mothers stay with their babies continuously for 6 days ("the up sitting") after which bed linens would be changed on the 10th day and the mother would be allowed to perform housekeeping duties.
- Burmese women rest for a 40-day period ("the quarantine" time) for purification and rest.
- In many cultures, postnatal women are believed to be dirty and weak (Japan, China, Canadian Intuits, Turkey, and Bangladesh).
- In England, the postnatal time is called the "lying-in period."
- In Germany, the period is called the wochenbett or "child bed."
- US customs are guided by self-help books that indicate it takes 6 weeks for the uterus to return to a nonpregnant size and bleeding to abate; similar guidelines are used for UK moms.
- Nepal and Mayan women get postpartum massages.
- China found that the 40-day seclusion period can adversely affect woman's mental health (postpartum depression).

- The Church of England has a thanksgiving and cleansing ritual to welcome new mothers back to church.
- In the Scottish highlands, churches hold a cleansing ritual ("kirking") to allow women polluted by childbirth to come back to church.
- The Greek orthodox Archdiocese in the United States states, "woman may stay home for 6 weeks after birth according to Leviticus XII: ...."
- Jewish women are allowed back into temple 33 days after the birth of son and 66 days after the birth of daughter.
- Laotian women believe that advance preparation of baby clothes would lead to the newborn's death.

Nutrition and Breastfeeding

- Special foods may be given during the postnatal period: kwati (beans and meat), dahi-chura (curd and beaten rice with curry meat), and gudpak (a sweet cake, rich in calories made with flour, clarified butter, cashews, and coconut).
- Newborns are given hamma ghuti, balmrita (Ayurvedic medicine herbs), and Jaiphal (nutmeg).
- Women who adhere to traditional foods in Burma and Turkey are not given any water to drink for 2 to 3 days after birth.
- For Cantonese Chinese, the pregnant mother is considered cold and the fetus hot. In Vietnam, both mother and fetus change from cold in the first trimester to hot in the last. The concept of hot and cold also exists in Laos.
- In Nepal, India, and other places in South Asia, colostrum is not given to an infant until the priest approves it, as it is considered pus.

(continued)

BOX 5-6	Childbirth and Postnatal Cultural Practices in Nepal and Other Countries (continued)

- In Bangladesh, breastfeeding is poor, and colostrum is not given, as it is considered "dirty milk." In the first 40 days, breast milk is given along with sweet water (misi pani); wealthier houses give babies goat or cow milk after 40 days.
- In Cairo, breastfeeding last 40 days.
- In one study, most participants discarded their colostrum, which they felt was inadequate in nutritional value.
- In contrast, the WHO recommends breastfeeding in the 1st hour after birth.

Alcohol Plays an Important Role in the Birth and Postpartum Periods in Nepal

- Alcohol and pregnancy are linked culturally; some women are allowed to sip it during labor.
- Alcohol is given to Akan and Igbo children.
- It is used for celebration at the naming ceremony; it also is thought to confer protection on children.
- Mayans bathe babies in stout (beer) to protect them from jaundice.

Source: Sharma, S., van Teijlingen, E., Hundley, V., Angell, C., & Simkhada, P. (2016). Dirty and 40 days in the wilderness: Eliciting childbirth and postnatal cultural practices and beliefs in Nepal. *BMC Pregnancy and Childbirth, 16*(1), 147. doi: 10.1186/s12884-016-0938-4

by 72% (from 0.87 in 2004 to 1.50 in 2014) (MacDorman & Declercq, 2016). Prior to labor, nurses should discuss with clients any specific things they would like to do during their labor and birth to determine what, if any, accommodations need to be made (see Evidence-Based Practice 5-5).

Cultural Expression of Labor

A woman's culture and religious beliefs can include taboos that can affect how a woman responds to labor. It is important to assess clients' comfort/pain level to determine if she needs a comfort intervention. Some women who believe it is a taboo to scream during labor may appear stoic with the pain of contractions. Ghanaian women's cultural beliefs are that crying out might delay the birth and taking pain medication may not be beneficial. Some cultures believe that shouting and crying with pain is a sign of weakness (Raman et al., 2016). Other cultures view childbirth pain as natural, and therefore the stronger the pain, the better. Because stoicism often is culturally expected, it is important to assess the mother's needs throughout the course of labor.

Birth Positions

In the United States, women birthing in hospitals with obstetricians typically deliver in the lithotomy position. In contrast, women receiving midwifery care in the United States deliver in a variety of positions: lithotomy, side lying, squatting, and hands and knees. Birth positions influenced by culture include sitting, squatting, or kneeling. Bangladeshi women favor all three positions, Mexican American women tend to favor birthing chairs, and Laotian Hmong women generally prefer a squatting position. Boxes 5-5 and 5-6 show specific birthing positions related to different cultures. During prenatal care, preparation for birth should include conversation about the mother's birthing expectations, including the desired birthing position. Do not assume that a client delivering in a hospital expects to deliver in a lithotomy position. It is important that the nursing staff and delivery provider offer culturally sensitive care during the birthing process.

Cultural Meaning Attached to Infant Gender

Infant gender preferences vary from culture to culture. Historically in Western culture, families

World Health Organizations Recommendations: Intrapartum Care for a Positive Childbirth Experience

The WHO's intrapartum care recommendations are encouraged globally, regardless of the setting or the birthing environment's level of health care. The recommendations are neither country nor region specific but designed for use with all birth-ing women. The 56 guidelines are geared toward woman-centered care to optimize the labor and childbirth experience for women and their babies through a holistic, human rights–based approach. Listed below are a few of the recommendations.

Care Option	Recommendation	Category of Recommendation
Care throughout labor and birth		
Respectful maternity care	Respectful care—which refers to care organized for and provided to all women in a manner that maintains their dignity, privacy, and confidentiality—ensures freedom from harm and mistreatment and enables informed choice and continuous support during labor and childbirth are recommended	Recommended
Effective communication	Effective communication between maternity care providers and women in labor, using simple and culturally acceptable methods, is recommended	Recommended
First stage of labor		
Oral fluid and food	For women at low risk, oral fluid and food intake during labor is recommended	Recommended
Second stage of labor		
Method of pushing	Women in the expulsive phase of the second stage of labor should be encouraged and supported to follow their own urge to push	Recommended
Third stage of labor		
Delayed umbilical cord clamping	Delayed umbilical cord clamping (not earlier than 1 minute after birth) is recommended for improved maternal and infant health and nutrition outcomes	Recommended
Controlled cord traction (CCT)	In settings where skilled birth attendants are available, CCT is recommended for vaginal births if the care provider and the parturient woman regard a small reduction in blood loss and a small reduction in the duration of the third stage of labor as important	Recommended

(continued)

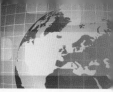

World Health Organizations Recommendations: Intrapartum Care for a Positive Childbirth Experience (continued)

Care Option	Recommendation	Category of Recommendation
Uterine massage	Sustained uterine massage is not recommended as an intervention to prevent postpartum hemorrhage (PPH) in women who have received prophylactic oxytocin	Not recommended
Newborn care		
Routine nasal or oral suction	In neonates born through clear amniotic fluid who start breathing on their own after birth, suctioning of the mouth and nose should not be performed	Not recommended
Skin-to-skin contact	Newborns without complications should be kept in skin-to-skin contact with their mothers during the first hour after birth to prevent hypothermia and promote breastfeeding	Recommended
Breastfeeding	All newborns, including low birth weight babies who are able to breastfeed, should be put to the breast as soon as possible after birth when they are clinically stable and the mother and baby are ready	Recommended

Reference: World Health Organization (WHO). (2018a). WHO recommendations: Intrapartum care for positive childbirth experience. Retrieved from http://www.who.int/reproductivehealth/publications/intrapartum-care-guidelines/en/

prefer males as the first born to solidify male inheritance of the family finances and property, carry on the family name, and assume the head-of-household role if the needs arise. With females legally able to inherit family property and having the ability and desire to take responsibility for caring for aging family members, modern society reports family preferences for a mix of genders among children.

According to Dubuc and Devinderjit (2017), son preference and prenatal sex selection against females have resulted in a significant imbalance in birth–sex ratio in several Asian countries, including India and China. The development of prenatal sex determination techniques by ultrasound screening has made sex-selective abortion possible. In addition, IVF combined with prefertilization selection of male spermatozoa (sperm sorting) allows sex selection of offspring.

Male child preference is still common in South Asia, Africa, the Middle East, China, and Turkey. Rouhi, Rouhi, Vizheh, and Salehi (2017) hypothesized that maternal perception of a family's male child preference was a risk factor for antenatal depression. Their study included a sample of 780 pregnant Iranian women and used the Iranian version of the Edinburgh Postnatal Depression Scale. Maternal perception of male child preference was common and associated with an antenatal depression value of 20.1%. Women who had a daughter from previous pregnancy were more likely to experience depression during the present pregnancy. Even when women and their families preferred female children but were content with having a boy, they feared being criticized by their husbands and his family if they had a female child.

To address these concerns, nurses should consider a woman's cultural background when discussing fetal/newborn gender. Additionally, establishing a trusting relationship with the woman may allow her to verbalize her feelings related to the selected gender. Assessment of antenatal or postpartum anxiety and depression related to gender preference also should be evaluated during the antenatal and postpartum periods.

Culture and the Postpartum Period

Most women who deliver in a US hospital are discharged 48 hours after a vaginal birth and 72 hours after a cesarean section. Nurses provide a great deal of teaching during this period, including providing information about breastfeeding and newborn care. With help from the nursing staff, the mother should be able to rest, take care of her newborn, and reflect on her birthing experience. It is important for nurses to observe a new mother's interaction with her newborn. A nurse who is unfamiliar with the practice of the mother-in-law acting as the dominant caregiver might think that the mother is not interested in the child. However, it is important to assess and be aware of cultural practices in which it may be taboo for the mother to handle the child and instead one of the baby's grandmothers assumes this role.

In some Muslim cultures, the postnatal seclusion period traditionally lasts 40 days. Performance of religious rituals on the 40th day may include shaving of the newborns hair, due to the unclean passage of the infant through the

vagina (Sharma et al., 2016). The Punjabi cultural tradition of *Sawa Mahina* is their period requiring 40 days of complete rest—however by their choice, mothers can take part in a few domestic chores after several weeks (Qamar, 2017). Japanese women may return to their mother's home during the birth period to receive care by their mother. This tradition is known as *gae ri bunben* (home to the village to give birth). In China, the women "do the month," a resting period expected to restore balance (Withers et al., 2018).

Filipino and Hispanic cultural belief systems include the practice of *balancing opposites*—that there are natural, external factors that must be kept in balance to maintain health. In other words, to restore a disrupted balance, you must apply the opposite. For example, to treat a "hot" condition such as a fever, the person eats cold food (fresh vegetables, meats, and dairy products). Conversely, hot foods (chocolate, aromatic beverages, cheese, and eggs) are consumed to treat a "cold" condition such as a headache (Withers et al., 2018).

Adams and Smith (2018) conducted an integrative review of 13 studies that identified factors affecting postpartum care in the developing countries of Nigeria, Uganda, the Philippines, Jordan, Pakistan, Nepal, Cameroon, South Africa, Egypt, Indonesia, and Bangladesh. Some cultures that regard childbirth as a natural process do not view postpartum care as a standard practice. In Ugandan culture, normalization of the birth process prevented clients from participating in postpartum visits. In Bangladesh, a woman must stay in a private room for 7 to 10 days after birth and therefore cannot leave for care. However, according to Adams et al. (2017), 34% to 50% of rural Malawi women receive a postpartum assessment (including having their blood pressure and temperature measured and their abdomen, vagina, and breasts examined) before discharge from a health care facility. Adams and Smith's (2018) review also found that women exposed to mass media were more likely to attend postpartum care appointments. In addition, women and men with higher educational and income levels who were not farm workers were more likely to seek postpartum care. The WHO (2015) noted that 99% of global maternal mortality occurs in developing countries, with more than half in sub-Saharan Africa. Nurses are in the best position to inform women about the importance of postpartum care and assess the family's understanding of its importance. See Boxes 5-5 and 5-6 to review cultural practices and rituals for the postpartum period.

Postpartum Depression

Postpartum depression (PPD) is associated with adverse infant and maternal outcomes such as less breastfeeding and poor maternal–infant bonding (Centers for Disease Control and Prevention [CDC], 2017; Wouk, Stuebe, & Meltzer-Brody, 2016). According to Alexander, LaRosa, Bader, Garfield, and Alexander (2017), PPD is commonly seen in women with a history of depression, relationship issues, a lack of social support, and negative life experiences. According to Ko, Rockhill, Tong, Morrow, and Farr (2017), PPD affects about one of every nine women in the United States. Greenberg, Fournier, Sisisky, Pike, and Kessler (2015) estimated that the economic burden of depression in the United States is $210.5 billion and can be attributed to workplace-, health care–, and suicide-related costs. Clearly, the prevalence of PPD means that it contributes to these costs.

The American College of Obstetricians and Gynecologists (ACOG) (2015) recommends women be screened at least once during the prenatal period using a standardized tool such as the *Edinburgh Postnatal Depression Scale*. Nurses should include information about PPD in their discharge teaching and have family members present to inform them of the condition. The women's support system needs to be identified and documented in her care plan. Additionally, women who experience signs or symptoms of PPD must be given follow-up information.

Treatment for PPD must be individualized, taking into account each women's unique preferences and cultural needs. Nyguyen (2017) conducted a literature review of alternative PPD therapies. In the review of 27 RCTs, 15 showed significant improvement in the intervention group over the control group, and 10 behavior therapies were found to be effective. Several studies demonstrated the efficacy of Internet- or telephone-delivered interventions, indicating that these modes of delivering education and counseling can be valid solutions that also increase health care access (Nyguyen, 2017).

Nurses must be cognizant of the signs and symptoms of PPD. Inquiring about a woman's history of PPD, depression, anxiety, and any other mental health issues is an important part of perinatal and postpartum care. For minority groups that are part of a subculture, such as immigrants, nurses should assess the support offered by their community groups to ensure they are not isolated when they return home.

In Western culture, PPD treatment typically involves prescribing pharmaceuticals. This approach may not be culturally appropriate for all groups. The health care team must find culturally acceptable treatments that will support the woman while addressing the problem's underlying cause.

Postpartum Dietary Prescriptions and Activity Levels

Despite being in a hospital setting, women often follow cultural practices related to the postpartum period. For example, Hispanics see pregnancy and childbearing as a hot state that requires the ingestion of cold foods during the postpartum period. In contrast, people in Asian cultures will not drink cold water, instead consuming only hot drinks during this period. In many Asian cultures, the woman does not leave the house for 28 to 40 days, during which time the mother-in-law is responsible for food preparation and infant care. African Americans may have an older female family member in charge of the room environment, monitor visitors, and care for the baby and new mother. It is common to have multiple visitors who bring food to the hospital for the new mother.

Nurses need to observe and inquire what foods are desired and taboo during this period to ensure the mother is receiving sufficient nutrition and fluid intake. The importance of continuing prenatal vitamins should be discussed. If certain foods are not customarily eaten due to cultural beliefs or likes and dislikes, the nurse should formulate a dietary guide of acceptable foods in order to support a healthy postpartum diet. See Box 5-4 for pregnancy and postpartum food taboos.

Postpartum Rituals

Placental burial rituals are part of postpartum traditions in several sub-Saharan African countries. The ritual also is found in Asian cultures and among some members of the African American community. Postpartum clients may request a container to use for the ritual burial of their placenta. It would be helpful if this request is incorporated in their care plan and supported by the facility. If placental burial is a cultural practice, health care facilities need to have guidelines about how to store placentas until patient discharge. Nurses working in postpartum areas should be aware of the cultural rituals of their surrounding community. Even though placental burial may seem out of the ordinary to those in Western culture, supporting cultural differences remains important. See Boxes 5-5 and 5-6 for a list of postpartum rituals.

Cultural Influences on Breastfeeding and Weaning

Several organizations recommend exclusive breastfeeding for the first 6 months of a baby's life (AAFP, 2014; Association of Women's Health, Obstetric and Neonatal Nurses [AWHONN], 2015a; Committee on Health Care for Underserved Women & ACOG, 2007). Research documents the advantages of breast milk for infants (development and immune support) and mothers (decreased risk of breast and ovarian cancers) (Victoria et al., 2016). Even when exclusive breastfeeding is not possible, even a small amount of breast milk consumed in the first few days of life is beneficial.

The breastfeeding initiation rate is 81.1% in the United States (CDC, 2014). African American women initiate breastfeeding at a much lower rate (66.3%) compared to White (84.3%) and Hispanic (83.0%) women (CDC, 2015) (see Evidence-Based Practice 5-6).

Alghamdi, Horodynski, and Stommel (2017) conducted an RCT with 540 low-income mothers of non-Hispanic White, African American, and Hispanic ethnicity to examine the racial and ethnic differences in their maternal knowledge, self-efficacy, and propensity to breastfeed. Data analysis showed that White mothers had the highest mean knowledge scores followed by African American and then Hispanic mothers. The results also indicated that Hispanic mothers had significantly lower self-efficacy in infant feeding than did Whites and African Americans, while White and African American mother's scores were similar in this category. After adjusting for mother's age and education, marital, and working status, the odds of breastfeeding was significantly higher among Hispanic mothers than among White and African Americans. The authors attributed the Hispanic mothers' higher odds of breastfeeding despite having the lowest infant feeding knowledge and self-efficacy scores to their social and cultural breastfeeding expectations (Hohl, Thompson, Escareno, & Duggan, 2016).

Shin et al. (2018) conducted an RCT of 150 pregnant women of Mexican descent to examine the influence of acculturation and cultural values on their breastfeeding practices. The results showed that a higher score on the Anglo orientation subscale of the Acculturation Rating Scale for Mexican Americans instrument was associated with less breastfeeding at 1-month postpartum and less exclusive breastfeeding. The researchers concluded that if an Anglo orientation is present

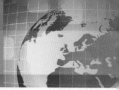

A Qualitative Study of Social, Cultural, and Historical Influences on African American Women's Infant-Feeding Practices

DeVane-Johnson, Giscombe, Williams, Fogel, and Thoyre (2018) described the cultural factors influencing African American mothers' perceptions about infant feeding. The participants were a purposive sample of 39 African American woman of diverse ages (26 to 45 years), educational backgrounds, and socioeconomic status. Six focus groups were conducted with a non-breastfeeding group (NBFG) and a breastfeeding group (BF), resulting in the following themes listed below with participant comments.

Theme 1: It Takes a Village

- "I grew up thinking breastfeeding was a White thing, I never saw a black woman breastfeed." "Everyone in my family bottle feeds, it's just been generationally. That's the way Grandma did it and continued." "But it's just like my aunts are old-fashioned. They're like, no, we're not allowed to do in front of family members." (NBFG)

Theme 2: Real-World Issues

- Work—"I think I feel more working moms, a lot of us really couldn't breastfeed. But I think by us being working, we didn't really have a choice to breastfeed." Other women described the inability to advance in the workplace while pumping and having no place to store milk. (NBFG)
- Pain—"I guess my boobs were really sore, so when my baby started to suck on them, they were really tender, so I stopped, I didn't want him to be on me."

Theme 3: Personal Realities

- "I wanted to make sure someone else could help." "I wanted a little bit of freedom, the bottle was easier." Artificial supplementation gave a sense of "empowerment." Formula feeding was described on social messaging as normal, convenient, and natural. (NBFG)
- "It's enough that you already have the spotlight because you are Black. If you are Black and you nurse, it's an additional, 'Oh my gosh, look at that person with that baby.'" "There's newer formulas that can replicate what's coming out of me, I have a choice today…"
- "Breast milk adjusts based on the needs of the baby, I want to be as natural as possible. I do not know what's in formula" (BFG)

Theme 4: Historical Stigma

- "The stealing of breast milk from the slaves. They put them down on their stomach and they will squeeze their breast into the jugs until they were empty."
- "Breastfeeding was what they had to do because the economy at that time for Blacks it was not that good. So mother, she breastfeed because she had to."
- "This day and time Black women have a better choice. So that is why I chose to bottle-feed, because I did have a better choice."
- "Some just associate breastfeeding with slavery, wet-nursing, and the lack of choice. So they feel like a formula will be a step up."

Theme 5: Negative Body Image (Breast-Related Self-Esteem and Body Image Issues Affect Infant-Feeding Decisions)

- "I was not happy with my breasts. I got boobs early and I would hunch to try and hide them." One-group member shared her satisfaction with her breasts because they were large yet reported disappointment that they did not produce milk, "I prayed to God every night for big breasts. I really do love my breasts, I just wish they would have done right for my babies." (NBFG)

A Qualitative Study of Social, Cultural, and Historical Influences on African American Women's Infant-Feeding Practices (continued)

Theme 6: Breastfeeding Described as "Nasty" (This Description Was Shared by Both Groups)

- "I chose to bottle-feed because I thought breast-feeding was nasty." "I thought it was nasty like 'Ooh, she got the baby sucking her breast!'" (NBFG)
- One woman said she received a message from her family that breastfeeding was nasty: "Breastfeeding is like taboo. I have a sister that's older than me and when she found out that I was breastfeeding, I wasn't allowed to do it at her house because she said it was nasty." (BFG)

Clinical Implications

- Nurses and health care professionals working with African American women must be made aware of the underlying historical stigma that can be related to breastfeeding by some members of this community (e.g., referencing slavery and wet nurses) compared to other racial/ethnic clients.
- Nurses should begin discussing the benefits of breastfeeding early during prenatal care.
- Nurses can promote breastfeeding demonstrations with the use of a shawl or blanket to decrease breast exposure and protect modesty.
- Health care professionals should prioritize culturally sensitive care while avoiding cultural or racial stereotypes that limit their ability to provide the highest quality of services.

Reference: DeVane-Johnson, S., Giscombe, C. W., Williams, R., Fogel, C., & Thoyre, S. (2018). A qualitative study of social, cultural, and historical influences on Africa American women's infant-feeding practices. *Journal of Perinatal Education*, 27(2), 71–85. doi: 10.1891/1058-1243.27.2.71

among mothers of Mexican descent, the nurse can emphasize the fact that breastfeeding is experiencing increasing acceptance in mainstream society and is congruent with Anglo norms.

Pérez-Escamilla, Martinez, and Segura-Pérez (2016) conducted a narrative, systematic review to examine the impact of the Baby-Friendly Hospital Initiative (BFHI) on breastfeeding and child health outcomes in 19 different countries located in South America, North America, Western Europe, Eastern Europe, South Asia, Eurasia, and sub-Saharan Africa. The BFHI is a key component of the WHO/United Nations Children's Fund's Global Strategy for Infant and Young Child Feeding, whose aim is to improve short, medium, and long-term breastfeeding outcomes. Community support was found to be a key factor for long-term breastfeeding sustainability.

Breastfeeding in several Asian cultures can include exclusive breastfeeding for 6 months and continuing breastfeeding for up to 2 years of age. While the practice of breastfeeding to age 2 is not common in Western society, it is common in indigenous societies. Nurses must remember to be culturally sensitive by not judging women breastfeeding a toddler, instead supporting their right to breastfeed.

Cultural Issues Related to Intimate Partner Violence

In the United States, homicide is one of the leading causes of death for women aged ≤44 years, resulting in the death of 3,519 girls and women in 2015 (Petrosky et al., 2017), and while the rate for homicide of females varies by race/ethnicity, nearly half of all victims are killed by current or former male intimate partners. **Intimate partner violence** (IPV) refers to behavior by an intimate partner or ex-partner that causes physical, sexual, or psychological harm, including physical aggression, sexual coercion, psychological abuse, and controlling behaviors. Analysis of 2003–2014 homicide data from the National Violent Death Reporting System indicated that among 10,018 women homicide victims ≥18 years in 18 states, more than half (55.3%) were related to IPV (Petrosky et al., 2017).

IPV is a serious social problem and public health issue. Existing data from more than 80 countries indicate that one in three women (35%) has experienced physical and/or sexual violence by an intimate partner or nonpartner sexual violence (WHO, 2017). IPV affects all countries. IPV prevalence estimates vary 23.2% in high-income countries, 24.65% in the Western Pacific region, 37% in the Eastern Mediterranean region, and 37.7% in the Southeast Asian region (WHO, 2017).

According to Chen et al. (2017), the incidence of IPV during pregnancy is estimated to be between 0.9% and 26%, depending on the IPV definition and study design used. Pregnant women are more vulnerable to the harmful effects of IPV because violence affects both maternal and fetal health and outcomes. Significant outcomes related to IPV are pregnancy-related death, inadequate antenatal care, labor complications, emotional distress, anxiety, depression, physical injury, preterm delivery, low birth weight, fetal death/miscarriage, and the need for neonatal intensive care (Chen et al., 2017; Malan, Spedding, & Sorsdahl, 2018).

Psychological and verbal intimate partner abuse (PIPA) during pregnancy is defined as the use of threats, jealousy, possessiveness, humiliation, constant destructive criticism, insults, belittling, ridiculing, and instigating false accusations (Debono, Borg Xuereb, Scerri, & Camilleri, 2017). PIPA during pregnancy is under the umbrella of IPV and rarely analyzed as a construct on its own merit. It is estimated that only 6% to 43.2% of such incidents are reported. Gentry and Bailey (2014) found a significant association between threat exposure during pregnancy and low birth weight.

Lee and Lee (2018) conducted a cross-sectional study of 250 pregnant South Korean married women to identify factors predictive of IPV. In South Korea, about 12% of married women report having an IPV experience during their lifetime. The results indicated that 34% of the pregnant women had experienced some form of IPV including psychological, physical, or sexual violence in the previous 12 months. Non-IPV group participants had a higher rate of employment and intended pregnancy compared to the IPV group. In addition, the non-IPV group had a significantly higher social support score than did the IPV group. IPV was more common among women with a graduate school education than among high school graduates. Unemployment also was significantly associated with IPV. The authors indicated that no investigation of IPV among pregnant women was previously conducted in South Korea. South Korean cultural norms dictate that women avoid exposing IPV. The authors suggested the need to screen and report violence toward pregnant women by their partners and provide social support during prenatal examinations. They also advocated for the legal system to mandate reporting of IPV cases in prenatal care settings (Lee & Lee, 2018).

Rogathi et al. (2017) conducted a prospective cohort study of 1,013 Tanzanian women to determine if PPD is associated with IPV experienced during the perinatal period. The results indicated that one out of three participants was exposed to IPV during pregnancy, and these events were strongly associated with the development of PPD. The authors indicated that seeking help from professionals, family members, or friends for depression is not typically part of the Tanzanian culture. For this reason, it is detrimental to train health care workers to assess for IPV as it creates awareness about the depression.

The WHO's multicountry study instrument was developed to identify women exposed to IPV (WHO, 2005). Rasch et al.'s (2017) study aim was to develop and determine the validity of a screening instrument in pregnant women in Tanzania and Vietnam. For the study, 1,309 Vietnamese women and 1,116 Tanzanian women were interviewed before 24 weeks of pregnancy and again between their 30th and 34th weeks. In the evaluation of the question combinations' performance, the researchers determined that asking three, simple questions allowed them to identify women exposed to IPV during pregnancy in two different countries. The authors stressed that a screening tool's cultural transferability should be considered, as they might perform differently according to the setting in which they were developed (Rasch et al., 2017).

In the United States, the Pregnancy Risk Assessment Monitoring System collects data from postpartum women regarding various health indicators including IPV. Findings from the most recent survey showed that 2.6% of women had experienced IPV in the 12 months before pregnancy and 2.2% were abused during pregnancy (Petrosky et al., 2017). According to AWHONN (2015b), "Women should be universally screened for IPV in private, safe settings where healthcare is provided" (p. 405). However, a survey of nurse practitioners, nurses, and primary care clinicians in California found that only 14% of providers always screened for IPV and 34% rarely or never performed screenings. Participants stated two reasons for not screening: they lacked confidence to screen for IPV and did not know how to assist women who had experienced violence (Tavrow, Bloom, & Withers, 2016).

For their hospital quality improvement project, Bermele, Andresen, and Urbanski (2018) implemented an IPV protocol for screening and case management on a Midwestern hospital's intrapartum unit. All unit nurses were trained about IPV and abuse during pregnancy, and RNs completed learning modules and participated in role-play scenarios. Women who needed support were referred to the unit's social worker. The scores indicated a significant increase in nurses' knowledge from the pretest (75%) to the posttest mean score (94%). Of the patient respondents, 64% reported experiencing abuse ($n = 25$) and were referred to the social worker (Bermele et al., 2018). Health care workers caring for childbearing women should screen them for IPV in a private place using culturally sensitive questions tailored to the community's population.

Hispanic Pregnant Women

As an ethnic group, Hispanics share a heritage that includes strong family and religious elements. As with any cultural group, differences exist, with subgroups maintaining distinct cultural beliefs and customs. For Hispanics, relatives and older family members are respected and often consulted on decisions involving health and illness (see Figure 5-7).

The incidence of IPV among Hispanics, including pregnant women, is not addressed in the literature. The National Intimate Partner and Sexual Violence Survey State Report (Petrosky et al., 2017) measures IPV in up to 21 states in the United States, but not all states report this data. The latest reporting on IPV prevalence by race/ethnicity indicates that 34.4% of Hispanic women experienced some form of lifetime contact sexual violence, physical violence, and/or stalking by an intimate partner.

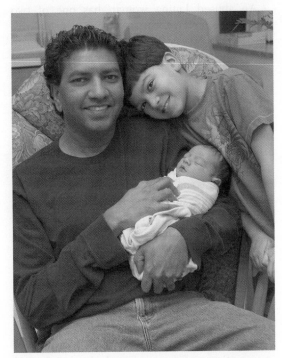

Figure 5-7. Hispanic dad, brother, and newborn (Glenda/https://www.shutterstock.com).

Several external factors can contribute to IPV among Latinos: immigration status, lower socioeconomic status, acculturation stress, and *machismo* (a term used in Latin America to describe male domination in the relationship) (Alvarez, Davidson, Fleming, & Glass, 2016). Additionally, due to cultural expectations not to express anger, Latinas may internalize their fears and conceal IPV because they feel everything must be done to keep the family together.

The aforementioned factors put abused Hispanic pregnant women at a disadvantage for accessing prenatal care, particularly if their partner is not amenable. Unfortunately, other factors also can affect Latina women's access to prenatal health care where they might get help for IPV: lack of health insurance coverage or knowledge of how to obtain insurance, language barriers, low education levels, and low-paying jobs. In addition, she may feel she lacks access to legal and social services, as well as not having any extended family or other support networks.

An abused Latina woman has one of two choices. Stay and try to make the relationship with the abuser work, or leave. Latinas often prefer to tell family members, female friends, or neighbors about IPV, while non-Latinas may be more likely to tell health care workers or clergy. Therefore, if the women's family is not in the United States and she does not have a supportive community, the situation becomes even more difficult. Low-acculturated Latinas are less likely to seek and use formal social services than their more acculturated counterparts. Additionally, Latinas often hesitate leaving their abuser, to keep with traditional norms of staying in a marriage.

Latina victims may be less likely to call the police due to undocumented immigration status, heightened immigration enforcement policies, and increased fear of deportation. Immigration status has been reported to be a control mechanism used by partners to make sure their victims do not leave or report the violence. This control mechanism is well supported by the realities of immigration enforcement and the heightened incidence of deportation.

Nurses and other health care providers are in good position to establish a trusting relationship with abused women so they can effectively screen for IPV. Hospitals and health care clinics should realize the advantage of employing qualified health care professionals and staff members who represent members from the Latino community. A Spanish-speaking health care provider might be able to form a trusting relationship with Latina women more quickly, enabling her to confide about experiencing IPV. Since the first sign of abuse is not always an admission of the problem, good assessment skills are vital. Physical signs of trauma should be discussed using a concerned and supportive approach. Even if IPV is denied, discussing the topic with clients and presenting statistics will inform them that they are not alone in this situation. Assisting abused Latina women can include involving the family and ethnic community structure (if applicable), notifying shelters, and providing referrals for legal counsel and community social services for emergency health care and resources. The best approach will involve helping the woman recognize that she is not to blame for the IPV and providing support to help her find her own strength.

Indigenous Peoples/Native American Pregnant Women

There are 560 federally recognized Indigenous People/Native American tribes in the United States with a concentration of 229 tribes in Alaska (see Figure 5-8). Unfortunately, far too many Indigenous women are experiencing IPV. The National Council of American Indians considers IPV as one of the most important issues facing Indigenous women today. According to the National Institute of Justice (Rosay, 2016), four in five Indigenous women experience violence in their lifetimes. In her qualitative research study, Matamonasa-Bennett (2015, p. 2) stated, "Most Native American scholars agree that IPV was almost non-existent in pre-contact cultures, and that, if it did occur, it was severely sanctioned." Before European colonization, IPV was rare among Native Americans, as Indigenous

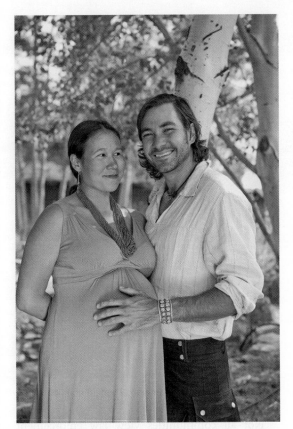

Figure 5-8. Native American pregnant couple (Mona Makela/https://www.shutterstock.com).

communities were familial, social, and spiritual organizations that had flexible, egalitarian gender roles and afforded women power (Burnette & Renner, 2017). According to the National Congress of American Indians Policy Insights Brief (2013), Indigenous women on tribal lands lack the most government protections from the threat of violence against them. While each reservation is considered a sovereign nation, tribal courts currently do not have jurisdiction to prosecute nontribal members for sexual assault and rape, even if they occur on a tribal land. Additionally, federal and state authorities often claim that the reservation is outside their jurisdiction (Weitz, 2017). This fact is significant because in 67% of rape or sexual assault cases, Indigenous women describe their offenders as non-Native.

For her qualitative study, Matamonasa-Bennett (2015) interviewed nine Indigenous men to examine their IPV-related beliefs, perspectives, and experiences. In this culture, alcohol—introduced by Europeans—is a symbol of destruction, colonization, and foreign invasion. The men related IPV to the use of substances including alcohol and drugs. According to Burnette and Renner (2017), structural inequalities and internalized dominant beliefs are risk factors for suboppression in which minority males oppress women and children to regain some level of control because striking out directly at the oppressor would be too risky. Therefore, Indigenous males may lash out at those with less power, such as women and children, through lateral violence.

The purpose of Burnette and Renner's (2017) study was to understand the evolution of victimization in the lives of Indigenous women. They interviewed 29 Indigenous women who experienced family violence and maltreatment as children. Five themes were revealed: overlapping and cumulative victimization experiences, pregnancy as vulnerability for IPV, jealousy fueled by insecurity, patriarchal gender norms disadvantaging women, and substance abuse.

Indigenous women may not discuss their situations, as they may be embarrassed about IPV in their communities. Strong physical assessment skills in nurses are crucial for detecting any physical signs of abuse. Once detected, nurses always should offer information about and support for IPV. Most domestic violence services within Indigenous communities are modeled after those used with the general population. It is extremely important to develop community- and culture-specific support programs for this vulnerable group.

An Indigenous woman may decide to speak with a family member or female elder prior to speaking with a health care team member. Several strategies can be used to help identify Indigenous women who require IPV supportive services. These strategies include increasing provider awareness of high IPV rates among this population and involving community elders and spiritual leaders in facilitating healing circles at the health care center with women's health-related topics including domestic violence. An IPV victim who decides to stay with her husband/partner must be continually supported by nurses who remain compassionate and empathetic while ensuring the client understands the nurses' concern for her and her unborn child's safety.

African American Pregnant Woman

Many African Americans participate in a culture that focuses on the importance of family and church. Family includes not only mother, father, sister, and brother but also the extended kinship of grandparents, aunts, uncles, cousins, and close individuals who, while not "blood" related, play an important role in the family system. The church has traditionally been a sanctuary for members of the African American community, offering spiritual worship, fellowship, education, guidance, and counseling (see Figures 5-9 and 5-10).

The IPV rate among the African American population is 43.7% compared with 37.1% for non-Hispanic Whites. After examining depression and IPV among African American women living in impoverished inner-city neighborhoods, Mugoya et al. (2017) found that 97.3% of participants (n = 295) experienced IPV, with most women experiencing minor psychological abuse and about half experiencing both physical assault and psychological aggression. Eighty-eight percent of the participants reported receiving economic assistance, and women with low education levels were significantly more likely to experience IPV. Research indicates that IPV is associated with depression, posttraumatic stress symptoms, and suicidal ideation in low-income African American women (Fincher et al., 2015). Alhusen, Frohman, and Purcell (2015) conducted a study of predominately African American (93%) pregnant women that found depressive symptomatology and experiencing IPV were associated with increased risk of suicidal ideation.

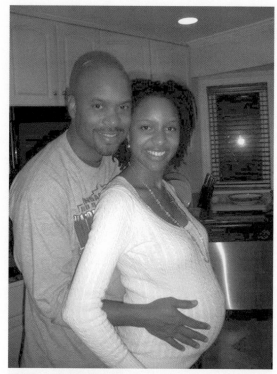

Figure 5-9. African American pregnant couple.

Not all communities view law enforcement agencies in the same way. Calling the police to the African American community for a domestic violence situation can be viewed as problematic, due to the incidences of police shooting unarmed people of color, particularly African American men.

Despite its prevalence, IPV is not considered an acceptable action in African American culture. As with other marginalized minority groups, African Americans may feel disengaged from the dominant society due to poor educational attainment, low incomes, job stress, or unemployment. In addition, drug and alcohol use also is common among abusers.

Nurses who work in the prenatal setting have an opportunity to initiate a caring, trusting relationship with the pregnant woman while gathering information. To protect her man, the abused woman may not reveal she is a victim because in her eyes he also is a "victim of society" as an African

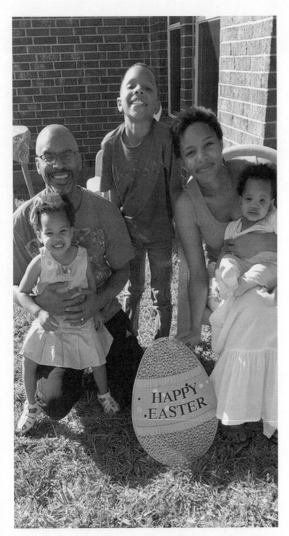

Figure 5-10. African American family.

American man. She may choose to remain in the relationship due to emotional attachment, financial dependence, shame, child custody issues, and anxiety about family and community responses to a separation. Nurse-provided education must stress the detrimental effects abuse can have on her and her unborn child's health. Even if she sees her partner as a "victim," she needs to learn that this is not a valid reason for accepting abuse. The client should be given information about community support systems and shelters and offered a referral to a social worker. Additionally, if applicable, the nurse should encourage her to speak with a trusted family or clergy member who can help improve interactions between the partners. Moreover, the nurse should help the women develop an escape plan should she feel unsafe and need to leave. This plan should indicate where she should go, what she should take, and whom she should call. Finally, nurses should ask follow-up questions and offer support at each visit.

Summary

As the United States moves toward a heterogeneous society, health professionals who work with childbearing women must incorporate cultural practices into their care plans. Health care providers should perform honest self-evaluations to assess their personal cultural beliefs and biases. All patients deserve compassion, support, and the best health care possible, regardless of their race, ethnicity, and socioeconomic status. As nurses and health care providers, we are taught to be nonjudgmental when caring for our patients. Providing cultural competent care is crucial for our patient's well-being.

REVIEW QUESTIONS

1. Describe the special needs of an African American childbearing family due to the health disparities of infant mortality and maternal morbidity.
2. How would you assess the obstetrical history and culture needs of a pregnant woman arriving at your clinic for prenatal care who does not speak English, however she has her 12-year-old son with her for interpretation of her native language of Spanish?
3. How do you assist your community health care center to be more involved in providing culturally centered care for the Native American women who fear coming for care due to the community perception of unnecessary labor interventions?

4. How would you describe a typical birthing option in a Westernized hospital to an immigrant woman that had two previous home births in her native country of Tibet? How could you assist her with a birth plan?

5. What nursing intervention would you use for a pregnant Asian woman (who speaks some English) who presents to the prenatal clinic with bruising on her left arm and abdomen (found on the initial physical exam)? When you inquire about the bruising, she begins to cry and tells you that she is alone in this country and her family is in Thailand. How do you provide culturally supportive care?

CRITICAL THINKING ACTIVITIES

1. Critically analyze and describe the culturally competent nursing intervention for an African American postpartum female who

desires to breastfeed but is concerned that her sisters and aunt think it is a bad choice. How would you support her decision?

2. Discuss the responses a postpartum nurse would make when she notices an Asian woman refuses to shower and is not eating her breakfast of cereal and orange juice or drinking cool water from the pitcher.

3. You are the labor nurse with a Ghanaian patient who refuses pain medication in labor. She is having strong palpable contractions every 2 minutes and tears are running down her face. What can you do to ensure her comfort?

4. Describe and analyze how the nurse might alter her care approach for a patient whose culture requires the father of the newborn to whisper a prayer in the infants' ear as the first sound they hear initially after birth?

REFERENCES

Abadi, A. S., Zandi, M., Shiva, M., Pourshirvani, A., & Kazemnejad, A. (2018). Effect of preparation for maternal role program on self-esteem of women undergoing in-vitro fertilization. *Evidence Based Care Journal, 7*(4), 63–72.

Adams, Y. J., & Smith, B. A. (2018). Integrative review of factors that affect the use of postpartum care services in developing countries. *Journal of Obstetric, Gynecologic, & Neonatal Nursing, 47*(3), 371–384. doi: 10.1016/j.jogn.2018.02.006

Adams, Y. J., Stommel, M., Ayoola, A., Horodynski, M., Malata, A., & Smith, B. (2017). Use and evaluation of postpartum care services in rural Malawi. *Journal of Nursing Scholarship, 49*(1), 87–95. doi: 10.1111/jnu.12257

Alexander, L. L., LaRosa, J. H., Bader, H., Garfield, S., & Alexander, W. J. (2017). *New dimensions in women's health* (7th ed.). Burlington, MA: Jones & Bartlett Learning.

Alghamdi, S., Horodynski, M., & Stommel, M. (2017). Racial and ethnic differences in breastfeeding, maternal knowledge, and self-efficacy among low-income mothers. *Applied Nursing Research, 37*, 24–27. doi: 10.1016/j.apnr.2017.07.009

Alhusen, J. L., Frohman, N., & Purcell, G. (2015). Intimate partner violence and suicidal ideation in pregnant women. *Archives of Women's Mental Health, 18*(4), 573–578. doi: 10.1007/s00737-015-0515-2

Alvarez, C. P., Davidson, P. M., Fleming, C., & Glass, N. (2016). Elements of effective interventions for addressing intimate partner violence in Latina women: A systematic review. *PLoS One, 9*(11), e0160518. doi: 10.1371/journal.pone.0160518

American Academy of Family Physicians. (2014). Breastfeeding, family physicians supporting [Position paper]. Retrieved from http://www.aafp.org/about/policies/all/breastfeeding-support.html

American College of Nurse Midwives (ACNM). (2016). Factsheet CNM/CM-attended Birth Statistics in the United States. Retrieved from www.midwife.org/acnm/files/ccLibraryFiles/filename/000000005950/CNM-CM-AttendedBirths-2014-031416FINAL.pdf

American College of Obstetricians and Gynecologists (ACOG). (2015). The American College of Obstetricians and Gynecologists committee opinion no. 630. Screening for perinatal depression. *Obstetrics and Gynecology, 125*(5), 1268–1271. doi: 10.1097/01.AOG.0000465192.34779.dc

Arousell, J., & Carlbom, A. (2016). Culture and religious beliefs in relation to reproductive health. *Best Practice & Research Clinical Obstetrics & Gynaecology, 32*, 77–87. doi: 10.1016/j.bpobgyn.2015.08.011

Association of Women's Health, Obstetric and Neonatal Nurses (AWHONN). (2015a). AWHONN position statement. Breastfeeding. *Journal of Obstetric, Gynecologic, and Neonatal Nursing, 44*(1), 145–150. doi: 10.1111/1552-6909.12530

Association of Women's Health, Obstetric and Neonatal Nurses (AWHONN). (2015b). AWHONN position statement. Intimate partner violence. *Journal of Obstetric, Gynecologic, and Neonatal Nursing, 44*(3), 405–408. doi: 10.1111/1552-6909.12567

Banu, K. K., Prathipa, A., Anandarajan, B., Ismail Sheriff, A. M., Muthukumar, S., & Selvakumar, J. (2016). Food taboos during antenatal and postpartum period among the women of rural and urban areas of Tamilnadu. *International Journal of Biomedical and Advance Research, 7*(8), 393–396. doi: 10.7439/ijbar.v7i8.3539

Barot, S. (2017). In a state of crisis: Meeting the sexual and reproductive health needs of women in humanitarian situations. *Guttmacher Policy Review, 20*. Retrieved from https://www.guttmacher.org/gpr/2017/02/state-crisis-meeting-sexual-and-reproductive-health-needs-women-humanitarian-situations

Berkatsky, N., (2015). The most common childbirth practice in America is unnecessary and dangerous. Why do doctors and patients insist on using electronic fetal monitoring? *The New Republic.* Retrieved from https://newrepublic.com/article/122532/most-common-childbirth-prac

Bermele, C., Andresen, P. A., & Urbanski, S. (2018). Educating nurses to screen and intervene for intimate partner violence during pregnancy. *Nursing for Women's Health, 22*(1), 79–86. doi: 10.1016/j.nwh.2017.12.006

Biggs, M. A., Neuhaus, J. M., & Foster, D. G. (2015). Mental health diagnoses 3 years after receiving or being denied an abortion. *American Journal of Public Health, 105*(12), 2557–2563. doi: 10.2105/AJPH.2015.302803

Bowlby, J. (1999). *Attachment and loss* (2nd ed., Vol 1). New York, NY: Basic Books.

Brown S. S., & Eisenberg, L. (1995). *The best intentions: Unintended pregnancy and the welling of children and families.* Washington, DC: National Academies Press.

Burnette, C. E., & Renner, L. M. (2017). A pattern of cumulative disadvantage: Risk factors for violence across indigenous women's lives. *British Journal of Social Work, 47*, 1166–1185.

Carson, L. D., Henderson, J. N., King, K., Klesznki, K., Thompson, D., & Mayer, P. (2015). American Indian diabetes beliefs and practices: Anxiety, fear, and dread in pregnant women with diabetes. *Diabetes Spectrum, 28*(4), 258–263. doi: 10.2337/diaspect.28.4.258

Centers for Disease Control and Prevention (CDC). (2010). *Guidelines for the identification and management of lead exposure in pregnant and lactating women.* Atlanta, GA: U.S. Department of Health and Human Services. Retrieved from https://www.cdc.gov/nceh/lead/publications/leadandpregnancy2010.pdf

Centers for Disease Control and Prevention (CDC). (2014). Breastfeeding report card United States/2014. Retrieved from https://www.cdc.gov/breastfeeding/pdf/2014breastfeedingreportcard.pdf

Centers for Disease Control and Prevention (CDC). (2015). Hospital actions affect breastfeeding. Retrieved from https://www.cdc.gov/vitalsigns/breastfeeding2015/index.html

Cesario, S. K. (2017). Immigration basics for nurses. *Nursing for Women's Health, 21*(6), 499–505. doi: 10.1016/j.nwh.2017.10.004

Chen, P. H., Rovi, S., Vega, M. L., Barrett, T., Pan, K. Y., & Johnson, M. S. (2017). Birth outcomes in relation to intimate partner violence. *Journal of the National Medical Association, 109*(4), 238–245. doi: 10.1016/j.jnma.2017.06.017

Committee on Health Care for Underserved Women, American College of Obstetricians and Gynecologists (ACOG). (2007). ACOG Committee Opinion No. 361: Breastfeeding: maternal and infant aspects. *Obstetrics and Gynecology, 109*(2 Pt 1), 479–480.

Costa, P., Pereira, H., & Leal, I. (2018). Through the lens of sexual stigma: Attitudes toward lesbian and gay parenting. *Journal of GLBT Family Studies, 1*–18. doi: 10.1080/1550428X.2017.1413474

Cutler, A., McNamara, B., Qasba, N., Kennedy, H. P., Lundsberg, L., & Gariepy, A. (2018). "I just don't know": An exploration of women's ambivalence about a new pregnancy. *Women's Health Issues, 28*(1), 75–81. doi: 10.1016/j.whi.2017.09.009

Debono, C., Borg Xuereb, R., Scerri, J., & Camilleri, L. (2017). Intimate partner violence: Psychological and verbal abuse during pregnancy. *Journal of Clinical Nursing, 26*(15–16), 2426–2438. doi: 10.1111/jocn.13564

Desai, G., Anand, A., Shah, P., Shah, S., Dave, K., Bhatt, H., ..., Modi, D. (2017). Sickle cell disease and pregnancy outcomes: A study of the community-based hospital in a tribal block of Gujarat, India. *Journal of Health, Population and Nutrition, 36*(1), 3. doi: 10.1186/s41043-017-0079-z

DeVane-Johnson, S., Giscombe, C. W., Williams, R., Fogel, C., & Thoyre, S. (2018). A qualitative study of social, cultural, and historical influences on Africa American women's infant-feeding practices. *Journal of Perinatal Education, 27*(2), 71–85. doi: 10.1891/1058-1243.27.2.71

Downe, S., Finlayson, K., Oladapo, O., Bonet, M., & Gulmezoglu, A. M. (2018). What matters to women during childbirth: A systematic qualitative review. *PLoS One, 13*(4), e0194906. doi: 10.1371/journal.pone.0194906

D'Souza, L., Jayaweena, H., Pickett, K. (2015) Pregnancy, diets, migration, and birth outcomes. *Health Care for Women International, 37*(9), 964–978. http://dx.org/10.1080/07399332.201.1102208

Dubuc, S., & Devinderjit, S. S. (2017). Gender preferences and fertility effects on sex-composition. Linking behavior and macro-level effects. Paper presented at the Annual Meeting of the Population Association of America, April 27–29, 2017, Chicago, IL.

Eichelberger, K., Doll, K., Edpo, G. E., & Zerden, M. (2016). Black lives matter: Claiming a space for evidence-based outrage in obstetrics and gynecology. *American Journal of Public Health, 106*(10), 1771–1772. doi: 10.2105/AJPH.2016.303313

Ekwochi, U., Osuroah, C. D. I., Ndu, I. K., Ifediora, C., Asinobi, I. N., & Eke, C. B. (2016). Food taboos and myths in South Eastern Nigeria: The belief and practice of mothers in the region. *Journal of Ethnobiology and Ethnomedicine, 12*, 7. doi: 10.1186/s13002-016-0079-x

Fikree, F. F., Lane, C., Simon, C., Hainsworth, G., & MacDonald, P. (2017). Making good on a call to expand method choice for young people—Turning rhetoric into reality for addressing Sustainable Development Goal Three. *Reproductive Health, 14*(1), 53. doi: 10.1186/s12978-017-0313-6

Fincher, D., VanderEnde, K., Colbert, K., Houry, D., Smith, L. S., & Yount, K. M. (2015). Effect of face-to-face interview versus computer-assisted self-interview on disclosure of intimate partner violence among African American women in WIC clinics. *Journal of Interpersonal Violence, 30*(5), 818–838. doi: 10.1177/0886260514536280

Finer, L. B., & Zolna, M. R. (2016). Declines in unintended pregnancy in the United States, 2008–2011. *The New England Journal of Medicine, 374*(9), 843–852. doi: 10.1056/NEJMsa1506575

Gentry, J., & Bailey, B. A. (2014). Psychological intimate partner violence during pregnancy and birth outcomes: Threat of violence versus other verbal and emotional abuse. *Violence and Victims, 29*(3), 383–392. doi: 10.1891/0886-6708.VV-D-13-00020

Gram, L., Skordis-Worrell, J., Manandhar, D., Strachan, D., Morrison, J., Saville, N, ..., Heys, M. (2018). The long-term impact of community mobilization through participatory women's groups on women's agency I the household: A follow-up study to the Makwanpur trial. *PLoS One, 13*(5), e0197426. doi: 10.1371/journal.pone.0197

Greenberg, P. E., Fournier, A., Sisisky, T., Pike, C. I., & Kessler, R. C., (2015). The economic burden of adults with major depression disorder in the United States (2005 and 2010). *Journal of Clinical Psychiatry, 76*(2), 155–162. doi: 10.4088/JCP.14m09298

Guerra-Reyes, L., & Hamilton, L. J. (2017). Racial disparities in birth care: Exploring the perceived role of African-American women providing midwifery care and birth support in the United States. *Women and Birth, 30*(1), e9–e16. doi: 10.1016/j.wombi.2016.06.004

Guttmacher Institute. (2015). Unintended pregnancies cost federal and state governments $21 billion in 2010. Retrieved from https://www.guttmacher.org/news-release/2015/unintended-pregnancies-cost-federal-and-state-governments-21-billion-2010

Guttmacher Institute. (2016). Unintended pregnancy in the United States. Retrieved from https://www.guttmacher.org/fact-sheet/unintended-pregnancy-united-states

Guttmacher Institute. (2018). Contraceptive use in the United States. Retrieved from https://www.guttmacher.org/fact-sheet/contraceptive-use-united-states

Hayman, B., Wilkes, L., Halcomb, E., & Jackson, D. (2015). Lesbian women choosing motherhood: The journey to conception. *Journal of GLBT Family Studies, 11*(4), 395–409. doi: 10.1080/1550428X.2014.921801

Herd, P., Higgins, J., Sicinski, K., & Merkurieva, I. (2016). The implications of unintended pregnancies for mental health in later life. *American Journal of Public Health Perspectives, 106*(3), 421–429. doi: 10.2105/AJPH.2015.302973

Hippocrates. (1849). *The genuine works of Hippocrates.* London, UK: Sydenham Society.

Hohl, S., Thompson, B., Escareño, M., & Duggan, C. (2016). Cultural norms in conflict: Breastfeeding among Hispanic immigrants in rural Washington state. *Maternal and Child Health Journal, 20*(7), 1549–1557. doi: 10.1007/s10995-016-1954-8

Holland, A. C., Strachan, A. T., Pair, L., Stallworth, K., & Hodges, A. (2018). Highlights from the U.S. selected practice recommendations for contraceptive use. *Nursing for Women's Health, 22*(2), 181–190. doi: 10.1016/j.nwh.2018.02.006

Kabakian-Khasholian, T., Bashour, H., El-Nemer, A., Kharouf, M., Sheikha, S., El Lakany, N., ..., Portela, A. (2017). Women's satisfaction and perception of control in childbirth in three Arab countries. *Reproductive Health Matters, 25*(Suppl. 1), 16–26. doi: 10.1080/09688080.2017.1381533

Kim, T. Y., Dagher, R. K., & Chen, J. (2016). Racial/ethnic differences in unintended pregnancy evidence from a national sample of U.S. Women. *American Journal of Preventive Medicine, 50*(4), 427–435. doi: 10.1016/j.amepre.2015.09.027

Klaus, M., & Kennell, J. (1982). *Parent-infant bonding* (2nd ed.). St. Louis, MO: Mosby.

Ko, J. Y., Rockhill, K. M., Tong, Y. T., Morrow, B., & Farr, S. L. (2017). Trends in postpartum depressive symptoms—27 states, 2004, 2008, and 2012. *Morbidity and Mortality Weekly Report, 66*(6), 153–158. http://dx.doi.org/10.15585/mmwr.mm6606a1

Lake, R. (Executive Producer), & Epstein, A. (Director). (2008). The business of being born [Indie Film/Documentary]. Retrieved from http://www.thebusinessofbeingborn.com/the-business-of-being-born/

Lee, I. S., Chang, M. H., Hwang J. I., Joo, J. S., & Chung, S. Y. (2016). *The domestic violence survey in 2016.* Seoul, Republic of Korea: Ministry of Gender Equality and Family. Retrieved from http://www.mogef.go.kr/eng/lw/eng_lw_s001d.do?mid=eng003

Lee, S., & Lee, E. (2018). Predictors of intimate partner violence among pregnant women. *International Journal of Gynecology & Obstetrics, 140*(2), 159–163. doi: 10.1002/ijgo.12365

MacDorman, M. F., & Declercq, E. (2016). Trends and characteristics of United States out-of-hospital births 2004–2014: New information on risk status and access to care. *Birth, 43*(2), 116–124. doi: 10.1111/birt.12228

MacDorman, M. F., Mathews, T. J., & Declercq, E. (2014) Trends in out-of-hospital births in the United States, 1990–2012. *NCHS Data Brief, 144*, 1–8.

Malan, M., Spedding M. F., & Sorsdahl, K. (2018). The prevalence and predictors of intimate partner violence among pregnant women attending a midwife and obstetrics unit in the Western Cape. *Global Mental Health*, 5, e18. doi: 10.1017/gmh.2018.9

Matamonasa-Bennett, A. (2015). "A disease of the outside people" Native American men's perceptions of intimate partner violence. *Psychology of Women Quarterly*, *39*(1), 20–36. doi: 10.1177/0361684314543783

Mugoya, G. C. T., Witte, T., Bolland, A., Tomek, S., Hooper, L. M., Bolland, J., & Dalmida, S. (2017). Depression and intimate partner violence among African American women living in impoverished inner-city neighborhoods. *Journal of Interpersonal Violence*, 88626051769151. doi: 10.1177/0886260517691519

Mutumba, M., Wekesa, E., & Stephenson, R. (2018). Community influences on modern contraceptive use among young women in low and middle-income countries: A cross-sectional multi-country analysis. *BMC Public Health*, *18*(1), 430. doi: 10.1186/s12889-018-5331-y

Myunghee, J., Thongpriwan, V., Choi, J., Choi, K. S., & Anderson, G. (2018). Decision-making about prenatal genetic testing among pregnant Korean-American women. *Midwifery*, *56*, 128–134. doi: 10.1016/j.midw.2017.10.003

Nakajima, M., Jebena, M. G., Taha, M., Tesfaye, M., Gudina, E., Lemieux, A., …, al'Absi, M. (2017). Correlates of khat use during pregnancy: A cross-sectional study. *Addictive Behaviors*, *73*, 178–184. doi: 10.1016/j.addbeh.2017.05.008

National Congress of American Indians. (2013). Policy insights brief—Statistics on violence against Native women. Retrieved from http://www.ncai.org/resources/ncai_publications/policy-insights-brief-statistics-on-violence-against-native-women

National Partnership for Women & Families. (2018). Black women's maternal health: A multifaceted approach to addressing persistent and dire health disparities, Issues brief. Retrieved from http://www.nationalpartnership.org/research-library/maternal-health/black-womens-maternal-health-issue-brief.pdf

Nyguyen, J. (2017). A literature review of alternative therapies for postpartum depression. *Nursing for Women's Health*, *21*(5), 348–359. doi: 10.1016/j.nwh.2017.07.003

Osterman, M. J. K., & Martin, J. A. (2014). Recent declines in induction of labor by gestational age. *NCHS Data Brief*, *155*, 1–8.

Osterman, M. J. K., & Martin, J. A. (2018) Timing and adequacy of prenatal care in the United States, 2016. *National Vital Statistics Reports*, *67*(3). Retrieved from https://www.cdc.gov/nchs/data/nvsr/nvsr67/nvsr67_03.pdf

Parente, S. (2018). Factors contribution to higher health care spending in the United States compared with other high-income countries. *JAMA*, *319*(10), 988–990. doi: 10.001/jama.2018.1149

Pérez-Escamilla, R., Martinez, J. L., & Segura-Pérez, S. (2016). Impact of the Baby-friendly Hospital Initiative on breastfeeding and child health outcomes: A systematic review. *Maternal & Child Nutrition*, *12*(3), 402–417. doi: 10.1111/mcn.12294

Petrosky, E., Blair, J. M., Betz, C. J., Fowler, K. A., Jack, S. P., & Lyons, B. H. (2017). Racial and ethnic differences in homicides of adult women and the role of intimate partner violence—United States, 2003–2014. *Morbidity and Mortality Weekly Report*, *66*(28), 41–746. http://dx.doi.org/10.15585/mmwr.mm6628a1

Qamar, A. (2017) The postpartum tradition of Sawn Mahina in rural Punjab, Pakistan. *Journal of Ethnology and Folkloristics*, *11*(1), 127–150. doi: 10.1515/jef-2017-0008

Raman, S., Nicholls, R., Ritchie, J., Razee, H., & Shafiee, S. (2016). How natural is the supernatural? Synthesis of the qualitative literature from low and middle income countries on cultural practices and traditional beliefs influencing the perinatal period. *Midwifery*, *39*, 87–97. doi: 10.1016/j.midw.2016.05.005

Rasch, V., Van, T. N., Nguyen, H. T. T., Manongi, R., Mushi, D., Meyrowitsch, D. W., … Wu, C. S. (2018). Intimate partner violence (IPV): The validity of an IPV screening instrument utilized among pregnant women in Tanzania and Vietnam. *PLoS One*, *13*(2), e0190856. doi: 10.1371/journal.pone.0190856

Rogathi, J. J., Manongi, R., Mushi, D., Rasch, V., Sigalla, G. N., Gammeltoft, T., & Meyrowitsch, D. W. (2017). Postpartum depression among women who have experienced intimate partner violence: A prospective cohort study at Moshi, Tanzania. *Journal of Affective Disorders*, *218*, 238–245. doi: 10.1016/j.jad.2017.04.063

Rosay, A. B. (2016). Violence against American Indian and Alaskan Native. Retrieved from https://nij.gov/journals/277/Pages/violence-against-american-indians-alaska-natives.aspx

Rosenthal, L., & Lobel, M. (2018). Gendered racism and the sexual and reproductive health of Black and Latina Women. *Ethnicity & Health*, 1–26. doi: 10.1080/13557858.2018.1439896

Rouhi, M., Rouhi, N., Vizheh, M., & Salehi, K. (2017). Male child preference: Is it a risk factor for antenatal depression among Iranian women? *British Journal of Midwifery*, *9*(25), 572–578. doi: 10.12968/bjom.2017.25.9.572

Roy, A., Furentes-Afflick, E., Fernald, L., Young, S. (2018). Pica is prevalent and strongly associated with iron deficiency among Hispanic pregnant women living in the United States. *Appetite*, *120*, 163–170. doi: 10.1016/j.appet.2017.08.033

Salari, M. (2018) The impact of intergenerational cultural transmission on fertility decisions. *Economic Analysis and Policy*, *58*, 88–99. doi: 10.1016/j.eap.2018.01.003

Schmidt, N. C., Fargnoli, V., Epiney, M., & Irion, O. (2018). Barriers to reproductive health care for migrant women in Geneva: A qualitative study. *Reproductive Health*, *15*, 43. doi: 10.1186/s12978-018-0478-7

Sharma, S., van Teijlingen, E., Hundley, V., Angell, C., & Simkhada, P. (2016). Dirty and 40 days in the wilderness: Eliciting childbirth and postnatal cultural practices and beliefs in Nepal. *BMC Pregnancy and Childbirth*, *16*(1), 147. doi: 10.1186/s12884-016-0938-4

Shaw, D., Guise, J., Shah, N., Gemzell-Danielsson, K., Joseph, KS., Levy, B., …, Main, E. (2016). Drivers of maternity care in high-income countries: can health systems support women-centered care? *Maternal Health, 4*. Retrieved from http://dx.doi.org/10.1016/S0140-6736(16)31527-6

Shin, C.-N., Reifsnider, E., McClain, D., Jeong, M., McCormick, D. P., & Moramarco, M. (2018). Acculturation, cultural values, and breastfeeding in overweight or obese, low-income, Hispanic women at 1 month postpartum. *Journal of Human Lactation, 34*(2), 358–364. doi: 10.1177/0890334417753942

Smith, I., Bentley-Edwards, K. L., El-Amin, S., & Darity, W., (2018). Fighting at birth: Eradicating the Black-White infant mortality gap. Retrieved from https://socialequity. duke.edu/sites/socialequity.duke.edu/files/site-images/ EradicatingBlackInfantMortality-March2018%20FINAL. pdf

Tavrow, P., Bloom, B. E., & Withers, M. H. (2016). Intimate partner violence screening practices in California after passage of the Affordable Care Act. *Violence Against Women, 23*(7), 871–876. https://doi.org/10.1177/1077801216652505

UNICEF. (2016). Female genital mutilation/cutting: A global concern. Retrieved from https://www.unicef.org/media/ files/FGMC_2016_brochure_final_UNICEF_SPREAD(1). pdf

United Nations Population Fund. (2017). Humanitarian action 2017 Overview. Retrieved from https://www.unfpa. org/sites/default/files/pub-pdf/Humanitarian_2017_ Overview_2017-01-18_web_0.pdf

Victoria, C. G., Bahl, R., Barros, A. J. D., Franca, G.V.A., Horton, S., Krasevec, J., …, Rollins, N. C. (2016). Breastfeeding in the 21st century: Epidemiology, mechanisms, and life-long effect. *Lancet, 387*(10017), 475–490. doi: 10.1016/ S0140-6736(15)01024-7

Weitz, E. (2017). Native American Women have been saying a lot more than #METOO for years. *Vice Impact*. https:// impact.vice.com/en_us/article/evbeg7/native-american-women-have-been-saying-a-lot-more-than-metoo-for-years

Westoff, C., & Bietsch, K. (2015). Religion and reproductive behavior in Sub-Saharan Africa. *DHS Analytical Studies 48*. Rockville, MD: ICF International. Retrieved from https://dhsprogram.com/pubs/pdf/AS48/AS48.pdf

Wilson, B., Kuha, J. (2017). Residential segregation and the fertility of immigrants and their descendants.

Population, Space and Place, 24(3), e2098. doi: 10.1002/ psp.2098

Withers, M., Kharazmi, N., & Lim, E. (2018). Traditional beliefs and practices in pregnancy, childbirth and post-partum: A review of the evidence from Asian countries. *Midwifery, 56*, 158–170. doi: 10.1016/j.midw.2017. 10.019

World Health Organization (WHO). (2005). WHO multi-country study on women's health and domestic violence against women. Report—Initial results on prevalence, health outcomes and women's responses. Retrieved from http://www.who.int/reproductivehealth/publications/ violence/24159358X/en/

World Health Organization (WHO). (2015). Maternal mortality. Retrieved from http://www.who.int/news-room/ fact-sheets/detail/maternal-mortality

World Health Organization (WHO). (2016). WHO recommendations on antenatal care for a positive pregnancy experience. Retrieved from http://www.who.int/repro-ductivehealth/publications/maternal_perinatal_health/ anc-positive-pregnancy-experience/en/

World Health Organization (WHO). (2017). Violence against women. Retrieved from https://www.who.int/news-room/ fact-sheets/detail/violence

World Health Organization (WHO). (2018a). WHO recommendations: Intrapartum care for positive childbirth experience. Retrieved from http://www.who.int/reproductivehealth/ publications/intrapartum-care-guidelines/en/

World Health Organization (WHO). (2018b). Female genital mutilation. Retrieved from http://www.who.int/news-room/fact-sheets/detail/female-genital-mutilation

Wouk, K., Stuebe, A. M., & Meltzer-Brody, S. (2016). Postpartum mental health and breastfeeding practices: An analysis using the 2010–2011 pregnancy risk assessment monitoring system. *Maternal and Child Health Journal, 21*(3), 636–647. doi: 10.1007/s10995-016-2150-6

Yoder, H., Hardy, L. (2018). Midwifery and antenatal care for Black women: A narrative review. *SAGE Open, 8*(1). doi: 10.1177/2158244017752220

Zurynski, Y., Sureshkumar, P., Phu, A., & Elliot, E. (2015). Female genital mutilation and cutting: A systematic literature review of health professionals' knowledge, attitudes and clinical practice. *BMC International Health and Human Rights, 15*, 32. doi: 10.1186/s12914-015-0070-y

Transcultural Perspectives in the Nursing Care of Children

Chapter 6

• Margaret M. Andrews

Key Terms

Bed sharing
Blended family
Conjugal family
Cosleeping
Curandero
Extended family
Infant attachment
Nuclear family
Parent–child relationship
Premasticate

Learning Objectives

1. Understand the composition of children as a population across cultures in the United States and Canada.
2. Explore child-rearing practices, both specific and universal across cultures, and their impact on the development of children.
3. Analyze the impact of selected cultural beliefs and practices on the development of children.
4. Examine the biocultural aspects of selected acute and chronic conditions affecting children.
5. Synthesize the transcultural concepts and evidence-based practices that support the delivery of culturally competent care for children and adolescents.

Children in a Culturally Diverse Society

Cultural survival depends on the transmission of values and customs from one generation to the next; this process relies on the presence of children for success. This interdependent nature of children and society reinforces the need for the greater society to nurture, care for, and socialize members of the next generation. In this chapter, the composition of children as a population, the effect of child-rearing practices both specific and universal across cultures, and the cultural influences on child growth, development, health, and illness are examined as well as an understanding of how transcultural concepts

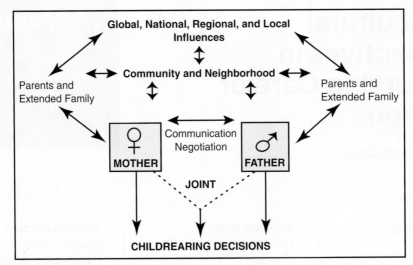

Figure 6-1. Model depicting the interrelation of culture, communication, and parental decisions about child-rearing practices.

and evidence-based practices support the delivery of culturally competent care for children and adolescents. Figure 6-1 provides a visual representation of the interrelationship among culture, communication, and parental decisions/actions during child-rearing. This schematic representation also serves as a model for understanding culturally significant decisions that affect the care of children and, therefore, will be evident throughout this chapter.

Most children are cared for by their natural or adoptive parents. In this chapter, the term *parent* refers to the primary care provider whether natural, adoptive, or relational (grandparents, aunts, uncles, cousins) or those who are unrelated but who function as primary providers of care and/or parent surrogates for varying periods of time. In some cases, the primary provider of care looks after the infant, child, or adolescent for a brief time, perhaps for an hour or two, while the parents are unable to do so. In other cases, this person might function as a long-term or permanent parent substitute even though legal adoption has not occurred. For example, a grandparent might assume responsibility for a child in the event of parental death, illness, disability, or imprisonment.

Children as a Population

When defining children as a population, it is important to consider various elements that shape this population as a whole, such as its racial and ethnic makeup, the impact of poverty on this population, and the health status of children and adolescents in the United States and Canada. Other important considerations when examining this population are cross-cultural differences in growth and development, infant attachment, and crying.

Racial and Ethnic Composition

According to the Forum on Child and Family Statistics (2018a), there are 73.7 million people under the age of 18 who live in the United States; of these, 50.7% are White, 25.2% Hispanic (of any race), 13.7% Black, and 6.0% Asian/Pacific Islander/Native American/Alaska Native. The proportion of children who are ethnically Hispanic has been growing steadily over the last few decades, from 9.0% in 1980 to 25% in 2016, and it is projected to reach 26% by the year 2020 (Child Trends, 2018). The ethnically Asian group has also been steadily growing and is now close to outnumbering the Hispanic group. It is estimated that by 2020, 40% of school-aged children in the United States will represent federal minority groups. In 2016, approximately 18 million children, under age 18, lived with at least one immigrant parent. These children accounted for 26% of the 73.7 million children under age 18 in the United States (Zong, Batalova, & Hallock, 2018). Many of these children constitute the more than 12.1 million school-aged children who speak a language other than English at home (National Kids Count, 2018). Approximately two-thirds of these children come from Spanish-speaking homes, and a large percentage of the remainder speaks a variety of Asian languages. Many children of immigrants live in linguistic isolation in the 4.5% of households where no member aged 14 or older speaks English "very well" (U.S. Census Bureau, 2017a). It is evident from the vast amount of statistics presented that the racial and ethnic composition of children in the United States is growing, and shifting, as the years unfold.

Although immigrants and their children are found throughout the United States and Canada, they tend to cluster in certain geographic areas. California, Nevada, New York, Texas, Florida, New Jersey, Illinois, and Massachusetts are homes for almost two-thirds of all foreign-born children. Georgia, Virginia, Washington, Arizona, and Maryland also have relatively high numbers of children whose parents recently immigrated to the United States (Migration Policy Institute, 2018). In Canada, most immigrants reside in one of the major metropolitan areas: Toronto, Vancouver, and Montreal are home for the majority of children of recent immigrants (Statistics Canada, 2018).

Poverty

The impact of poverty on children's health is cumulative throughout the life cycle, and disease in adulthood frequently is the result of early health-related episodes that become compounded over time. For example, when poverty leads to malnutrition during critical growth periods, either prenatally or during the first 2 years of life, the consequences can be catastrophic and irreversible, resulting in damage to the neurologic and musculoskeletal systems. If the brain fails to receive sufficient nutrients during critical growth periods, the child is likely to experience diminished cognitive development, leading to poor academic performance and later poorer job performance, lower pay, and thus perpetuation of the cycle of poverty and poor health.

Throughout the last few decades, child poverty rates have fluctuated, with a peak most recently in 2010. In 2016, the poverty threshold for a family with two adults and two children was deemed $24,339 (Forum on Child and Family Statistics, 2018b). As of 2016, 18% of all children aged 0 to 17 were living in poverty, in families with incomes below 100% of the poverty threshold, which is down from 22% in 2010. Numbers continue to fluctuate for those living in extreme poverty, defined as families below 50% of the poverty threshold, where numbers were as high as 10% in 2010 and have decreased to 8% as of 2016 (Forum on Child and Family Statistics, 2018b). In 2017, nearly 5.9 million children, which breaks down to around 1 in 12 children, lived in extreme poverty, defined as an annual income of less than half the poverty level. To put that into perspective, that is $12,642 for a family of four, which amounts to about $1,053 a month, $243 a week, or $35 a day (Children's Defense Fund, 2017b)—a shocking number when you consider the high cost of living in the United States.

In 2017, the Children's Defense Fund reported that more than two-thirds of children in poverty lived in working family households of US citizens, and more than 3.9 million children under 18 were uninsured as of 2017. A disproportionate number of children in poverty are from African American and Latino backgrounds. Children in mother-only families are nearly four times as likely to be in poverty as those in married-couple families. Research links poverty to numerous risks and disadvantages for children, including increased abuse, neglect, lower reading scores, overall less success in the classroom, failure, delinquency, malnutrition, and violence (Chaudry & Wimer, 2016; Children's Defense Fund, 2017a, 2017b). One out of every five Canadian children lives in poverty, which amounts to 1.3 million children, and among children from Aboriginal heritage, a group that constitutes 4% of the total Canadian population, 25% of children are poor (Canada Without Poverty, 2018; Statistics Canada, 2015).

Children's Health Status

Indicators of child health status include birth weight, infant mortality, and immunization rates. In general, children from diverse cultural backgrounds have less favorable indicators of health status than do their white counterparts. Health status is influenced by many factors, including access to health services. There are numerous barriers to quality health care services for children, such as poverty, geography, lack of cultural competence by health care providers, racism, and other forms of prejudice. Families from diverse cultures might have trouble in their interactions with nurses and other health care providers, and these difficulties might have an adverse impact on the delivery of health care. Because ethnic minorities are underrepresented among health care professionals, parents and children often have different cultural backgrounds from their health care providers.

Growth and Development

Although the growth and development of children are similar in all cultures, important racial, ethnic, and gender differences can be identified. For example, there is cross-cultural similarity in the sequence, timing, and achievement of developmental milestones such as smiling, separation anxiety, and language acquisition. However, from the moment of conception, the developmental processes of the human life cycle take place in the context of culture. Literature and research on culture–health interactions in behavioral medicine, medical anthropology, cross-cultural psychiatry/ psychology, and cultural neuroscience suggest

that cultural norms and practices influence the perception and maintenance of health, as well as the incidence, presentation, diagnosis, and treatment of illness (Losin, 2017). Throughout life, culture exerts an all-pervasive influence on the developing infant, child, and adolescent. Developmental researchers who have worked in other cultures have become convinced that human functioning cannot be separated from the cultural and more immediate context in which children develop (Chen & Eisenberg, 2012). For example, during a study of children aged 0 to 6 years from three different Aboriginal groups in Canada, researchers discovered that although the participants' gross motor developmental milestones were achieved earlier when compared to the general population of Canadian children, language skills were developed later (Findlay, Kohen, & Miller, 2014).

Although it is difficult to separate nongenetic from genetic influences, some populations are shorter or taller than others are during various periods of growth and in adulthood. African American infants are approximately three-fourths of an inch shorter at birth than Whites. In general, African American and White children are tallest, followed by Native Americans; Asian children are the shortest. Children of higher socioeconomic status are taller in all cultures. Data on African American and White children between 1 and 6 years old show that at age 6, African Americans are taller than Whites. Around age 9 or 10 years, White boys begin to catch up in height. White girls catch up with their African American counterparts around 14 or 15 years of age. African American children have longer legs in proportion to height than other groups (Overfield, 2017). During puberty, growth in African American children begins to slow down, and White children catch up so that the two races achieve similar heights in adulthood.

The growth spurt of adolescence involves the skeletal and muscular systems, leading to significant changes in size and strength in both sexes but particularly in boys. White North American youths aged 12 to 18 years are 22 to 33 pounds heavier and 6 inches taller than Filipino youths of the same age. African American teenagers are somewhat taller and heavier than White teens up to age 15 years. Japanese adolescents born in the United States or Canada are larger and taller than Japanese adolescents who are born and raised in Japan, primarily due to differences in diet, climate, and social milieu (Overfield, 2017). To provide consistent comparisons of height and weight of children, in 2006, the World Health Organization (WHO) published the results of a study aimed at developing universally approved benchmarks for age-appropriate height/weight measures for children up to age 5 years. The WHO Multicentre Growth Reference Study, which was a longitudinal study that took place from 1997 through 2003, produced growth charts derived from growth data of children from six countries with widely different ethnic backgrounds. Many countries have adopted these charts as an essential tool to monitor child development, and other countries are comparing their data in order to find the best fit nationally. There are articles and studies that have been published since 2006 comparing the WHO data to both broad ethnic data from up to 55 different countries, and more narrow data sets comparing nation-specific data to the WHO growth charts (Natale & Rajagopalan, 2014; Scherdel et al., 2015; World Health Organization, 2006). Based on the wide variation in head circumference data gathered in the more broad comparative study by Natale and Rajagopalan (2014), findings indicated that the use of a single international standard for head circumference was not justified in an effort to avoid misdiagnosis of microcephaly or macrocephaly.

Certain growth patterns appear across cultural boundaries. For example, regardless of culture, neuromuscular activities evolve from general to specific, from the center of the body to the extremities (proximal-to-distal development), and from the head to the toes (cephalo-caudal development). Adult head size is reached by the age of 5 years, whereas the remainder of the body continues to grow through adolescence. Physiologic maturation of organ systems, such as the renal, circulatory, and respiratory systems, occurs early, whereas maturation of the central nervous system continues beyond childhood. Tooth eruption occurs earlier in Asian and African American infants than in their White counterparts.

In terms of child development, many developmental theories are based on observations of Western children and, therefore, may not have cross-cultural generalization. Investigations of the universality of the stages of development proposed by Piaget, the family role relations emphasized by Freud, and patterns of mother–infant interaction suggested by Bowlby to indicate security of attachment have resulted in modifications of the theories to reflect newer cross-cultural data.

Other growth and development patterns seem to be specific to cultural groups. For example, in some cultures, the standard Western mobility pattern of sitting–creeping–crawling–standing–walking–squatting is not followed. The Balinese infant goes from sitting to squatting to standing. Hopi (Native American) children begin walking 1 to 2 months later than do Anglo-American children.

Infant Attachment

Cross-cultural differences are apparent when examining **infant attachment**, the relationship that exists between a child and its primary caregiver, which provides "a secure base from which to explore and, when necessary, as a haven of safety and a source of comfort" (Benoit, 2004, p. 1). Many researchers have discussed the role of culture and ethnicity in shaping caregiver behaviors, such as infant attachment. In Western countries, mothers of ethnic majority groups are frequently found to be more sensitive to their infants than mothers of ethnic minority groups, and they are said to have more individualistic cultural beliefs. In an individualistic culture, there is more weight put on independence, pursuit of self-interest, and authoritative parenting and more object-directed play (Heng et al., 2018). In contrast, individuals of

Hispanic, African, or Asian descent are thought to hold more collectivistic cultural ideals, which value interdependence, the inhibition of personal desires, and respect to others. In addition, those in these cultures tend to be more authoritarian, or strict, to demand greater compliance, and to engage in more proximal aspects of parenting such as physical contact and stimulation with their children (Heng et al., 2018).

Researchers have discovered that German and Anglo-American mothers expect early autonomy in the child and have fewer physical interventions as the child plays, thus encouraging exploration and independence (Dewar, 2017a, 2017b). Japanese children are seldom separated from their mother, and there is close physical interaction with the child (Dewar, 2017a, 2017b). Similarly, Puerto Rican and Dominican mothers display close mother–child relationships with more verbal and physical expression of affection than do European American parents. Anglo-American mothers tend to give greater emphasis to qualities associated with individualism such as autonomy, self-control, and activity (Dewar, 2017a, 2017b). In many studies, cultural anthropologists have found, and continue to find, that an overriding goal of American parents is to make a child independent and self-reliant (Bernstein, 2016). Puerto Rican mothers describe children in terms congruent with Puerto Rican culture: emphasis is placed on relatedness (e.g., affection, dignity, respectfulness, responsiveness to mother) and proximity seeking (Dewar, 2017a, 2017b).

Studies suggest that differences in infant attachment are linked to cultural variations in parenting behavior and life experiences. Parental socialization, values, beliefs, goals, and behaviors are determined in large measure by how a culture defines good parenting and preferred child behaviors for each gender. Other factors include the move from rural to urban residences and the associated social, economic, and lifestyle changes that shift children to more independent and autonomous behaviors. Some researchers argue that contemporary urbanization has created complex and highly technological societies that simultaneously foster children's autonomous, cooperative, and prosocial behavior (Chen & Eisenberg, 2012; Keller, 2013).

Crying

Cultural differences exist in the way mothers perceive, react, and behave in response to their infants' cues, behaviors, and demands. Knowledge of cultural differences in parental responses to crying is relevant for nurses because assessment of the severity of an infant's distress is often based on the parent's interpretation of the crying. The seriousness of a problem may be overestimated or underestimated because of cultural variations in perception of the infant's distress. The degree of parental concern toward an infant may be misinterpreted if one's cultural beliefs and practices differ from those of the parent (Dewar, 2017a, 2017b). For example, in Asian and Latino cultures, the male child is expected to maintain strong control over his emotions and not cry in the presence of others; therefore, a child crying in pain may be interpreted one way by a nurse and dismissed as inappropriate gender-related behavior by a parent.

Culture-Universal and Culture-Specific Child-Rearing

The values, attitudes, beliefs, and practices of one's culture affect the way parents and other providers of care relate to a child during various developmental stages. In all cultures, infants and children are valued and nurtured because they represent the promise of future generations. Figure 6-2 presents a model summarizing the cultural factors that influence parental beliefs and practices related to child-rearing. Influences on the parents include cultural and socioeconomic factors, educational background, political and legal considerations, religious and philosophical beliefs, environmental factors, contemporary technologies, personal attributes, and individual preferences. These influences, in turn, shape and form parental beliefs about normal growth and development, nutrition

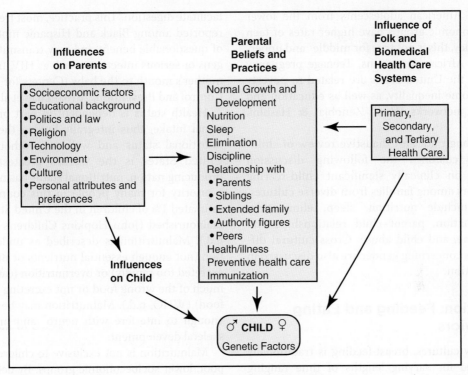

Figure 6-2. Model depicting cultural perspectives of child-rearing.

and diet, sleep, toilet training, communication patterns, and parent–child interactions and relationships, including beliefs and practices concerning parental authority. Beliefs and practices also influence discipline and culturally appropriate relationships with siblings, extended family members, nurses, physicians, teachers, law enforcement and other authority figures, and peers. Similarly, parental cultural beliefs and practices influence behaviors and interventions that promote the child's health (immunizations, foods, exercise/activity) and the manner in which he/she is cared for during illness, how parents know when their child is sick or injured, the perceived seriousness of the illness or injury (and the need for primary, secondary, or tertiary care), type(s) of healers, and interventions used to cure or heal the child. Lastly, factors inherent in the child, such as genetic and acquired conditions, gender, age, and related characteristics.

Throughout infancy, childhood, and adolescence, girls and boys undergo a process of socialization aimed at preparing them to assume adult

roles in the larger society into which they have been born or to which they have migrated. As children grow and develop, their communications and interactions occur within a cultural context. That which is considered acceptable is strongly influenced by parental education, social expectation, religious background, and cultural ties. However, all parents want their children to treat them respectfully and to show respect toward others, thus becoming a source of pride and honor to their family and cultural heritage.

There are many universal child-rearing practices, but most research has focused on specific cultural differences rather than on similarities. It is important to distinguish between cultural practices and those that reflect the economic well-being of the family, for example, the stereotypes that suggest that teenage pregnancy is more common and more acceptable among African Americans than among counterparts in other cultures. When socioeconomic factors are considered, the myth is shattered. Although

African American adolescents from the lower socioeconomic groups have higher rates of teen pregnancy, this is not true for middle- and upper-income African Americans. Teenage pregnancy rates in the United States are related to poverty and income inequality, as well as education and support networks (Hadi, Zenobia, & Hasbini, 2016).

Although not an exhaustive review of child-rearing customs, the following discussion focuses on clinically significant child-rearing behaviors among families from diverse cultures. These include nutrition, sleep, elimination, menstruation, parent–child relationships and discipline, and child abuse. Cross-cultural differences concerning gender are also discussed in this section.

Nutrition: Feeding and Eating Behaviors

In many cultures, breast-feeding is traditionally practiced for varying lengths of time ranging from several weeks to several years. The growing availability and convenience of extensively marketed prepared formula have resulted in a decrease in the number of women who attempt to breast-feed, especially among recent migrants to the United States who may culturally find it inappropriate to breast-feed in public. Many nursing mothers immigrating to the United States or Canada may be separated from female family members who could assist them with successful breast-feeding, and lack of an interpreter during prenatal and postnatal visits with health professionals can become a barrier to breast-feeding (Jones et al., 2015).

Some cultural feeding practices might result in threats to the infant's health. The practice of propping a bottle filled with milk, juice, or carbonated beverages to quiet a child or lull it to sleep is known in many cultures and can result in dental caries; this practice should be discouraged (American Academy of Pediatrics, 2015). In some cultures, mothers **premasticate**, or chew, food for young children in the belief that this will

facilitate digestion. This practice, most frequently reported among Black and Hispanic mothers, is of questionable benefit and may transmit pathogens or serious infections, such as HIV, from the mother's mouth to the baby (Centers for Disease Control and Prevention, 2018a; Zhao et al., 2017).

Health status is dependent in part on nutritional intake, thus integrally linking the child's nutritional status and wellness. Although the United States is the world's greatest food-producing nation, nutritional status has not been a priority for many people in this country. An estimated 1% of children in the United States are malnourished (John Hopkins Children's Center, n.d.). Malnutrition is described as undernutrition (not enough essential nutrients or nutrients excreted too rapidly) or overnutrition (eating too much of the wrong food or not excreting enough food) (WHO, n.d.). Malnutrition may be serious enough to interfere with neuro- and musculoskeletal development.

Malnutrition is not exclusive to children from poor, lower socioeconomic groups. By definition, many middle- and upper-income families have obese children who are also malnourished. Obesity frequently begins during infancy, when some mothers succumb to cultural pressures to overfeed (Moreno, Johnson-Shelton, & Boles, 2013; Yavuz & Selcuk, 2018). For example, among many who identify themselves as Filipino, Vietnamese, Somali, Hispanic American, and Mexican, to name a few cultures, fat babies generally are considered healthy babies (Bresnahan et al., 2014; Cachelin & Thompson, 2014; Cartagena et al., 2014; Rachmi, et al., 2017; Shader, 2018). Among some African tribes, such as the Igbo and Yoruba in Nigeria, overweight babies are considered healthy, and mild to moderate obesity in children is considered a sign of affluence. Similar beliefs have been identified among Somali and Berber women (Liamputtong, 2011) as well as some Hispanic mothers who subscribe to a long-standing cultural belief that "a chubby baby is a healthy baby" (Ramirez, 2016). Evidence-Based Practice 6-1 describes racial and ethnic differences in childhood obesity.

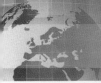

Racial and Ethnic Differences in Childhood Obesity

The World Health Organization warns that the increasing prevalence of obesity in children during the past 30 years has reached epidemic levels. Childhood obesity is a global problem affecting many low- and middle-income countries. In the United States alone, in children and adolescents aged 2 to 19 years, the prevalence of obesity in 2014 was 17.0% and extreme obesity was 5.8% (Ogden et al., 2016). The number of overweight or obese infants and young children, aged 0 to 5 years, increased from 32 million globally in 1990 to 41 million in 2016 (World Health Organization, 2017). The majority of overweight or obese children live in developing countries, where the rate of increase has been more than 30% higher than that of developed countries. These children are at risk for remaining obese into adulthood, at which time they are more likely to develop diabetes and cardiovascular diseases (World Health Organization, 2017, n.d.). Children at highest risk for obesity live in the United States, the United Kingdom, and Mexico.

Measuring Overweight and Obesity in Children

It is difficult to develop one simple index for the measurement of overweight and obesity in children and adolescents because their bodies undergo a number of physiologic changes as they grow. Measurement is further compounded by the child's race; African Black children carry less body fat than do White counterparts, and Hispanic and Asian children typically have a higher percentage of body fat. Given the wide variation in the level and distribution of body fat between different racial and ethnic groups, different benchmarks for defining overweight and obesity are used in different countries. Cowie (2014) reports on various tools and strategies used to measure and assess overweight and obesity in children and identifies what is currently considered to be the most reliable and effective. Different methods to measure a body's healthy weight, depending on the age, are available from the World Health Organization. In the United States, the Centers for Disease Control's reference data are based on a sample of boys and girls aged 2 to 20 years (CDC, 2017).

Factors Contributing to Obesity in Early Childhood

Weden, Brownell, and Rendall (2012) studied differences in the likelihood of early childhood obesity between Black and White US children using data from the Early Childhood Longitudinal Study directed by the National Center for Education Statistics. The sample consisted of a nationally representative cohort with $n = 1,515$ children and their mothers (age 14 to 21 years) who were assessed in waves at 9 months, at 2 years, at 4 years, and upon entry into kindergarten using computer-assisted, in-home interviews with children, mothers, fathers, or guardians. The investigators examined differences in Black and White children's prevalence of socioeconomic, prenatal, perinatal, and early life risk and protective factors relative to their likelihood of obesity in early childhood. Black children's mothers were only one-third as likely as White children's mothers to have completed high school, a strong indicator of socioeconomic disadvantage. Black children were 3 to 3.5 times as likely as White children to live in a family or household whose annual income was below $25,000, and their mothers were three to four times as likely to be unmarried. In analyzing prenatal and perinatal risk factors, almost half of Black children's mothers, compared to one-third of White children's mothers, were overweight or obese before pregnancy. Prepregnant obesity was the strongest risk factor for early childhood obesity, with Black children's mothers being more likely to be obese than White counterparts, thus perpetuating "a troubling cycle of intergenerational transmission of racial disparities in body mass index" (Weden et al., 2012, p. 2062). The investigators also studied racial differences in protective factors that would decrease the likelihood of early childhood obesity, for example, long-duration breast-feeding (greater than 8 months), frequency and quality of meals, children's television viewing, and exercise/physical activity care (Bresnahan et al., 2014; Cachelin & Thompson, 2014; Kirby, Liang, Hsin-Jen, & Wang, 2012; Moreno et al., 2013).

(continued)

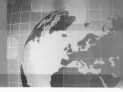

Racial and Ethnic Differences in Childhood Obesity (continued)

Protective Factors Contributing to Prevention of Obesity in Early Childhood

Among early life protective factors to reduce the likelihood of obesity, Black children were less likely than White children to be breast-fed for 1 to 7 months and only one-third as likely to be breast-fed for 8 months or longer. Black children were also less likely than White children to have daily family meals. Twice as many Black children as White children watched television for 4 or more hours per day during the daytime at 4 years of age. Black children's mothers were more likely to be employed full time than White children's. Black children also were more likely to be cared for by relatives or in a day care center and less likely to be cared for by a nonrelative or exclusively by their parents. In the statistical analyses, it was revealed that younger children's television watching was not correlated with obesity, as has been reported elsewhere in the literature, perhaps because television-related sedentary behavior is a more critical determinant in obesity at older ages.

Clinical Implications

The study findings provide insights into potentially modifiable determinants of racial disparities in early childhood obesity among Black and White preschool-aged children. Disparities among Black children are concerning because early childhood obesity often develops into adult obesity, which, in turn, has implications for adult cardiovascular disease and diabetes, the leading causes of premature death in African Americans. Eliminating Black–White differences in early childhood obesity provides an opportunity to reduce racial disparities in the overall health and longevity of both Black and White populations. The study findings also have implications for nurse–midwives, obstetric nurses, obstetricians, doulas, and others who assist with deliveries and engage in parent education programs about the benefits of breast-feeding, proper nutrition, and exercise/activity, for employers who establish workplace policies related to breast-feeding, for teachers responsible for exercise and activity programs in preschools and kindergartens, for dieticians who are responsible for nutrition and diet education programs for the parents and other caregivers for preschool-aged children, and for federal, state, foundation, and corporate funding for the prevention of childhood obesity.

References: Centers for Disease Control and Prevention. (2017). *Clinical Growth Charts.* Retrieved from https://www.cdc.gov/growthcharts/clinical_charts.htm

Cowie, J. (2014). Measurement of obesity in children. *Primary Health Care, 24*(7), 18–23.

Kirby, J. B., Liang, L., Hsin-Jen, C., & Wang, Y. (2012). Race, place, and obesity: The complex relationships among community racial/ethnic composition, individual race/ethnicity, and obesity in the United States. *American Journal of Public Health, 102*(8), 1572–1578.

Moreno, G., Johnson-Shelton, D., & Boles, S. (2013). Prevalence and prediction of overweight and obesity among elementary school children. *Journal of School Health, 83*(1), 157–163.

Ogden, C. L., Carroll, M. D., Lawman, H. G., et al. (2016). Trends in obesity prevalence among children and adolescents in the United States, 1988–1994 through 2013–2014. *JAMA, 315*(21), 2292–2299. doi: 10.1001/jama.2016.6361

Weden, M. M., Brownell, P., & Rendall, M. S. (2012). Prenatal, perinatal, early life, and sociodemographic factors underlying high body mass index in early childhood. *American Journal of Public Health, 102*(11), 2057–2065.

World Health Organization. (2017). Facts and figures on childhood obesity. Retrieved November 26, 2018 from https://www.who.int/end-childhood-obesity/facts/en/

World Health Organization. (n.d.). Global strategy on diet, physical activity: Childhood overweight and obesity. Retrieved November 26, 2018 from http://www.who.int/dietphysicalactivity/childhood/en/

The popularity of fast-food restaurants and "junk" foods has resulted in a high-calorie, high-fat, high-cholesterol, and high-carbohydrate diet for many children. Parents and children are frequently involved in numerous activities outside the house and have less time for traditional tasks such as cooking or seating the family together for a meal. Because fast foods have some

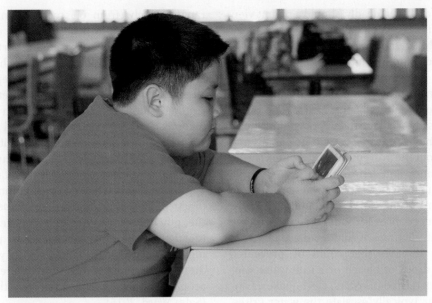

Figure 6-3. Widespread use of cell phones and other electronic devices contributes to childhood obesity (Phawat/Shutterstock.com).

intrinsic nutritional value, their benefit should be evaluated based on age-specific requirements. Poverty forces some parents to provide inexpensive substitutes for the expensive, often unavailable, essential nutrients. These lower nutrients, high-fat, high-calorie foods are referred to as "empty calories" and have led to the epidemic of childhood obesity. The prevalence of childhood obesity among various cultural and ethnic groups within the United States was described by Ogden, Carroll, Kit, and Flegal (2014). The reported weight-for-age imbalance among preschool, school-age, and adolescent African American and Hispanic children was especially disturbing and purports serious complications of hypertension, diabetes, and cardiovascular disease for young Black and Hispanic adults (see Figure 6-3). Since 2014, data continue to show increases in childhood obesity rates, with Min, Wen, Xue, and Wang (2018) echoing the ethnic disparities in obesity rates. The researchers reported that Hispanic boys and African American girls have unfavorably higher BMI and obesity rates when compared to other groups, and parenting

practice and socioeconomic status contribute to the disparities.

The extent to which families retain their cultural practices at mealtime varies widely. However, when a child is hospitalized, their recovery might be enhanced by familiar foods, and nurses should assess the influence of culture on eating habits. For example, most Asian parents believe that children should be fed separately from adults and that they should acquire "good table manners" by the time they are 5 years old; these practices can be supported during hospitalization. For hospitalized children, nurses can foster an environment that closely simulates the home (e.g., use of chopsticks rather than silverware). Family members can be encouraged to visit during mealtime to encourage the child to eat. As the child's condition allows, food may be brought from home, and/or the family can be encouraged to eat with the child if this is appropriate.

In many cultures, illness is viewed as a punishment for an evil act, and fasting (abstaining from solid food and sometimes liquids) is viewed as penance for evil. A situation may become dangerous, and even deadly, should a parent view the child's illness as an "evil" event and consequently withhold food and/or water. Dehydration occurs rapidly and malnutrition may quickly follow. These dangerous issues may require legal intervention to protect the child and may produce difficult, culturally insensitive outcomes. Nurses must be vigilant to support cultural eating habits and be prepared to educate parents and children about the prevention of and intervention for malnutrition and dehydration.

Safe drinking water is not always available in many regions of the world. Contaminated water is found in all countries at some time and in some countries at all times. Children die daily from waterborne diseases that could be prevented with a few drops of bleach or a safe water supply. Weather-related disasters, earthquakes, famine, and war typically escalate the water crises. In cases of vomiting, diarrhea, and dehydration, contaminated water supplies should always be investigated as a possible source.

Sleep

Although the amount of sleep required at various ages is similar across cultures, differences in sleep patterns and bedtime rituals exist. The sleep practices in a family household reflect some of the deepest moral ideals of a cultural community. Nurses working with families of young children in both community and inpatient settings frequently encounter cultural differences in family sleeping behaviors.

Community health, psychiatric, and pediatric nurses who work with young children and their families often assess the family's sleep and rest patterns. **Bed sharing** is the practice of a child sleeping with another person on the same sleeping surface for all or part of the night. Although bed sharing may be born out of financial necessity, it is a cultural phenomenon in many societies that emphasize closeness, togetherness, and interdependence (Jain, Romack, & Jain, 2011; Mileva-Seitz, Bakermans-Kranenburg, Battaini, & Luijk, 2017). Globally, bed sharing prevalence

ranges widely, from 6% to 70%; an estimated 15% of US children bed share, but rates could be higher. The CDC released a report that sampled data from 2009 through 2015, showing that around 60% of caregivers sampled reported bed sharing with their infant (Bombard et al., 2018). Among children in households with an annual income less than $20,000/year, bed sharing is 1.5 times more likely than those with incomes greater than $20,000/year. On the issue of family cosleeping, nurses traditionally have taken a rigid approach that excludes this common cultural practice. Although some degree of **cosleeping**— the practice of parents and children sleeping together in the same bed for all or part of the night—is common in families with young children, there are marked cultural differences in the proportion that regularly implement this practice (Salm Ward, 2015).

Research has found that the majority of parents bring their children into bed with them at some time. Parents bring their children into bed with them to facilitate breast-feeding, to comfort the child, to improve the child's sleep or parent's sleep, to monitor the child, to improve bonding or attachment, and for other reasons; the constellation of reasons for bed sharing depends largely on the culture of the family, particularly parental values and beliefs (Bailey, 2016; Huang et al., 2013; Salm Ward, 2015).

Cosleeping, or bed sharing, is more common and occurs most frequently among African American families (Gaydos et al., 2015). Most White middle-class North American and European families believe that infants and children should sleep alone. Studies suggest there are no negative associations between cosleeping during the toddler years and behavior and cognition at 5 years of age (Barajas, Martin, Brooks-Gunn, & Hale, 2011). Yet, there are some researchers that present the opposite view, reporting that while bed sharing is a common practice, it is associated with impaired child mental health at the age of 6 years (Santos et al., 2017).

The type of bed in which a child sleeps might vary considerably. In a traditional American

Samoan home, infants sleep on a pandanus mat covered with a blanket, and sometimes, a pillow is used. The cradleboard is used by several Native American nations. Constructed by a family member, a cradleboard is made of wood and might be decorated in various ways depending on the affluence of the family and tribal customs (see Figure 6-4). The cradleboard helps the infant feel secure and is easily moved while the family engages in work, travel, or other activities. Although cradleboards have been blamed for exacerbating hip dysplasia in Native American infants, diapering counterbalances this by causing a slight abduction of the hips (International Hip Dysplasia Institute, 2018).

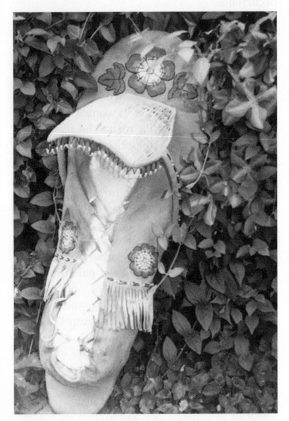

Figure 6-4. The cradleboard, created many centuries before the car seat, helps to promote infant mobility and safety and its use is still prevalent among some Native Americans.

In the United States and Canada, the common developmental milestone of sleeping for 8 uninterrupted hours by age 4 to 5 months is regarded as a sign of neurologic maturity. In many other cultures, however, the infant sleeps with the mother and is allowed to breast-feed on demand with minimal disturbance of adult sleep. In such an arrangement, there is less parental motivation to enforce "sleeping through the night" or having the infant sleep in solidarity, and the infants continue to wake up frequently during the night to be fed (Shimizu & Teti, 2018; St James-Roberts, Roberts, Hovish, & Owen, 2017). Thus, it appears that this developmental milestone, in addition to its biologic basis, is a function of context.

A common transition from sleeping in a crib to a bed without side rails is a developmental marker that is important to the child. This transition usually occurs during preschool years, depending upon the physical space in the home, the parental attitude toward the child's independence, and the child's neuromuscular development/coordination. For the hospitalized child, caregivers need to identify the child's usual bedtime routines. For example, once children have gained the independence of leaving a crib, it may be emotionally traumatic for them to be placed into a hospital bed with side rails of any kind. Health care providers need to be sensitive to this situation and reassure both child and parent that any regressive behavior that occurs as a result of reverting to a bed with side rails will be short-lived. Bedtime routines and preparation for sleep might include a snack, prayers, and/or a favorite toy or story. Common bedtime routines should be continued in the hospital as much as possible.

Homelessness presents many problems, one of which is the lack of a consistent place for a child to sleep. Although nomadic tribes have for centuries moved their habitat on a daily basis, even they generally had a consistent tent or covering. Today, it is estimated that a staggering 2.6 million children experience homelessness each year, which represents 1 in every 30 children in the United States. These children face daily issues of not having a permanent, safe, or secure place in which to lay their head (American Institutes for Research, 2018). Whether because of poverty, disease, war, or disaster, children with or without families nightly wander without a safe place to sleep. The toll of the massive number of homeless children that are the result of recent natural disasters, war, and famine has yet to be estimated. Lack of a safe place to sleep is only one of many issues to be considered.

Elimination

Elimination refers to ridding the body of wastes. It is a function that is accomplished by the combined work of the gastrointestinal, genitourinary, respiratory, and integumentary systems of the body. Of primary concern to parents of toddlers and preschoolers is bowel and bladder control. Toileting or toilet training is a major developmental milestone and is taught through a variety of cultural patterns.

Most children are capable of achieving dryness by 2½ to 3 years of age. Bowel training is more easily accomplished than bladder training. Daytime (diurnal) dryness is more easily attained than nighttime (nocturnal) dryness. Some cultures start toilet training a child before his or her first birthday and consider the child a "failure" if dryness is not achieved by 18 months. Often, there is significant shaming, blaming, and embarrassment of the child who has not achieved dryness by the culturally acceptable timetable. The nurse should remember that due to spinal cord/nerve development, maintenance of dryness is not physiologically possible until the child is able to walk without assistance. In some cultures, children are not expected to be dry until 5 years of age. Generally speaking, "Girls typically acquire bladder control before boys, and bowel control typically is achieved before bladder control" (Kliegman et al., 2016, p. 2581). Constipation in a child is a persistent concern among parents who expect a ritualistic daily pattern of bowel movements. In some cultures, infants are given herbs aimed at purging them when they are a few days, weeks, or months old to remove evil spirits from the body. Parents should be advised against using purgatives in infants because fluid and electrolyte imbalance occurs and dehydration can ensue rapidly.

The role of the nurse is to acknowledge that toilet training can be taught through a variety of cultural patterns but that physical and psychosocial health are promoted by accepting, flexible approaches. A previously toilet-trained child might become incontinent as a result of the stress of hospitalization, but will generally regain control quickly when returned to the familiar home environment. Parents should be reassured that regression of bowel and bladder control frequently occurs when a child is hospitalized; this is normal and is expected to be a short-term occurrence.

Menstruation

Ethnicity is the strongest determinant of the duration and character of menstrual flow, although diet, exercise, and stress are also known to influence menstruation in women of all ages. In most cultures globally, menarche signals that a girl's body is physiologically becoming ready for motherhood. The age at which it is culturally appropriate for a young woman to bear children is highly variable; in some cultures, menstruation signals the preparation for marriage (Hartmann, Rivadeneyra, & Toro-Morn, 2016; Lahme, Stern, & Cooper, 2016). As indicated in Figure 6-5, in some cultures, motherhood occurs in the early teens, which results in children parenting children, often with encouragement and support from an extended family, including other wives in polygamous cultures. In other cultures, adolescent pregnancy is discouraged.

Attitudes toward menstruation are often culturally based, and the adolescent girl might be taught many folk beliefs. For example, in some traditional cultures such as Italian, Filipino, Mexican, or Chilean, girls and women are not permitted to walk barefooted, wash their hair, or take showers or baths during menses. In encouraging hygienic practices, respect cultural directives by

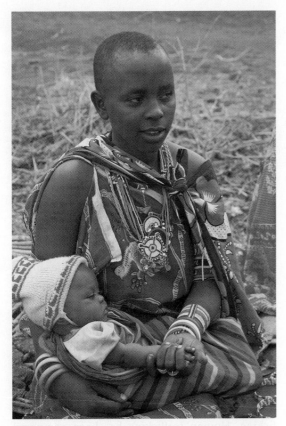

Figure 6-5. Menarche sets the developmental stage for girls to become mothers: children parenting children (Giancana/Shutterstock.com).

encouraging sponge bathing, frequent changing of sanitary pads or tampons, and other interventions that promote cleanliness (Dammery, 2016; Farange, Miller, & Davis, 2011). Some Mexican Americans believe that sour or iced foods cause the menstrual flow to thicken, and some Puerto Rican teenagers have been taught that drinking lemon or pineapple juice will increase menstrual cramping. The nurse should be aware of these beliefs and should respect personal preferences concerning beverages. The teenager might have been taught the folk practices by her mother or by another woman in her family who might be watchful during the girl's menstrual periods. If menstruation coincides with hospitalization, nurses should respect the teenager's preferences

and reassure the mother or significant other that cultural practices will be respected.

Many cultural groups treat menstrual cramping with herbs and a variety of home remedies. Health care providers should ask the adolescent whether she takes anything special during menstruation or in the absence of menstrual flow. Verify the amount and type of home remedies used to determine possible interactive effect with prescribed medications.

Adolescent girls of Islamic religious backgrounds have cultural and/or religious prohibitions and duties during and after menstruation. In Islamic law, blood is considered unclean. The blood of menstruation, as well as blood lost during childbirth, is believed to render the female impure. Because one must be in a pure state to pray, menstruating girls and women are forbidden to perform certain acts of worship, such as touching the Koran, entering a mosque, praying, and participating in the feast of Ramadan. During the menstrual period, sexual intercourse is forbidden for both men and women. When the menstrual flow stops, the girl or woman performs a special washing to purify herself. In Islam, sexual pollution applies equally to men and women. For men, sexual intercourse and the discharge of semen is an act that renders a man impure and requires a ritual washing before being able to perform the prayer. Buddhist and Hindu women do not enter the kitchen and may sleep in separate/special rooms during menses (Dammery, 2016; Farange et al., 2011).

Parent–Child Relationships and Discipline

In some cultures, both parents assume responsibility for the care of children, whereas in other cultures, the relationship with the mother is primary and the father remains somewhat distant. With the approach of adolescence, the gender-related aspects of the **parent–child relationship** might be modified to conform to cultural expectations.

Some cultures encourage children to participate in family decision-making and to discuss or even argue points with their parents. Some African American families, for example, encourage children to express opinions verbally and to take an active role in all family activities. Many Asian parents value respectful, deferential behavior toward adults, who are considered experienced and wise; therefore, children are discouraged from making decisions independently. The witty, fast reply that is viewed in some US, Canadian, European, and Australian cultures as a sign of intelligence and cleverness might be punished in some non-Western circles as a sign of rudeness and disrespect.

The use of physical acts, such as spanking or various restraining actions, is connected with discipline in many groups, but can sometimes be interpreted by those outside the culture as inappropriate and/or unacceptable. Physical punishment of Native North American children is rare. Instead of using loud scolding and reprimands, Native North American parents generally discipline with a quiet voice, telling the child what is expected, and orienting the child toward the needs and feelings of others. During breast-feeding and toilet training, or toilet learning, Native North American children are typically permitted to set their own pace, and parents tend to be permissive and nondemanding. Some African American parents' discipline in a "no-nonsense" style where they tend to point out negative behaviors of a child and may use spanking and physical punishment as a strategy to quickly gain the child's attention and rapidly get him or her to behave, especially in public (Streit, Carlo, Ispa, & Palermo, 2017, p. 1013; Whaley, 2013).

With the approach of adolescence, parental relationships and discipline generally change. Teens are usually given increasing amounts of freedom and are encouraged to try out adult roles in a supervised way that enables parents to retain considerable control. In many cultures, adolescent boys are permitted more freedom than girls of the same age. Among some religious groups, such as the American Amish, adolescents are given a period of time (a month to a year) of a more independent lifestyle prior to commitment to specific religious life rules.

Child Abuse

Child abuse and neglect have been documented throughout human history and are evident across cultures. Current data show that over one billion children worldwide experience some type of violence annually, with five children dying each day due to child abuse. International attention to child maltreatment emerged in the late 1970s, and the International Society for the Prevention of Child Abuse and Neglect (ISPCAN) held an international congress to explore physical abuse and neglect, molestation, child prostitution, nutritional deprivation, and emotional maltreatment from a cross-national perspective. This congress led to the formation of a multicountry study of child maltreatment/abuse and the United Nations–WHO joint publication "Enhancing the Rights of Adolescent Girls." This publication focused on priorities that include educating adolescent girls, improving health, keeping them free from violence, promoting girl leaders, and counting adolescent girls in data to advance their well-being (WHO, 2010). Currently, the ISPCAN and other agencies, such as Homeland Security, are also reaching out to educate on human trafficking. Human trafficking has been compared to modern-day slavery, is a form of abuse, and involves the use of force, fraud, or coercion to obtain some type of labor or commercial sex act from not only men and women, but children and adolescents as well (International Society for the Prevention of Child Abuse and Neglect, 2017; U.S. Department of Homeland Security, 2018).

Cross-cultural variability in child-rearing beliefs and practices has created a dilemma that makes the establishment of a universal standard for optimal child care, as well as definitions of child abuse and neglect, extremely difficult. In defining child maltreatment across cultures, the WHO and UNICEF have included Korbin's (1991) classic three characteristics: (1) cultural differences in child-rearing practices and beliefs, (2) departure from one's culturally acceptable behavior, and (3) harm to children.

Practices that are acceptable in the culture in which they occur may be considered abusive or neglectful by outsiders; some examples follow. In many Middle Eastern cultures, despite warm temperatures, infants are covered with multiple layers of clothing and might be observed to sweat profusely because parents believe that young children become chilled easily and die of exposure to the cold. Many African nations continue to practice rites of initiation for boys and girls, usually at the time of puberty. In some cases, ritual circumcision—of both boys and girls—is performed without anesthesia, and the ability to endure the associated pain is considered to be a manifestation of the maturity expected of an adult. In the United States and Canada, some Southeast Asian folk healing practices such as coining, cupping, and burning that produce marks on the body are used for treatment of upper respiratory illnesses, pain relief, and various other illnesses. In some Middle Eastern and Mexican societies, fondling of the genitals of infants and young children is used to soothe them or encourage sleep; however, such fondling of older children or for the sexual gratification of adults falls outside of acceptable cultural behaviors.

Although African American children are three times more likely than White children to die of child abuse (U.S. Department of Health and Human Services, 2016), there is considerable disagreement about whether race differences exist in the prevalence of child abuse independent from socioeconomic factors such as income, education, and employment status. Health care providers need to become knowledgeable about folk beliefs, child-rearing practices, and cultural variability in defining child maltreatment.

Gender Differences

From the moment of birth, differentiation between the sexes is recognized. Physical differences between boys and girls appear early in life and form the basis for adult roles within a culture. Normal newborn boys are larger, are more active, and have more muscle development than newborn girls. Normal newborn girls react more positively to comforting than do newborn boys.

Physiologically, adult men differ from adult women in both primary and secondary sex characteristics. On average, men have a higher oxygen-carrying capacity in the blood, a higher muscle-to-fat ratio, more body hair, a larger skeleton, and greater height.

Behaviorally, there are also differences between the two sexes, especially in the division of labor. The early differentiation of gender roles is manifested in gender-specific tasks, play, and dress. For children, gender differences can be identified cross-culturally in six classes of behavior: nurturance, responsibility, obedience, self-reliance, achievement, and independence (Barry, Bacon, & Child, 1967). Variability in gender role behavior is common. Most people in a society adopt common behaviors defined as appropriate to their biologic sex, but there are many exceptions. Gender roles are themselves highly variable by age, social class, religious orientation, and sexual preference. The stringency of expectations also varies: girls and women in the United States, Canada, Australia, Israel, and many parts of Europe can violate gender role norms with fewer explicit sanctions than their counterparts in other regions of the world.

Health and Health Promotion

The concept of health varies widely across cultures. Regardless of culture, most parents desire health for their children and engage in activities that they believe to be health promoting. Because health-related beliefs and practices are such an integral part of culture, parents might persist with culturally based beliefs and practices even when scientific evidence refutes them, or they might modify them to be more congruent with contemporary knowledge of health and illness.

Illness

The family is the primary health care provider for infants, children, and adolescents. It is the family that determines when a child is ill and when to seek help in managing an illness. The family also determines the acceptability of illness and sick-role behaviors for children and adolescents. Societal and economic trends influence the cultural beliefs that are passed from generation to generation. Health, illness, and treatment (care/cure) are part of every child's cultural heritage. Every society has an organized response to defined health problems. Certain people are designated as being responsible for deciding who is sick, what kind of sickness the person has, and what kind of treatment is required to restore the person to health.

Research has consistently demonstrated that African American and Hispanic children are less likely to have seen a physician than are Whites. They also have a lower average number of ambulatory visits than their White counterparts. Even when children are hospitalized, minorities receive fewer services than do Whites. As a record high, 95% of children in America have health coverage, yet 1 in 19 children is uninsured. The Children's Defense Fund (2017c) states that "poor children and children of color have worse access to health care and worse outcomes than their higher-income, white counterparts" and continues by saying "children with unmet health needs fall behind developmentally and have trouble catching up physically, socially and academically" (Children's Defense Fund, 2017c, The Problem section, para. 1).

Health Belief Systems and Children

Among many cultural groups, traditional health beliefs coexist with Western medical beliefs. Members of a cultural group choose the components of traditional (Western) medicine, Eastern medicine, or folk beliefs that seem appropriate to them. A Mexican American family, for example, might take a child to a physician and/or a traditional healer (curandero). After visiting the physician and the curandero, the mother might consult with her own mother and then give her sick child the antibiotics prescribed by the physician and the herbal tea prescribed by the traditional healer. If the problem is viral in origin, the child will recover because of his or her own innate immunologic defenses, independent of either treatment. Thus, both the herbal tea of the curandero and the penicillin prescribed by the physician might be viewed as folk remedies; neither intervention is responsible for the child's recovery.

Belief systems about specific symptoms are culturally unique. These are referred to as cultural illnesses. In Hispanic culture, susto is caused by a frightening experience and is recognized by nervousness, loss of appetite, and loss of sleep. Mexican American babies must be protected from these experiences. Pujos (grunting) is an illness manifested by grunting sounds and protrusion of the umbilicus. It is believed to be caused by contact with a woman who is menstruating or by the infant's own mother if she menstruated sooner than 60 days after delivery.

The evil eye, mal ojo, is an affliction feared throughout much of the world. The condition is said to be caused by an individual who voluntarily or involuntarily injures a child by looking at or admiring him or her. The individual has a desire to hold the child, but the wish is frustrated, either by the parent of the infant or by the reserve of the individual. Several hours later, the child might become listless, cry, and/or experience fever, vomiting, and/or diarrhea. The most serious threat to the infant with mal ojo is dehydration; the nurse encountering this problem in the community setting needs to assess the severity of the dehydration and plan for immediate fluid and electrolyte replacement. Parents should be taught the warning signs and the potential seriousness of dehydration. A simple explanation of the causes and treatment of dehydration should be provided. If the parents adhere strongly to traditional beliefs, respect their desire for the curandero to participate in the care. Parents or grandparents might wish to place an amulet, talisman, or religious object such as a crucifix or rosary on the child or near the bed.

For the Mexican American family, caida de la mollera, or fallen fontanelle, can be attributed to a number of causes such as failure of the midwife to press preventively on the palate after delivery, falling on the head, abruptly removing the nipple from the infant's mouth, and failing to place a cap on the infant's head. The signs of this condition include crying, fever, vomiting, and diarrhea. Given that health care providers frequently note the correspondence of these symptoms with those of dehydration, many parents see *deshidratacion* (dehydration) or *carencia de agua* (lack of water) as synonymous with *caida de la mollera*. Although regional differences exist, parental treatment usually is directed at rehydration, thus raising the fontanelle.

Empacho is a digestive condition believed by Mexicans to be caused by the adherence of undigested food to some part of the gastrointestinal tract. This condition causes an "internal fever," which cannot be observed but which betrays its presence by excessive thirst and abdominal swelling believed to be caused by drinking water to quench the thirst. Children who are prone to swallowing chewing gum are believed to experience *empacho*, but it can affect persons of any age.

Among some Hindus from northern India, there is a strong belief in ghost illness and ghost possession. These culture-bound syndromes, or folk illnesses, are based on the belief that a ghost enters its victim and tries to seize the soul. If the ghost is successful, it causes death. Illness and the supernatural world are linked by the concepts of fever and the ghost, which is a supernatural being discussed in Hindu sacred scriptures. One sign of ghost illness is a voice speaking through a delirious victim; this may occur in children and adults. Other signs are convulsions and body movements, indicating pain and discomfort, and choking or difficulty breathing. In the case of an infant, incessant crying is a sign. The psychological state of the parents is often involved in the diagnosis, and some believe that ghosts might be cultural scapegoats for the illness and death of children. When an infant or small child becomes ill and dies, a mother or father might be relieved of psychic tension from feelings of personal guilt by transferring the blame for the death to a ghost.

Biocultural Influences on Childhood Disorders

Children may be born with genetic traits inherited from their biologic parents, who have inherited their own genetic compositions. The child's genetic makeup affects his or her likelihood of both contracting and inheriting specific conditions. In both children and adults, genetic composition has been demonstrated to affect the individual's susceptibility to specific diseases and disorders. It is often difficult to separate genetic influences from socioeconomic factors, such as poverty, lack of proper nutrition, and poor hygiene, and environmental conditions, such as lack of ventilation, sanitary facilities, and heat during cold weather and clothing that is insufficient to provide protection during the various seasons. Other factors responsible for differing susceptibilities to specific conditions are variations in natural and acquired immunity, intermarriage, geographic and climatic conditions, ethnic background, race, and religious practices. Some studies have attempted to explain differences in susceptibility solely on the basis of cultural heritage, but they have not succeeded in doing so. This section examines some common conditions in which genetic constitution seems to be a factor influencing child health.

Immunity

Perhaps one of the most frequently cited examples of the connection between immunity and race is that of malaria and the sickle cell trait in Africans. Black Africans possessing the sickle cell trait are known to have increased immunity to malaria, a serious endemic disease found in warm, moist climates. Thus, Blacks with the sickle cell trait survived malarial attacks and reproduced offspring who also possessed the sickle cell trait.

The transfer of immunity to many contagious diseases via injection/ingestion of live or attenuated viruses has been a major factor in decreasing childhood deaths. However, there is no evidence of culture-bound positive or negative effects where vaccines are available. Some religious groups refuse immunizations and often experience outbreaks of preventable communicable diseases within their community. Other parents refuse immunizations based on the belief of a connection between childhood autism and vaccines, which has not been supported by clinical research to date.

Intermarriage

Intermarriage among certain cultural groups has led to a wide variety of childhood disorders. For example, there is an increased incidence of ventricular septal defects (VSDs) among the Amish, amyloidosis among Indiana/Swiss and Maryland/German families, and intellectual disability in several other groups (Kliegman et al., 2016).

Ethnicity

Although the role of socioeconomic factors in tuberculosis—such as overcrowding and poor nutrition—cannot be disregarded, ethnicity also appears to be a factor in this disease. Groups with a relatively high incidence of tuberculosis are Native North Americans living in the Southwest United States and in northern and prairie regions of Canada, Mexican Americans, and Africans and refugees from third world countries. Ethnicity is also linked to several noncommunicable conditions such as Tay–Sachs disease, a neurologic condition affecting Ashkenazi Jews of Northeastern European descent, and phenylketonuria (PKU), a metabolic disorder primarily affecting Scandinavians (Kliegman et al., 2016).

Race

Race has been linked to the incidence of a variety of disorders of childhood. For example, the endocrine disorder cystic fibrosis primarily affects White children, and sickle cell anemia has its primary influence among Blacks and those of Mediterranean descent. Black children are known to be at risk for inherited blood disorders, such as thalassemia, G6PD deficiency, and hemoglobin C disease. In addition, the inability to digest lactose, the predominant sugar in dairy products, varies by race. For primary lactose intolerance, about 75% to 90% of Native Americans, Blacks, Latinos, Asians, Mediterraneans, and Jewish peoples are affected. Yet, only 5% of northern and central European descendants are affected (Glaser, 2016).

Beliefs Regarding the Cause of Chronic Illnesses and Disabilities

Chronic illnesses and disabilities in children and adults have become the dominant health care problem in North America and are the leading causes of morbidity and mortality (Centers for Disease Control and Prevention, 2018b). Illness is viewed by many cultures as a form of punishment. The child and/or family with a chronic illness or disability might be perceived to be cursed by a supreme being, to have sinned, or to have violated a taboo. In some cultural groups, the affected child is seen as tangible evidence of divine displeasure, and its arrival is accompanied throughout the community by prolonged private and public discussions about what wrongs the family might have committed.

Inherited disorders and illnesses are frequently envisioned as being caused by a family curse that is passed along from one generation to the next through blood. Within such families, the nurse's desire to determine who is the carrier for a particular gene might be interpreted as an attempt to discover who is at fault and might be met with family resistance.

Folk beliefs mingled with eugenics have resulted in the realization that many chronic conditions, particularly intellectual disability, are the products of intermarriage among close relatives, otherwise known as a consanguineous relationship (Lakhan, Bipeta, Yerramilli, & Nahar, 2017). The belief that a chronically ill or disabled child might be the product of an incestuous relationship can further complicate attempts to encourage parents to seek assistance.

Among those who believe that chronic illness and disability are caused by an imbalance of hot and cold (as in Latino cultures) or yin and yang (as in Southeast Asian cultures), the cause and potential cure lie within the individual. He or she must try to reestablish equilibrium through regaining balance. Unfortunately for those with permanent disabilities who cannot be fully healed, their community might perceive them as living in a continually impure or diseased state.

Traditional beliefs can be tenacious and tend to remain even after genetic inheritance or physiologic patterns of chronic disease progression are explained to the family. However, new information is quickly integrated into the traditional system of folk beliefs more often, as is evidenced by the addition of currently prescribed medications to the hot/cold classification system embraced by many Hispanic families. An explanation of the genetic transmission of disease might be given to a family, but this does not guarantee that the older, traditional belief in a curse or "bad blood" will disappear.

When disability is seen as a divine punishment, an inherited evil, or the result of a personal state of impurity, the very presence of a child with a disability might be something about which the family is deeply ashamed or with which they are unable to cope. In addition to suffering from public disgrace, some parents or families, especially immigrant groups from Eastern Europe and Southeast Asia, also fear that disabled children will be taken away and institutionalized against their will.

Some cultural explanations of the cause of chronic disease or disability are quite positive. For example, some Mexican American parents of chronically ill children believed that a certain number of ill and disabled children would always be born into the world. Many Mexican American parents who embrace Roman Catholicism believe that God has singled them out for the role because of their past kindnesses to a relative or neighbor who was disabled and view the birth of the disabled infant as God's will.

The number of chronically ill children in industrialized nations has increased markedly over the past decade, particularly those from minority and low-income households who are at high risk for health disparities (American Academy of Pediatrics, 2016). This increase is primarily due to dramatic changes in obesity, environmental pollutants responsible for asthma and other respiratory illnesses, accidents, and injuries. Adolescent pregnancy among low-income populations is often accompanied by poor nutrition before and during pregnancy, failure to seek prenatal care (or waiting until the third trimester to do so), and low-birth-weight infants who are at high risk for respiratory illnesses and failure to thrive (Johnson & Moore, 2016; Kim et al., 2016; Kliegman et al., 2016). In the United States, extensive medical resources are used to save the lives of very low–birth-weight infants; however, the lifesaving efforts often leave a child with multiple chronic illnesses; in countries with fewer medical resources, such as Uganda and Haiti, these same very low–birth-weight babies will not survive infancy (see Figure 6-6).

Special Health Care Needs of Adolescents

There are almost 46 million adolescents aged 10 to 19 in the United States and Canada (Statistics Canada, 2017; U.S. Census Bureau, 2017b). Teenagers are in a process of evolving from childhood to adulthood, and they belong not only to the cultural groups that have formed the basis for their values, attitudes, and beliefs but also to the subculture of adolescents. This subculture links the adolescent with other adolescents through a system of socially transmitted behaviors and belongings, such as brand-named clothing, music, and status symbols. The adolescent subculture has its own set of values, beliefs, and practices that may or may not be in harmony with those of the cultural group that previously guided their behaviors.

The adolescent subculture is vaguely structured and lacks formal written rules or codes. Conformity with the peer group behavior is expected. One of the most outstanding characteristics of the adolescent subculture is preoccupation with clothing, hairstyles, and grooming. Clothing mirrors the personal feelings of the adolescent and facilitates identity with the peer group.

Some young men and women prefer to dress in traditional clothing. In the hospital setting, gowns might stifle the individual's sense of identity, so the adolescent should be permitted to wear familiar clothing whenever the style does

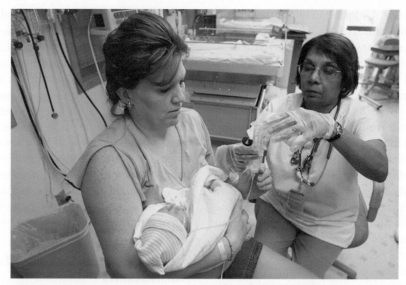

Figure 6-6. Many low-birth-weight infants are "saved" by the availability of hi-tech health care, only to experience multiple chronic illnesses later in life. (Reprinted from *Broadribb's Introductory Pediatric Nursing* (p. 244), by N. Hatfield, 2008, Philadelphia, PA: Wolters Kluwer Health | Lippincott Williams & Wilkins.)

not interfere with safety, comfort, or hygiene. In a clinical setting, there is no harm in allowing a reasonable amount of makeup, jewelry, or other items of apparel that might be important to the adolescent. Body piercing, prominent in some culture for years, has become widely accepted to the adolescent subculture worldwide. The nurse must assess the placement of the piercing to determine whether it may safely remain in place or must be removed. Piercing of the tongue may prove a hygienic issue and must be discussed with the teen before requiring removal.

There is a relationship between some diseases and socioeconomic status; consequently, low-income teenagers may have a wide range of diagnosed and undiagnosed diseases. During the transition from dependent children to independent adults, some disorders might interfere with the adolescent's development of a positive body image, sexual and personal identity, and value system. The entrance of HIV/AIDS as a global health issue has caused adolescents and adults worldwide to seriously evaluate their sexual behavior. Countries are increasingly acknowledging the importance of equipping adolescents with the knowledge and skills to make responsible choices in their lives, with sex education having a central role. Over the years, government and private companies have partnered to educate young people on safe sex practices. One such educational tool for adolescents was teaching the ABCs of sex: *A*bstinence, *B*e Faithful, and use *C*ondoms (The ABCs of Sex Education, 2017). Currently, the United Nations and the World Health Organization are promoting the Global Education 2030 Agenda and using comprehensive sexuality education (CSE). CSE is a curriculum-based process of teaching and learning about the cognitive, emotional, physical, and social aspects of sexuality (United Nations Educational, Scientific and Cultural Organization, 2018). However, condoms are not always used, and unplanned pregnancies and/or unwanted diseases such as HIV, AIDS, pelvic inflammatory disease, chlamydia, and others often follow in adolescents globally (Centers for Disease Control and Prevention, 2018c). Evidence-Based Practice 6-2 identifies effective ways to assist Latina adolescents prevent rapid repeat births.

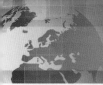

Preventing Rapid Repeat Births Among Latina Adolescents: The Role of Parents

Nationally, up to 50% of adolescent mothers become pregnant again within 24 months of a previous birth; this is known as a *rapid repeat birth* (Damle et al., 2015). Latina adolescents have the highest rate of rapid repeat births in the United States. Although not all adolescent births have adverse outcomes for the Latina mother, they have been associated with an increased rate of sexually transmitted infections and HIV, reduced educational attainment, and decreased financial independence. Adolescent childbearing can also influence future generations. Children born to adolescent mothers have lower levels of cognitive development in childhood, experience less academic achievement, and face a statistically higher probability of becoming adolescent parents themselves, thereby perpetuating a cycle of rapid repeat births among the Latino community.

Several effective pregnancy prevention and parent-based interventions to prevent rapid repeat births among Latino youths from engaging in risky sexual behavior have been developed:

- National Campaign to Prevent Teen and Unplanned Pregnancy
- National Council of La Raza
- Families Talking Together
- Familias Unidas (Families United)
- Cuidalos (Take Care of Them)
- Rompe el Silencio (Break the Silence)
- Steps to Success

In a national random-digit dial telephone survey of greater than 1,000 adolescents aged 12 to 19 years, investigators found that the majority of Latino youths (55%) identified their parents as the greatest influence on their sexual decision-making, a proportion significantly greater than reported by their White (42%) and African American (50%) peers. Among pregnant and parenting Latina adolescents, parents are often the primary source of social, emotional, and financial support, and most adolescent parents live at home after giving birth to a child. Research reveals that parents can influence a range of significant behaviors and outcomes among pregnant and parenting teens, including participation in prevention programs, encouragement

to pursue higher education, improved contraception knowledge and use, and reduced likelihood of future pregnancies.

Clinical Implications

- Latina adolescent parents are an underserved population with complex reproductive and sexual health needs.
- Nurses should recognize the importance of the Latino family in guiding adolescent sexual behavior.
- Parent-based interventions should take into account that adolescents have already engaged in sexual activity and are likely to do so again.
- Intervention programs for adolescent mothers can reduce the risk of rapid repeat pregnancy by providing a combination of individualized support services and improved access to effective contraception (Kisker, Berman, Blasberg, & Wood, 2016). Interventions should also examine the pregnancy intentions of pregnant and parenting Latina adolescents, specific issues in having a partner who is older, various forms of effective contraceptive use, integration of secondary prevention with sexually transmitted infections and HIV prevention, and support for further education and/or pursuit of a career or technical training that will enable the adolescent to be financially self-sufficient.

References: Bouris, A., Guiliamo-Ramos, V., Cherry, K., Dittus, P., Michael, S., & Gloppen, K. (2012). Preventing rapid repeat births among Latina adolescents. *American Journal of Public Health*, 102(10), 1842–1847.

Damle, L. F., Gohari, A. C., McEvoy, A. K., Desale, S. Y., & Gomez-Lobo, V. G. (2015). Early initiation of postpartum contraception: Does it decrease rapid repeat pregnancy in adolescents? *Journal of Pediatric and Adolescent Gynecology*, 28(1), 57–62.

Kisker, E. E., Berman, J., Blasberg, A., & Wood, R. G. (2016). Preventing rapid repeat births among adolescent mothers: Implementing steps to success in San Angelo, Texas. Retrieved November 26, 2018 from https://www.acf.hhs.gov/sites/default/files/opre/prep_hfsa_implementation_report_oct_2016_b508.pdf

Culturally Competent Nursing Care for Children and Adolescents

A few principles of care for specific cultural groups have been provided to illustrate the practical ways in which culturally competent nursing care should be provided. The examples are intended to be illustrative, not exhaustive.

Nursing Assessment of the Family

When assessing the family of a child or adolescent in a clinical setting, nurses should consider the cultural background of the family, the belief systems of the family, as well as the relationship between the child and their family. Each of these components plays a vital role in the cultural assessment of the family and their ability to provide culturally competent care.

Cultural Background

Culture, like language, is acquired early in life, and cultural understanding is typically established by age 5. Every interaction, sound, touch, odor, and experience has a cultural component that is absorbed by the child even when it is not taught directly. Lessons learned at such early ages become an integral part of thinking and behavior. Table manners, the proper behavior when interacting with adults, sick-role behaviors, and the rules of acceptable emotional response are anchored in culture. Many beliefs and behaviors learned at an early age persist into adulthood.

Over time, culture has influenced family functioning in many ways, including marriage forms and ceremonies; choice of mates; postmarital residence; family kinship system; rules governing inheritance, household, and family structure; family obligations; family–community dynamics; and alternative family formations. These traditions have given families a sense of stability and support from which members draw comfort, guidance, and a means of coping with the problems of life, including physical and mental illness, handicaps, disabilities, dying, and death.

Each family modifies the culture of the larger group in ways that are uniquely its own. Some beliefs, practices, and customs are maintained, whereas others are altered or abandoned. Although it is helpful for you to have a basic knowledge of children's cultural backgrounds, it is also necessary to view each family on an individual basis. Assumptions or biased expectations cannot be allowed to replace accurate assessment. It is essential for the nurse to remember that not all members of a cultural group behave in the same fashion. For example, although many Chinese North American children behave in a manner congruent with the stereotype—showing respect for authority, polite social behavior, and a moderate-to-soft voice—some are disrespectful, impolite, and boisterous, and illness only exaggerates the differences. Individual differences, changing norms over time, the degree of acculturation, the length of time the family has lived in a country, and other factors account for variations from the stereotype.

Family Belief Systems

The behavior of children and adolescents is influenced by child-rearing practices, parental beliefs about involvement with children, and the type and frequency of disciplinary measures. Although both parents exert an influence on the child's orientation to health, research indicates that a wide cultural variability exists, with the mother being the most influential parent in many cultural groups; this is easily verified in most single-parent households and also very visible in matriarchal societies of African and African American families. Identifying the attitudes, values, and beliefs about health and illness held by the parents and other providers of child care is an important part of the cultural assessment of the family.

Mothers' attitudes toward health and illnesses are related to their educational level. Mothers with little formal education tend to be more fatalistic about illness and less concerned with detecting clinical manifestations of disease in their children than are well-educated mothers. The former are also less likely to follow up on precautionary measures suggested by health care providers. A mother who believes that people have no control over whether they become sick is more likely to seek care in an emergency facility and less likely to have a preventive approach to health. She is also less likely to seek preventative education and might not comply with recommended immunization schedules. Nursing interventions with a mother who believes that there is much a person can do to keep from becoming ill will be different with regard to the nature of health education and counseling provided.

Assessment data related to the belief system(s) of the family provide the nurse with facts from which to choose approaches and priorities. For a mother who is not oriented to prevention of illness or maintenance of health, focusing energies on teaching might not be productive; it might be more useful to spend time designing family follow-up care or establishing an interpersonal relationship that invites the parent to follow recommended immunization schedules, well-child care, and other aspects of health promotion.

Family Structures

Families have become increasingly diverse and complex in recent decades, and there are many ways that social scientists have classified them. A trend of population growth can be seen with the number of children under age 18 with at least one foreign-born parent increasing from 15.7 million in 2006 to 17.7 million in 2014, and the population is projected to become even more ethnically diverse in the future (Woods & Hanson, 2016). The number of children under age 18 living in **nuclear** or **conjugal** families, those with two married biologic parents and one or more children, is 47.7 million or 69% of all children (U.S. Census Bureau, 2016). Among families worldwide, the nuclear family is a rarity. In only 6% of the world's societies are families as isolated

and nuclear as in the United States and Canada. Approximately 22.4 million children, or 27% of all US children, live in a **single-parent family**, most of whom live with a single female parent (Grall, 2018). An additional 3.8 million children, or 5% of children, live with two unmarried parents. In 2015, estimates showed that 3.9% of children do not live with either parent; rather, they reside with a guardian, such as another relative or nonrelative acting as a guardian for the child in the absence of a parent (Child Trends, 2015). Fifty-five percent of children (1.83 million) who do not live with a parent live with a grandparent or other extended family member. If children coreside with members of their mother's family, this is referred to as a matrifocal family constellation; if the children coreside with members of their father's family, it is called a patrifocal family constellation.

Blended families include children from a previous marriage of the wife, husband, or both parents or families formed outside of marriage. Lastly, there are **extended families** in which parents and children coreside with other members of one parent's family. The most recent published estimates indicate that 16% of children live with extended family, including around 10% of children coresiding with a grandparent (Cross, 2018). The extended family is far more universally the norm. Kin residence sharing, for example, has long been acknowledged as characteristic of many African American, Chinese American, Mexican American, Amish, and other groups who place a great emphasis on familism (Cross, 2018; Laughlin, 2014).

Early in the nurse–parent relationship, it is necessary to identify members of the family who play a significant role in the care of the child. In societies where the extended family is the norm, parents—particularly those who married at a young age—might be considered too inexperienced to make major decisions on behalf of their child. In these groups, key decisions are frequently made in consultation with more mature relatives such as grandparents, uncles, aunts, cousins, or other kin. Sometimes, nonkin is considered to be part of the extended family.

In many religions, the members of one's church, synagogue, temple, or mosque are viewed as extended family members who might be relied on for various types of support, including child care. Not coincidentally, members of some congregations refer to one another as brothers and sisters. The Amish family pattern is referred to as *friendscraft*, or three-generational family structure. Amish parents know that they can rely on the support of their entire church community. For example, a young Amish couple might turn to that community for assistance with decision-making, finances, and emotional and spiritual support when a child is ill. The nurse should ask the parents if anyone else will be participating in the decision-making that affects their child. Once that information is known, the person(s) identified by the parents should be included in the child's plan of care.

The influence of the extended family or the social support network on the child's development becomes particularly important when the number of single-parent families in some culturally diverse groups is considered. The nuclear family is the unit for which most health care programs are designed. Consider the implicit message about the family when two or three chairs for visitors are placed in hospital rooms, physician or nurse practitioner offices, and other health care settings, for example. Although a handful of rural hospitals make special accommodations for the extended and church family of clients, few provide a place for the Amish to hitch their horses and buggies adjacent to the facility. With the advent of family-centered care in the United States, all children's hospitals provide more flexible visiting hours and extend visiting privileges to include siblings, extended family, and friends (see Evidence-Based Practice 6-3).

Nursing Interventions

Care of the hospitalized child's body is the primary domain of the nurse. Principles related to personal hygiene, including bathing, shaving, and hair care, apply to children of all racial and ethnic backgrounds, but the specific manner in which care is given might vary widely. Despite its importance, hair care is sometimes omitted for Black children because White, Hispanic, Asian, and Native American nurses might be unfamiliar with proper care. The hair of black children varies widely in texture and is usually fragile. Hair might be long and straight or short, thick, and kinky. The hair and scalp have a natural tendency to be dry and to require daily combing, gentle brushing, and application to the scalp of a light oil such as Vaseline or mineral oil. The hair might be rolled on curlers, braided, or left loose, according to personal preference. Bobby pins or combs might be used to keep the hair in place. If an individual has cornrow braids or shaved, sculptured hair, the scalp might be massaged, oiled, and shampooed without unbraiding the hair. Some Blacks prefer straightened hair, which might be obtained chemically or thermally. Hair that has been straightened with a pressing comb will return to its naturally kinky state when exposed to moisture or humidity or when hair growth occurs. Children of Asian descent tend to have straight hair that does not require the same amount of care as the hair of most African Americans or Whites.

Textural variations also are found in the facial hair of culturally diverse boys and men during adolescence and adulthood. Many Asian teenage boys have light facial hair and require infrequent shaving, whereas African American boys and men tend to have a heavy growth of facial hair requiring regular attention. Some Black teenage boys have tightly curled facial hair, which, when shaved, curls back upon itself and penetrates the skin. This may result in a local foreign-body reaction on the face that can lead to the formation of papules, pustules, and multiple small keloids. Some African American teens and men might prefer to grow beards rather than shave, particularly when they are ill. Before shaving a teen, determine his usual method of facial grooming and attempt to shave or apply depilatories (agents that remove hair) in a similar manner. When using depilatories, protect the skin from irritation by

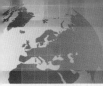
When Health Care Provider Decisions Clash with Parental Preference

Each year, health care research unravels the mystery of previously unknown diseases and conditions; recently, expanded knowledge about Proteus syndrome has been revealed. This rare congenital and progressive disorder causes soft tissue overgrowth (nonmalignant tumors), resulting in swelling that compresses nerves, vessels, and organs. Asymmetrical growth of skeletal and soft tissue also produces spinal deformities and respiratory compromise. It was a 12-year-old with Proteus syndrome who attracted the attention of the health care team. Turner (2010) provides unique insight into 2 years in the life of this child. These 2 years reflected a situation in which the care perceived necessary for the longevity of the child was in direct conflict with the traditional cultural beliefs of a Chinese family who immigrated to the United States. Over several years, the child deteriorated from attending school regularly to a nonverbal, agitated child exhibiting self-injurious behavior (head banging, scratching, and banging of extremities); she was hospitalized seven times. The mother had difficulty physically managing the child; the family had limited financial resources, lived in a small apartment that could not accommodate needed care equipment, was unable to communicate in English, and had no extended family available; the parents voluntarily placed the child in medical foster care.

Over nearly 2 years in foster care, the child improved significantly. Consistent pain management helped to eliminate the self-injurious behavior; mobility improved; she demonstrated the understanding of simple words and began smiling. Since the course/progression of Proteus syndrome is unknown and hospitalizations were becoming more frequent, the primary medical team requested a palliative care consultation.

To determine the outcome of the ethical dilemma, the health care team utilized a four-quadrant ethical decision-making tool taking into consideration medical indications (principles of beneficence and nonmalfeasance), patient preference (respect for autonomy), quality of life (principles of beneficence, nonmalfeasance, and autonomy), and contextual features (loyalty and fairness). When the decisions were made and presented to the parents, they determined it was their familial duty to take the child out of foster care and back to their home to provide a dignified death. The health care team was severely divided about this decision: some felt, for the child's well-being, she should return to the foster care home where she was showing emotional improvement, and others believed it was a parental decision related to the care of a minor child. This dilemma was taken to the hospital ethics committee for decision. The committee determined that the rights of the parents superseded the other factors and the child was discharged to the parental home with a home care and pain management plan.

This was clearly a difficult decision; however, the solution has ended being a correct one. Once again in her home environment, the child began to thrive, smile, make eye contact with her family, and even walk as few feet. She has been at home for 2 years and her parents seemed quite comfortable with the results: supported by strong cultural ties, her mother never stops smiling.

Reference: Turner, H. N. (2010). Parental preference or child well-being: An ethical dilemma. *Journal of Pediatric Nursing,* 25(1), 58–63.

---

keeping the chemical from contacting the client's nose, mouth, eyes, and ears. Straight and safety razors are contraindicated when depilatories are used because they can cause local irritation to the skin.

Nurses should ask the child's parent or extended family member how personal hygiene is carried out at home if in doubt. Children might feel more secure if a parent or close family member actually provides the care. If you determine that the child would benefit from care by a familiar caregiver from home, the rationale for requesting family intervention should be explained. Comments that the nursing staff is too busy or uninterested in providing personal hygiene or hair care should be avoided; rather, the benefit to the child's security and sense of well-being should be emphasized.

When bathing a client, remember that the washcloth removes some parts of the outermost skin layer. Such sloughed skin, which will be evident on the washcloth and in the bathwater, will vary in color depending on the ethnic group of the person being bathed. The sloughed skin of a darkly pigmented child, for example, will be a brownish black color. This does not mean that the child was dirty; the normal sloughing of skin is simply more evident in darkly pigmented people when compared with lightly pigmented groups. The more melanin that is present, the darker the skin color will be. Because dryness is more evident on darkly pigmented skin, Vaseline, baby oil, lanolin cream, and lotions can be applied after the bath to give the skin a shiny, healthy appearance.

Communicating with the Hospitalized Child and Family

Communicating with the child and the family is a key component in a successful hospitalization and recovery. Verbal communication is especially difficult when the child–family–health care provider do not speak the same language. The nurses may obtain the services of an interpreter, although they should be aware of gender- and age-related customs before doing so. For instance, an adolescent girl might be uncomfortable with an older male interpreter, and an older boy might prefer a friend to translate rather than an interpreter connected to the health agency. Attention should also be paid to the correct national origin of the child before seeking an interpreter; for example, an individual from Southeast Asia may speak Vietnamese, Cambodian, or Laotian— vastly different languages. Approximately 15% of migrant/immigrant families speak English in the home; this factor should be included in the nursing assessment. Most children and adolescents involved in the American school system learn English quickly and may serve as interpreters for family members. Even in families who have mastered English as a second language, the stress of illness and hospitalization may cause them to have difficulty communicating with English. Therefore, using a formal or informal interpreter is recommended.

Nonverbal expressions can be powerful communication tools. Nurses should take their cues from observing the family interactions. Some Italian parents/families are very demonstrative with facial expressions and arm/hand gestures while the children may remain quiet. On the other hand, Asian parents and children both remain quiet and often wear "masked faces" showing very little emotional expression. Nurses must be aware of their own nonverbal expressions or actions, as they are often interpreted as disrespect or dislike of the individual rather than a situation.

Evaluation of the Nursing Care Plan

Obtaining a thorough cultural assessment, including use of folk remedies, during the initial encounter with the child/adolescent and parents is essential. It is upon this basis that the plan of care is developed, negotiated, and evaluated. To evaluate the effectiveness of the nursing care plan in providing culturally competent care, first ask a few probing questions to determine whether the plan was successful in achieving the desired outcomes, including the mutual goals established with the child and parents. Second, if the goals were not met, ask a few probing questions to determine the reasons for failure. Were the child and parents included in the planning and implementation of the nursing care? Were extended family members included in the plan? Did the true decision-maker in the family participate in the care plan? Third, if the goals were met, the reasons for their success should be evaluated and communicated to other members of the health care team for future reference.

Application of Cultural Concepts to Nursing Care

Two case studies are presented here to demonstrate the application of transcultural nursing concepts, theories, and research findings to clinical nursing practice. The first, Case Study 6-1, focuses on a very young child from an American Amish family and the second, Case Study 6-2, on a dying child from a Buddhist family. Each case exemplifies the need for involvement of extended families of varying types. Each also reflects how the response of the nursing team affected the end result of the

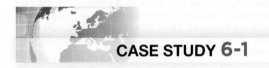

CASE STUDY 6-1

Presence of Immediate and Extended Family

A rural Amish community is located about 50 miles from an urban medical center, the only facility available for care of an acutely ill child. An enthusiastic new RN emphatically presents her case to allow the presence of family/**extended family** of a 6-month-old Amish child who has been admitted for the repair of a cardiac VSD. The nurse is passionate about the issue, rational in her approach, and assured that she can prevail to change existing visitation policies.

The problem of overnight accommodation for the extended community family has become a topic of debate among the nursing staff. Sensitive to the cultural practices and beliefs of the Amish child and his family, the new RN begins stating her position on behalf of the family's right to adhere to Amish cultural practices to her supervisor. The supervisor listens impatiently and quickly interrupts with her decision. "These people are such a nuisance. The child wouldn't even have the VSD if they didn't insist on intermarriage within their own community. Then they come here in droves and think we have to give them a place to sleep. This isn't a hotel. They can just go back to their horses and buggies and old-fashioned ways. The answer is NO! The natural, biologic mother and father may spend the night. Everyone else is to go home. And that's final."

child's care. In addition, a specific, individualized plan of care for the Amish family is presented. As shown, the nursing issues in each case are complex and multifaceted. The interconnectedness of the various components of the child's situation with the larger system is often minimized or disregarded. The values and beliefs of both the nurses within the health care delivery system and the family's extended social network must be considered. For the purpose of analysis, some fundamental conflicts in values and beliefs have been identified. Similarities and differences also have been indicated in the nursing plan of care.

The nurse leaves the discussion with her supervisor feeling dejected; however, she completes her data collection. Using Leininger's transcultural model (1991), she examines the underlying attitudes, values, and beliefs among the Amish parents and those of the health care providers and then develops an individualized, culturally congruent plan of care. Prior to discharge, the nurse, in collaboration with the parents and other significant members of the extended family, evaluates the effectiveness of the nursing care from a transcultural nursing perspective. The young nurse must also review the process in which change can be accomplished within the agency. She needs to determine what parts of the system can/should be manipulated to bring about desired change and who are the formal and informal leaders who can effect change.

Outcome: There are no definitive solutions or answers for this dilemma. The case study is intended to demonstrate the complexity of the cross-cultural issues and to emphasize the necessity for thoughtful analysis of various facets of the problem. The ability to synthesize information from previous learning—psychology, anthropology, religion and theology, history, economics, sociology, principles of leadership, and others—to the nursing care of children from culturally diverse backgrounds is invaluable.

The cultural assessment is the foundation of excellent transcultural care and cannot be overlooked even in the face of major obstacles of attitudes of others or limited time. A cultural assessment must become an integral part of the admission assessment of all children and adolescents, thus enabling excellent, individualized, family-centered care.

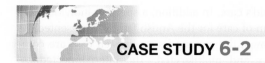

CASE STUDY 6-2

End-of-Life Care for a Buddhist Adolescent

Ving, 16 years of age, was born in Vietnam and immigrated to Australia with her family 15 years ago. She is a devout Buddhist. Ving was born hepatitis B positive, which is now complicated by advanced liver cancer. Over the past few weeks, Ving's pain has become unmanageable at home, and her family has her admitted to the hospital for better pain management. Her family is concerned that appropriate preparations be made for her death.

In collaboration with Buddhists monks, the nurses of the inpatient unit agree that Ving would be cared for through the final hours of her life with minimal noise and minimal activity in her room; this was to ensure that her soul was as untroubled as possible. Her family remained with Ving around the clock and agreed to notify the nurses when she died; the health care team agreed not to touch the body until the family agreed it was appropriate.

Outcome: On the day of her death, family, close friends, and spiritual advisors were present to oversee the process. Eight hours after her death, it was determined that Ving's consciousness had departed; she was then examined by the health care team, and the time of death was documented.

Adapted with permission from The Royal Australian College of General Practitioners from Clark, K., & Phillips, J. (2010). End of life care—The importance of culture and ethnicity. *Australian Family Physician*, *39*(4), 210–213. Retrieved from www.racgp.org.au/afp/2010/april/end-of-life-care-%E2%80%93-the-importance-of-culture-and-ethnicity

In the case involving the Amish child, the young nurse was clearly advocating for a patient, in a situation requiring change in hospital practice, if not policy. It is assumed that this facility had not yet implemented principles of family-centered care, which are common practice in most agencies that care for children. Given the negative response of the nursing supervisor, it would seem the nurse needs to reassess her approach to the problem. She would be wise to first gather data from her colleagues to help her understand the immediate, inflexible response of the supervisor and then determine whether there are possible compromises that would be acceptable to both family and supervisor. She will need to present the risk versus benefits of having the extended family remain with the child: consider factors from agency perspective, the legal perspective, perspective of other patients, and the child/family perspective (see Box 6-1). A review of the literature will reveal significant data that support involvement of extended family in hastening recovery of the child by supporting the entire family.

BOX 6-1 | Nursing Plan of Care: Hospitalization of an Amish Child: Conflicting Cultural Values

Goal: Child's recovery and ultimate discharge from the hospital (return to parents) in an optimal state of health. This is a mutual goal of the Amish child's parents and of the health care providers within the health care system. In order to plan care for this child, the nurse needs to examine the underlying attitudes, values, and beliefs of the two groups that are in conflict. Points on which there is agreement must be identified as well.

Amish–Rural, Agricultural Lifestyle	Urban Health Care Providers
Family	
Large families, extended sociocultural–religious network of community members who assist the natural parents	Small family units, urban lifestyle, nuclear family

BOX 6-1	Nursing Plan of Care: Hospitalization of an Amish Child: Conflicting Cultural Values (continued)

Cooperation and support among extended family, especially in stressful "crisis" times such as hospitalization of a child

Individual responsibility by members of a nuclear family; mother and father primarily responsible

Child generally not left alone when away from community; someone from the community visits or stays in the absence of parents

Visiting by grandparents and siblings accepted but only two at any given time and only parents can remain overnight

Concept of family includes "nonblood relatives."

Concept of family includes only biologically related persons.

Parental Obligations

Children are a part of a larger cultural group; adult members of the larger community have various relationships and obligations to the children and parents even though they are not biologically related.

Mother and father are responsible for children; only they may stay with the child overnight. Physical size of hospital facilities does not allow for a large number of visitors, who clutter rooms, violate fire safety rules by blocking doorways, and hinder delivery of care. Responding to requests for information from every visitor is time-consuming and violates HIPAA policies.

Economic Considerations

Communal sharing of resources; hospital bill is paid from a common fund; the entire bill is paid in cash upon discharge.

Rely on private or state-subsidized health insurance coverage for payment of all costs related to patient care; sense of anonymity and impersonal involvement

Traditional and Religious Values

Religious values permeate all aspects of daily living; time set aside daily for prayer and reading of scripture.

Religion is important and adherence to practices often varies based on severity of illness; worship is usually limited to a single day of the week, such as Saturday or Sunday.

Belief that illness afflicts both the "just" and the less righteous and is to be endured with patience and faith.

Illness is part of a cause–effect relationship; science and technology will one day conquer illness.

Protestant work ethic (in an agricultural, rural sense)

Protestant work ethic (in an urban sense)

Dress is according to 19th-century traditions; specific colors and styles indicate marital status.

Fashions occur in trends; wide range of "acceptable" dress

Married men wear beards; single men are clean-shaven.

Whether a man shaves is a matter of personal preference.

Simple, rural lifestyle; family-oriented living. For religious reasons, avoid "modern" conveniences such as electricity; use candles/kerosene lights and outdoor sanitary facilities.

Use hi-tech electronic equipment, electricity, and nuclear energy. Indoor plumbing is the norm; autoflush toilets and water that runs with the wave of a hand are "ordinary."

Summary

Culture exerts an all-pervasive influence on infants, children, and adolescents and determines the nursing interventions appropriate for the individual child, parents, and extended family members. Knowledge of the cultural background of the child and family is necessary for the provision of excellent transcultural nursing care. Cross-cultural communication must convey genuine interest and allow for expression of expectations, concerns, and questions.

Culture influences the child's physical and psychosocial growth and development. Basic physiologic needs such as nutrition, sleep, and elimination have aspects that are culturally determined. Parent–child relationships vary significantly among families of different cultures, and individual differences among those with the same background add to the complexity. Cultural beliefs and values related to health and illness influence health-seeking behaviors by parents and determine the nature of care and cure expected.

Regardless of the cultural background of an adolescent, the transition from childhood to adulthood must be accomplished. This can be complicated when the adolescent's values, beliefs, and practices conflict with traditional cultural values or with those of the dominant culture in which the teenager lives. Acculturation of an adolescent presents multiple issues for the family as well as for the teen.

REVIEW QUESTIONS

1. Compare and contrast the child-rearing practices of three cultural groups. For each of the three groups, also discuss the role of extended family members in raising children, and describe the ways in which extended family members can assist parents during a child's illness.

2. Critically examine the perceived causes of chronic illness and disability in children from diverse cultures. Describe how the parental philosophic and religious beliefs affect their reaction to and explanations for the child's chronic illness and/or disability.

3. Describe the symptoms associated with the following Hispanic cultural illnesses affecting children:

   a. *Pujos* (grunting)
   b. *Mal ojo* (evil eye)
   c. *Caida de la mollera* (fallen fontanelle)
   d. *Empacho* (a digestive disorder)

CRITICAL THINKING ACTIVITIES

1. Arrange for an observational experience in a culturally diverse classroom. Compare and contrast the behaviors observed. Does the student–teacher interaction vary according to cultural background? What culturally based attitudes, values, and beliefs are reflected in the children's behaviors? The teacher's attitude? Ask the teacher(s) to describe the cultural similarities and differences in the classroom.

2. When caring for a child from a cultural background different from your own, spend time talking with the child's parents or primary provider of care, and discuss the child-rearing beliefs and practices specifically related to the child's nutrition, sleep, elimination, parent–child relationship, discipline, growth, and development. Compare and contrast the parental responses with your own beliefs and practices.

3. When assigned to the pediatric unit, observe the number and relationship of visitors for children from various cultures. Who visits the child? If nonrelated visitors come, how do they interact with the child? With the parent(s)?

4. When caring for a child from a cultural background different from your own, ask the parent(s) or primary provider(s) of care to tell you what they believe causes the child to be healthy and unhealthy. To what cause(s) do they attribute the current illness or hospitalization? What interventions do they believe will help the child to recover? Are there any healers outside of the professional health care system (e.g., folk, indigenous, or traditional healers) whom they believe could help the child return to health?

REFERENCES

ABC's of Sex Education. (2017). The ABCs of sex education: Kufanya Uamuzi Bora (making wise decisions). Retrieved November 24, 2018 from http://abcsofsex-ed.org/wp-content/uploads/2018/03/ABCs-Training-Manual-August-2017.pdf

American Academy of Pediatrics. (2015). How to prevent tooth decay in your baby. Retrieved from healthychildren. org: https://www.healthychildren.org/English/ages-stages/baby/teething-tooth-care/Pages/How-to-Prevent-Tooth-Decay-in-Your-Baby.aspx

American Academy of Pediatrics. (2016). Percentage of U.S. children who have chronic health conditions on the rise. Retrieved November 21, 2018 from https://www. aap.org/en-us/about-the-aap/aap-press-room/pages/Percentage-of-U-S--Children-Who-Have-Chronic-Health-Conditions-on-the-Rise.aspx

American Institutes for Research. (2018). National Center on family homelessness. Retrieved November 19, 2018 from https://www.air.org/center/national-center-family-homelessness

Aruda, M. M. (2011). Predictors of unprotected intercourse for female adolescents measured at their request for a pregnancy test. Journal of Pediatric Nursing, 26(3), 216–223. doi: 10.1016/j.pedn.2010.02.005

Bailey, C. (2016). Breastfeeding mothers' experiences of bedsharing: A qualitative study. Breastfeeding Review, 24(2), 33–40. Retrieved from http://libproxy.umflint.edu/login?url=http://search.ebscohost.com/login.aspx?direct=true&db=ccm&AN=117003990&site=ehost-live&scope=site

Barajas, R. G., Martin, A., Brooks-Gunn, J., & Hale, L. (2011). Mother-child bed-sharing in toddlerhood and cognitive and behavioral outcomes. Pediatrics, 128(2), e339–e347. doi: 10.1542/peds.2010-3300

Barry, H., Bacon, M. K., & Child, I. L. (1967). Definitions, ratings, and bibliographic sources of child-training practices of 110 cultures. In C. S. Ford (Ed.), Cross-cultural approaches (pp. 293–331). New Haven, CT: HRAF Press.

Benoit, D. (2004). Infant-parent attachment: Definition, types, antecedents, measurement and outcome. Paediatrics & Child Health, 9(8), 541–545.

Bernstein, R. (2016). Parenting around the world: Child-rearing practices in different cultures. Retrieved November 14, 2018 from https://www.tuw.edu/content/health/child-rearing-practices-different-cultures/

Bombard, J. M., Kortsmit, K., Warner, L., et al. (2018). Vital signs: Trends and disparities in infant safe sleep practices—United States, 2009–2015. Morbidity and Mortality Weekly Report, 67(1), 39–46. http://dx.doi.org/10.15585/mmwr.mm6701e1

Bresnahan, M., Zhuang, J., & Park, S. (2014). Cultural differences in the perception of health and cuteness of fat babies. The International Journal of Communication and Health (4), 52–58.

Cachelin, F. M., & Thompson, D. (2014). Impact of Asian American mothers' feeding beliefs and practices on child obesity in a diverse community sample. Asian American Journal of Psychology, 5(3), 223–229.

Canada Without Poverty. (2018). Basic statistics about poverty in Canada. Retrieved November 11, 2018 from http://www.cwp-csp.ca/poverty/just-the-facts/

Cartagena, D. C., Ameringer, S. W., McGrath, J., Jallo, N., Masho, S. W., & Myers, B. J. (2014). Factors contributing to infant overfeeding with Hispanic mothers. Journal of Obstetric, Gynecologic, and Neonatal Nursing, 43(2), 139. doi: 10.1111/1552-6909.12279

Centers for Disease Control and Prevention. (2014). Strategies for reducing health disparities: Selected CDC-sponsored interventions, United States, 2014. Morbidity and Mortality Weekly Report, Supplement, 63(1), 1–47.

Centers for Disease Control and Prevention. (2018a). HIV among pregnant women, infants, and children. Retrieved from Centers for Disease Control and Prevention: https://www.cdc.gov/hiv/group/gender/pregnantwomen/index.html

Centers for Disease Control and Prevention. (2018b). Deaths: Leading causes for 2016. Retrieved November 21, 2018 from https://www.cdc.gov/nchs/data/nvsr/nvsr67/nvsr67_06.pdf

Centers for Disease Control and Prevention. (2018c). Sexual risk behaviors: HIV, STD, & teen pregnancy prevention. Retrieved November 24, 2018 from https://www.cdc.gov/healthyyouth/sexualbehaviors/

Chaudry, A., & Wimer, C. (2016). Poverty is not just an indicator: The relationship between income, poverty, and child well-being. Academics Pediatrics, 16(3), S23–S29. https://doi.org/10.1016/j.acap.2015.12.010

Chen, X., & Eisenberg, N. (2012). Understanding cultural issues in child development: Introduction. Child Development Perspectives, 6(1), 1–4.

Child Trends. (2015). Living arrangements of children under 18 years old, percentages by race and Hispanic origin: Selected years, 1960–2015. Retrieved November 26, 2018 from https://www.childtrends.org/wp-content/uploads/2014/07/59_appendix1.pdf

Child Trends. (2018). Racial and ethnic composition of the child population. Retrieved November 9, 2018 from https://www.childtrends.org/indicators/racial-and-ethnic-composition-of-the-child-population

Children's Defense Fund. (2017a). Overview of the State of America's Children 2017. Washington, DC: Author. Retrieved from https://www.childrensdefense.org/wp-content/uploads/2018/06/state-of-americas-children-overview.pdf

Children's Defense Fund. (2017b). Child poverty in America 2016: National analysis. Retrieved November 11, 2018 from https://www.childrensdefense.org/wp-content/uploads/2018/06/child-poverty-in-america-2016.pdf

Children's Defense Fund. (2017c). Health. Retrieved November 20, 2018 from https://www.childrensdefense.org/policy/policy-priorities/health/

Clark, K., & Philips, J. (2010). End of life care: The importance of culture and ethnicity. *Australian Family Physician*, *39*(4), 210–213.

Cowie, J. (2014). Measurement of obesity in children. *Primary Health Care*, *24*(7), 18–23.

Cross, C. J. (2018). Extended family households among children in the United States: Differences by race/ethnicity and socio-economic status. *Population Studies*, *72*(2), 235–251. doi: 10.1080/00324728.2018.1468476.

Dammery, S. (2016). *First blood. A cultural study of menarche.* Victoria, Australia: Monash University Publishing.

Dewar, G. (2017a). Infant crying, fussing, and colic: An anthropological perspective on the role of parenting. Retrieved from Parenting Science: http://www.parenting-science.com/infant-crying.html

Dewar, G. (2017b). The science of attachment parenting. Retrieved from Parenting Science: http://www.parenting-science.com/attachment-parenting.html

Farange, M. A., Miller, K. W., & Davis, A. (2011). Cultural aspects of menstruation and menstrual hygiene in adolescents. *Expert Review of Obstetrics & Gynecology*, *6*(2), 127. http://dx.doi.org.libproxy.umflint.edu/10.1586/eog.11.1

Findlay, L., Kohen, D., & Miller, A. (2014). Developmental milestones among aboriginal children in Canada. *Paediatrics & Child Health*, *19*(5), 241–246.

Forum on Child and Family Statistics. (2018a). America's children in brief: Key national indicators of well-being, 2018. Retrieved November 9, 2018 from https://www.childstats.gov/pdf/ac2018/ac_18.pdf

Forum on Child and Family Statistics. (2018b). Child poverty and extreme poverty. Retrieved November 9, 2018 from https://www.childstats.gov/americaschildren/poverty.asp

Gaydos, L. M., Blake, S. C., Gazmararian, J., Woodruff, W., Thompson, W. W., & Dalmida, S. G. (2015). Revisiting safe sleep recommendations for African-American Infants: Why current counseling is insufficient. *Maternal Child Health Journal*, *19*(1), 496–503. doi: 10.1007/s10995-014-1530-z

Glaser, K. (2016). Lactose intolerance. Retrieved November 21, 2018 from https://academic-eb-com.libproxy.umflint.edu/levels/collegiate/article/lactose-intolerance/627368

Grall, T. (2018). Custodial mothers and fathers and their child support: 2015. Current Population Reports, U.S. Census Bureau, 60-262. Retrieved November 26, 2018 from https://www.census.gov/content/dam/Census/library/publications/2018/demo/P60-262.pdf

Hadi, D., Zenobia, B., & Hasbini, T. (2016). Targeting unintended teen pregnancy in the U.S. *International Journal of Childbirth Education*, *31*(1), 28–31. Retrieved from http://libproxy.umflint.edu:2048/login?url=https://search-proquest-com.libproxy.umflint.edu/docview/1789782798?accountid=14584

Hartmann, K., Rivadeneyra, R., & Toro-Morn, M. (2016). A study of Mexican immigrant mothers and adolescent daughters in the heartland: "mi mamá nada más me dice que me cuide mucho" (my mom just tells me to take care of myself a lot). *The Journal of Latino-Latin American Studies*, *8*(1), 55–76. Retrieved from http://libproxy.umflint.edu:2048/login?url=https://search-proquest-com.libproxy.umflint.edu/docview/1781649104?accountid=14584

Heng, J., Quan, J., Sim, L. W., Sanmugam, S., Broekman, B., Bureau, J., ..., Rifkin-Graboi, A. (2018) The role of ethnicity and socioeconomic status in Southeast Asian mothers' parenting sensitivity. *Attachment & Human Development*, *20*(1), 24–42. doi: 10.1080/14616734.2017.1365912

Huang, Y., Hauck, F. R., Signore, C., Yu, A., Raju, T. N., Huang, T. T., & Fein, S. B. (2013). Influence of bedsharing activity on breastfeeding duration among U.S. mothers. *JAMA Pediatrics*, *137*(11), 1038–1044. doi: 10.1001/jamapediatrics.20132632

International Hip Dysplasia Institute. (2018). Causes of DDH. What causes hip dysplasia? Retrieved November 18, 2018 from https://hipdysplasia.org/developmental-dysplasia-of-the-hip/causes-of-ddh/

International Society for the Prevention of Child Abuse and Neglect. (2017). International Society for the Prevention of Child Abuse and Neglect, Impact of ISPCAN. Retrieved November 20, 2018 from https://www.ispcan.org/

Jain, S., Romack, R., & Jain, R. (2011). Bed sharing in school-age children: Clinical and social implications. *Journal of Child and Psychiatric Nursing*, *24*, 185–189.

John Hopkins Children's Center. (n.d.). Malnutrition. Retrieved November 16, 2018 from https://www.hopkins-medicine.org/healthlibrary/conditions/adult/pediatrics/malnutrition_22,Malnutrition

Johnson, W., & Moore, S. E. (2016). Adolescent pregnancy, nutrition, and health outcomes in low- and middle-income countries: What we know and what we don't know. *BJOG, An International Journal of Obstetrics and Gynaecology*, *123*(10), 1589–1592. https://doi-org.libproxy.umflint.edu/10.1111/1471-0528.13782

Jones, K. M., Power, M. L., Queenan, J. T., & Schulkin, J. (2015). Racial and ethnic disparities in breastfeeding. *Breastfeeding Medicine: The Official journal of the Academy of Breastfeeding Medicine, 10*(4), 186–196. doi: 10.1089/bfm.2014.0152

Keller, H. (2013). Attachment and culture. *Journal of Cross-Cultural Psychology, 44*(2), 175–194.

Kim, J., van Priscilla Reddyrt, D. B., Sewpaul, R., Nyembezi, A., Naidoo, P., & Crutzen, R. (2016). Predictors of nurses' and midwives' intentions to provide maternal and child healthcare services to adolescents in South Africa. *BMC Health Services Research, 16*(1), 658. http://dx.doi.org.lib-proxy.umflint.edu/10.1186/s12913-016-1901-9

Kirby, J. B., Liang, L., Hsin-Jen, C., & Wang, Y. (2012). Race, place, and obesity: The complex relationships among community racial/ethnic composition, individual race/ethnicity, and obesity in the United States. *American Journal of Public Health, 102*(8), 1572–1578.

Kliegman, R. M., Stanton, B. F., Saint Geme, J. W., Schor, N. F., & Behrman, R. E. (2016). *Nelson textbook of pediatrics* (20th ed.). Philadelphia, PA: Elsevier Saunders.

Korbin, J. E. (1991). Cross-cultural perspectives and research directions for the 21st century. *Child Abuse and Neglect, 15*(Suppl. 1), 67–77.

Lahme, A. M., Stern, R., & Cooper, D. (2016). Factors impacting on menstrual hygiene and their implications for health promotion. *Global Health Promotion, 25*(1), 54–62. doi: 10.1177/1757975916648301

Lakhan, R., Bipeta, R., Yerramilli, S., & Nahar, V. K. (2017). A family study of consanguinity in children with intellectual disabilities in Barwani, India. *Journal of Neurosciences in Rural Practice, 8*(4), 551–555. doi: 10.4103/jnrp.jnrp_104_17

Laughlin, L. (2014). *A child's day: Living arrangements, nativity, and family traditions: 2011 (selected indicators of child well-being).* Current Population Reports, 70-139. Washington, DC: U.S. Census Bureau.

Leininger, M. M. (1991). *Culture care delivery and universality: A theory of nursing.* New York, NY: National League for Nursing Press.

Liamputtong, P. (2011). *Infant feeding practices: A cross-cultural perspective.* New York, NY: Springer Science + Business Media.

Losin, E. A. R. (2017). Culture, brain, and health: Introduction to the special issue. *Culture and Brain, 5*(1), 1–3. https://doi-org.libproxy.umflint.edu/10.1007/s40167-017-0049-8

Migration Policy Institute. (2018). U.S. immigrant population by state and county. Data from the U.S. Census Bureau's pooled 2012–2016 American Community Survey. Retrieved from https://www.migrationpolicy.org/programs/data-hub/charts/us-immigrant-population-state-and-county

Mileva-Seitz, V. R., Bakermans-Kranenburg, M. J., Battaini, C., & Luijk, M. (2017). Parent-child bed-sharing: The good, the bad, and the burden of evidence. *Sleep Medicine Reviews, 32*(1), 4–27. https://doi.org/10.1016/j.smrv.2016.03.003

Min, J., Wen, X., Xue, H., & Wang, Y. (2018). Ethnic disparities in childhood BMI trajectories and obesity and potential causes among 29,250 US children: Findings from the Early Childhood Longitudinal Study-Birth and Kindergarten Cohorts. *International Journal of Obesity, 42*(1), 1661–1670. https://doi-org.libproxy.umflint.edu/10.1038/s41366-018-0091-4

Moreno, G., Johnson-Shelton, D., & Boles, S. (2013). Prevalence and prediction of overweight and obesity among elementary school children. *Journal of School Health, 83*(1), 157–163.

Natale, V., & Rajagopalan, A. (2014). Worldwide variation in human growth and the World Health Organization growth standards: A systematic review. *British Medical Journal Open, 8*(1), e003735. Retrieved from http://www.pubfacts.com/detail/24401723/Worldwide-variation-in-human-growth-and-the-World-Health-Organization-growth-standards:-a-systematic

National Kids Count. (2018). Children who speak a language other than English at home. Retrieved November 9, 2018 from https://datacenter.kidscount.org/data/tables/81-children-who-speak-a-language-other-than-english-at-home#detailed/1/any/false/871,870,573,869,36,868,867,133,38,35/any/396,397

Ogden, C. L., Carroll, M. D., Kit, B. K., & Flegal, K. M. (2014). Prevalence of childhood and adult obesity in the United States, 2011–2012. *JAMA, 311*(8), 806.

Overfield, T. (2017). *CRC revivals: Biologic variation in health and illness: Race, age and sex differences* (2nd ed.). New York, NY: CRC Press.

Rachmi, C. N., Hunter, C. L., Li, M., & Baur, L. A. (2017). Perceptions of overweight by primary carers (mothers/grandmothers) of under five and elementary school-aged children in bandung, indonesia: A qualitative study. *International Journal of Behavioral Nutrition and Physical Activity, 14*(1), 101. doi:http://dx.doi.org.libproxy.umflint.edu/10.1186/s12966-017-0556-1.

Ramirez, M. (2016). Childhood obesity, malnutrition connected to mom's perception of child's weight. Retrieved November 16, 2018 from The University of Houston: https://www.uh.edu/news-events/stories/2016/April/420HHPimmigrantmoms.php

Salm Ward, T. C. (2015). Reasons for mother-infant bed sharing: A systematic narrative synthesis of the literature and implications for future research. *Maternal and Child Health Journal, 19*(3), 675–690. doi: 10.1007/s10995-014-1557-1

Santos, I. S., Barros, A. J., Barros, F. C., Munhoz, T. N., Da Silva, B., & Matijasevich, A. (2017). Mother–child bed-sharing trajectories and psychiatric disorders at the age of 6 years. *Journal of Affective Disorders, 208*, 163–169. doi: 10.1016/j.jad.2016.08.054

Scherdel, P., Botton, J., Rolland-Cachera, M. F., Léger, J., Pelé, F., Ancel, P. Y., ..., Heude, B. (2015). Should the WHO growth charts be used in France? *PLoS One, 10*(3), e0120806. doi: 10.1371/journal.pone.0120806

Shader, R. I. (2018). Baby Fat or a Fat Baby? *Clinical Therapeutics, 40*(10), 1621–1625. Retrieved from https://doi.org/10.1016/j.clinthera.2018.09.001

Shimizu, M. & Teti, D.M. (2018). Infant sleeping arrangements, social criticism, and maternal distress in the first year. *Infant and Child Development, 27*(3), 1–16. Retrieved from https://onlinelibrary-wiley-com.libproxy.umflint.edu/doi/pdf/10.1002/icd.2080

St James-Roberts, I., Roberts, M., Hovish, K., & Owen, C. (2017). Video evidence that parenting methods predict which infants develop long night-time sleep periods by three months of age. *Primary Health Care Research & Development, 18*(3), 212–226. http://dx.doi.org.libproxy.umflint.edu/10.1017/S1463423616000451

Statistics Canada. (2015). Aboriginal peoples: Fact sheet for Canada. Retrieved November 11, 2018 from https://www150.statcan.gc.ca/n1/pub/89-656-x/89-656-x2015001-eng.htm

Statistics Canada. (2017). Population estimates on July 1st, by age and sex. Retrieved November 21, 2018 from https://www150.statcan.gc.ca/t1/tbl1/en/tv.action?pid=1710000501

Statistics Canada. (2018). Immigration and ethnocultural diversity in Canada. Retrieved November 9, 2018 from https://www12.statcan.gc.ca/nhs-enm/2011/as-sa/99-010-x/99-010-x2011001-eng.cfm

Streit, C., Carlo, G., Ispa, J. M., & Palermo, F. (2017). Negative emotionality and discipline as long-term predictors of behavioral outcomes in African American and European American children. *Developmental Psychology, 53*(6), 1013–1026. https://doi-org.libproxy.umflint.edu/10.1037/dev0000306

Turner, H. N. (2010). Parental preference or child well being: An ethical dilemma. *Journal of Pediatric Nursing, 25*(1), 58–63.

United Nations Educational, Scientific and Cultural Organization. (2018). International technical guidance on sexuality education. An evidence-informed approach. Retrieved November 24, 2018 from http://unesdoc.unesco.org/images/0026/002607/260770e.pdf

U.S. Census Bureau. (2016). The majority of children live with two parents, census bureau reports. Retrieved from U.S. Census Bureau: https://www.census.gov/newsroom/press-releases/2016/cb16-192.html

United States Census Bureau. (2017a). *Limited English Speaking Households, 2013-2017 American Community Survey 5-Year Estimates.* Retrieved from https://factfinder.census.gov/faces/tableservices/jsf/pages/productview.xhtml?src=bkmk

U.S. Census Bureau. (2017b). Annual estimates of the resident population for selected age groups by sex for the United States, States, Counties, and Puerto Rico Commonwealth and Municipios: April 1, 2010 to July 1, 2017. Retrieved November 21, 2018 from https://factfinder.census.gov/faces/tableservices/jsf/pages/productview.xhtml?src=bkmk

U.S. Department of Health and Human Services. (2016). Child maltreatment, 2014. Retrieved November 20, 2018 from https://www.acf.hhs.gov/cb/resource/child-maltreatment-2014

U.S. Department of Homeland Security. (2018). What is human trafficking? Retrieved November 20, 2018 from https://www.dhs.gov/blue-campaign/what-human-trafficking

Weden, M. M., Brownell, P., & Rendall, M. S. (2012). Prenatal, perinatal, early life, and sociodemographic factors underlying high body mass index in early childhood. *American Journal of Public Health, 102*(11), 2057–2065.

Whaley, A. (2013). Sociocultural differences in the developmental consequences of the use of physical discipline during childhood. *Cultural Diversity and Ethnic Minority Psychology, 6*(1), 5–12.

Woods, T., & Hanson, D. (2016). Demographic trends of children of immigrants. Retrieved November 26, 2018 from https://www.urban.org/sites/default/files/publication/85071/2000971-demographic-trends-of-children-of-immigrants_2.pdf

World Health Organization. (2006). WHO child growth standards, methods and development. Retrieved November 13, 2018 from https://www.who.int/childgrowth/standards/Technical_report.pdf

World Health Organization. (2010). Accelerating efforts to advance the rights of adolescent girls. Retrieved November 20, 2018 from http://www.who.int/mediacentre/news/statements/2010/joint_statement_20100303/en/

World Health Organization. (n.d.). WHO child growth standards. Retrieved November 16, 2018 from http://www.who.int/childgrowth/4_double_burden.pdf

Yavuz, H. M., & Selcuk, S. (2018). Predictors of obesity and overweight in preschoolers: The role of parenting styles and feeding practices. *Appetite, 120*(1), 491–499. https://doi.org/10.1016/j.appet.2017.10.001

Zhao, A., Zheng, W., Xue, Y., Li, H., Tan, S., Zhao, W., ... Zhang, Y. (2017). Prevalence of premastication among children aged 6–36 months and its association with health: A cross-sectional study in eight cities of China. *Maternal & Child Nutrition, 14*(1), e12448. Retrieved from https://doi-org.libproxy.umflint.edu/10.1111/mcn.12448

Zong, J., Batalova, J., & Hallock, J. (2018). Frequently requested statistics on immigrants and immigration in the United States. Retrieved November 9, 2018 from https://www.migrationpolicy.org/article/frequently-requested-statistics-immigrants-and-immigration-united-states#Children

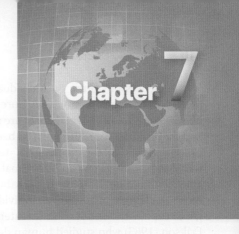

Chapter 7

Transcultural Perspectives in the Care of Adults

- Joyceen S. Boyle and John W. Collins

Key Terms

Adulthood
Caregiving
Developmental crises
Developmental tasks
Generativity

Health/illness situational
  crises
"High blood"
HIV/AIDS
Middle adulthood
Midlife crisis
"Nerves"

Physiologic development
Psychosocial development
Sandwich generation
Social age
Social roles
Stroke belt
Young adulthood

Learning Objectives

1. Evaluate how culture influences adult development.
2. Explore how health-related situational crises or transitions might influence adult development.
3. Analyze the influences of culture on caregiving in the African American culture.
4. Analyze the influences of culture on women's development in the African American family.
5. Evaluate cultural influences in adulthood that assist individuals and families to manage during health-related situational crises or transitions.
6. Explain how gender and specific religious beliefs and practices might influence an adult's health and/or illness during situational crises or transitions.

This chapter discusses transcultural perspectives of health and nursing care associated with developmental events in the adult years. The focus is primarily on young and middle adulthood. The first section of this chapter presents an overview of cultural influences on adulthood, with an emphasis on how health/illness situational crises or transitions might be influenced by cultural variations. The second section provides the context for and gives an example of a health-related situational crisis.

The influences of culture on individual and family responses to health problems, caregiving, and health/illness transitions and crises are discussed.

Health/illness transitions have been referred to in the past as developmental tasks, those transitions that occur in a normal successful adulthood. A health/illness situational crisis refers to changes or turmoil as individuals struggle to cope with a sudden life-threatening illness. Erikson (1963) who studied human development used the term "developmental tasks" or "developmental crises" to describe those times in an individual's life when changes occur, such as marriage or the birth of a child. Nursing theorist A. I. Meleis chose the term "transitions" believing that term more adequately describes life changes and is a conceptually more appropriate term for nursing theory (Im, 2014). In this chapter, transitions refer to those health or illness events that occur within adulthood and require an individual to make lifestyle modifications. Transitions can occur gradually over a period of time or they may be preceded by a situational crisis. A situational crisis includes a greater level of turmoil and anxiety and is more threatening to an individual and family. An example of a health/illness situational crisis might be a sudden myocardial infarction experienced by a 48-year-old man. Until his condition is stabilized, both he and his family will be in a crisis situation, worried and very anxious about his life. When his condition stabilizes and is no longer life threatening, both he and his family members will experience a more gradual health/illness transition. This transition will include changes in behavior such as appropriate exercises, dietary changes that promote weight reduction, and the addition of prescribed medications. Whether the client experiences a crisis or a transition, he or she will need culturally competent and contextually meaningful nursing care.

Overview of Cultural Influences on Adulthood

Health/illness crises and/or transitions during adulthood are of interest to nursing because they include responses to health and illness. In addition, health/illness transitions influence how individuals respond to health promotion and wellness by shaping individual lifestyles including eating habits, exercise, work, and leisure activities. Consider, for example, how pregnancy (a transition into motherhood) influences many young adult women to improve their diet, begin moderate exercise, abstain from alcohol and generally take better care of themselves for the health of the baby.

The adult years are a time when gradual physical and psychosocial changes occur and reflect the normal processes of aging. These physical changes, or physiologic development, are evident in the hormonal changes that take place in adulthood in both men and women. Psychosocial development, or the development of personality, may be more subtle but is equally important. Both physiologic development and psychosocial development are influenced by cultural values and norms, and they occur throughout a lifetime.

Physiologic Development During Adulthood

Women undergo menopause, one of the more profound physiologic changes that results in a gradual decrease in ovarian function with subsequent depletion of progesterone and estrogen. While these physiologic changes occur over time, the psychosocial concepts of self-image and self-concept may also change. The influence of culture is relevant because women learn to respond to menopause within the context of their families and culture. The *perception* of menopause and *aspects* of the experience of menopausal symptoms appear to vary across cultures. It has sometimes been assumed that non-Western women do not experience the menopausal problems seen in Western society because their status increases as they age; however, this assumption has been challenged. In Western cultures such as Canada and the United States, youth and beauty are valued and aging is viewed with trepidation. Western medicine has tended to treat the symptoms of menopause with hormone replacement therapy, surgical interventions, and/or pharmaceutical products. Although there are not many studies on the perimenopausal transition across cultural groups, there seem to be cultural differences in the reporting of symptoms associated with treatments for menopausal symptoms. One recent study has shown that such factors as family income, perceived general health, and perimenopausal status were factors associated with and predictors of depressive symptoms among women of four major ethnic groups. Further, sports and exercise activities were negatively associated with depressive symptoms, while occupational and household and caregiving physical activity were associated positively with depressive symptoms (Im, Ham, Chee, & Chee, 2015). This reinforces an earlier statement that women and their families respond differently to menopause and aging within the context of their families and culture.

Men also have physical and emotional changes from the decreased levels of hormones. Loss of muscle mass and strength and a possible loss of sexual potency occur slowly. However, developmental differences among both adult men and women have not been extensively examined cross-culturally, and most existing theoretical and conceptual models of adult health do not provide insight into cultural variations. The cultural belief that aging, however gradual, is a normal process and not a cause for medical and/or surgical intervention may be more apparent in diverse cultural groups.

Psychosocial Development During Adulthood

Adulthood was termed the "empty middle" by Bronfenbrenner (1977). A recognized developmental psychologist, his use of this term was an indication of Western culture's lack of interest in the adult years. Traditionally, these years were viewed as one long plateau that separates childhood from old age. It was assumed that decisions affecting marriage and career were made in the late teens and that drastic changes in developmental processes seldom occurred afterward. For many years, most developmental theorists saw adulthood as a period to adapt to and come to terms with aging and one's own mortality. Western thinking has changed considerably since Bronfenbrenner's observations. Psychosocial development in middle age is now viewed as a vigorous and changing stage of life involving many challenges and transformations.

Sociocultural factors in Western society have precipitated tremendous changes, producing crises, changes, and other unanticipated events in adult lives. Divorce, remarriage, career changes, and increased mobility, as well as other societal changes (the sexual revolution, the women's movement), have had a profound impact on the adult years. Further, many middle-aged adults may be caught in the **sandwich generation**, the years where they still have concerns with older children (and sometimes grandchildren) while also increasingly concerned with the care of aging parents. Middle life can be a time of reassessment, turmoil, and change. Society acknowledges this with common terms such as **midlife crisis** or even *empty nest syndrome*, along with other terms that imply stress, dissatisfaction, and unrest. However, adulthood is not always a tumultuous, crisis-oriented state; many middle-aged persons welcome the space, time, and independence that middle age often brings. Midlife can be a time of challenge, enjoyment, and satisfaction for many persons. According to Meleis, we now tend to view a "midlife crises" as a time of transition that can be a positive experience, including the mastery of new skills and behaviors that helps an individual change and grow in response to a new environment (Im, 2014).

Chronologic Standards for Appropriate Adult Behavior

Much of the contemporary work on adult development was done in the 1960s and 1970s by developmental psychologists such as Bronfenbrenner (1977), Havighurst (1980), and Neugarten (1968), all of whom proposed different theories about adult development. We still rely on some of this early work as we attempt to understand the complexities of adult development. Neugarten (1968) observed that each culture has specific chronologic standards for appropriate adult behavior and that these cultural standards prescribe the ideal ages at which to leave the protection of one's parents, choose a vocation, marry, have children, and, in general, get on with life. The events associated with these standards do not necessarily precipitate crises, but they do bring about change. What is more important is the timing of these events. As a result of each culture's sense of social time, individuals tend to measure their accomplishments and adjust their behavior according to a kind of social clock. Awareness of the social timetable is frequently reinforced by the judgments and urging of friends and family, who may say, "It's time for you to…" or "You are getting too old to…" or "Shouldn't you act your age." However, an example of recent societal change is seen as late baby boomers and Generation Xers have touted that "50 is the new 30" emphasizing that the typical roles and responsibilities once thought to be anchored to specific decades of life are subject to change (Mapes, 2016).

Problems often arise when social timetables change for unpredictable reasons. An example is the recent trend of adult children, frequently divorced, unemployed, or both, returning to live with their parents, often bringing along their own children. This arrangement is very common in Western society with one in three 18- to 34-year-olds living with parents in their parents' home. Grandparents caring for grandchildren is now a common phenomenon in Western society (Sandberg-Thoma, Snyder, & Jang, 2015; Vespa, 2017). Also, being widowed in young adulthood and losing one's job in midlife due to an economic downturn are examples of events in adulthood that are likely to cause stress and conflict because they occur outside of the anticipated social timetable.

Culture exerts important influences on human development in that it provides a means for recognizing stages in the continuum of individual development throughout the lifespan. It is culture that defines **social age**, or what is considered appropriate behavior in each stage of the life cycle.

In nearly all societies, adult role expectations are placed on young people when they reach a certain age. Several cultures have defined rites of passage that mark the line between youth and adulthood. In the United States, markers of beginning adulthood may include reaching the legal age to obtain a driver's license, to drink alcohol, or to join the military forces, but coming of age is rarely tied to a defined moment or event among many Western populations.

Menarche is a milestone in a young girl's physiologic development and a psychologically significant event that provides a rather dramatic demarcation between girlhood and womanhood. However, this is not an event that is celebrated openly in Western culture; most girls are too embarrassed to talk openly about it with anyone but their mothers or close friends. There are no definitive boundaries that mark adulthood for either young girls or young boys, although legal sanctions confer some rights and responsibilities at the ages of 18 and 21 years. There is no single criterion for the determination of when Western young adulthood begins, given that different individuals experience and cope with growth and development differently and at different chronologic ages. A young boy who joins the military forces at age 18 and serves in Iraq or Afghanistan may "grow up" more quickly than the 18-year-old who lives with his parents, has a part-time job, and attends a local community college.

Adulthood is usually divided into **young adulthood** (late teens, 20s, and 30s) and **middle adulthood** (40s and 50s), but the age lines can be fuzzy. Generally, a **young adult** in his or her late teens and early 20s struggles with independence and issues related to intimacy and relationships outside the family. Role changes occur when the young adult is pursuing an education, experiencing marriage, starting a family, and establishing a career. A **middle adult** most often concentrates on career and family matters. However, as previously mentioned, adulthood is not necessarily an orderly or predictable pattern. Experiences at work have a direct bearing on the middle-aged adult's development through exposure to job-related stress, levels of physical and intellectual activity, and social relationships formed with coworkers. "Recareering" or changing careers during middle adulthood is becoming more common as old careers are eliminated due to increasing technology and automation, while new high demand career fields are popping up overnight. Additionally, recent societal changes being observed are that baby boomers and Generation Xers in middle age are voluntarily changing careers or are retooling their education and pursuing second careers in the fourth and fifth decade of life. It is clear that the transition from middle age into retirement for many is delayed as boomers and Xers continue in the active workforce beyond traditional retirement age, thereby impacting societal changes, global economic and political issues, as well as family dynamics (Kojola & Moen, 2016).

Resultant of both forced and voluntary career changes, the sometimes required relocation, educational retooling, and financial impacts can make family life chaotic, with role changes and other developmental transitions occurring with dizzying frequency. Some life changes can lead to developmental crises (McLeod, 2018). According to Erikson (Erikson, 1963), developmental crisis occurs when an individual experiences normal and expected challenges that are age appropriate. Examples of adult developmental crises are:

- A young adult may have difficulties separating from his or her parents and establishing independence. This is usually resolved as "homesickness" and dissipates as the young adult gains the ability to adjust to a new lifestyle such as college, the military, or employment away from home. The major developmental task of young adulthood is the resolution of intimacy versus isolation, with intimacy being the goal of happy relationships and being comfortable with one's commitments.
- Middle adults may experience difficulty in adjusting to career, marriage and parenthood, but these usually resolve with time and the development of a trusting intimate

relationship. A new normal of balancing career and family develops as the individual adapts to the middle adult years. The major developmental task of middle adulthood is the resolution of **generativity** versus stagnation. Resolution of the "crises" or conflict between these two conflicting forces results in attainment of generativity, or the feeling of having created things that will outlast one's lifetime through parenting, working in one's career, participating in community activities, or working cooperatively with peers, spouse, family members, and others to reach mutually determined goals.

- Older adults may find the "golden years" difficult as they are faced with the realization that they are getting older and may feel like they have made some wrong choices or have left many things still undone. Further, they may find it difficult to experience not being productive and contributing to society via their career. Resolution of the "crises" or conflict between ego integrity versus despair is successfully resolved as the senior adult develops integrity about the level of accomplishment and life success they have achieved. Mature adults having resolved this crisis have a well-developed philosophy of life that serves as a basis for stability in their lives, and the numerous **social roles**, such as spouse, parent, child of aging parent, worker, friend, organization member, and responsible citizen they have attained (McLeod, 2018).

A health/illness situational crisis is often focused and specific and can occur at any time during any developmental stage. Sometimes, a situational crisis can be precipitated by an illness, such as a diagnosis of type 2 diabetes, or the death of a family member. A situational health/illness crisis usually is time limited, although additional transitions may occur. How well individuals cope with and manage the challenges of health/illness crises and transitions in adulthood is influenced by cultural values, traditions, and backgrounds.

Developmental Tasks

Throughout life, each individual is confronted with developmental tasks, those responses to life situations encountered by all persons experiencing physiologic, psychological, spiritual, and sociologic changes (Erikson, 1963). Although the developmental tasks of childhood are widely known and have long been studied, the developmental tasks of adulthood are less familiar to most nurses.

Several theorists have studied and defined the developmental or *midlife* tasks of adulthood. Among others, personality theorists Erikson and Fromm cite maturity as the major criterion or task of adulthood (Erikson, 1963; Fromm, 1969). These various theories have implications for how we define "development," "maturity," and "wisdom." Each of these social roles involves expected behaviors established by the values and norms of society. Through the process of socialization, the individual is expected to learn the behaviors appropriate to the new role. It is important to note that many developmental theories have connotations of stability and blandness associated with adulthood, although this probably is not the case. The constellation of characteristics enumerated by Erikson and other theorists has been attributed to predominantly White Anglo-Saxon Protestant (WASP) views and behaviors. For many cultural groups in Western society, the mastery of Erikson's developmental tasks is not easily managed and is not always applicable, and in some cases, it may even be undesirable. For some groups, developmental tasks may be accomplished through culturally defined patterns that are different from or outside of the norm of what is expected in the dominant culture.

Evidence-Based Practice 7-1 discusses how an observant Jewish woman and her family, in labor, delivery, and postpartum, should have nursing care that allows her to abide by Jewish laws, customs, and practices that influence everyday life as well as those that pertain to childbearing. Childbearing is a special time for most cultures, and there are cultural prescriptions to ensure the well-being of both the mother and the child. Childbearing that occurs in young and middle adulthood is a prime example of the interface between culture, religion, childbearing practices, and transcultural nursing care.

Studies focusing on the developmental experiences of women have led some authors to suggest that developmental stages and the associated developmental tasks of adulthood often published have been derived primarily from studies of men (Belenky, 1997), suggesting that women experience adult development differently. Women's traditional location of responsibility was in the home, nurturing children and husbands as well as parents. Hollis-Sawyer and Dykema-Engblade (2016) point out that this view is changing, prompted by societal changes and informed by scholars who are addressing women's psychosocial development in new ways.

Culture and Adult Transitions

More recent theories on adulthood (Demick & Andreoletti, 2003; Kjellstrom & Stalne, 2017) suggest that development is an evolutionary expanse involving different eras and transitions. Within nursing, Meleis proposed a framework to study life transitions (Im, 2014). The focus is on transitions that are developmental and situational, including those brought about by an illness.

The next section discusses several important adult life transitions and examines how culture and life events influence adult growth and change during these transitions. The successful progression through developmental tasks and/or life transitions may occur slowly over many years and is important in terms of quality of life and life satisfaction. Culture influences these transitions, and it is important that nurses be able to evaluate their adult clients and help them adjust and change in culturally appropriate ways. These adult life transitions are often based on what we could call "middle-class, White American culture." Diverse cultures may experience different life transitions or experience life transitions in different

Some Characteristics of Immigrant and Refugee Families

1. Traditional family values are evident; for example, roles of men and women are differentiated. Women's role is in the home, with the family. Men are heads of the household and family providers.
2. Families tend to be extended; if members do not actually live in the same household, they visit and contact each other frequently. New immigrants and refugees tend to keep in fairly close contact with family members in the home country.
3. Many immigrants come to the United States because they already have family members here.
4. Most immigrants and refugees are poor and struggle to earn an adequate income. Often, men in refugee communities have been professionals in their home country but are unable to be employed in the same capacity in their new host country. Women are often more easily employed outside of the home, and they often find employment as domestic or service workers. For many refugee or immigrant women, working outside of the home is a new experience for them. To earn a salary and provide for their families can be very empowering for these women.
5. Refugees may be fleeing war and political persecution. Many may experience symptoms of posttraumatic stress syndrome.
6. Traditional health and illness beliefs may influence behavior. Immigrant and refugee families may combine traditional health practices with modern Western health care. The use of traditional practices is fairly common in some groups.
7. Language is a significant barrier for the first few years that immigrants and refugees live in the United States and Canada. Children tend to learn English and become acculturated faster than their parents.

---

ways depending on the cultural group (Baird, 2012; Baird & Boyle, 2012). The following section focuses on various cultural groups and how they might experience adult life transitions. The terms "transitions" and "developmental tasks or goals" are used interchangeably and refer to selected activities at a certain period in life that are directed toward a goal. According to Erikson, unsuccessful achievement of a goal is thought to lead to inability to perform tasks associated with the next period or stage in life (Erikson, 1963); thus, successful development transitions are important.

Developmental Transitions: Achieving Career Success

Many persons in traditional Western culture define career success in financial terms, while others may see it as providing service or making a contribution to the lives of their fellow citizens. Achieving success in one's career, including adequate financial remuneration as well as satisfaction and enjoyment, is considered an important developmental task or goal in adulthood. However, there are many groups who struggle to attain this goal. Immigrants to the United States, Canada, or Europe may find it very difficult to find employment that pays an adequate salary or offers opportunities for advancement or job satisfaction. North America and Europe, as well as other parts of the world, have experienced a tremendous influx of immigrants and refugees from Southeast Asia, Latin America, Eastern Europe, the Middle East, Africa, and other geographical areas over the last 30 years ("U.S. immigration trends," 2017). Although immigrants and refugees may aspire to career success or to earn a higher salary, those may be difficult goals to attain. They may have difficulty with the language, with the skills, and with the educational level required, as well as other factors necessary for holding a good job in their new country.

Other factors, such as gender, also influence the attainment of satisfaction in career choices. More women are working outside of the home, and there may be a different division of time and energy for both spouses that pose challenges. Women's presence in the workforce has increased dramatically, from 29.7 million in 1970 to 70.9 million in 2016, and this has had a significant impact on childcare and family finances. Although women have made significant gains in certain occupations, many women continue to be employed in low-paying jobs with little chance for advancement. Many are employed in occupations that have been traditionally oriented toward women (*Women in the labor force: A databook*, 2017), and the salaries are less than men earn in similar positions. Working in a low-paying job that does not offer opportunities for advancement or intellectual challenges does not lead to career success or recognition from one's peers.

Many immigrant and refugee families experience role conflict and stress as gender roles begin to change during contact with Western culture. For example, sometimes, the male head of household who has immigrated is unable to find employment; if he was a professional in his former country, he may be reluctant to accept the menial jobs that are traditionally filled by immigrants or refugees when they first migrate to another country. Frequently, low-status jobs are more available to immigrant women, yet their traditional roles are closely tied to the home and family. When an immigrant or refugee woman begins to work outside of the home, her role changes and those changes alter the traditional power structure and the roles within the family. The lack of adequate social supports, such as affordable daycare for children and adequate compensation for work, and the additional physical and emotional stress result in an unacknowledged toll on immigrant and refugee families. Box 7-1 lists some characteristics of immigrant and refugee families.

At present, to expect members of certain groups, such as poor or ethnic minorities, newly arrived immigrants or refugees, the homeless, the mentally ill, or the unemployed, to achieve satisfaction from jobs that interest them or from status derived from succeeding in a career is unrealistic and indicates a lack of sensitivity to the problems faced by these groups. Thus, although the work role is valued in American society, the attainment of a successful career that includes financial success and personal fulfillment may not be realistic for some minority groups, immigrants, or even certain individuals within the majority culture, some of whom are returning to school in the hope of preparing for a second career.

Developmental Transition: Achieving Social and Civic Responsibility

Social and civic responsibilities are in part culturally defined. Generally speaking, American and Canadian cultures value the voluntary contributions of their citizens in various agencies and organizations that contribute services to the community or society in general. For this discussion, achieving social and civic responsibilities can be viewed as participation in those activities in adulthood that contribute to the "good of society." Usually, this means activities and commitments outside of the immediate family. It can vary considerably, from serving as a board member for a community agency, such as a homeless shelter, to volunteering to teach in a literacy program or donating blood at the local blood bank. Not all members of dominant Western cultures value achieving an elected office in, for example, the local parent–teacher association (PTA) or Rotary Club; other cultures may find these goals baffling and, instead, emphasize activities and contributions within the cultural group. For example, in some groups, religious obligations are given priority over civic responsibilities. Usually, traditional religious groups have not encouraged the emergence of women in leadership roles within the church structure or the wider society, although this is now being challenged by women within several religious groups.

Sometimes within traditional cultures, women who seek roles outside the family are criticized because recognition and acknowledgment outside the family group may conflict with the

BOX 7-1	Jewish Laws, Customs, and Practice in Labor, Delivery, and Postpartum Care

This article provides a comprehensive and thorough guide to specific laws, customs, and practices of traditionally, religious observant Jewish people that assist the transcultural nurse or midwife to provide culturally congruent and sensitive care during labor, delivery, and the postpartum period. Providing culturally congruent care includes cultural knowledge; in this case, the nurse or midwife needs to understand the Jewish laws, customs, and practices that guide everyday life, as well as those that pertain to childbearing. These cultural issues include adherence to the laws that influence intimacy issues between husband and wife, or *niddah*; dietary laws, or *kashrut*; and observance of the Sabbath. Detailed tables are provided that list the following: (1) observant Jewish customs, laws, and practices during labor, delivery, and postpartum; (2) annual Jewish holidays and fast days; and (3) a cultural assessment for Jewish clients in labor, delivery, and postpartum. Case studies are presented that describe cultural competence challenges for nurses who want to learn about the Jewish culture and how to provide culturally competent care to Jewish women during childbirth.

Clinical Implications

- Recognize that observant Jewish couples are committed to maintaining their religious laws, customs, and practices as much as possible throughout the labor, delivery, and postpartum experiences.
- Understand that childbirth is a time that is highly influenced by cultural values and beliefs.
- The religious laws, customs, and practices that will be most apparent during labor, delivery, and postpartum will pertain to prayer, communication between husband and wife, dietary laws, the Sabbath, modesty issues, and labor and birth customs.
- The culturally competent nurse follows the cues of the religious family, tailoring his or her health and nursing care in a manner that allows the family to practice their traditions in their specific designed manner while employing professionalism and creativity in providing quality patient care.

Reference: Noble, A., Rom, M., Newsome-Wicks, M., Engelhardt, K., & Woloski-Wruble, A. (2009). Jewish laws, customs, and practice in labor, delivery and postpartum care. *Journal of Transcultural Nursing, 20*, 323–333.

traditional role of women. Some religious and ethnic or cultural groups believe that a woman's place is in the home, and women who attempt to succeed in a career or participate in activities outside the home or group are frowned on by other members of the group. Civic responsibilities that relate to children or domestic matters may be viewed as more appropriate for women to assume, whereas other civic activities may be viewed as more within the opportunities and obligations of men. However, Middle Eastern and Southeast Asian cultures emphasize and value responsibilities and contributions to the extended family or clan rather than to the wider society. Numerous researchers (Baird, 2012; Baird & Boyle, 2012)

have reported that refugee women in the United States continue to socialize almost exclusively with other refugee women, often extended family/clan or tribe members. They are more comfortable with others who not only share their traditional culture and language and life events, but who are also going through similar situational transitions (the immigrant experience).

Many refugee women are single or widowed with children. Women whose husbands have been killed or have stayed behind to fight in various conflicts are often forced to flee with children and/or elderly family members. Women refugees carry a substantial burden during the migration process and are essential in helping the family members settle into a new country. Coping with life in a new country becomes the focus of their daily lives. Finding a job, getting children into school, learning English, and other resettlement activities become challenging transitions for them. Many refugee women are justifiably very proud of their accomplishments. They learn new job skills, a new language, and how to drive a car, all accomplishments that are not always recognized by members of their new society. For the refugee women and her family, these are significant achievements; however, they can be quite stressful. Often, informal social networks, such as having family members and friends nearby, are very helpful and supportive. The social and civic responsibilities that we have associated with adulthood in Western cultures may not be appropriate for many other cultural groups. Concepts such as social connectedness and integration, resilience, and strength might help us better understand adult development and transitions in refugee and immigrant families (Salo & Birman, 2015).

Developmental Transition: Marriage and Raising Children to Adulthood

Marriage and raising children usually take place in early to middle adulthood. The age at which young persons marry and become independent varies by custom or cultural norm, as well as by socioeconomic status. Generally speaking, in Western culture, young adults of lower socioeconomic status leave school, begin work, marry, and become parents and grandparents at earlier ages than middle-class or upper-class young adults. Indeed, many North American families encourage early independence by urging their children to attend college or to find employment away from home. Other cultural groups, such as those from the Middle East and Latin America, place more emphasis on maintaining the extended family. Even after marriage, a son and his new wife may choose to live very close to both families and to visit relatives several times each day. Families from some cultural groups, such as Hispanics, or traditional religious groups, such as the Hutterites or the Amish, may be reluctant to

allow their young daughters to leave home until they marry. In many Muslim families, girls do not leave home until they are married.

Increased mobility in American and Canadian societies has impacted family life as many young families now live far away from grandparents, and the traditional influences of grandparents on young grandchildren are decreasing. Sometimes, because of geographical distance, grandparents barely know their grandchildren, although digital photos via Internet access, cell phones, video calling, and other technological devices are helping to keep grandparents up to date with the growth and activities of their grandchildren.

Changes in terms of women's participation in the workforce began in the 1960s and 1970s when it became increasingly difficult for a single-income household to support a comfortable, middle-class lifestyle (Burke, 2017; *Women in the labor force: A databook*, 2017). In addition, many young women attend college or universities and want to become established in their careers before they marry or have children. With both mothers and fathers working, children are often placed in childcare facilities. These factors have had a tremendous impact on men and women's roles and responsibilities within the marriage and on how children are raised.

Developmental Transition: Changing Roles and Relationships

Relationships between marriage partners, between and among genders, within social networks of family and friends, between parents and children, and the roles men and women play within these relationships are all influenced by cultural norms and traditions. In Western culture, the relationship between a wife and husband is often enhanced in middle adulthood, although divorce at this time is not infrequent in the United States. The frequent need for both spouses to work may conflict with traditional roles and cause feelings of guilt on the part of both the husband and wife. Some women continue to assume all responsibility for domestic chores while working outside the home, and they experience considerable stress and fatigue as a result of multiple role demands. If either or both spouses are working in low-paying jobs and still struggling to make ends meet, or if the jobholder is laid off or loses his or her job, adulthood may not be a time of enjoyment and leisure activities. Some adults may experience what is known as a "midlife jolt," a particularly dramatic life event such as an accident, divorce, death of a spouse, or other life-changing event. The struggle to adjust to such an event and make meaning out of it often inspires profound and lasting personal growth and change. Of course, not everyone experiences transformative growth after a traumatic event; for some individuals, such an event might trigger depression, a sense of despair, and a downward trajectory in terms of quality of life.

The relationship between married adults can vary considerably by culture. For example, not all cultures emphasize an emotionally close inter-personal relationship between spouses. In some Hispanic cultures, women develop more intense relationships or affective bonds with their children or relatives than with their husbands. Latin men, in turn, may form close bonds with siblings or friends—ties that meet the needs for companion-ship, emotional support, and caring that in other cultures might be expected from their wives.

Gender roles and how men and women go about establishing personal ties with either sex are heavily influenced by culture. Touch between men (walking arm in arm) and between women is acceptable in many societies. In contemporary American society, women are more likely to have intimate, self-disclosing friendships with other women than men have with other men; a man's male friends are likely to be working, drinking, or playing "buddies." In Southern Europe and the Middle East, men are allowed to express their friendship with each other with words and embraces; expressions of affection between men are less common in American culture or might be attributed to homosexuality.

Affiliation and friendship needs in adulthood and the satisfaction of these needs are facilitated or hindered by cultural expectations. Social support, family ties, and friendship needs can be met through the extended family and kinship system or through other culturally prescribed groups such as churches, singles bars, work, and civic associations. Social networking websites are an increasingly popular way to connect with friends and family as well. An individual's health may be affected by these social ties: persons who have a reliable set of close friends and an extensive network of acquaintances are usually healthier emotionally and physically than persons without supportive networks and close friends. Facebook, LinkedIn, and other Internet sites might meet social needs of younger persons or even older adults.

Roles and relationships change between adult children and their parents as both become older. Caring for and launching their own children and caring for their own aging parents place some middle-aged adults between the demands of caregiving from parents and those from children. Primarily, caregivers have been women, and the stress resulting from the demands of caregiving places them at increased risk of health problems (*Caregiving in the U.S. 2015*, 2015). In traditional cultures that value and maintain extended family networks, the responsibilities of caring for both children and older parents can be shared with other family members (see Figure 7-1). This decreases the responsibilities being placed on any one family member.

Adjusting to the aging of parents and the associated responsibilities, as well as finding appropriate solutions to problems created by aging parents, is a challenge created by situational, developmental, and even health–illness transitions. Placing an aged mother or father in a nursing home or extended care facility may be a decision made with reluctance and only when all other alternatives have been exhausted. Such actions may be totally unacceptable to some members of other cultural groups, in which family and community networks would facilitate the complex care required by an aged ill person. Such cultural norms would exert a great deal of social pressure on an adult son, or especially a daughter, who failed in this obligation.

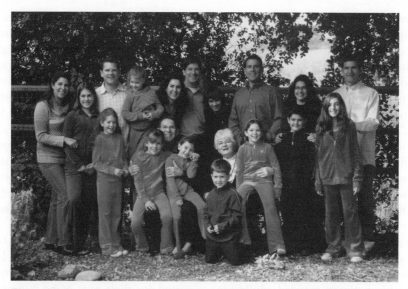

Figure 7-1. The extended family of Teresa and Neil Cooper of Carlsbad, California. This family is multiethnic in each generation, yet maintaining close family ties is a priority that has continued through three generations.

Cultural values also influence professional health care roles and relationships. How individuals are approached and greeted as well as the kind and type of relationship established may be closely tied to cultural expectations and norms. A casual, first-name basis has become the norm in many health care situations, with medical receptionists and often other health professionals calling patients by their first names. While this may be appropriate at the check-in desk because of HIPPA regulations, it can be inappropriate in other instances. Health care professionals should always inquire about the appropriate manner to use in approaching clients and their family members. Table 7-1 provides some suggestions and guidelines to use in approaching clients and using their names in professional relationships.

Health-Related Situational Crises and Transitions

Situational transitions often occur when a serious illness is diagnosed or other traumatic events occur to individuals and their families. Some developmental theorists refer to the initial period as a "situational crisis" when a serious illness is diagnosed or traumatic event occurs. Such a diagnosis or event often leads to fear and anxiety in the client and family members. As clients and family members learn more about the precipitating condition, they realize that many of their fears are unfounded as they gain more confidence in managing the illness condition. The "crisis" dissipates but still the illness remains and must be managed appropriately. The client and family must "transition" to living with a chronic illness. It is not uncommon for a situational transition, precipitated by an illness event, to occur in middle age or late adulthood. The leading causes of death in the United States are heart disease, cancer, chronic lower respiratory diseases, accidents, cerebrovascular disease, Alzheimer's disease, and diabetes, and they are usually diagnosed in adults ("Leading causes of death," 2017; Murphy, Xu, Kochanek, Curtin, & Arias, 2017). These conditions affect individuals, but they also occur within a family system and affect children, spouses, aging parents, and other close relatives. Because middle-aged adults may be caring for aging parents, adult children, and even grandchildren,

Table 7-1	Guidelines for Names
Culture	**Guidelines**
Arab	Both male and female children are given a first name. The father's first name is used as the middle name; the last name is the family name. Usually, a person is called formally by the first name, such as Mr. Mohammed or Dr. Anwar.
Chinese	The family name is stated or written first followed by the given name (the opposite of European and North American tradition). Only very close friends use the given name. Politeness and formality are stressed; always use the whole name or family name. Use only the family name to address men, for example, if the family name is Chin and the man's given name is Wei-jing, address the man as Chin. Women in China do not use their husband's name after marriage.
	Many Chinese take an English name that they use in their North American host country. Use the title Mr. or Mrs. preceding the English name; using only the first name is considered rude.
Latin American	The use of surnames may differ by country. Many Latin Americans use two surnames, representing the mother's and father's sides of the family. "Maria Cordoba Lopez" indicates that her father's name is Cordoba and her mother's surname is Lopez. When Maria marries, she will retain her father's name and add the last name of her husband, becoming Maria Cordoba de Recinos.
	Many Latin American immigrants drop their mother's surnames after they immigrate to the United States because having two last names can be inconvenient. In approaching clients of traditional Latin cultures, it is appropriate to use the Spanish terms *señor* or *señora*, followed by the primary surname (the husband's), if the nurse is comfortable with those terms.
Native North American	Native North American names differ by tribal affiliation. Many tend to follow the dominant cultural norms. In the Navajo culture, a health care provider may call an older Navajo client "grandfather" or "grandmother" as a sign of respect. In the past, some tribes have tended to convert traditional names into English surnames, for example, Joe Calf Looking and Phyllis Greywolf.

The abovementioned examples are very general. If in doubt, always ask: it can be embarrassing for both the nurse and the client if the nurse uses a name in an inappropriate manner. Generally speaking, it is *always best and most appropriate* to be formal and to use the surname with the appropriate title of Mr. or Mrs. (or other culturally appropriate titles) preceding the name, unless the client has indicated that he/she prefers to be called by his/her first name.

Adapted from Purnell, L. D. (2013). *Transcultural health care: A culturally competent approach* (4th ed.). Philadelphia, PA: F.A. Davis.

the illness of any one individual must be evaluated carefully for the myriad of ways in which it affects all members of the family. Evidence-Based Practice 7-2 describes the experiences of Latina wives as their husbands recovered from radical prostatectomy. The shock of the cancer diagnoses and the long-term effects of the surgery precipitated a situational transition that affected both husbands and wives.

Cultural beliefs and values influence health promotion, disease prevention, and the treatment of illness. Families influence the health-related behavior of their members because definitions of health and illness, and reactions to them, form during childhood within the family context. When an illness has social and/or cultural connotations, or involves sexual issues, shame, and/or stigma, the response from the client and the family may be more pronounced. Sexual education has sometimes been a "flash point" in numerous communities, and many parents have objected to such programs in the school setting. Shambley-Ebron, Dole, and Karikari (2016) conducted a study with preadolescent African American girls

Purposeful Normalization When Caring for Husbands Recovering from Prostate Surgery

This study describes the experiences of Latina women as their husbands recovered from radical prostatectomies. Purposeful normalization can be viewed as a situational transition. The women's lives changed dramatically when their husbands were diagnosed with cancer. Cultural beliefs related to gender roles and sexual functioning are some of the strongest values and traditions within a cultural system. The husbands' depression, irritability, and erectile dysfunction posed special challenges to the Latina women in this study.

Prostate cancer is the most frequently diagnosed noncutaneous cancer in men in the United States.

Despite high incidence rates, overall survival rates are very high and increasing all of the time. Issues such as postsurgical incontinence and erectile dysfunction, along with the fact that many prostate survivors are married men, have prompted many to describe prostate cancer as a *couple's disease.* Partnered men have significantly better mental health, lower symptom distress, and less urinary problems than unpartnered men. Still, many wives experience significant distress when faced with their partner's diagnosis and treatment. This study interviewed 28 partners of *Latino* men who had a radical prostatectomy. The primary aim was to describe the experiences of low-income *Latinas* as their husbands recovered from radical prostatectomies. The overarching process was identified as normalization with some themes working against normality while others worked toward it.

Working Against Normality: Threats to normality of the women's lives began immediately when their husbands were diagnosed with cancer. Some concerns diminished with time, such as the initial shock and fear and dealing with the side effects. They feared losing their husband. Dealing with the symptoms and the side effects caused the women to feel anxious and frustrated. The husbands' depression and irritability, as well as erectile dysfunction, posed special challenges.

Working Toward Normality: The Latina women described many themes that kept them feeling a sense of "normal." They worked hard to conceal their own emotions and to show their husbands that they had everything under control. They tried to move forward, putting changes brought about by their husband's illness behind them. They tried to make dietary changes that they believed were helpful—such as eating more vegetables and fruits and cutting down on sugar. Their families were supportive with the grown children visiting and making frequent phone calls. Grandchildren visited and were a source of joy and comfort. Women found great support in their religious faith that helped them make changes in a positive way.

Clinical Implications

- Understand that caregiving can be extremely stressful and that caregivers need support, understanding, and help in this role. Simply acknowledging the emotional impact of both the illness itself and of caring for the patient can be helpful.
- Talk to wives/caregivers about actively shaping the emotional responses they feel and how they can help their husbands deal with the changes they are experiencing.
- Encourage caregivers to contribute to recovery by empowering them to make healthy changes in their lifestyle, such as eating healthy food, getting appropriate amounts of sleep, and perhaps simple exercise such as walking short distances together with their husband.
- Become comfortable when discussing symptoms such as erectile dysfunction and helping clients and their partners consider alternative forms of intimacy.
- Actively encourage family members to visit and to telephone frequently. Help clients plan for grandchildren to spend the night.

Reference: Williams, K. C., Hicks, E. M., Chang, N., Connor, S. E., & Maliski, S. L. (2014). Purposeful normalization when caring for husbands recovering from prostate surgery cancer. *Qualitative Health Research, 24*(3), 306–316.

and included their mothers. A targeted 8-week educational program tapped into the cultural and gender beliefs and practices to educate girls about human immunodeficiency virus/acquired immune deficiency syndrome (**HIV/AIDS**) prevention. Input for educational intervention was solicited from women in the community, including the mothers of the young girls. The findings from these studies indicate that culture and gender influences play a critical role in how young African American girls develop culturally appropriate strategies to deal with sexuality and healthy womanhood. Further, these studies are an example of how education about sensitive topics such as HIV/AIDS prevention can be conducted.

The content in this section provides the context for and gives an example of a health-related situational crisis (which is detailed in Case Study 7-1). The influences of culture on individual and family responses to health problems, caregiving, and health/illness transitions and crises are discussed.

Caregiving

Caregiving occurs when a (typically) unpaid person, usually a family member, helps another family member who has a chronic illness or disease. Many caregivers are women who are caring for their aged and ill parents or husbands. Caregiving, as used in this chapter, implies the provision of long-term help to an impaired family member or close friend. Caregiving is usually labor intensive, time consuming, and stressful; the exact effects on the physical and emotional

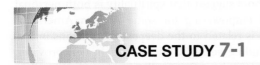

CASE STUDY 7-1

Mrs. Ernestine Pollard, a 57-year-old African American woman, lives in a small town in rural Georgia. Mrs. Pollard cares for her older sister, Ethel, who is now 65 years old. Mrs. Pollard explains that her sister "can't talk, and her mind's not good." Mrs. Pollard says that even as a little girl, she knew that Ethel would be her special responsibility, and when she (Mrs. Pollard) married, Ethel came to live with her and her new husband. Mr. Pollard died a few years ago following a stroke. Recently, Ethel's health has been deteriorating because of a series of what Mrs. Pollard calls "little strokes." Additionally, just a few months ago, Mrs. Pollard's 26-year-old daughter, Tywanda, returned home to live with her. Tywanda was living and working in New Jersey, where she had become ill. She was taken by friends to the emergency department and admitted to a local hospital. During this hospitalization, she tested positive for HIV. Tywanda has been a great worry to her mother for a number of years; Mrs. Pollard has suspected that Tywanda was occasionally using drugs. Although Mrs. Pollard welcomed Tywanda home again, she worried about her past high-risk behaviors and

hoped they would not continue. When Tywanda told her mother about her HIV status, Mrs. Pollard was very upset and worried.

Mrs. Pollard explains that sometimes with the stress of caregiving for Ethel and worrying about Tywanda, her "pressure goes sky high." She tells the nurse that she has had "high blood" for several years. Her physician prescribed medication for her blood pressure, and she tries to take it on a regular basis, but sometimes, she forgets. Other times, she decides that she just does not have the money for medication. Lately, Tywanda has been staying away from home and acting secretively, so Mrs. Pollard is not sleeping well and she is worried that Tywanda may be taking drugs again. She told her doctor that she has bad "nerves" and explained that she is unable to sleep at night. The physician prescribed sleeping pills for her, but Mrs. Pollard is unwilling to take them because she fears that she will not hear Ethel if she gets up during the night. Ethel seems to be getting more confused and disoriented, especially at night. Mrs. Pollard's other grown children, two daughters, live in Atlanta, several hours' drive from the small town where Mrs. Pollard lives. Mrs. Pollard is experiencing a health/illness situational crisis resulting from the stress of caregiving, the challenges of managing ongoing chronic diseases, and anxiety about her young adult daughter who is HIV positive and engages in risky behaviors.

health of caregivers are still being documented. Although positive outcomes, such as feelings of reward and satisfaction, do occur for caregivers, caregivers still experience negative psychological, emotional, social, and physical outcomes (*Caregiving in the U.S. 2015*, 2015). When caregiving for other family members takes place during middle adulthood, the roles for both the caregiver and the recipient may change as new challenges emerge. The caregiver may be forced to quit his or her job as caregiving responsibilities increase when the person being cared for becomes more infirm or ill and the need for assistance in tasks of daily living increases.

Culture fundamentally shapes how individuals make meaning out of illness, suffering, and dying. Cultural beliefs about illness and aging influence the interpretation and management of caring for the ill and aged, as well as the management of the trajectory of caregiving. Family members provide care for the vast majority of those in need of assistance. The demands of caregiving can result in negative emotional and physical consequences for caregivers. How they cope with stress, social isolation, anxiety, feelings of burden, and the challenges of caregiving will all be influenced by cultural values and traditions.

Shambley-Ebron et al. (2016) have documented that these general problems and characteristics of caregivers are compounded for African American women by the special circumstances of their lives and the lives of the men and children for whom they care. In the case of African American caregivers, prejudice, discrimination, health disparities, and poverty often all interact to increase stress and pose challenges that frequently result in poor health. Like other caregivers, African American caregivers are mostly female; most recipients of care from African American caregivers are females as well (e.g., mothers, grandmothers, aunts) (*Caregiving in the U.S. 2015*, 2015).

Culture and ethnicity can influence beliefs, attitudes, and perceptions related to caregiving, including how often individuals engage in self-care versus seeking formal health services, how many medications they take, how often they rest and exercise, and what types of foods they consume when ill. Ethnic and/or cultural differences have rarely been analyzed in caregiver research; only recently have nurse researchers and others focused on specific cultural groups to study caregiving (*Caregiving in the U.S. 2015*, 2015) and the ethnocultural factors that are so important in planning support for caregivers (Crist, Montgomery, Pasvogel, Phillips, & Ortiz-Dowling, 2018).

Studies of African American caregivers have found that they tend to use religious beliefs and/or spirituality to help them cope with the stress of caregiving; Collins and Hawkins (2016) found that a major source of support for African American caregivers was their personal relationships with "Jesus," "God," or "the Lord." These authors suggest that spirituality is both personal and empowering for some African Americans and is related to the deepest motivations in life, including seeing God as their healer, provider, and sustainer. Spirituality is often expressed in the context of the daily life, not necessarily by formal attendance at religious events. Numerous researchers have noted that the specific nature of the religion–health connection among African Americans is of great interest to health professionals as it holds promise for integrating church-based health interventions.

The Context of HIV/AIDS and the African American Community

HIV/AIDS disproportionately affects African Americans and has had a devastating effect on African American communities. According to CDC data, at every stage from HIV diagnosis through the death of persons with AIDS, the hardest-hit racial or ethnic group is African Americans. Even though African Americans make up only approximately 13% of the US population, 44% of the estimated new cases of HIV/AIDS diagnoses in the United States in 2010 were in African Americans (*HIV among African Americans fact sheet*, 2014). In 2014, women accounted for about one in four new HIV/AIDS cases in the United States. Of these newly infected women, about two in three are African American. Most of these women contracted HIV from having unprotected sex with a man. The rate of AIDS diagnosis for African American women was 16 times the rate of White women in 2015. In 2016, 44% of all new AIDS cases were among African Americans despite representing only 12.7% of the US population (*HIV among African Americans fact sheet*, 2014, 2017).

Prevention Challenges

From a public health standpoint, preventive education about HIV/AIDS has been hindered by an unwillingness to talk frankly about behaviors surrounding sex and drug use, and this has been a substantial barrier in effective HIV-preventive programs. In essence, the AIDS epidemic has forced society to examine and attempt to alter cultural behaviors and values that were largely ignored in the past; as a society, we have not always been comfortable with this frankness. Over the past three decades in the United States, the practice of high-risk HIV behaviors has changed from selected populations of White homosexual men with no history of drug use to heterosexuals having multiple sex partners and/or using drugs. HIV/AIDS disproportionately affects selected groups, especially Blacks and Hispanics, and risk patterns are different for men and women. African American women (adolescents and adults) are especially at risk.

The CDC points out that the African American community faces numerous barriers that impact HIV prevention efforts. Among these factors are biological vulnerabilities as well as the unique characteristics and nuances of heterosexual relationships in African American culture. Also contributing to increased HIV transmission in African American communities are poverty, unemployment, substandard education, and incarceration (*HIV among African Americans fact sheet*, 2014, 2017; "HIV and AIDS," 2018). Implementing intervention programs has proven

extremely difficult. Evidence-Based Practice 7-3 describes a study with African American mothers to understand how they talked to their young daughters about sexual health. This knowledge is helpful when developing culturally relevant prevention programs for sexual health, including the prevention of HIV/AIDS.

Influential Factors

Numerous explanations have been offered about the factors that influence the high rate of HIV/AIDS in African American communities. Poverty is a major factor. Denial, drug use, and homophobia and concealment of homosexual behavior also influence HIV/AIDS rates.

Poverty

The poverty rate is higher among African Americans than other racial/ethnic groups; likewise, the poverty rate among African Americans is higher than the rate among the general population. The poverty rate for all African Americans in 2016 was 22.0%, compared with 9.0% for White Americans ("Poverty rate by race/ethnicity," 2016). Black families with children under 18 headed by a single mother have the highest rate of poverty, at 34.2% ("Historical poverty tables: People and families—1959 to 2016," 2017; "Poverty rate by race/ethnicity," 2016). The socioeconomic issues associated with poverty, including limited access to high-quality health care, housing, and HIV prevention education directly and indirectly increase the risk for HIV infection. The CDC (*HIV among African Americans fact sheet*, 2017) suggests that these factors may explain why African Americans have worse outcomes on the HIV continuum of care, including lower rates of linkage to care, retention in care, prescription HIV treatment, and viral suppression. Accessing health care services is a problem if an individual does not have health insurance; further, not all community health departments offer high-quality care and follow-up for clients.

In addition, for many African Americans, day-to-day living activities (long working hours,

Cultural Preparation for Womanhood in Urban African American Girls: Growing Strong Women

Poor sexual health is a significant contributor to morbidity in young African American women. Human immunodeficiency virus/acquired immune deficiency syndrome (HIV/AIDS) and other sexually transmitted infections (STIs) are tragic and costly in all populations; however, African Americans bear an excess burden of poor health due to these conditions. Understanding how knowledge about sexual health is transmitted to African American girls is needed to develop effective and culturally relevant preventive interventions.

This study explored the ways that African American mothers transmitted sexual values and information to their daughters. The author interviewed 14 mothers who had young daughters, 8 to 16 years of age. The data were qualitatively analyzed, and three major themes about *Growing Strong Black Women* were identified: truth-telling, building strength through self-esteem, and spirituality as helper.

Helping their daughters grow into strong, successful, and healthy women was viewed by the mothers as a task that was primarily their responsibility. This responsibility was enacted through an ongoing process of providing truthful answers and open communication, helping their daughters develop a healthy self-esteem that would promote independence, and providing a foundation of spirituality and religious beliefs to enable their daughters to deal with the societal issues that face young African American girls and women. Mothers were honest with their daughters with regard to sexuality, their changing bodies, and relationships with men. Sometimes, mothers told their daughters painful stories of their own experiences. Other times, they sought out literature to explain how their bodies worked or how STIs occurred. Mothers reinforced their daughters' self-esteem and helped them develop confidence in their own abilities to be successful in life. They encouraged them to become active in church and school activities, to develop a faith and belief in God, and to participate in religious practices such as prayer and attendance at religious services.

Clinical Implications

- Supportive networks for young African American girls can be broadened and strengthened by involving teachers, nurses, and women from their church groups as support persons to help them achieve their goals relative to age-appropriate relationships and sexual behaviors.
- African American mothers (indeed, all mothers) of teenage girls need accurate information about sexual health and STIs. Nurses can work with churches and various community groups to provide information and support to parents.
- Culture and gender are unique and distinct aspects of the lives of young African American girls and must be taken into account when planning preventive interventions for health and well-being.
- Nursing interventions that focus on building self-esteem and supporting the future aspirations of young African American girls can be useful to reinforce parental teachings and help young girls move into adulthood successfully.
- The use of spirituality and religiosity appears consistently in the literature as ways to help young African American girls deal appropriately with life experiences.

Reference: Shambley-Ebron, D., Dole, D., & Karikari, A. (2016). Cultural preparation for womanhood in urban African American girls: Growing strong women. *Journal of Transcultural Nursing, 27,* 25–32. doi: 10:1177/1043659614531792

low pay, family responsibilities) often take precedence over whether an individual has the time and energy to access educational information about HIV and AIDS. Poverty or lack of money, stigma, and lack of access to high-quality health care influence access to HIV testing and state-of-the-art treatment if an individual is diagnosed with HIV. Often, stigma, racism, and fear are associated with poverty, and they too play a part in delaying appropriate up-to-date treatment, complying with medication regimens and other appropriate care. Delay in diagnosis until late in the course of HIV infection is too common for African Americans, and this delay results in missed opportunities for early medical intervention and prevention of transmission to others (*HIV among African Americans fact sheet*, 2017).

Denial

Denial and lack of awareness of HIV/AIDS have frequently led to late diagnoses and treatment for many rural African Americans. They know that HIV/AIDS is a problem in urban population centers like Atlanta or New York City, but they find it hard to believe that HIV/AIDS is a problem in rural Georgia or Alabama. This lack of awareness of HIV presence can affect HIV rates within communities. Talking about HIV/AIDS may be met with disapproval as some African Americans may feel that it is not an appropriate subject for discussion. Talking frankly about sexual behavior with new partners and insisting on the use of condoms may be very difficult for African American women. They may be afraid to ask a male partner about his sexual history or his use of or experience with drugs for fear of abruptly ending their relationship. The nuances of African American male–female relationships are rarely understood by health care providers. Shambley-Ebron et al. (2016) suggest that problematic relationships between black males and females are complex in nature and are reflections of institutional racism, political and economic oppression, and internalization of negative stereotypes on the parts of both men and women (Shambley-Ebron et al., 2016). These disabling relationships often lead to denial about HIV; this may be why many African Americans who are HIV infected do not seek early testing and do not know they are HIV positive. Persons who do not know that they are HIV infected are more likely than those with a diagnosis to engage in risky behavior and to unintentionally transmit HIV to others (*HIV among African Americans fact sheet*, 2014; "HIV and AIDS," 2018). The denial of risks of HIV/AIDS can affect HIV rates. Approximately one in five

adults and adolescents in the United States living with HIV do not know their HIV status. Late diagnosis of HIV infection is common; this creates missed opportunities to obtain early medical care and prevent transmission to others. The sooner an individual is diagnosed and linked to appropriate care, the better the outcome (*HIV among African Americans fact sheet*, 2014; "HIV and AIDS," 2018).

Drug Use

Most new HIV infections among African American women (87% or 5,300) are attributed to heterosexual contact (*HIV among African Americans fact sheet*, 2014). Injecting drugs is the second leading cause of HIV infection for African American women and the third leading cause of HIV infection for African American men. In addition to the danger from contaminated needles, syringes, and other drug paraphernalia, persons who use drugs are more likely to take other risks, such as unprotected sex, while under the influence of drugs (*HIV among African Americans fact sheet*, 2014). An early study of HIV-infected women found that women who used drugs, compared with women who did not, were also less likely to take their antiretroviral medicines exactly as prescribed or to attend clinic appointments on a regular basis (Zhang et al., 2017).

Homophobia and Concealment of Homosexual Behavior

Homophobia and stigma can cause some homosexual African American men to identify themselves as heterosexual or to not disclose their sexual orientation, presenting challenges to prevention programs (Garcia et al., 2016). The CDC indicated that in 2010, African American gay, bisexual, and other men who have sex with men represented an estimated 72% of new infections among all African American men and 36% of an estimated 29,800 new HIV infections among all gay and bisexual men (*HIV among African Americans fact sheet*, 2014). It is extremely important to involve African American community stakeholders in developing and implementing programs to address sensitive topics and behaviors associated with homosexual sex. Confronting homophobia is necessary to achieve significant reductions in HIV/AIDS and ultimately to end this epidemic among African Americans. Involving community stakeholders will mobilize African American communities to become more aware of the need to develop strategies that address broader social and cultural factors such as homophobia, drug use, stigma, and denial (*HIV among African Americans fact sheet,* 2014, 2017).

Adult Development in an African American Family: The Convergence of Developmental and Health-Illness Situational Transitions

Case Study 7-1 provides an example of a middle-aged African American woman who provides care to her developmentally delayed sister and to her 26-year-old daughter, who has HIV/AIDS. This case study points out the complex situation of three adult women, each facing significant life changes brought about by health/illness situational crises. Issues related to caregiving, aging, chronic diseases, drug use, and HIV are described. Each woman faces difficult issues that require different kinds of responses to stabilize and improve their health as they are experiencing myriad transitions that are significantly influencing their lives. Culturally appropriate ways in which the nurse might implement nursing care are suggested.

Health Promotion Interventions for Health/Illness Situational Crises

African American women are at high risk for cardiovascular diseases, particularly hypertension and stroke. Mrs. Pollard lives in the area of the South known as the **stroke belt** because morbidity and mortality from cardiovascular diseases, especially among African Americans, are quite high in the region ("Stroke death rates, 2014–2016," 2018). The nursing management priorities for Mrs. Pollard will be to support her caregiving

role and provide health promotion strategies to control her blood pressure and help reduce the stress she is currently experiencing. In terms of blood pressure management, a nurse might advise Mrs. Pollard to lose weight by incorporating changes in eating habits and regular exercise into her lifestyle. However, social and cultural factors, as well as the caregiving situation, may compromise these health goals. Nurses can become more sensitive to cultural norms and values of clients like Mrs. Pollard by listening carefully, being empathetic, recognizing the client's self-interest and needs of her family members, being flexible, having a sense of timing, appropriately using the client's and family's resources, and giving relevant information at the appropriate time.

Although Mrs. Pollard does have a private physician and tries to seek care when appropriate, she considers Ethel's and Tywanda's needs before her own. Mrs. Pollard does not have health insurance and therefore access to quality care is compromised. Tywanda attends an infectious disease clinic about 50 miles from where her mother lives. Her medications are provided through the Ryan White HIV/AIDS Program, a federal program focused exclusively on HIV/AIDS care. The program is for those who do not have sufficient health care coverage or financial resources for coping with HIV disease ("HIV/AIDS Bureau," 2018). Mrs. Pollard does not accompany Tywanda when she visits the clinic because Tywanda acts as if she does not want her mother to go with her and Mrs. Pollard does not wish to leave her sister alone. The nurses at the clinic wonder if anyone in Tywanda's family really cares about her because she always comes alone to the clinic appointments. However, Tywanda does not always attend the clinic, nor does she tell her mother when she misses an appointment. Mrs. Pollard does not know about the medications that Tywanda takes for HIV/AIDS. Tywanda does not readily disclose information, and Mrs. Pollard tries to be sensitive to her daughter's wishes.

Mrs. Pollard is concerned about Ethel's appetite because she believes that the proper food will promote and enhance her health. Like many other adults, Mrs. Pollard has fairly definite preferences about food and the way it is prepared and served. The Pollard family frequently eats foods that are high in fat; for example, they enjoy servings of bacon or fatback for breakfast once or twice during the week. Breakfast is an important meal for them. They prefer their vegetables cooked with bacon, fatback, or ham for flavoring. Symbolism is attached to food in every culture, and Mrs. Pollard believes that both Ethel and Tywanda's health will improve by eating what Mrs. Pollard considers "healthy" foods. With her concern for Tywanda and the time she spends with her sister, Mrs. Pollard neglects her own diet or eats whatever is convenient, often "fast foods" or those high in fat, cholesterol, and sodium.

Mrs. Pollard needs to be gently reminded by the nurse that it is important for her to pay attention to her own nutrition also. The nurse could initiate a discussion about the kinds of nutritious foods that would be appropriate for the three of them and the different ways of preparing food. For example, vegetables can be cooked without the addition of fatback. Young-Mason (2009, 2018) suggested that understanding the art and culture of food of those we seek to help is paramount to being and becoming an astute and learned nurse. Campinha-Bacote (2013) observed that food can have many roles, in addition to providing physical nourishment. For example, food can serve as a means of enhancing interpersonal relationships or communicating love and caring. Historically, African American rites revolve around food. Being able to prepare food that her daughter and sister will eat and enjoy is a source of satisfaction for Mrs. Pollard and a reinforcement of her successful role as caregiver. It is an act of caring and love for her to prepare a meal for her family. At the same time, she must maintain her own health to continue to provide care for Tywanda and her sister.

Nurses providing care to clients like Mrs. Pollard will need to consider other cultural factors that ultimately influence the nursing goals. Rural African Americans often have cultural ways to view health and illness; these patterns of beliefs and behaviors can be viewed as culture-bound syndromes. Many of these patterns are indigenously considered to be "illnesses" or at least afflictions and most have local names. **"High blood"** is an illness condition or affliction that is associated with African American culture in the rural South. Many health care professionals make the wrong assumption that "high blood" is the same as high blood pressure, and although there are similarities, the cultural explanation of "high blood" is different from the biomedical explanation of high blood pressure. "High blood" is conceptualized in terms of blood volume, blood thickness, or even elevations of the blood in the body (e.g., "blood rushes to your head").

"High blood" is believed to be caused primarily by factors that "run blood up," such as salt, fat, meats, and sweets. This condition can result in an increased "pressure" or high blood pressure. Sometimes, "high blood" leads to a feeling of faintness that may cause the afflicted person to "fall out" or faint. Other causal factors that result in "high blood" are emotional upsets, troubling experiences, or prolonged stress. Sometimes, it is thought to be caused by a falling out with God or by eternal forces such as enemies putting a "hex" on someone. Many older African American clients believe that eating slightly acidic foods, such as collard greens with vinegar or dill pickles, will lower "high blood." Thus, although there are similarities between "high blood" and high blood pressure, the explanations and treatments are not always the same in the cultural prescriptions as in the biomedical model.

Mrs. Pollard tries to be conscientious about taking her blood pressure medication, but she sometimes forgets to take it and sometimes does not get around to promptly renewing the prescription, so she might go without her medication for several days or a couple of weeks. The nurse should acknowledge Mrs. Pollard's active involvement in her own health promotion, encourage her to take her blood pressure medication as prescribed, and remind her to renew it promptly before she is completely out of medication. The nurse can also discuss "high blood" with

Mrs. Pollard, and if there are no contraindications, she can encourage her to eat collard greens with vinegar or dill pickles. She can listen carefully to Mrs. Pollard's explanation of "high blood," and if Mrs. Pollard believes she has somehow offended God, the nurse should encourage her to talk with her church pastor.

Nerves or even **bad nerves** while not unique to the rural South are commonly described by many Southerners. "Bad nerves" are often equated with anxiety and worry but may refer to something as serious as a "mental breakdown" or severe emotional disorder. Mrs. Pollard uses the term to refer to her worry, concern, and anxiety about Tywanda and Ethel. Sometimes, she has "crying spells" that she describes as "just crying and crying, and not being able to stop." She gets up several times at night to answer her sister's call or to check on Tywanda and make certain that they are sleeping well. Lack of sleep and continued worry and anxiety accelerate her psychological distress. Again, recognition and acknowledgment from the nurse that she is providing excellent care for her sister and her daughter will be reassuring for her. She should be encouraged to rest and should be assured that crying and feeling sad are normal reactions to her sister's deteriorating condition and Tywanda's HIV/AIDS.

In her seminal work, Clark-Hine described common socioeconomic issues impacting African American women's lives, including insufficient economic resources, and stressful life events such as job and marital instability, lack of male companions as heads of households, erratic income, and frequent changes and relocations (Clark-Hine, 1998). Because she has worked in small local businesses (dry cleaners, restaurants) most of her life, Mrs. Pollard lacks health insurance. She has experienced many life stresses related to the lack of economic resources. Mrs. Pollard was working as a clerk in a local dry-cleaning establishment when Tywanda returned home and told her mother that she had HIV/AIDS. However, as Ethel's health deteriorated and Tywanda's risky behaviors became more obvious and problematic, Mrs. Pollard decided to stop working for a while, thinking that if she stayed home, she could provide closer supervision and care to Ethel and be available to Tywanda when she needed her mother. Mrs. Pollard faces numerous situational crises: Tywanda's illness and high-risk behaviors, the poor health and aging of her sister, and economic hardship because she is the family provider and is not working at the present time. Her own health is also a concern.

Stress and anxiety are normal reactions in the lives of middle-aged adults like Mrs. Pollard. However, limited resources and lack of access to high-quality health care compound the stress and complicate a situational crisis. Mrs. Pollard's physician prescribed sleeping medication for her, assuming that would take care of her inability to sleep. The nurse can reinforce Mrs. Pollard's decision not to take this medication and explore with her how to set aside time during the day when she might be able to take a nap. Mrs. Pollard's anxiety and inability to sleep well are directly related to the stress of caregiving. Some ways to support and help Mrs. Pollard deal with stress and anxiety may be family support and participation in religious activities. The nurse might suggest that Mrs. Pollard set aside some time during the day to quietly read the Bible or other appropriate reading material and listen to religious music. Mrs. Pollard told the nurse that she used to enjoy crocheting; she could be encouraged to try crocheting again.

Close family and spiritual ties within the African American family and community support the caregiving role. Extended and nuclear family members willingly care for sick persons and assume these roles without hesitation. Mrs. Pollard's two daughters try to help their mother and Tywanda as much as possible, but they live several hours' drive away. They try to visit one weekend each month and bring their children with them. Tywanda enjoys the company of her sisters, and Mrs. Pollard notices that on weekends when one of the sisters is expected, Tywanda's mood seems improved as she obviously looks forward to the visit. Ethel is always excited to see her nieces and looks forward to their visits. While Mrs. Pollard's daughters know that Tywanda has been diagnosed with HIV/AIDS, they are reluctant to disclose the diagnosis to others outside the family because the stigma of disclosure in a small community can affect all members of the family. Mrs. Pollard's minister is aware of Tywanda's condition, as are a few members of Mrs. Pollard's "church family." One of the primary stressors of women during the midlife years is the loss of relationships and friendship networks, often because of competing demands on time. Caregivers, like Mrs. Pollard, have very little time for their own needs. It is extremely important for Mrs. Pollard's health and coping abilities that she continue to participate in church activities as much as possible and to maintain those friendships and networks.

Spiritual beliefs form a foundation for Mrs. Pollard's daily life. Like other African Americans who live in the same rural community, Mrs. Pollard attends a small Protestant church whose membership is exclusively African American. Many, but not all, African Americans strongly believe in the use of prayer for all situations they may encounter. They use prayer and reading the Bible as a means of dealing with everyday problems and concerns. Mrs. Pollard relies a great deal on prayer, and her religious beliefs and practices provide her with support and strength in her caregiving role. Encouraging Mrs. Pollard to take even 15 minutes each day to read familiar biblical verses or listen to religious music might be one of the most helpful interventions the nurse could suggest.

Mrs. Pollard has a lifetime of experience with her church; the church has been the center of activities for African Americans for decades (Campinha-Bacote, 2013). Mrs. Pollard's religious beliefs are integrated into her daily life as a caregiver, and her belief in God enhances her ability to care for Ethel and Tywanda. She, like many other African Americans, has a personal relationship with God and is able to share her worries and concerns through prayer. Her traditional spirituality and church support provide a foundation for an active approach to coping with problems.

Adult Health Transitions and Nursing Interventions

Mrs. Pollard is distressed about the deterioration of her sister's physical condition and Tywanda's diagnosis of HIV/AIDS and drug use. In addition, Mrs. Pollard is dealing with several health problems of her own. While there are certain "crisis dimensions" to this situation, the conditions are not life threatening. Overtime, the crises lessen and the situation slowly develops a transitory nature. The health/illness transitions occur over a longer period of time. They can best be dealt with by the provision of culturally relevant health promotion and risk reduction strategies. The health teaching and nursing interventions provided to the Pollard family should focus on wellness and health promotion. In addition to the nursing interventions that are important for health promotion, there are several interventions that will help Mrs. Pollard navigate the transitions and changes of caregiving.

An important priority of nursing care for Mrs. Pollard and her family is to help them understand and adjust to the impact of HIV disease. This includes urging Tywanda to seek help for her drug use. The nurse can refer Mrs. Pollard to the social services available for patients who have HIV/AIDS and their family members. Mrs. Pollard may want to talk to a mental health counselor about the fears and concerns she has about Tywanda and drug use. In addition, the nurse can encourage Tywanda to keep clinic appointments and to seek appropriate counseling and follow-up, not only for her HIV status but also for the use of illicit drugs. While the nurse is not a trained mental health counselor, she or he can recommend that Tywanda seek mental health services, and the nurse can be supportive and encourage health-seeking behaviors. Medications now available for treating HIV can lower viral counts and transmission of the virus to others; helping Tywanda find appropriate services and follow-through treatment is a priority in providing nursing care for this family. Of particular concern is the timing of Tywanda's illness. A serious health condition in a young, previously healthy adult child will cause unique trauma and conflict because of society's expectations that young adults will outlive their older parents. In addition, as a person diagnosed with HIV/AIDS, Tywanda has a condition that often generates shame and stigma. It is important that these issues be acknowledged by both Mrs. Pollard and Tywanda.

Achieving career success is one of the developmental transitions that Western culture emphasizes. Mrs. Pollard has worked successfully outside the home most of her adult life; because rural African American culture does not place the same kind of value on work and career as does the larger culture, career "success" is not necessarily viewed as an important accomplishment. Family ties and providing for her family are highly valued in African American culture and are emphasized over women's successful careers outside the home. Mrs. Pollard's ties of love and affection to Tywanda and to her sister, Ethel, are reinforced by African American cultural values. In a historical study of African American women in America, Hine and Thompson (1998) suggested that Black women have always been the financial providers in Black families and that women's work roles have been culturally viewed as an inherent part of Black motherhood, not as individual careers. Mrs. Pollard has always been proud that she was able to take care of her family and that she could "make do" with very little. These values are important to family integrity and they can be positively reinforced by the nurse.

Many African American women of Mrs. Pollard's generation obtain meaning in their lives by caring for family members. Their feelings, behaviors, and attitudes go beyond a simple sentiment of affection or of family ties. In explaining why she cares for her older developmentally challenged sister, Mrs. Pollard says, "We were little girls together. I always knew that I was going to take care of her." In many societies, women disproportionally provide caregiving services and social policies, and home-based programs are organized around the assumption of women's availability and willingness to provide care. At the same time, it is important to understand that Mrs. Pollard values the traditional caregiving role, and she needs support and assistance in providing the care she believes her family members need. It is important for the nurse to acknowledge that Mrs. Pollard is valued, recognized, and respected for her competence and expertise as a caregiver and as a caring and generous sister.

The nurse could begin by including Mrs. Pollard, Tywanda, and her sisters in developing mutual goals for Tywanda's progress and care. At the same time, they can discuss Ethel's deteriorating condition and the realistic expectations for her future. Mrs. Pollard should be encouraged in her role of providing help and care to family members and in promoting the health of her daughter and sister. It is also important that her attention be directed toward her own needs on occasion, considering that she tends to focus on meeting the needs of Tywanda and Ethel before her own.

Social and civic responsibilities among rural, older African Americans in the South are met almost entirely at the level of the extended family and the African American church. These ties and associations are very strong, are often complex, and are not readily understood by outsiders. African American pastors are key players in the lives of their congregants and in their communities. Mrs. Pollard should be encouraged to attend church services and to seek the help and support available to her through this important cultural resource. Mrs. Pollard sings in the church choir and tries to attend choir practice every Wednesday evening. Tywanda has agreed to stay home with her aunt Ethel on Wednesday evenings while Mrs. Pollard is away for the evening. This should be positively reinforced by the nurse. The Black church has been a traditional source of support, and congregations are frequently made up of middle-aged or older adults. Coping strategies such as prayer, singing, or reading the Bible and resources such as family and church support may help mediate Mrs. Pollard's reaction to stressful situations. A culturally competent nurse understands that spirituality is a traditional cultural value that can be supportive during a health crisis.

Mrs. Pollard's life revolves around her family and church. The nurse must acknowledge and support cultural ties with kin and others. It is not uncommon for adult African Americans to cope with little social support from others, relying instead on internal spiritual resources. However, the support provided by close personal relationships is crucial when health conditions deteriorate or an illness develops and is necessary for successful health promotion and maintenance in caregiving activities. Mrs. Pollard's Atlanta-based daughters are crucial for support and assistance during this stressful time. The nurse should actively seek to meet them and acknowledge and encourage their contributions. They should be encouraged to participate in mutual goal setting with the members of the Pollard family.

The nurse can continue to encourage Mrs. Pollard to attend church services because her social life is derived from her participation in the activities of her church. Providing positive reinforcement for Tywanda's decision to stay with her aunt Ethel while Mrs. Pollard attends church services and choir practice would be appropriate. It is the church family who will be instrumental in providing emotional support and help as Ethel's condition continues to decline, as well as the opportunity for Mrs. Pollard to find meaning and to cope with her loss and grief if Ethel predeceases her. If Tywanda continues risky drug and sexual behavior, Mrs. Pollard will need continued support and counseling from health care professionals to continue her caregiving role. Nursing interventions at the individual and family level are extremely important in maintaining and extending quality of life.

Summary

All individuals are confronted with life transitions, crises, and/or changes. All cultures have acceptable and defined ways of responding to these life situations. Adulthood is a busy and productive time and should no longer be considered a stable "slide" toward old age. A situational health transition was presented: an African American woman, Mrs. Pollard, who cared for her developmentally delayed sister, Ethel, and her 26-year-old daughter who has HIV/AIDS. Ethel's health was deteriorating and Mrs. Pollard was fearful that her daughter was using illicit drugs. Mrs. Pollard's own health problems were exacerbated by this situational transition, and her normal development through adulthood was disrupted. How nurses can understand such situations and provide culturally appropriate care was described.

REVIEW QUESTIONS

1. Describe examples of health transitions in your family members and friends. Which types of transitions can you identify in your clients/patients? Do you think it is helpful to think of "transitions" as opposed to "developmental tasks or stages?" Why?

2. How does culture influence transitions of adulthood? For example, explain how a woman from a traditional culture such as those in the Middle East might experience adulthood differently.

3. Discuss how gender might influence adult development in a white, middle-class family.

4. Describe how social factors such as mobility, increased education, and changes in the economy have influenced adult development in American and Canadian cultures.

5. How might caregiving for a family member bring about a situational transition for a middle-aged adult? Would this differ in cultural groups such as Chinese Americans or Mexican Americans? How?

6. Describe how culture influences the role of the caregiver in some African American cultures. What can you find in the literature about caregiving in other cultural groups?

CRITICAL THINKING ACTIVITIES

1. Interview a middle-aged colleague, a client, or a person from another cultural group. Ask about adult roles within the family and how they are depicted. How are these role descriptions typical of traditional roles that are described in the literature? If not, how are they different? What are some of the reasons why they have changed?

2. Interview a middle-aged client from another cultural group. Ask about the client's experiences within the health care system. What were the differences the client noted in health beliefs and practices? Ask the client about his or her health needs during middle age.

3. Using the Andrews/Boyle Transcultural Nursing Guide for Individuals and Families provided in Appendix A, conduct a cultural assessment of a middle-aged client of another cultural group. Critically analyze how the client's culture affects the client's role within the family and the timing of developmental

transitions. How might the assessment data differ if the client were older? Younger?

4. Review the literature on Mexican American culture. Describe the traditional Mexican American family. What are the cultural characteristics of Mexican Americans to consider in assessing the developmental transitions of adulthood in this group?

5. You are assigned a new patient, a 24-year-old man, from El Salvador named Jose Calderon. At morning report, you learn that he has been a gang member in El Salvador, and because he wanted to stop all gang-related activities, his life was threatened. He fled to the United States and has been granted political asylum. You are told that he has extensive tattoos on his body. What do you know about gang membership in Central America? In the United States? How does membership in a gang address the needs of adolescents? What are the cultural factors that are important to consider when you are planning nursing care for a patient like Jose? For example, how do you view body tattoos? What are the issues related to political asylum, immigration, and the like? How might you assist Jose to meet his developmental needs? What might be the problems he will encounter in the US society or in our health care system?

REFERENCES

Baird, M. B. (2012). Well-being in refugee women experiencing cultural transition. *ANS. Advances in Nursing Science, 35*(3), 249–263. doi: 10.1097/ANS.0b013e31826260c0

Baird, M. B., & Boyle, J. S. (2012). Well-being in Dinka refugee women of southern Sudan. *Journal of Transcultural Nursing, 23*(1), 14–21. doi: 10.1177/1043659611423833

Belenky, M. F. (1997). *Women's ways of knowing: The development of self, voice, and mind* (10th anniversary ed.). New York, NY: Basic Books.

Bronfenbrenner, U. (1977). Toward an experimental ecology of human development. *American Psychologist, 32*(7), 513–531. doi: 10.1037/0003-066X.32.7.513

Burke, A. (2017, December 5). 10 facts about American women in the workforce. Retrieved from https://www. brookings.edu/blog/brookings-now/2017/12/05/10-facts-about-american-women-in-the-workforce/

Campinha-Bacote, J. (2013). People of African American heritage. In L. D. Purnell (Ed.), *Trancultural health care: A culturally competent approach* (4th ed.). Philadelphia, PA: F. A. Davis Company.

Caregiving in the U.S. 2015. (2015). Retrieved from https://www.aarp.org/content/dam/aarp/ppi/2015/caregiving-in-the-united-states-2015-report-revised.pdf

Clark-Hine, D. (1998). African American women. In W. Mankiller, G. Mink, M. Navarro, B. Smith, & G. Steinem (Eds.), *The reader's companion to U.S. women's history.* Boston, MA: Houghton Mifflin.

Collins, W. L., & Hawkins, A. D. (2016). Supporting caregivers who care for African American elders: A pastoral perspective. *Social Work and Christananity, 43*(4), 85–103.

Crist, J. D., Montgomery, M. L., Pasvogel, A., Phillips, L. R., & Ortiz-Dowling, E. M. (2018). The association among knowledge of and confidence in home health care services, acculturation, and family caregivers' relationships to older adults of Mexican descent. *Geriatric Nursing, 39*, 689–695. doi: https://doi.org/10.1016/j.gerinurse.2018.05.005

Demick, J., & Andreoletti, C. (2003). *Handbook of adult development.* New York, NY: Kluwer Academic/Plenum Publishers.

Erikson, E. H. (1963). *Youth: Change and challenge.* New York, NY: Basic Books.

Fromm, E. (1969). *Escape from freedom.* New York, NY: Henry Holt and Company, LLC.

Garcia, J., Parker, C., Parker, R. G., Wilson, P. A., Philbin, M., & Hirsch, J. S. (2016). Psychosocial implications of homophobia and HIV stigma in social support networks: Insights for high-impact HIV prevention among black men who have sex with men. *Health Education & Behavior, 43*(2), 217–225. doi: 10.1177/1090198115599398

Havighurst, R. J. (1980). Life-span developmental psychology and education. *Educational Researcher, 9*(10), 3–8. doi: 10.2307/1174928

Hine, D. C., & Thompson, K. (1998). *A shining thread of hope: The history of Black women in America* (1st ed.). New York, NY: Broadway Books.

Historical poverty tables: People and families—1959 to 2016. (2017, September 8). Retrieved from https://www.census.gov/data/tables/time-series/demo/income-poverty/historical-poverty-people.html

HIV among African Americans fact sheet. (2014). Retrieved from https://www.hivlawandpolicy.org/sites/default/files/HIV%20Among%20African%20Americans.pdf

HIV among African Americans fact sheet. (2017). Retrieved from https://www.cdc.gov/nchhstp/newsroom/docs/factsheets/cdc-hiv-aa-508.pdf

HIV and AIDS. (2018). Retrieved from https://www.womenshealth.gov/hiv-and-aids

HIV/AIDS Bureau. (2018, July 2017). Retrieved from https://www.hrsa.gov/about/organization/bureaus/hab/index.html

Hollis-Sawyer, L., & Dykema-Engblade, A. (2016). *Women and positive aging: An international perspective.* Retrieved from https://www.sciencedirect.com/book/9780124201361/women-and-positive-aging. doi: 10.1016/C2013-0-13447-2

Im, A. (2014). Afaf Ibrahim Meleis: Transitions theory. In M. R. Alligood (Ed.), *Nursing theorists and their work* (8th ed., pp. 378–395). St. Louis, MO: Elsevier.

Im, E., Ham, O. K., Chee, E., & Chee, W. (2015). Physical activity and depressive symptoms in four ethnic groups of milife women. *Western Journal of Nursing Research, 37*(6), 746–766. doi: 10.1177/0193945914537123

Kjellstrom, S., & Stalne, K. (2017). Adult development as a lens: Applications of adult development theories in research. *Behavioral Development Bulletin, 22*(2), 266–278. doi: 10.1037/bdb0000053

Kojola, E., & Moen, P. (2016). No more lock-step retirement: Boomers' shifting meanings of work and retirement. *Journal of Aging Studies, 36*, 59–70. doi: 10.1016/j.jaging.2015.12.003

Leading causes of death. (2017). Retrieved from https://www.cdc.gov/nchs/fastats/leading-causes-of-death.htm

Mapes, D. (2016, October 14). America's favorite age? It's 50, new poll says. Retrieved from https://www.today.com/health/americas-favorite-age-its-50-new-poll-says-8C11144329

McLeod, S. (2018). Erik Erikson's stages of psychological development. *SimplyPsychology.* Retrieved from simplypsychology.org

Murphy, S. L., Xu, J., Kochanek, K. D., Curtin, S. C., & Arias, E. (2017). *Deaths: Final data for 2015.* (2018-1120). Hyattsville, MD: Center for Disease Control and Prevention Retrieved from https://www.cdc.gov/nchs/data/nvsr/nvsr66/nvsr66_06.pdf

Neugarten, B. L. (1968). Perspectives of the aging process. Developmental perspectives. *Psychiatric Research Reports American Psychiatric Association, 23*, 42–48. Retrieved from https://www.ncbi.nlm.nih.gov/pubmed/5667122

Noble, A., Rom, M., Newsome-Wicks, M., Engelhardt, K., & Woloski-Wruble, A. (2009). Jewish laws, customs, and practice in labor, delivery, and postpartum care. *Journal of Transcultural Nursing, 20*(3), 323–333. doi: 10.1177/1043659609334930

Poverty rate by race/ethnicity. (2016). *State health facts.* Retrieved from https://www.kff.org/other/state-indicator/poverty-rate-by-raceethnicity/?currentTimeframe=0&sortModel=%7B%22colId%22:%22Location%22,%22sort%22:%22asc%22%7D

Purnell, L. D. (Ed.) (2013). *Transcultural health care: A culturally competent approach* (4th ed.). Philadelphia, PA: F. A. Davis Company.

Salo, C. D., & Birman, D. (2015). Acculturation and psychological adjustment of vietnamese refugees: An ecological acculturation framework. *American Journal of Community Psychology, 56*, 395–407. doi: 10.1007/s10464-015-9760-9

Sandberg-Thoma, S. E., Snyder, A. R., & Jang, B. J. (2015). Exiting and returning to the parental home for boomerang kids. *Journal of Marriage and the Family, 77*(3), 806–818. doi: 10.1111/jomf.12183

Shambley-Ebron, D., Dole, D., & Karikari, A. (2016). Cultural preparation for womanhood in urban African American girls: Growing strong women. *Journal of Transcultural Nursing, 27*(1), 25–32. doi: 10.1177/1043659614531792

Stroke death rates, 2014–2016. (2018, May 21). Retrieved from https://www.cdc.gov/dhdsp/maps/national_maps/stroke_all.htm

U.S. immigration trends. (2017). Retrieved from https://www.migrationpolicy.org/about/contact-and-directions

Vespa, J. (2017). *The changing economics and demographics of young adulthood: 1975–2016.* (P20-579). Washington DC: United States Census Bureau. Retrieved from http://hispanicad.com/sites/default/files/p20-579.pdf

Williams, K. C., Hicks, E. M., Chang, N., Connor, S. E., & Maliski, S. L. (2014). Purposeful normalization when caring for husbands recovering from prostate cancer. *Qualitative Health Research, 24*(3), 306–316. doi: 10.1177/1049732314523842

Women in the labor force: A databook (1071). (2017). Retrieved from https://www.bls.gov/opub/reports/womens-databook/2017/pdf/home.pdf

Young-Mason, J. (2009). Understanding culture: The art of food from the annals of the Caliph's kitchen. *Nursing and the Arts, 23*(3), 175–176.

Young-Mason, J. (2018). Art, body, and soul: A converstation with Nawal Nasrallah. *Nursing and the Arts, 32,* 279–284. doi: 10.1097/NUR.0000000000000390

Zhang, Y., Wilson, T. E., Adedimeji, A., Merenstein, D., Milam, J., Cohen, J., & Golub, E. T. (2017). The impact of substance use on adherence to antiretroviral therapy among HIV-infected women in the United States. *AIDS Behavior, 22,* 896–908. doi: 10.1007/s10461-017-1808-4

Transcultural Perspectives in the Care of Older Adults

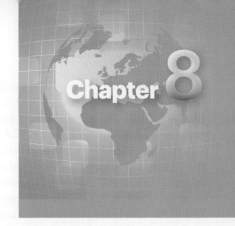

Chapter 8

• Margaret A. McKenna

Key Terms

Chronic conditions
Continuing care retirement
  communities

Health behavior
Illness behavior
Long-term care

Self-care
Successful aging

Learning Objectives

1. Demonstrate knowledge of the sociodemographic shift in the older adult population that affects the demand for nurses prepared to meet diverse clients' needs.
2. Identify how socioeconomic factors, including income level, as well as community resources will influence the interactions of older adults in the health care system.
3. Identify that the growing population of older adults has contributed to the development of expanded community residential options where nurses may have a variety of roles in caring for older adults.
4. Develop nursing interventions for older adults in different health care contexts that are based on the clients' cultural values and individual preferences.
5. Analyze factors affecting the needs of diverse older adults in a continuum of services from health promotion community-based services through care in long-term care facilities.

In 2035, the number of older individuals in the United States is expected to exceed that of children for the first time in our history with a projected 78 million older adults and 76.4 million children under 18 years of age (U.S. Census Bureau, 2018). Another first is that between 2020 and 2050, the increasing birth rate is not pro-jected to be totally offset by the pattern of rising deaths among the large population of aged individuals. This will lead to natural increases diminishing as a factor of population growth so that international migration becomes a bigger driver of our population growth. This shift will contribute to an increasingly ethnically and racially diverse older population with a declining proportion of non-Hispanic whites (58%) (U.S. Census Bureau, 2018). The population of 65 years and older is expected to more than double to 98 million in 2060. The older adult population includes the "young old" sometimes depicted as engaging in retirement travel and hobbies, while there is another sector of the "older old" aged 85 years and older. This latter sector is variously depicted in the media as possessing secrets of longevity or as a population sector that is facing inevitable decline (Rozanova, Miller, & Wetle, 2016). This older old sector is projected to double from 6.3 to 14.6 million by 2040 (USDHHS, 2017).

Most of the developed world countries have applied the age of 65 years to refer to an older person, since this is associated with the age when an individual is likely to be eligible to receive pension benefits. However, there is no universal agreement on the age at which a person becomes old; indeed, research tells us that the refugee or immigrant experiences of coming from a war-torn country or having posttraumatic stress disorder can be associated with an older subjective age (Avidor, Benyamini, & Solomon, 2016; Nielsen, Minet, Zeraig, Rasmussen, & Sodermann, 2018). Thus, some ethnically diverse adults may chronologically be 50 years old and be referred to as elders.

Older adults are diverse in their life experiences, education and employment histories, lifestyles, cultural backgrounds, family composition, as well as other social characteristics. Older adults also live in a variety of settings that may extend from independent residences, congregate care facilities, or adult family homes, to **long-term care** institutions typically referred to as nursing homes or skilled nursing facilities. In any of these settings, nurses and health care providers may interact with the older clients in different roles to provide preventive education, acute illness care, chronic illness management, therapeutic care, or hospice care coordination. Nurses may also engage with community-dwelling older adults in any number of ways as a case manager or care coordinator or direct care provider.

The increasing older adult population and the racial, ethnic, and cultural diversity of that population call for a diverse nursing workforce and a workforce prepared to deliver culturally competent care (Cayo, 2018). In any care settings, the nurse identifies that culture is a critical dimension in understanding the interactions of older clients within their families and in the encompassing health care system. The older clients' cultural traditions and values will influence how they interact with health care providers, whether they decide to follow health care regimens, and where they prefer to live and receive care. In assessing older adults, nurses consider how individuals have multiple roles—such as whether they are caregivers within their own families—to identify and determine the families' strengths, resources, and capacities for care of aging family members. One influence on delivering culturally appropriate care to clients is how available, affordable, and accessible are state and local health care resources for older adults. Many rural and urban locations differ in the range of information and referral sources, acute and extended care facilities, and community-based services that are available to older adults to support their quality of life. Box 8-1 highlights multiple factors that will affect the responses and interactions of older adult clients when they initiate or continue in seeking health care services to meet their acute and extended care needs.

This chapter is organized in three sections that describe the surrounding ecological domains that influence older adults' experiences as aging members of their families and in other roles: the encompassing societal context, local community settings, and the interpersonal and family level. Each of these areas contributes to and influences the older adult's overall well-being, help-seeking behavior, responses to illness, and age-related adjustments in carrying out activities:

1. Encompassing social and economic factors affect the affordability and accessibility of health care options for acute, chronic, and long-term care.
2. Available community resources such as informal and formal sources of help will

BOX 8-1	Factors that Influence Older Adults' Responses in Seeking Health Care

Societal Factors

- Clients' income and financial levels affect eligibility for assistance to pay for supplemental or Medicare gap insurance. The lack of insurance can limit older adults from receiving preventive care, acute care, or health care maintenance in the health care system.
- Changes to control Medicare expenditures force shorter hospital stays.
- Gaps in health care services put greater burdens on older patients for home- and community-based care.

Cultural Influences

- Cultural values, acculturation, access to traditional sources of health medicine, and logistical factors including language and transportation can all interact in determining when and where older adults will access the biomedical health care system.

- Different cultural values influence patterns in caring for older adult family members as they age and require more assistance.
- Younger family members become acculturated, and their availability to care for elders may differ from older adults' expectations to be cared for at home.

Individual and Family Characteristics

- Younger adult family members who are more accustomed to the range of health care options and services may conflict with older adult parents.
- Female family members who were once expected to be primary caregivers for older family members may be engaged in the workforce and unavailable as caregivers.
- Families' economic situations, proximity to the older adult, and sources of formal support in the community will determine options for residence and care needs of the older adult.

influence patterns of caregiving as well as when and where older clients interact in the biomedical health care system.

3. Personal and family values, culturally influenced behaviors and actions such as health-promoting or risk-taking behavior, and earlier experiences in the health care system affect the older client's decisions about health care and services.

The Older Adult in Contemporary Society: Factors Affecting Health Care

This section addresses societal influences on older adult clients: demographic factors of the aging population, socioeconomic conditions, and the theoretical frameworks that shape how older adults in Western society perceive growing older.

Demographics and Disparities

Nearly all older adults desire and strive to achieve **successful aging** without disease and disability and to maintain cognitive and physical functioning along with active social engagement (Rozanova et al., 2016). However, many older adults develop **chronic conditions** that may include diabetes, hypertension, arthritis, and other illnesses that require medication, diet modification, or symptom monitoring. Older adult clients may also develop risks for heart disease and conditions including stroke, chronic respiratory diseases, Alzheimer's, and diabetes. National health care costs are expected to increase by 25% by 2030 with the growing numbers of older adults who have chronic illnesses (Centers for Disease Control and Prevention (CDC), 2017). The cost of caring for each adult aged 65 or older is estimated to be three to five times higher than that for younger adults. There are an estimated 5.7 million individuals living with Alzheimer's dementia, and the number is projected to grow to 13.8 million by 2050 (Alzheimer's Association, 2018). Deaths resulting from Alzheimer's dementia increased 123% from 2000 to 2015, while during that time, the deaths resulting from stroke, heart disease, and prostate cancer decreased.

There are many racial and ethnic disparities in the prevalence of chronic conditions that are underlying the older patient's entry and trajectory in health care services. Among adults aged 60 to 79 years, the prevalence of diabetes alone or diabetes with cardiovascular disease was twice as high among Hispanics and non-Hispanic blacks as among non-Hispanic whites (CDC, 2017). The rate of diagnosed diabetes is 77% higher among non-Hispanic blacks, 66% higher among Hispanics, and 18% higher among Asians than among non-Hispanic whites (CDC, 2016). Cardiovascular disease affects black adults much more consistently than it does other racial groups, and non-Hispanic blacks are less likely to have hypertension under control, regardless of differences in socioeconomic status (see Figure 8-1). Native Hawaiians who have been studied have patterns of diet and physical inactivity associated with the highest prevalence of diabetes compared with Latinos, African Americans, Japanese, and Caucasians (Wong & Kataoka-Yahiro, 2017). These disparities exist for interrelated reasons, including lower income levels; lack of insurance, including supplemental insurance to Medicare; barriers in access to care; lower quality of care for some health conditions even when the individual is insured and care is received; and individual decisions to not seek care.

Both ethnicity and income level affect the older adults' health status and need for care. Older White males with the highest incomes can generally expect to live more than 3 years longer than those in the lowest income levels. Among adults aged 65 years or older, Hispanics and Native Americans experience 25% and 50% more physically unhealthy days, respectively, than do non-Hispanic whites (CDC, 2016). Elderly African Americans often suffer functional declines at earlier ages than do White

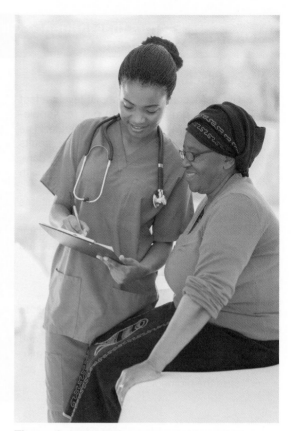

Figure 8-1. A nurse assesses an older adult client (michaeljung/Shutterstock.com).

Americans. There are 2 to 4 million Americans aged 60 years or older who are historically disadvantaged, including individuals who have been marginalized and have very low incomes and who more frequently have higher levels of disability. Thus, there is no simple correlation between the need for care and increased age; care needs and health status are affected by many dimensions in an older person's life, including socioeconomic level, ethnicity, and lifestyle risk factors (e.g., dietary habits).

Socioeconomic Status Affects Health Care Options

Most older adults who retire usually live on a fixed income, but many have increased health-related expenses and may cope with the death of a spouse or life partner that also affects their personal financial resources including health care costs. Some older adults, especially minority ethnic elders, who endured the societal constraints of discrimination on the basis of gender, race, or social class may have limited available resources or financial security to face the economic demands of aging (Rozanova et al., 2016). Older adults who had occupational experiences of marginalization or exclusion are likely to be financially disadvantaged and rely on public benefits or safety net funding to meet basic needs. Among ethnic older adults, including Hispanics and African Americans, 40% have no private savings for their retirement and will look to state and federal reimbursement programs for health and social service needs. The reality is that many ethnic elderly of color have accumulated fewer financial assets; that is, they have a lower household income and have less income from private pensions than do elderly Whites.

The majority of older adults prefer to age in place, that is, to stay in their family homes and in their familiar neighborhoods as long as possible (Cramm, Van Dijk, & Nieboer, 2018). Frail elderly who live alone, especially those who have dementia, and who have no support are particularly vulnerable and are more likely to not be able to age in place (Epps, Weeks, Graham, & Luster, 2018). Older adults who have good health status, mobility, and cognitive functioning have options to remain in their homes or might decide to live in a retirement community. **Continuing care retirement communities** (CCRC) have developed as a one-stop option with a continuum of services in an environment with safe outdoor space, transportation, social and civic engagement activities, and health services. There is a wide variety of assisted living programs in terms of size, structure, sponsorship, amenities, cost, and service availability. High-functioning older adults may decide to initially live in their own apartment (Schafer, 2016). At some point when the older adult requires more care, the resident may move to an assisted living unit to receive help with activities of daily living. When more intensive care is needed or following

an acute illness or injury, the resident may transition to a skilled nursing care unit on the CCRC campus. Such communities with accessible levels of increasing intensity of care contribute to supporting older adults who are gradually becoming frailer to delay placement into a skilled nursing care facility.

One of the major problems that many older adults and their families face is that limited tangible assets and lower equity in their homes may limit possible care options because families cannot afford costly residential care of the older adult family member. Community-based services may include homemakers, modifying a home with safety equipment, adult day care, transportation, personal care, and respite care. These services may be provided to some frail elderly who meet eligibility criteria, and the support services will enable more elderly to reside longer in their preferred community residences. A community assessment of urban African Americans who have dementia found that family caregivers faced multiple challenges. These included the lack of affordable safe housing, high health care costs and inadequate health insurance, insufficient transportation, and feelings of shame and stigma that limited their reaching out to access resources and restricted home care of older family members (Epps et al., 2018).

An example from the caseload of a nurse who provides preventive health care and assessments in a low-income housing complex for older adults illustrates that individuals have different experiences using health care services and Medicare. An 82-year-old woman working as a housekeeper did not seek health care until she had a stroke related to untreated hypertension. She had limited contributions to Social Security owing to an episodic work history, and her illness depleted any savings. She receives Medicare-funded services and continues to receive home health care through Medicaid, which is state-funded health care coverage for individuals with low income. The home health nurse assessed that this patient and other older patients on her caseload would benefit from nursing visits and medication monitoring, but the patient's insurance and Medicare will not cover such services. Medicare pays only a small portion of home health care services, and the patient must be medically eligible to qualify. Older adults who have other insurance may have some coverage for additional home health services for a limited period. The care that older adults may receive will be influenced and determined by economic necessity as well as environmental situations such as resources for nursing services and homemaker resources. For example, community-based care has some limitations as frail older adults in very rural or remote areas may have to enter nursing homes as a safe housing option when there are too few community-based support services or assisted living centers to sustain the frail adult.

Older adults' needs for care, their requests for assistance, and the sources of caregivers are also dimensions that are culturally influenced. Nurses and health care professionals see numerous variations in community caregiving support resources, both formal and informal, that are provided for older adults. In addition to the demographic and economic factors that affect the older population, several theoretical assumptions underlie how people feel about aging adults and shape how resources are made available to care for older adults in communities.

Perspectives of Aging

There are several perspectives of aging that have been depicted in the media and influence how older adults are viewed in society. One social construction of aging refers to the growing population of older adults as a burden that will likely consume a large share of limited societal health care resources (Pulkki & Tynkknen, 2016). For others who accept the disengagement theory, older adults' status is linked to employment so they perceive less self-worth in retirement when relieved of their roles and responsibilities. Activity theory describes that older adults may substitute recreational and meaningful opportunities to take the place of previous occupations and careers. Many older adults are actively con-

tributing as family caregivers and as volunteers for community organizations and in other productive activities. Continuity theory focuses on supporting adults to remain engaged by adapting patterns of behavior from their younger adulthood to keep them involved into older adulthood. One explanatory view of aging is the life course perspective that stresses how progressive developmental processes culminate in health outcomes in older adults. This perspective emphasizes the importance of time, context, and meaning on human development and focuses on the ways that external forces and the meanings individuals ascribe to these forces shape older adults' experiences, outcomes, and responses (Phillips et al., 2015).

A classic developmental theory by Erickson advances that older adults may struggle with the tension between maintaining the integrity of their experience while facing the reality of declining physical and mental functions. In late older adulthood, individuals may despair with the perception that life is too short and with old age comes less authority and power (Erickson & Erickson, 1997), but they may also find joy in being a keeper of meaning and holding enduring relationships. Older adults participating in community center activities are shown in Figure 8-2.

The Older Adult in the Community: Cultural Influences

In community settings, we observe differences in how culturally and ethnically diverse older adults' life experiences will shape their **health behavior** and illness behavior. Older adults may carry out positive health behavior, such as not smoking, eating healthy foods, or maintaining regular exercise. Older immigrants or refugees could have walked daily when living in their home countries and eaten diets high in vegetables. When they are relocated into an urban setting, they may no longer feel safe to walk in unfamiliar areas, and

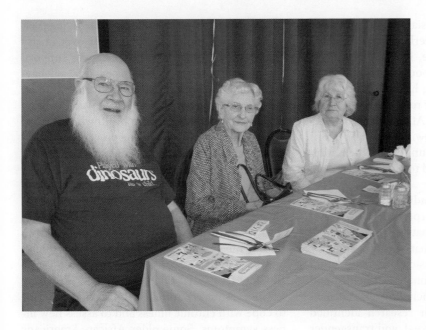

Figure 8-2. Active seniors enjoy a birthday celebration at a community center.

they may alter their diets to include available pre-pared and packaged foods. Among refugees from different regions, including Eritrea and Ethiopia in East Africa, as well as immigrants from Eastern bloc nations, many have lived through civil wars, ethnic tensions, and political revolution, and they feel depleted in trying to cope with more changes in their lives after leaving their homelands. As aging adult immigrants, they may experience adjustment problems that warrant care in the health and mental health care system, but at the same time, they may distrust the system or have very limited experience in seeking biomedical health care.

Nurses who are providing care to clients whose backgrounds differ from their own need to be sensitive to assessing the client's culture. Individuals who have immigrated from the same country or region will differ in their needs and in the ways that their cultural background influences their health- and illness-related actions. These differences are based on a number of factors:

- Regional or religious identity
- Situation in their homeland that may have prompted them to emigrate

- Length of time they have spent in the country where they resettled or immigrated, and degree of acculturation
- Proximity to immediate family or extended family members
- Network of friends and social support from their homeland
- Link with ethnic, social, and health-related institutions

As an example, there are intragroup differences in the Hispanic/Latino population, where persons of Mexican descent are approximately half of the population, Cubans represent 14%, Puerto Ricans 9%, and other Spanish-speaking countries represent 24%. Many educated and professionally well-established Cubans immigrated to the United States in the 1960s, remained, and are now retired. In contrast, families emigrating from Mexico have been younger, some older Mexican immigrants returned to their homeland, and older Mexican Americans do not have as long a life expectancy as their Cuban American peers. The life experiences of the individuals, including their occupations and education, and their acculturation will affect their expectations for care in their advancing years.

Among more than 40 Asian American ethnic groups, the immigrant elderly represent a rich diversity including Chinese, Japanese, Filipinos, Koreans, Vietnamese, Cambodians, Laotians, and Hmong who have had long histories of occupational migration and family relocation to various regions of North America. At this time, the percent of Asian Indians is growing in some regions as elder family members reunite with their adult children who have relocated to North America in skills-based immigration.

Culture influences how individuals view aging, define health, manage interpersonal crises, and face alterations in health that accompany aging. Nurses should consider that for older adults, health has multiple dimensions: physical functioning, social and emotional well-being, and quality-of-life measures, including life satisfaction and happiness. Earlier research identified that older lesbian, gay, bisexual, and transgender (LGBT) adults have distinct health care needs, yet there is very limited research and even less on the care of LGBT older adults who may reside in extended care facilities (Simpson, Almack, & Walthery, 2018). Older adults differ in their perceptions of health but generally regard their physical activity and psychological well-being as indicators of health. Poor health refers to self-reported problems with physical functioning or a need for assistance to complete daily activities.

Older adults are inclined to seek health information and to make behavioral changes to maintain their independence into old age. Older adults who use self-help strategies to maintain their health generally report better psychological well-being and physical functioning than do older adults who do not use these approaches. Nurses typically provide information about the risks of not exercising as well as the benefits of increasing activity, stopping smoking, or adopting healthy eating habits. Nurses may also ask older clients about the circumstances that lead to a lack of exercise and then help clients to take small steps such as seeing how others fit exercise into their lives. Nurses who are aware of cultural variations can appreciate that older individuals will

have different value orientations underlying their decisions to adopt healthy behavior over at-risk behaviors. Older adults who have peer support, anticipate a possible setback in changing a behavior and plan how to get past a challenge, and use incentives through self-talk and rewards will be more likely to make positive health changes. See health promotion goals for the prevention of cardiovascular disease in older adults in Table 8-1.

Interventions should take into account older adults' cognitive ways of coping and practical strategies and support these strategies. For example, the matriarch of an extended family who has always valued the social benefits that come from sharing meals with family members may be reluctant to stop that practice and substitute exercise and low-fat meals. Older adults will also have learned responses in their help-seeking behavior to cope with chronic illness and to assess new illness symptoms. Some older African Americans have been more resourceful in their problem solving, planning, and coping, which may be due in part to the lack of access to health care including mental health services that they may have experienced over time (Epps et al., 2018).

As nurses prepare to care for older clients, they must assess the heterogeneity of the population as ethnicity, cultural traditions, social and economic situations, living arrangements, employment status, and migration history of older adults are as varied as they are for younger adults. These background factors contribute to older adults' varied responses to illness and to their illness behavior that brings them to the health care system. **Illness behavior** refers to how individuals identify that they are ill, accord symptoms significance, decide to seek care or take action to reduce their symptoms, and decide whether or not to comply with a recommended regimen or option for treatment.

Culture will influence the older person's expectations of what constitutes illness and will also influence whether the older adult uses traditional sources of health care, such as practices conducted by healers or actions that are known as family remedies. Researchers have described the simultaneous use of Western medicine and

Table 8-1	Health Promotion Goals to Reduce Cardiovascular Disease in Older Adults		
Goal	**Health Professionals' Actions**	**Indicators of Success**	
Reduce the number of older Americans who need cardiovascular treatment by increasing health-promoting behaviors and health-protective actions to reduce disease risks	**PROTECT** residents of multiunit housing from secondhand smoke exposure by (1) educating everyone about the benefits of smoke-free housing, (2) offering free or low-cost cessation services.	Increase in the number of older adults completing health education programs offered in their communities. Reduction in numbers of older adults who smoke.	
	IMPROVE community access to healthy food by improving public transit for low-income older adults to healthy food retail outlets.	Diverse groups of older adults complete wellness programs that are tailored to be culturally appropriate to encourage all individuals with different lifestyles to reduce their disease risks through increasing exercise and eating healthy.	
	REDUCE rates of death and disability due to diabetes, heart disease, and stroke by 3%.		
	BUILD local partnerships to enhance the effectiveness and efficiency of efforts to prevent heart attack and stroke (CDC, 2017).	Communities respond by creating safe and accessible walking paths to increase use by older adults.	

Source: Centers for Disease Control and Prevention, 2017.

traditional Chinese health practices that focus on restoring harmony and balance in the body and spirit among some groups of Chinese immigrants. Many older clients could have grown up with limited preventive care and associate health care only with emergent conditions, so nurses should assess the older client's previous experiences in the health care system.

Traditional Beliefs and Practices

Older adults may have strong recollections of traditional beliefs and related remedies from their childhood. As an example, while the origins of their beliefs are very different, some Somali patients may believe illness is caused by spirit possession while some Hmong patients may believe that an illness can be caused by evil spirits if one's own spirit has left the body. Some Hindu and Sikh patients may believe that illness is due to karma, one's actions in past lives. Some older Asian Indian immigrants might follow Ayurveda, which includes the use of spices and herbs for

cold, congestion, diabetes, and heart problems. Older Chinese adults experiencing chronic pain, musculoskeletal problems, and headaches might follow traditional practices including herbal medicine, massage, acupuncture, or dietary therapy. Some older Vietnamese immigrants may also use traditional remedies as well as biomedicine, but they may not disclose the use of traditional medicine to a provider, so the nurse should ask a patient what he or she does to relieve symptoms such as the ingestion of certain foods for medicinal properties. An example of eliciting information from a patient is given in Case Study 8-1.

The patient in the case study immigrated as a young woman, but not all immigrants are young. Many immigrants who migrated after the age of 50 experience more depression, which is associated in part with their increased dependence. Depressed older adults are more likely to have lower self-rated health and may have more functional impairment. The older adult usually does not have an option to work, nor is public assistance an option, so the family must provide for

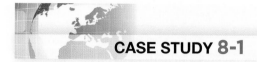

CASE STUDY 8-1

Using Traditional Medicine

Sopha Danh, as a young mother in her 20s, fled with her two young children from Cambodia, settled first in the southeast United States, and then relocated to the Pacific Northwest in the late 1970s. Prior to fleeing from Cambodia, members of Sopha's extended family were tortured and died during a decade of genocide. The extended trauma resulted in patterns of posttraumatic stress disorder and depression being common among older Cambodian refugees. More Cambodian refugees also rate their health as poor and have poor physical functioning when compared to Pacific Islanders who were similar in age and other demographic features.

When Sopha becomes acutely ill and her adult children bring her to a biomedical provider, she does not trust a male health care provider and is very reluctant to adhere with the biomedical care. Sopha is more familiar with traditional medicine, and her experience in help seeking is with traditional healers who took time to develop a relationship with patients. When the biomedical provider starts to elicit Sopha's history, and acknowledges how trauma affects health behavior, and when Sopha's younger family members help to interpret the cultural differences, the provider develops care recommendations that Sopha accepts.

---

the older adult members. Older family members may reciprocate services for younger family members. As part of a nursing assessment, the nurse should note if older adults are primary care providers for grandchildren or other family members and if an illness episode in the older adult disrupts the family.

Older adult clients may also use traditional medicine or practices from their family of origin as a means to prevent illness. Traditional preventive measures as well as actions to treat symptoms may include a magical or religious element, burning a candle, offering cornmeal to the spirits, wearing an amulet, or reciting a prayer. The individual may also consult a traditional healer, someone who is well respected for demonstrating unique abilities to relate to a person seeking help and decrease the person's discomfort. To assess the older adult's cultural beliefs and practices, the nurse can demonstrate a nonjudgmental attitude and develop culturally appropriate communication as shown in Box 8-2.

Adults aged 65 years or older are much more likely than young and middle-aged adults to have low health literacy skills, which means they are more likely to misunderstand medical tests, end up in the emergency room, and have a harder time managing chronic diseases. A majority of

older adults have trouble understanding everyday health information available in health care facilities, which indicates nurses have a role to make information and instruction understood by all patients. A study of older adults from several minority communities who had a recent hospital stay found that when these patients had a language barrier and could not understand what was happening to them or share information they had increased feelings of fear, anxiety, and loneliness (Ellins & Glasby, 2016). Overcoming language barriers with the aid of skilled interpreters and translated instructions, or by involving family members to interpret and advocate for the older patients contributed to perceived higher quality of care. All of the study patients from diverse backgrounds also desired personalized and humanistic approaches when receiving care in the hospital and transitional services at home. Older patients typically wish to build a trusting relationship, receive clear information, and be respected in their interactions with health care providers.

The use of traditional sources of health care concurrently with or in place of the biomedical health care system is not limited to members of recently migrated cultural groups but is common to nearly all individuals. Several chronic

BOX 8-2 | Guidelines for Communicating with Older Adult Clients

- Elicit the client's views on why the client thinks he or she has symptoms.
- Ask what home remedies or treatment the client has used and what treatment the client expects.
- Respond with information about the biomedical model using words the client can understand.
- Negotiate with the client what he or she accepts about the biomedical health care model and will likely comply with.
- Create a positive environment by being patient, inviting, and sitting close to the client so the client can hear you (avoid standing above the client). If working with an interpreter, position yourself so the client sees you. Typically, address the client in formal terms.
- Ask the client if a family member can also be present to help the client remember or participate in any client teaching.

- Have printed instructions in the client's native language, if possible. Have nonverbal methods of communication, including photographs or symbols to convey instructions, especially for clients who do not read their home language or English.
- Be aware if the client wants to make decisions or defer to family members as the decision makers about care issues.
- Demonstrate new skills that the client has to learn and discuss medications in words the client will understand. Show the client medications and help the client identify how to remember to take medications. Ask the client to repeat instructions to you.

conditions that often accompany age, including osteoarthritis or diabetes, increase the likelihood that older adults will use traditional sources or self-care to treat their symptoms. An older adult doing self-care may choose an over-the-counter medication and may use other popular remedies before, during, or after the use of prescribed sources of care. Nurses can show an interest in the client and ask them about any actions they take to treat their conditions, in order to assess the older client's concurrent use of traditional practices, folk medicine, or popular medicine. Case Study 8-2 illustrates that assessing the client's use of alternative sources of treatment is useful in developing a care plan that the client will accept.

Understanding Culture Change

Some older adults have relocated to different regions of the country or have made a significant transition in their late adult years to be close to younger family members or for other reasons.

Some older refugees have fled their home countries to escape political oppression and trauma. Older clients may have the common experience of relocating or migrating, but they may vary in adjusting to new settings and to a new social environment (Nielsen et al., 2018). Older adults may clash with their grown children who have acculturated to their new cultural contexts and adopted new behaviors. Cultural change can contribute negatively to mental health, and this psychological stress is more intense for older refugees. For example, among some Central American immigrants living in a metropolitan area in the United States, their perceived stress was correlated with their psychological health. An example of a refugee making many social and financial adjustments is in Case Study 8-3.

The nurse in this case study assesses several areas that are relevant for any older adult client to maintain good health; these are listed in Box 8-3. For many Burundian refugees and other refugees and immigrants, low socioeconomic status could be a barrier to health care, especially

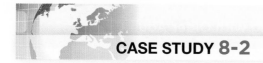

CASE STUDY 8-2

How an Older Client Treats Pain

Mrs. Teadora Matthews is an 83-year-old retired seamstress who has hypertension, high cholesterol, obesity, and degenerative joint disease, which makes her joints painful and limits her mobility. She was raised in Romania, immigrated to the United States as a young woman, married a man in the mid-western United States, raised a family, and now lives in the same home as her daughter and grandchildren. She has been the primary caregiver for her grandchildren and remains active as a volunteer receptionist at her church. Her joint pain causes her to miss her planned volunteer work, and she uses over-the-counter remedies including ointments, topical applications, and pain relief patches to reduce her pain.

The nurse assesses that Mrs. Matthews tolerates a great deal of pain while carrying out her usual activities and remaining as active as possible. Her occasional use of the topical remedies does not interfere with Mrs. Matthews' prescribed medications for her other conditions. Mrs. Matthews believes that self-medicating and using a rubbing compound decreases her pain, which allows her to participate in her preferred family and volunteer activities. The nurse will continue to assess whether the use of an alternative source of treatment would interfere with a prescribed care plan.

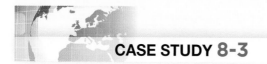

CASE STUDY 8-3

Older Adult Adopts New Practices

Mr. Sylvestre Longo is very proud to have been born in Burundi, in central Africa. However, due to the strife, ethnic conflict, and genocide, he had to flee his native country. He lived in refugee camps in Tanzania for almost 30 years before he was relocated by an international relief agency to Washington State. The Burundian refugees initially received financial assistance upon arrival in the United States, but after months of limited support, members of the community sought work in order to pay rent, meet their basic needs, and partially repay the costs of their relocation. Several of the Burundians learned of a social service organization that was recruiting refugees and immigrants to participate in a pilot project to develop their employment and English language skills while learning farming. The Burundians learned English vocabulary and improved their diet by eating homegrown lettuce, beans, kale, chard, and root vegetables. The Burundians also became more physically active when they were planting and harvesting their plots and working in the fields, which contributed to the new farmers developing peer relationships.

When Mr. Longo experiences shortness of breath and seeks treatment through a neighborhood health clinic, a nurse elicits basic information about his health history, his social network, and his life transitions. Although he is only 50 years old, he is regarded as an elder among the other Burundians, who are in their 30s, some of whom lived their entire lives in refugee camps. Mr. Longo often attends monthly get-togethers of the local Burundians in which the younger, more acculturated members help to explain the cultural practices of their adopted country, such as completing applications to get entry-level jobs, buying food in large markets, and making appointments to request financial assistance.

Mr. Longo's nurse identifies several of his health-promoting behaviors. His informal social network could offer him some informational support to comply with his prescribed medications. She also assesses that he eats a diet high in fresh vegetables. This is in contrast to many immigrants and older adults who have income only from public benefits; typically, they have very limited access to fresh food when they live in neighborhoods without grocery stores. The nurse also assesses that Mr. Longo walks daily because he cannot afford other transportation, and this regular exercise contributes to his overall health and decreased risk factors for chronic conditions.

BOX 8-3 | Assessing Older Adults' Social Roles

- Family relationships and social interaction of the older client within the family—that is, the role the older adult has with a spouse, partner, adult children, and grandchildren as well as the role of the elder with peers and others in a social network
- Environment to which the older client will return
- Adherence of the client and the family to traditional values including the preferences of the patient to prepare, cook, or eat traditional foods. Adoption of new nutritional patterns of eating prepared and packaged foods in place of traditional foods
- Linguistic or social isolation of the older client
- Desire to maintain a moderate level of activity
- Ability to take personal responsibility for one's health
- Access to services and amenities including a safe place to exercise, senior center, and transportation
- Significance of spirituality and religious practices to health

for early diagnosis and treatment of chronic conditions. Access to affordable health insurance is increasing for many low-income individuals, but paying insurance premiums often remains a challenge. Some of the older immigrants from East Africa experience mild declines in their health when they gradually become less active and modify their diets to eat more of the prepared high carbohydrate foods that are abundant in their new country. Supplemental nutrition programs including community lunches high in fresh vegetables and a protein serve several purposes of supporting positive mental health through peer interaction and stimulating healthy eating practices. These communal meals often increase the participants' intake of healthy foods and decrease their risks for poor nutritional status, which are associated with some older adults' functional limitations, cognitive dysfunction, decreased physical activity level, social isolation, alcohol or substance abuse, or other factors.

Caregiving of Older Adults

Older family members are part of the informal social support in their families, so they may be the caregivers for grandchildren or younger family members and they may receive assistance and support from other family members (see Figure 8-3). If the older adult becomes ill, then families may have to adapt to find an alternate caregiver. Older adults in their family social support networks may also be in need of assistance and nurturing. Consider the preferences of the older person and his or her family members, as well as the capacities of the older adult for self-care and the willingness and capabilities of the family to offer support and assistance with care. The type and duration of support that can be provided by family members must be considered in relation to sources of formal support from home health workers, hospice care, and visiting nurses and therapists that could be used to sustain the family care.

The roles that family members take in caring and supporting their elders vary according to cultural, socioeconomic, and demographic characteristics. All families have culturally influenced patterns of responsibility to care for older family members, but these patterns vary across cultures and among individuals in any cultural group. As an example, in a study of *familismo* in a Latino sample, younger family members were more inclined to provide instrumental support regardless of their understanding of the patient's control over their illness but caregivers were not as ready to provide any emotional support when they perceived the older adult's controllability of their illness (Villalobos & Bridges, 2016).

Nurses and health care professionals are often aware of how family members may differ in

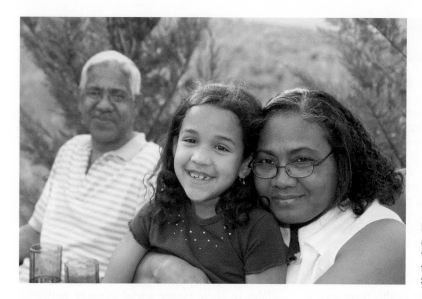

Figure 8-3. Grandparents are often the primary caregivers for grandchildren or younger family members (Rob Marmion/Shutterstock.com).

whether they retain traditional values or blend other competing demands with their underlying values that affect caring for older family members. Nurses working with older adults should be sensitive to the evolving needs of family caregivers that will be influenced by the caregivers' acculturation and their time since immigration, factors that place the caregiver between value systems. The economic necessity that two adults in many households must work to provide adequate household income has contributed to a decline in the availability of adult children as caregivers to parents and grandparents. Adult children and other family members may be available to provide episodic assistance, emotional support through short visits, or some financial assistance to purchase in-home services. Because it is not possible to talk about older adults or their families as if they were a homogeneous group, it is necessary to consider that cultural diversity and lifestyle choices may determine the options for care of the older adult. Several examples of community care options for older adults are highlighted in Table 8-2.

Community nurses may have to coordinate how families caring for older adult members can access and use formal support services (visiting nurse services, chore services, adult day care) and informal support services (family members who provide relief care, neighborhood volunteers, meal delivery). Families of older ethnic minority adults have had varying reactions to and access of formal services owing to their knowledge, confidence, and comfort in the use of service providers (Bonds & Lyons, 2018; Crist, Montgomery, Pasvogel, Phillips, & Ortiz-Dowling, 2018; Epps et al., 2018). Nurses typically also assess a caregiver's capacities, needs, and resources in planning for extended care of an older adult at home as well as assessing the well-being of the older adult client. For example, a nurse may support a caregiver who is a working parent sandwiched between the care of an older relative and also caring for adolescent children, or a caregiver may be a retired worker in their 60s who also has a chronic illness.

Dimensions of Social Support

Social support has been delineated in three ways: affective support, or expressions of respect, and love; affirmational support, or having endorsement for one's behavior and perceptions; and tangible support, or receiving some kind of aid

Table 8-2	Highlights of Selected Health Care Studies of Caregiving and Older Adults		
Study Author (Date) Topic or Group Studied	**Cultural Concepts Relevant in Care of Older Adult Client**	**Implications for Nursing Care**
Crist et al. (2018) • Mexican-descent older adults and their caregivers who lived in Arizona (74 dyads) were recruited during the older adults' hospitalization. Study participants responded to questionnaires on their knowledge of home health care services (HHCS), their confidence in using the services, and level of acculturation.	Among spousal caregivers, knowledge of services was associated with a higher Anglo-oriented social interaction and English language preference. However, these spouse caregivers also expressed fear of HHCS providers entering their home to care for their loved one. Offspring caregivers tended to have less fear of HHCS workers whom they expected to provide quality care to their relatives.	Mexican-descent families may tend to have a lower use of HHCS partially due to the cultural value of familismo. Because family caregivers may have some fear of HHCS nurses may want to engage family members during predischarge planning and ensure cultural competence in explaining services.
Pan, Jones, and Winslow (2017) • Caregivers to parent stroke survivors in China (n = 126) were surveyed at hospitals or in homes on mutuality, filial attitude and behavior, and depression scales. Mutuality referred to the relationship quality in the caregiving dyad.	As many as one-third of the caregivers of stroke patients in different studies conducted in Canada, Finland, and the United States have reported signs of depression. Caregivers have also expressed physical exhaustion, feelings of being ignored, and being deprived of socialization.	One finding that may be applied in the care of other families is to assess if mutuality and filial attitude may serve as protective factors that counter caregiver depression.
Wilks, Spurlock, Brown, Teegen, and Geiger (2018) • Secondary data analysis of a sample of 691 Alzheimer's disease caregivers, one-third of whom were reported as African American. African American caregivers have exhibited higher religiosity compared to Caucasian caregivers in response to caregiving stress.	The study examined spiritual support as religious or spiritual beliefs linked with psychological and social resources for coping with stress. A study aim was to describe if spiritual support could be viewed as a potential buffer in a manner similar to social support to moderate the negative effects of caregiving of a significant other with Alzheimer's.	Nurses interacting with clients in home-based settings may wish to consider that spiritual support did not buffer the caregiver burden risk but did affect caregiver resilience for both groups of African American and white study sample participants.

or physical assistance, such as accompanying a person to an appointment. Many older adults are deprived of the informal social supports due to losses:

• Separation from immediate family members because of geographic mobility
• Age-related segregation caused by increased nuclear families in neighborhoods
• Loss of spouse or partner because of death or illness

• Loss of leisure pursuits or entertainment due to illness, loss of income, or declining physical abilities

It is especially important for many older adults to have social, emotional, and physical sources of support to assist them to remain as independent as possible. We know that social support may mitigate the negative effects of social stress, but the exact mechanisms are unclear. We do understand variations in these patterns of support, which helps to prepare nurses who work in acute care, extended care, or community settings. Some minority older adult clients may have more connections to kin in their support networks, but they may also be more vulnerable to conflicts in tight-knit networks; this is less common for older adults who have multiple networks of family, friends, neighbors, and coworkers.

Culture may influence the types of social support family members offer to older clients, and nurses may assess that families' size and structure affect how informal support is provided. Some families, including German Americans and families of English heritage, often have a linear structure. The expectation is that adult children will assume care responsibilities for aging parents, and grandchildren will assume caregiving for aging parents and grandparents when needed. Another family structure is collateral, when the perceived bonds are more diffuse. Parents, aunts, uncles, grandparents, and family friends may be part of the collateral bonds of families. Among families with a collateral structure are some Irish, Polish, and African American families, who expect to receive and to provide informal support among all collateral contacts. The expectation for care among many Irish families is that relatives must assist each other when needed. Many Irish and Irish American families would agree that their relatives are obliged to enter into generalized reciprocity.

In addition to cultural variation in patterns of giving help and support, socioeconomic status will influence the amount and level of assistance that family members provide to older adult family members. Demographic factors, such as family size, migration patterns, rural/urban residence, and socioeconomic factors, including income level and educational level, affect patterns of family support to their older members. These factors may determine the availability of family members to offer assistance and may influence the type of support that is offered. Thus, nurses must assess the influence of these factors on the older adult's social support network and identify that demographic and socioeconomic factors may be

blended with culturally influenced patterns of behavior.

Many elder Native Americans tend to socialize less outside of their extended families and expect that the needs of extended family members will come before those of the individual. Native American values support the care of older family members in the home, but the pool of available caregivers is diminishing because of some of the same patterns observed for other families, such as employment mobility. Elder Native Americans and Alaska Natives living in multigenerational households are more likely than White peers to have significant disabilities (see Figure 8-4). A pattern that has been seen in some Native American and Alaska Native families is that each adult child, in birth order, assumes the burden of responsibility and cost of care for the aging parent, which may exhaust the adult child's personal financial resources.

Intragroup Differences

The large older Hispanic/Latino population includes very diverse individuals who not only represent different countries, traditions, and acculturation status but also have many variations in their patterns of social support from friends and family. While there are intragroup and intergroup differences, some patterns have been observed in studies of Hispanic/Latino elders.

The nurse may look for ways in the client's neighborhood or local community to support an older adult immigrant in making ties to his or her home country to enhance self-esteem and feelings of belonging. Nurses may ask if an older adult can talk to a group of children at an ethnic community center, such as the Ukrainian Community Center, El Centro de la Raza, or the Polish Association. The older adult can also tell the history of his or her immigration to adolescents who may be tracing their cultural heritage for an oral history project. Senior adults may also be connected to school-age children by walking them to and from school or tutoring them through an after-school project that may enhance the older adults' feelings of contributing and belonging.

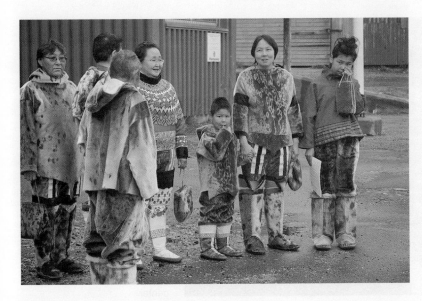

Figure 8-4. Three generations of an Inuit family (TeodorLazarev/Shutterstock.com).

The Older Adult: Caring for Individual Clients

At an individual level, older adults continue to meet developmental tasks similar to the ways of middle-aged adults as aging is a dynamic process and not a static event. Older adults work on developmental tasks that include satisfaction of basic needs, such as safety, security, and dignity, and the fulfillment of integrity and self-actualization. For the majority of older adults, meeting these needs is intertwined with the lifestyle and the residence of the older adult. The older adult also usually prefers to maintain self-esteem through exercising self-determination in planning where he or she will live. Older adults may confer with their family members in discussing what housing option provides a safe environment where risks for injury or falls are reduced and social and health supports are available for the older adult. Depending on whether older adults reside in a community setting or an institutional residence, the individual may find an outlet for individual or group activity, volunteer efforts, artistic activity, or socialization that are sources of self-esteem. For most older adult clients, participating in some meaningful activity contributes to the positive

fulfillment of the developmental tasks of aging (see Figure 8-5).

Across different cultural groups, aging is a developmental experience for individuals who are in a stage of reflecting on life experiences and finding meaning in their lives. Older adults may have many transitions that are chosen or are inevitable with growing older. These often include retirement, grandchildren, changed living arrangements, family mobility, declining health, and deaths of family members, including a spouse, siblings, or children.

Older adults may assume new roles, and nurses who work with older adults in community settings can reinforce changing roles as opportunities for positive growth. Nurses often view the strengths and residual abilities that older clients possess rather than dwelling on the losses, and in doing so, the nurse promotes optimal functioning for the older adult who may be experiencing unavoidable dependency.

Cultural factors, including the cultural group history, and life experiences, including immigration, will interact and determine the older client's efforts to achieve security, autonomy, and integrity. In achieving integrity, the older client has a need to bring closure to life and acceptance of eventual

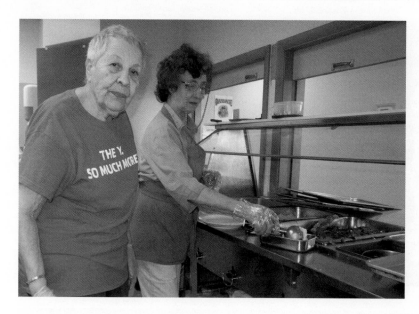

Figure 8-5. Older adults volunteering at a community center.

death. A nurse may assess this need in a client's family and be a sensitive listener when the client works through the steps of achieving integrity. Older clients need time for a purposeful life review. The older adult may relinquish some aspects of their typical responsibilities, such as paying bills, to an adult child, so they can be free to spend time on other activities or have more time to reflect.

Faith and Spirituality

Many older adults experience an increase in religion or spirituality, which is evident in showing increased humanistic concern for future generations, changing relationships with others, and spending time coming to terms with one's mortality. Older adults respond differently to these spiritual development tasks as influenced by their culture, life experiences, and individual qualities. Religion and spirituality may be a source of emotional support, a psychosocial resource, or a coping mechanism for older adults who experience challenging health conditions, losses in personal relationships and fulfilling roles, and stress.

Previous studies have found that older adults' immigration status and countries of origin influence different religious and spiritual participation

and devotion behavior. Some African American female elders have reported higher importance of religion and spirituality in their lives when compared to younger adults, and church-based social support was related to positive well-being and life satisfaction.

Decisions on a Continuum of Care

In the process of aging, many older adults will receive three types of care based on their evolving needs: (1) intensive personal health service, depending on the presence of acute and chronic conditions; (2) health maintenance and restorative care, depending on chronic conditions; and (3) coordinated nursing, social services, and ancillary services that may be provided on an episodic basis for older clients in the community. Many older adults will require care and assistance to manage chronic conditions; a public health goal is to encourage adults to adopt and follow health-promoting actions in their earlier years to minimize the occurrence of chronic conditions.

Older adults may experience loneliness linked with grieving the loss of loved ones, declining physical health or living alone. Older adults who live in their own apartments or who reside in retirement communities may develop loneliness associated with grieving personal losses, declining health or separation from social contacts such as friends or relatives. A study of older adults in age-restricted communities (typically at least 55 years of age) endorsed a wide range of activities such as shared meals with neighbors as well as events external to the community as a means to reduce social isolation, promote relationships, stimulate cognitive status, and help physical activity among residents to minimize their need for more intensive services (Gray & Worlledge, 2018).

Families have often developed culturally influenced patterns of caregiving and social support. The nurse may assess the following: Does the family modify the environment and assist in home care so that the older adult remains at home? Do children and grandchildren share tasks, provide meals, and run errands so the grandparents can live alone? Do family members have a plan to have relatives share responsibility to provide support and supervision for an older family member? Does the older family member have caregivers and alternates who can provide care as needed if the older adult wishes to remain at home?

Some differences have been noted in the patterns of living arrangements according to the families' ethnic and religious background. In a study of relocated refugees, Muslim elders in a northern European country expected their adult children to care for them as it was written in the Quran that if you raise your children well you will be well looked after when you are old (Nielsen et al., 2018). Even if adult children might wish to care for aged parents at home, their limited income, employment status, and crowded family living situation might limit that as an option. When family assistance and informal as well as formal sources of health care and social support are coordinated in a plan of care, some older adults may remain in a community setting longer before being cared for in long-term care facilities. The proximity of the older adult to younger family members who are willing and prepared to provide assistance with activities of daily living, transportation, nutrition, respite care, and social support may defer or delay nursing home

placement for older family members. Nurses must also assess that the values of independence and self-reliance may be very strong for some older clients, and they may refuse any assistance from family members, so the nurse should evaluate clients' behaviors relative to underlying values.

The interaction of factors including the availability, acceptability, and affordability of a skilled nursing facility that is in proximity to the ethnic populations also definitely impacts the overall residence patterns by members of cultural and ethnic groups. Older adults who do enter residential care facilities desire to maintain their dignity, and this can be evident in their personal care preferences including making choices on when to eat, what to eat, and whether to eat alone or with others (Ellins & Glasby, 2016). A nurse may ask questions on topics that were meaningful to the older client, for example, what was most important for them to maintain in their daily routines and what would they like to do so they could be as independent as possible. Older adults who for the majority, if not all, of their lifetime have spoken their native language and surrounded themselves with friends who also shared their customs might find it enormously difficult to enter a skilled nursing facility that would appear quite different in its practices. Nurses and other health care professionals are not always aware that certain behaviors, such as an insistence on schedules, order, and cleanliness, might not be valued equally by all older adults. Older adults may feel especially uncomfortable if they do not understand why they are awakened at a certain time, required to be dressed, and asked to participate in group socialization and may find the skilled nursing facility to be intrusive or unfriendly.

Some older adults, coping with terminal illnesses and debilitating and painful conditions, may choose to be cared for in hospice care in facilities or in their homes with professional, formal, and informal sources of care. Nurses preparing to care for and support hospice patients who experience chronic pain may refer to evidence-based practices in pain management as shown in Evidence-Based Practice 8-1.

Pain Management in Older Adults: Tailoring Nursing Interventions to Improve Patient Outcomes

A study of nearly 600 Medicare beneficiaries who experienced activity-limiting pain highlighted that racial and ethnic group differences existed among the study participants in their experience of pain self-efficacy and depressive symptoms (Murtaugh et al., 2017). The older adult patients were receiving part-time skilled nursing care in their homes through the Visiting Nurse Services of New York. The study participants were screened initially and then completed questionnaires on their pain presentation, pain-related disability, and the presence of psychosocial factors.

The study analysis found that the older Hispanics and non-Hispanic blacks reported a greater number of pain sites, worse pain intensity, and higher levels of pain disability than non-Hispanic whites. Since higher levels of pain intensity at the start of an older adult patient's therapy program are typically related to poorer outcomes, this could lead to ethnic minority older adults having a greater risk of decline than other patients.

The Hispanic older adults and non-Hispanic blacks also had higher levels of depressive symptoms and also had lower health literacy than the non-Hispanic whites. There was also a relationship of more modifiable psychosocial factors and higher pain intensity and pain-related disability among the Hispanic and non-Hispanic blacks than non-Hispanic whites. The high level of psychosocial risk factors among the racial and ethnic older adult patients demonstrates the importance of nurses to be aware of these disparities and potential effect on patient outcomes.

Clinical Implications

Nurses working in the community interact with patients and their caregivers to negotiate an acceptable pain management plan. This study affirms that nurses should assess for the signs of any depressive symptoms and to develop an acceptable and appropriate care plan tailored to the individual. Nurses should also assess for the patient's tolerance for pain, past and present experience with pain, effect of pain on quality of life, and the meaning attached to pain; these are all factors that can be influenced by the patient's cultural background and the patient's life experiences. The meaning that a patient may ascribe to pain will be affected by the patient's current perceptions and also past recollections of painful situations and treatments. The nurse who is striving to be culturally competent will assess the patient's culturally influenced model about the cause of the pain and the patient's expectations of treatments to relieve the pain. Spiritual support as well as behavioral therapies, which may include meditation, music, or imagery, were not described in this study but have been reported by groups of older patients to be effective. The nurse may assist in integrating the patient's preferences to use traditional and popular remedies including cold packs, herbal remedies, heat applications, or other therapies along with the prescribed medicines when the traditional or alternative sources would not harm the patient, give comfort to the patient, and do not interact with prescribed medications.

Clinical guidelines have been evolving that are based on evidence-based practices for care of the older adult client with acute and chronic conditions who reside in community and institutional settings. Several sources in print and visual media help guide the nurse in assessing the older client; see Table 8-3.

Community-Based Services for Older Adults

The developing array of home-based care organizations that offer personal care services by trained home health care aides as well as supportive services such as transportation are

Table 8-3	Clinical Guidelines for Caring for Older Adult Clients	
Reference for Practice	**Source**	**Evidence Base or Focus for Clinical Practice**
Nurses caring for older adults will find the concepts of geriatrics and cultural competence blended in Ethnogeriatrics that has been advanced by the Hartford Institute for Gerontological Nursing at New York University College of Nursing. The term Ethnogeriatrics and a curriculum on 11 ethnic groups was developed earlier through the Stanford Geriatric Education Center.	Resources include webinars, eLearning resources, mobile apps on geriatric concepts, and definitions of commonly used terms that can be accessed online at https://consultgeri.org/	The *Try This* series of evidence-based geriatric tools addresses a wide range of topics and refers to scales available on pain assessment, nutrition assessment, falls, functional decline, cognitive status, depression, confusion, activities of daily living, and caregiver strain.
The Stanford Geriatric Education Center (SGEC) set goals to increase knowledge of evidence-based practices for the elderly and has led conferences on research and developments in care of patients with dementia.	Resources include a list of Ethnogeriatric competencies for health care providers and a list of publications from partner organizations on communication and interactions with ethnically diverse older populations that can be accessed at: https://sgec.stanford.edu/competencies.html	The SGEC has provided topic-focused trainings, such as Assessment of Dementia in Diverse Groups, as well as trainings that were specific to the practices and beliefs of specific ethnic groups of older adults. Availability could be checked through the Web site: https://sgec.stanford.edu/competencies.html

presenting options for the growing population of older adults to live in their home communities. The levels and types of services that are available call for an expanded role for nurses and nursing consultants who work in ambulatory care settings to assess older clients to help determine the best care option. The terms screening, geriatric assessment, or health risk appraisal may be used for a systematic process when a nurse identifies the strengths and limitations in an older client's physical, mental, or social condition (Simpson & Pedigo, 2018). Nurses are prepared and accustomed to assess their patients' health care needs and to develop appropriate plans of care to improve patients' well-being. With older adult clients, a screening or appraisal is a comprehensive review of the client's abilities for self-care, independent mobility, continence, activities of daily living, medication management, as well as existing connections to a support system in neighbors, friends, or family members. The older client's receipt of services such as home-delivered meals, participation in any out-of-home group socialization, and plan for regular health care services should also be included.

Nurses can assess social and cultural factors that influence the care that older adults will need, the resources to meet those needs, and the locations for residence and care that are most acceptable to the client. Nurses must assess the physiologic status of the older adult and consider the safety of the client in a residential setting, including medication management. The nurse should assess for the older clients' understanding of medication directions, as the client's eyesight may be failing, and should clarify directions, which may be open to multiple interpretations. Nurses planning care for older adults may also interact with patient and family to help the patient to maintain their function and prevent injury. Studies have affirmed that early intervention that may reduce frail older adults' decline includes physical activity such as strength training and fall prevention, nutrition, cognitive training, social interaction, and cognitive stimulation (Shaw et al., 2018).

Nurses who work with individual clients and those who are assigned a caseload of groups of older adults in community settings, such as apartment complexes and assisted living centers, will assess the client's needs, available sources of support from the family, and formal sources of support to develop a total plan of care for each client. Community-based care typically includes a broad spectrum of services, often using formal and informal networks of caregivers, as well as resources such as home-delivered meals or older adult day care. Local programs through the Division of Aging, Aging Services, or a comparable agency may leverage available state or federal funds with innovative programs and local resources and donations to assist elderly clients so they can remain in the community.

Local or church-affiliated agencies that recruit and train volunteer visitors and caregivers to the elderly may be used in conjunction with the aging agency programs to enable the fragile older adult to function at home with formal sources of support. These organized sources of support that may include a weekly visitor or a person to do chores for the elderly client may supplement the care and support that family members may provide. For many older adults, the long-held value of independence is so strong that the person would rather live alone, even in poor health, than become a burden to his or her family. There are some older adults who feel stigmatized by residence in a congregate care facility and much prefer to live in an independent location such as an apartment in the community.

When other older adults choose to relocate to new smaller, safer residences late in their lives and gain security, these decisions can lead to increased unfamiliarity in new neighborhoods. These new residents must then decide to take the opportunity to interact with peers. For many older adults,

the option to participate in community activities, including cultural events or enrichment, or exploring nearby recreational sites becomes very fulfilling (see Figure 8-6). Other prospective residents might prefer the stimulation of intergenerational contact outside of an age-restricted residence and would prefer living on their own. Older adults deciding on any of these options are typically working through developmental tasks of discovering where they will feel satisfied and fulfilled and find meaning in their lives.

One challenge that the majority of older individuals will face is the high cost of paying for levels of care in residential communities or in skilled nursing facilities. As mentioned earlier, many older clients and their families assume that

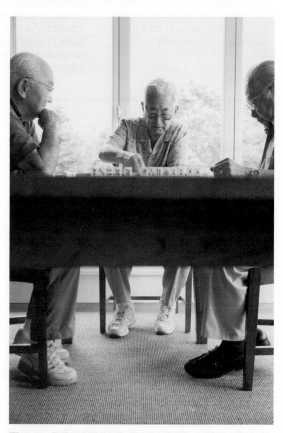

Figure 8-6. Retirees enjoy an activity in their residential community. (Blend Images/Shutterstock.com).

Medicare will be the means for paying for such care. However, Medicare has limitations for hospital care and posthospital rehabilitation and does not cover what is termed custodial care of the older client. Older individuals and their families may exhaust their personal resources to cover extended care needs.

There has been an increase in the development of day programs in communities that provide nursing assessment, physical or occupational therapy, group socialization, and nutrition to older adults. These programs may supplement the affective support and tangible assistance that families give, and the programs provide settings that affirm the older clients' dignity. The range of these services provided at each site varies according to the support of the local community, including volunteers and professional staff. Some sites provide group socialization and nutrition for a lunchtime meal. The older adults are usually ambulatory or able to be independent with assistive devices, so they may be transported to the sites by public or private transportation. Some adult day centers offer programs and services for older adults who may be caregivers for their grandchildren. The grandparent may bring the grandchild for well-child examinations and also access a health care provider for care, so two generations access health care at the same site.

The options are expanding for older clients to participate in community-based services such as adult day care, which may follow a social model, a health support model, or a combined service delivery approach. The number of adult day programs has more than doubled in the last two decades, but the increase is not keeping pace, nor are services being funded at an adequate level to meet the needs of ethnically diverse older adults trying to remain in their familiar settings as they grow older. Nurses working in health care facilities or in community settings may want to assess the availability of local health and social enrichment programs and encourage the older adult client to attend a program. Many mutual assistance associations or cultural affiliations may provide

programs for older adults to interact with young people and to share cultural traditions. These cultural center programs and similar church-affiliated programs provide a means for older clients to receive affirmational peer support and to reinforce their cultural identity in a way that restores self-esteem and dignity.

Other intergenerational programs support older adults becoming involved within the community and the educational system. These types of programs include the Older American Volunteer Program, the Retired and Senior Volunteer Program, and the Foster Grandparents Program. There are also intergenerational child care centers that are demonstrating that older volunteers are resources in the community, and the children and older adults benefit. Evaluations of multigenerational programs found that the older volunteers had a high level of life satisfaction, including psychosocial adjustment, positive social exchanges, and self-esteem.

Summary

A cultural approach to the older adult client recognizes that individuals are the products of, as well as the participants in, an encompassing societal framework. Within the societal framework, the cultural backgrounds of the older clients will influence their variations in their perceptions, behavior, and practices. Culture serves as a guide to the older client to determine what health-related choices and actions are appropriate and acceptable. Within cultural groups, individual variation is evident in responses to the physiologic signs and the psychosocial demands of increasing age. Examples of older immigrant clients demonstrate that the clients' views and perceptions may differ from those of family members and from the views of the nurse. The different attitudes, practices, and behaviors among older clients result from their heritage, experiences, education, acculturation, and socioeconomic status.

Nurses who are providing care in acute care settings or in the community often ask several questions as part of the nursing assessment:

1. Is the older adult isolated from culturally relevant supportive people, or is the older client enmeshed in a caring network of relatives and friends?
2. Has a culturally appropriate network replaced family members in performing some tasks for the older adult client?
3. Does the older adult expect family members to provide care, including nurturance and emotional support, which family members are unable to provide?
4. Does language create a barrier in the older client's receipt of services from formal resources?

Older adult clients have often developed their own informal support systems such as help from neighbors for coping with illness and with changes associated with age. Formal resources may be used to sustain the informal support systems to promote the lifestyle preferred by the older client. Nurses caring for older adult clients should give attention to the client's family and social roles and develop care plans that maintain and restore the individual to his or her usual roles and patterns of activity. In the future, nurses will assess and work with more older clients as they progress along a continuum of services and through more than one type of residence in the community.

Clients may be reluctant to use services for various reasons that include cultural and linguistic differences or prior negative experiences in health care settings. To overcome any of the barriers that are perceived by older clients, nurses may well serve as advocates and teach clients to be self-advocates for services for which they are eligible. Nurses may also assume a care coordinator role to link interdisciplinary services such as physical and occupational therapy, nutrition services, or social support services to safely sustain frail elderly in community settings (Shaw et al., 2018). Nurses can assume several approaches to interact effectively with older adults from diverse groups:

- Be sensitive to the life experiences and previous health care experiences of the older clients.
- Listen attentively to the older client's complaints, recollections, and strengths.
- Listen to related conversations to assess for underlying depression.
- Elicit information about the older client's preferences for care, including diet and use of self-care remedies, and include them when appropriate.
- Identify available sources of informal support and confirm availability.

REVIEW QUESTIONS

1. What resources, needs, and limitations should the nurse assess to develop a care plan for a recently discharged 82-year-old chronically ill man who is returning to a single-room occupancy hotel in a crowded inner city location?
2. As the nurse who does health assessments for frail older adults who attend a community comprehensive day program, what information should the nurse assess to identify culturally appropriate care plans or service delivery plans for older Filipino and Chinese American clients?
3. The short-term subacute unit where you are the nurse manager serves a multinational group of older clients who are admitted for orthopedic surgery. What cultural assessments do you teach the staff to use in identifying the needs of clients and their families?

CRITICAL THINKING ACTIVITIES

1. Many local communities offer adult day care for older adults with chronic health care problems who are residing alone or with family members. Services usually include health

screening by a nurse as well as occupational health and/or physical activity sessions for these community-based older adults. Request permission to attend an activity as an observer and attentive listener. Through observation and, if possible, conversation with a participant, try to assess the levels of self-care that session participants possess and identify the types of assistance that these clients require to remain in the community.

2. If you are a case manager for a managed care organization, you receive many authorization requests for in-home nursing services to assist older adults who have been discharged home following hospitalization for acute illnesses or surgery. List the factors that you will consider and the types of data that you need to make an informed decision about the nursing and health-related services and the duration of services that the older client should receive while at home.

3. In many communities, nurses provide hospice services to residents in long-term care facilities or to older adults living in other settings. Contact a community-based hospice nurse to request information about how the services meet older adults' needs for love and belongingness, as well as reflection and recollection that are expressed late in life.

4. With your awareness that cultural traditions and life experiences influence many older adults to prefer independent living, prepare a letter as a home health nurse to the appropriate official to request government-funded home health services for older adults.

REFERENCES

Alzheimer's Association. (2018). 2018 Alzheimer's disease facts and figures. *Alzheimer's & Dementia, 14*(3), 367–429.

Avidor, S., Benyamini, Y., & Solomon, Z. (2016). Subjective age and health in later life: The role of posttraumatic symptoms. *Journal of Gerontology B: Psychological Sciences and Social Sciences, 71*, 415–424. doi: 10.1093/geronb/gbu150

Bonds, K., & Lyons, K. S. (2018). Formal service use by African American individuals with dementia and their caregivers: An integrative review. *Journal of Gerontological Nursing, 44*, (6), 33–39.

Cayo, S. N. (2018). Care of older adults of color: Bridging the gap and building relationships. *Geriatric Nursing, 39*, 362.

Centers for Disease Control and Prevention. (2016). Racial and Ethnic Approaches to Community Health (REACH). Retrieved April 20, 2018 from https://www.cdc.gov/chronicdisease/resources/publications/aag/reach.htm

Centers for Disease Control and Prevention. (2017). Prevalence of single and multiple leading causes of death by race/ethnicity among people aged 60 to 70 years. Retrieved April 21, 2018 from https://www.cdc.gov/pcd/issues/2017/16_0241.htm

Cramm, J. M., Van Dijk, H. M., & Nieboer, A. P. (2018). The creation of age-friendly environments is especially important to frail older people. *Aging & Society, 38*(4), 700–720.

Crist, J. D., Montgomery, M. L., Pasvogel, A., Phillips, L. R., Ortiz-Dowling, E. M. (2018). The association among knowledge of and confidence in home health care services, acculturation, and family caregivers' relationships to older adults of Mexican descent. *Geriatric Nursing, 39*(6), 689–695. Retrieved from www.gnjournal.com

Ellins, J. & Glasby, J. (2016). "You don't know what you are saying 'Yes' and what you are saying 'No' to:" hospital experiences of older people from minority ethnic communities. *Aging & Society, 36*(1), 42–63.

Epps, F., Weeks, G., Graham, E., &Luster, D. (2018). Challenges to aging in place for African American older adults living with dementia and their families. *Geriatric Nursing, 39*(6), 646–652. Retrieved from www.gnjournal.com

Erickson, E. H., & Erickson, J. M. (1997). *The life cycle completed.* New York, NY: W.W. Norton & Company.

Gray, A. & Worlledge, G. (2018). Addressing loneliness and isolation in retirement housing. *Aging & Society, 38*(3), 615–644.

Murtaugh, C. M., Beissner, K. L., Barron, Y., Trachtenberg, M. A., Bach, E., Henderson, C. R., ... Reid, M. C. (2017). Pain and function in home care a need for treatment tailoring to reduce disparities. *Clinical Journal of Pain, 33*(4), 300–309.

Nielsen, D. S., Minet, L., Zeraig, L., Rasmussen, D. N., Sodermann, M. (2018). Caught in a generation gap: A generation perspective on refugees getting old in Denmark—A qualitative study. *Journal of Transcultural Nursing, 29*(3), 265–273. doi: 101177/1043659617718064

Pan, Y. P., Jones, P. S., & Winslow, B. W. (2017). The relationship between mutuality filial piety, and depression in family caregivers in China. *Journal of Transcultural Nursing, 28*(3), 455–463.

Phillips, L. R., Salem, B. E., Jeffers, K. S., Kim, H., Ruiz, M. E., Salem, N., & Woods, D. L. (2015). Developing and proposing the ethnocultural gerontological nursing model. *The Journal of Transcultural Nursing, 26*(2), 118–128.

Pulkki, J., & Tynkkynen, L. (2016). All elderly people have important service needs: a study of discourse on older people in parliamentary discussions in Finland. *Aging & Society, 36*(1), 64–78.

Rozanova, J., Miller, E. A., & Wetle, T. (2016). Depictions of nursing home residents in US newspapers: Successful aging versus frailty. *Aging & Society, 36*(1), 17–41.

Schafer, M. H. (2016). Health as status? Network relations and social structure in an American Retirement Community. *Aging & Society, 36*(1), 79–105.

Shaw, R. L., Gwyther, H., Holland, C., Bujnowska, M., Kurpas, D., Cano, A., ..., D'Avanzo, B. (2018). Understanding frailty: meanings and beliefs about screening and prevention across key stakeholder groups in Europe. *Aging & Society, 38*(5), 1223–1252.

Simpson, P., Almack, K., & Walthery, P. (2018). "We treat them all the same": The attitudes, knowledge and practices of staff concerning old/er lesbian, gay, bisexual and trans residents in care homes. *Aging & Society, 38*(5), 869–899.

Simpson, V., & Pedigo, L. (2018). Health risk appraisals with aging adults: An integrative review. *Western Journal of Nursing, 40*(7), 1049–1068.

U.S. Census Bureau. (2018). Older people projected to outnumber children for first time in U.S. history. March 13, 2018 Release Number: CB18-41. Retrieved from https://www.census.gov/newsroom/press-releases/2018/cb18-41-population-projections.html

U.S. Department of Social and Health Services. (2017). *2017 Profile of Older Americans.* Retrieved from https://acl.gov/sites/default/files/Aging%20and%20Disability%20in%20America/2017OlderAmericansProfile.pdf

Villalobos, B. T. & Bridges, A. J. (2016). Testing and attribution model of caregiving in a Latino samples: The roles of familismo and the caregiver-care recipient relationship. *Journal of Transcultural Nursing, 27*(4), 322–332.

Wilks, S. E., Spurlock, W. R., Brown, S. C., Teegen, B. C., & Geiger, J. R. (2018). Examining spiritual support among African American and Caucasian Alzheimer's caregivers: A risk and resilience study. *Geriatric Nursing, 39*(6), 663–668. Accessed online May 25, 2018 www.gnjournal.com

Wong, K. A., & Kataoka-Yahiro, M. R. (2017). Nutrition and diet as it relates to health and well-being of native Hawaiian Kupuna (elders): A systematic literature review. *Journal of Transcultural Nursing, 28*(4), 408–422.

Health Care Settings

PART

THREE

Health Care Settings

Chapter 9

Creating Culturally Competent Health Care Organizations

- Patti A. Ludwig-Beymer

Key Terms

Community-based participatory research
Cultural assessment tools
Culturally congruent services

Culturally responsive services
Culture of safety
Institutional racism
Limited English proficiency (LEP)

Magnet designation
Participatory action research
Transcultural nursing administration

Learning Objectives

1. Assess the need for culturally competent health care organizations.
2. Discuss how to achieve health equity, eliminate disparities, and improve the health of all groups.
3. Evaluate organizational cultures.
4. Describe how organizations can develop cultural competency.
5. Analyze culturally competent initiatives designed and implemented by health care organizations.

An individual's culture affects access to health care and health-seeking behaviors, as well as perceived quality of care. In addition to understanding the culture of clients, however, it is also essential to examine the culture of health care organizations. The interplay of client, provider, and organizational cultures may create barriers, lead to a client's lack of trust or reluctance to access services, cause cultural conflicts, and ultimately result in health care inequities. Conversely, organizational

culture may facilitate access that decreases health disparities.

This chapter serves to augment the current dialogue on creating culturally competent organizations. It defines a culturally competent organization, explains the need for culturally competent organizations, describes mechanisms for assessing organizational culture, and provides strategies for developing culturally competent organizations.

Defining a Culturally Competent Health Care Organization

Cultural competence refers to the ability of health care providers and organizations to understand and respond effectively to the cultural and linguistic needs of clients. Culturally and linguistically appropriate services are respectful of and responsive to the health beliefs, practices, and needs of diverse patients (Office of Minority Health, 2017). Cultural competence encompasses a variety of diversities, including age, culture, ethnicity, gender, language, race, religion, sexual preference, gender identity, and socioeconomic status. Culturally competent organizations provide services that are respectful of and responsive to the cultural and linguistic needs of the clients they serve.

The Need for Culturally Competent Health Care Organizations: External Motivation

Nursing has been at the forefront of cultural competence for individuals and organizations. The Transcultural Nursing Society was established in 1975; its mission is to enhance the quality of culturally congruent, competent, and equitable care that results in improved health and well-being for people worldwide (Transcultural Nursing Society, 2018). An expert panel identified 10 standards of practice for culturally competent nursing care. Salient to this chapter is Standard 6, Cultural Competence in Health Care Systems and Organizations. The standard holds that "Healthcare organizations should provide structures and resources necessary to evaluate and meet the cultural and language needs of their diverse clients" (Douglas et al., 2014, p. 113).

The American Nurses Association has also been proactive in addressing discrimination and racism in health care and promoting justice in access and delivery of health care to all people. ANA (2016) revised a position statement on ethics and human right to provide nurses with specific actions to protect and promote human rights in every practice setting. Box 9-1 contains a partial listing of their recommendations. In addition, they expanded the Nursing Social Policy Statement by creating Diversity Awareness materials that address nursing organizations; health insurance and health care access; the lesbian, gay, bisexual, and transgender (LGBT) communities; mental health; bariatric/obesity; racial and ethnic minority communities; the elderly, self-assessment; and culturally specific tools (ANA, 2018). Many other nursing organizations including the American Association of Colleges of Nursing (2018), Sigma Theta Tau (Wilson, Sanner, & McAllister, 2003), and the American Organization of Nurse Executives (2011) emphasize the need for culturally competent health care.

Regulatory agencies address the need for culturally competent organizations. The Centers for Medicare and Medicaid Services (2012) issued guidance to help health care providers become more effective and culturally aware of how they provide care to diverse populations. The Joint Commission (2018) provides resources on effective communication, cultural competence, patient- and family-centered care, and innovative ways to eliminate health disparities. They include standards to ensure that clients receive care that respects their cultural, psychosocial, and spiritual values, outlined in Box 9-2 (Joint Commission Resources, 2018).

The Institute of Medicine (IOM) report "Health Professions Education: A Bridge to Quality" (Greiner & Knebel, 2003) identified five core competencies for all health professionals: provide patient-centered care, work in interdisciplinary teams, employ evidence-based practice, apply quality improvement, and utilize informatics. Providing patient-centered care includes sharing power and responsibility with clients and caregivers; communicating with clients in a shared and fully open manner; taking into account clients'

BOX 9-1	American Nurses Association Recommendations Related to Cultural Competence

- Nurses promote the human rights of patients, colleagues, and communities.
- Health care agencies assess for human rights violations related to patients, nurses, health care workers, and others within their organizations.
- Nurses serve on ethics committees, discuss ethics and human rights with colleagues, and participate in policy development to increase care access and equality.
- Nurses collaborate to promote, protect, and sustain ethical practice and the human rights of all patients and providers.
- Nurse educators use the principles of justice and caring to teach students about ethics and human rights in health care delivery.
- Nurse educators help students identify nursing professional responsibilities to address unjust systems and structures. Educators demonstrate the profession's commitment to health and

social justice through class content, critical thinking exercises, and clinical experiences.
- Nurse researchers conduct research that is relevant to communities of interest. They invite communities to identify research problems and work to benefit patients, society, and professional nursing practice.
- Nurse executives implement ethics and human rights principles by monitoring the practice environment for actual or potential human rights violations of patients, nurses, and other health care providers.
- Nurse executives analyze policies and practices and identify risks for reduced safety and quality that may result from unacknowledged violations of human rights.
- Nurse executives promote a caring, just, inclusive, and collaborative environment in their organizations and communities.

Source: American Nurses Association. (2016). The nurse's role in ethics and human rights: Protecting and promoting individual worth, dignity, and human rights in practice settings. Retrieved May 15, 2018 from https://www.nursingworld.org/globalassets/docs/ana/nursesrole-ethicshumanrights-positionstatement.pdf

individuality, emotional needs, values, and life issues; implementing strategies for reaching those who do not present for care on their own, including care strategies that support the broader community; and enhancing prevention and health promotion. To accomplish the goal of meeting clients' individuality, emotional needs, values, and life issues, the IOM report further indicates that clinicians must provide care in the context of the culture, heath status, and health needs of the client.

Using the IOM competencies as a base, Quality and Safety Education for Nurses (QSEN, 2018) identified six core competencies for nurses: patient-centered care; teamwork and collaboration; evidence-based practice; quality improvement; safety; and informatics. These competencies require a knowledge of many dimensions, including

and understanding of diverse cultural, ethnic, and social backgrounds and patient, family, and community values.

The U.S. government has also addressed culturally appropriate health care systems. The National Standards for Culturally and Linguistically Appropriate Services in Health Care (CLAS Standards), outlined in Box 9-3, were developed by the U.S. Department of Health and Human Services' Office of Minority Health (2016a) to advance health equity, improve quality, and help eliminate health care disparities. All people entering the health care system should receive equitable and effective care in a culturally and linguistically appropriate manner. The CLAS standards are inclusive of all cultures and are especially designed to address the needs of racial,

BOX 9-2	2018 Joint Commission Standards That Address Cultural Competence

Leaders

- Create and maintain a culture of safety and quality throughout the hospital.
- Provide services that meet patient needs.
- Ensure that patients with comparable needs receive the same standard of care throughout the hospital.

Human Resources

- Confirm staff competency to perform their responsibilities.

Rights and Responsibilities of the Individual

- Respect, protect, and promote patient rights.
- Honor the patient's right to receive information in a manner he or she understands.
- Uphold the patient's right to participate in decisions about his or her care.
- Respect the patient's right to give or withhold informed consent.

- Protect the patient's rights during research, investigation, and clinical trials.
- Incorporate patient decisions about care received at the end of life.

Provision of Care

- Accept the patient for care and treatment based on its ability to meet the patient's needs.
- Plan and provide the patient's care.
- Effectively communicate with patients.
- Coordinate the patient's care based on the patient's needs.
- Prioritize the patient's comfort and dignity received during end-of-life care.
- Provide patient education and training based on each patient's needs and abilities.
- Address the patient's need for continuing care, treatment, and services after discharge or transfer.
- Inform and educate the patient about follow-up care, treatment, and services.

Source: Joint Commission Resources. (2018). The Joint Commission Edition. Retrieved May 21, 2018 from https://e-dition. jcrinc.com/MainContent.aspx

ethnic, and linguistic populations that experience unequal access to health services. Ultimately, the aim of the standards is to contribute to the elimination of racial and ethnic health disparities and to improve the health of all Americans.

The Need for Culturally Competent Organizations: Eliminating Health Disparities

Disparities in health have long been acknowledged; these racial and ethnic disparities document the reality of unequal health care treatment. Healthy People 2020 defines a health disparity as "a particular type of health difference that is closely linked with social, economic, and/or

environmental disadvantage. Health disparities adversely affect groups of people who have systematically experienced greater obstacles to health based on their racial or ethnic group; religion; socioeconomic status; gender; age; mental health; cognitive, sensory, or physical disability; sexual orientation or gender identity; geographic location; or other characteristics historically linked to discrimination or exclusion." At the most basic level, disparities are evident in life expectancies. For example, the Centers for Disease Control and Prevention (2017) reported that the overall US life expectancy at birth in 2015 was 78.8 years, a decrease from the previous year. However, life expectancy varies by race and ethnicity. Hispanic/Latino females had the highest life expectancy (84.3 years) followed by White females (81.1 years), Hispanic/Latino males

| BOX 9-3 | National Standards for Culturally and Linguistically Appropriate Services (CLAS) in Health Care |

Principal Standard

1. Provide effective, equitable, understandable, and respectful quality care and services that are responsive to diverse cultural health beliefs and practices, preferred languages, health literacy, and other communication needs.

Governance, Leadership, and Workforce

2. Advance and sustain organizational governance and leadership that promotes CLAS and health equity through policy, practices, and allocated resources.
3. Recruit, promote, and support a culturally and linguistically diverse governance, leadership, and workforce that are responsive to the population in the service area.
4. Educate and train governance, leadership, and workforce in culturally and linguistically appropriate policies and practices on an ongoing basis.

Communication and Language Assistance

5. Offer language assistance to individuals who have limited English proficiency and/or other communication needs, at no cost to them, to facilitate timely access to all health care and services.
6. Inform all individuals of the availability of language assistance services clearly and in their preferred language, verbally and in writing.
7. Ensure the competence of individuals providing language assistance, recognizing that the use of untrained individuals and/or minors as interpreters should be avoided.

8. Provide easy-to-understand print and multimedia materials and signage in the languages commonly used by the populations in the service area.

Engagement, Continuous Improvement, and Accountability

9. Establish culturally and linguistically appropriate goals, policies, and management accountability, and infuse them throughout the organization's planning and operations.
10. Conduct ongoing assessments of the organization's CLAS-related activities and integrate CLAS-related measures into assessment measurement and continuous quality improvement activities.
11. Collect and maintain accurate and reliable demographic data to monitor and evaluate the impact of CLAS on health equity and outcomes and to inform service delivery.
12. Conduct regular assessments of community health assets and needs, and use the results to plan and implement services that respond to the cultural and linguistic diversity of populations in the service area.
13. Partner with the community to design, implement, and evaluate policies, practices, and services to ensure cultural and linguistic appropriateness.
14. Create conflict- and grievance-resolution processes that are culturally and linguistically appropriate to identify, prevent, and resolve conflicts or complaints.
15. Communicate the organization's progress in implementing and sustaining CLAS to all stakeholders, constituents, and the general public.

Source: Office of Minority Health, Department of Health and Human Services. (2016). The National CLAS standards. Retrieved May 15, 2018 from https://minorityhealth.hhs.gov/omh/browse.aspx?lvl=2&lvlid=53

(79.3 years), Black females (78.1 years), White males (76.3 years), and Black males (71.8 years). In Canada, the 2017 overall life expectancy was reported as 79 years for males and 83 years for females but was only 64 years for male Inuit and 73 years for female Inuit (Statistics Canada, 2018).

Annually, the Agency for Healthcare Research and Quality (AHRQ) tracks disparities in health care delivery as it relates to racial and socioeconomic factors. These themes emerged from the 2016 National Healthcare Disparities Report (AHRQ, 2018a):

1. Although the rate of uninsured individuals decreased, 65% of the access measures did not demonstrate significant improvement.
2. Quality of health care improved overall, but the pace of improvement varied by priority area:
   a. Person-centered care: About 80% of person-centered care measures improved overall.
   b. Patient safety: Almost two-thirds of patient safety measures improved overall.
   c. Healthy living: About 60% of healthy living measures improved overall.
   d. Effective treatment: More than half of effective treatment measures improved overall.
   e. Care coordination: About half of care coordination measures improved overall.
   f. Care affordability: Only 30% of care affordability measures improved overall.
3. Disparities persist, especially for poor and uninsured populations in all priority areas:
   a. Most disparities have not changed significantly for any racial and ethnic groups.
   b. More than half of measures show that poor and low-income households have worse care than do high-income households; for middle-income households,

more than 40% of measures show worse care than high-income households.
   c. Nearly two-thirds of measures show that uninsured people had worse care than did privately insured people.

Access (getting into the health care system) and quality care (receiving appropriate, safe, and effective health care in a timely manner) are key factors in achieving good health outcomes. While many believe that access to high-quality care is a fundamental human right, the poor and racial and ethnic minorities often face more barriers to care and receive poorer quality of care when they access care.

The U.S. Department of Health and Human Services (HHS) uses a variety of measures to evaluate access to health care. Based on the 2016 National Healthcare Disparities Report (AHRQ, 2016), when compared to Whites, Blacks experienced worse access for 50% of measures and the same access for 50% of measures. When comparing Hispanics and non-Hispanic Whites, Hispanics experienced better access to care for 10% of the measures and worse access for 75% of the measures. When comparing the poor (those below the poverty level) to those with high incomes, the poor experienced worse access for 95% of the measures and the same access for 5% of the measures.

HHS also uses a variety of measures to evaluate the quality of health care. Compared to Whites, Blacks experienced better quality of care for 13% of the measures and worse quality of care for 40% of the measures. Compared to non-Hispanic Whites, Hispanics experienced better quality of care for 23% of measures and worse quality of care for 36% of measures. Compared to high-income households, those considered poor experienced the same quality of care for 45% of measures and worse quality of care for 55% of measures. Select disparities that are worsening over time are summarized in Box 9-4 (AHRQ, 2018b).

Canada's experience with universal access to care suggests that access may help to reduce health disparities between groups but does not eliminate them (Alter, Stukel, Chong, & Henry, 2011). Their longitudinal study followed nearly 15,000 people for over a decade and found that clients with lower incomes used more health care resources than did those with a higher socioeconomic status. Regardless, individuals with lower incomes had poorer health, including depression, hypertension, diabetes, cancer, and cataracts, and were more likely to die during the follow-up. These findings imply that factors in addition to access account for some health disparities. Potential barriers that contribute to the disparities may be related to demographics, culture, and the health care system itself. Potential barriers are summarized in Box 9-5.

While identifying disparities in care is important, it is not sufficient. To reduce health disparities, individuals must deliver culturally competent health care that focuses on risk reduction, vulnerability reduction, and promotion and protection of human rights (Flaskerud, 2007) within culturally competent health care settings. A culturally competent organization is extremely complex. Organizational culture may influence provider cultural competence, organizational cultural

| BOX 9-4 | Health Care Disparities That Have Worsened in the United States, 2000–2014 |

Group	Measures
Black compared to White	• Emergency department visits for asthma • Avoidable hospital admissions for hypertension
American Indian/Alaskan Native compared to White	• Disparities improving or unchanged
Asian compared to White	• Obstetric trauma per 1,000 instrument-assisted deliveries • Incidence of end-stage renal disease due to diabetes per million population
Hispanic compared to non-Hispanic White	• Disparities improving or unchanged
Poor compared to high-income*	• Emergency department visits with principal diagnosis of mental health only • Emergency department visits with principal diagnosis of substance abuse • Potentially avoidable emergency department visits for asthma

*Poor is defined as people whose individual or family income falls at or below 100% of the Federal Poverty Level (FPL), established annually by the U.S. Bureau of the Census based on family size and composition. Poverty rates vary by race and ethnicity, with 12.7% of individuals below the poverty level in 2016. Individual rates vary as follows: 22.0% of Black, 19.4% of Hispanic, 10.1% of Asian and Pacific Islander, and 8.8% of non-Hispanic White individuals are classified as poor in 2016.

Sources: Agency for Healthcare Research and Quality. (2018). 2016 National Healthcare Disparities Report. Retrieved May 15, 2018 from https://www.ahrq.gov/research/findings/nhqrdr/nhqdr16/index.html
U.S. Census. (2017). Income and poverty in the United States: 2016. Retrieved May 15, 2018 from https://www.census.gov/library/publications/2017/demo/p60-259.html

BOX 9-5 | Potential Demographic, Cultural, and Health System Barriers

Demographic Barriers

Age
Gender
Ethnicity
Primary language
Religion
Educational level and literacy level
Occupation, income, and health insurance
Area of residence
Transportation
Time and/or generation in the United States

Cultural Barriers

Age
Gender, class, and family dynamics
Worldview/perceptions of life
Time orientation
Primary language spoken
Religious beliefs and practices
Social customs, values, and norms
Traditional health beliefs and practices

Dietary preferences and practices
Communication patterns and customs

Health System Barriers

Differential access to high-quality care
Insurance and other financial resources
Orientation to preventive health services
Perception of need for health care services
Lack of knowledge and/or distrust of Western medical practices and procedures
Cultural insensitivity and incompetence in providers, including bias, stereotyping, and prejudice
Lack of diversity in providers
Western versus folk health beliefs and practices
Poor provider–client communication
Lack of bilingual and bicultural staff
Unfriendly and cold environment
Complex, fragmented, and uncoordinated health care organizations
Physical barriers (such as excessive distances)
Information barriers

competence, and health disparities. Within the health care setting, practitioners must be aware of the effects of organizational culture on individual behaviors.

Assessing Organizational Culture

Organizational culture has emerged as an important variable for behavior, performance, and outcome in the workplace. Organizations are complex, with multiple and competing subcultures. The subcultural systems have inherent values and beliefs, folklore, and language; these systems are organized in a hierarchy of authority, responsibilities, obligations, and functional tasks that are understood by members of the organization. Leininger (1996) defined organizational culture as the goals,

norms, values, and practices of an organization in which people have goals and try to achieve them in beneficial ways.

Organizational culture has been studied as it relates to accountability, change, emotional intelligence, effectiveness, implementation of best practices and research, leadership and management, Magnet recognition status, mentoring, and patient safety. Organizational culture affects not only people working in the institution, such as employees, physicians, and volunteers, but also those who access the institution's services, such as clients, families, and community members. The social organization of hospitals and other health care facilities has a profound effect on clients, both directly through the care provided and indirectly through organizational policies and philosophy.

Theories of Organizational Culture

A variety of definitions, methods of measurement, and theories for organizational culture exist. There is reasonable consensus on the following (Strasser, Smits, Falconer, Herrin, & Bowen, 2002):

- An organization's culture consists of shared beliefs, assumptions, perceptions, and norms leading to specific patterns of behaviors.
- An organization's culture results from an interaction among many variables, including mission, strategy, structure, leadership, and human resource (HR) practices.
- Culture is self-reinforcing; once in place, it provides stability, and changes are resisted by organizational members.

Bolman and Deal's Organizational Culture Perspective

Bolman and Deal (2017) describe four organizational culture perspectives or "frames" that affect the way in which an organization resolves conflicts: HR, political, structural, and symbolic. The HR frame strives to facilitate the fit between person and organization. When conflict arises, the solution considers the needs of the individual or group as well as the needs of the organization. The political frame emphasizes power and politics. Problems are viewed as "turf" issues and are resolved by developing networks to increase the power base. The structural frame focuses on following an organization's rules or protocols. This culture relies on its policies and procedures to resolve conflict. The symbolic frame relies on rituals, ceremony, and myths in determining appropriate behaviors.

To understand how these four perspectives will result in different outcomes, consider typical responses to the following situation. Hospital A is located on the border of two communities. One community is primarily African American. The other community is primarily Hispanic.

The hospital has traditionally provided care to African Americans and is well regarded by that community. The hospital has noted, however, that few members of the Hispanic community use its services. The hospital's board of directors realizes that, to survive, the hospital must expand its client base. The approach to this challenge will vary based on the organization's culture.

Hospital leaders with a HR perspective are likely to approach the situation by assessing the needs of both communities and the staff. For example, the hospital may convene focus groups with members of the Hispanic community to identify why the hospital's services are not used by that community. At the same time, the hospital will assess the African American community's perspective on the hospital's plan to expand its services and become a more inclusive organization. The hospital will also encourage staff members to provide input and to express their feelings about the goals of the organization. In the end, the hospital with a HR perspective will reach a decision that balances the needs of all the groups while enhancing the goal of expanding the client base.

Hospital leaders in a political culture will take a different approach. They will identify key "power" leaders in the Hispanic community. Perhaps they will invite a Hispanic leader to join their board of directors or serve in another advisory capacity; or they may ask a priest from a Hispanic congregation to serve as a hospital chaplain. In addition, they will actively recruit Hispanic physicians and other clinicians. They will build a Hispanic power base within the hospital and use it to reach out to the larger Hispanic community and expand the client base.

Hospital leaders in a structural culture will develop policies and procedures to attract more Hispanic clients. For example, they may make certain that all signage appears in both English and Spanish or develop a policy that requires all client educational materials to be available in both Spanish and English. They may require all staff to attend a session on Hispanic culture and may strongly encourage or mandate Spanish-language training for key personnel.

Hospital leaders in a symbolic culture will use ceremony to meet their goal. They will make physical changes to the environment to attract more Hispanics. For example, they may create or alter a chapel, inviting a priest from a Hispanic congregation to say mass. They may display other religious symbols, such as a crucifix or a statue of Our Lady of Guadalupe. They may alter their artwork to be more culturally inclusive. They may also include Hispanic stories and rituals in their internal communications. These leaders will draw on symbols and rituals that will help make persons of Hispanic cultures comfortable in the hospital environment and that will attract a larger Hispanic client base.

None of these organizational cultures are inherently good or bad, just different. Each perspective presents both strengths and weaknesses, and more than one culture may exist in an organization. For example, an organization may be guided primarily by both HR and symbolic perspectives.

Schein's Organizational Culture

Schein (2016) describes organizational culture at three levels: (1) observable artifacts, (2) values, and (3) basic underlying assumptions. Artifacts are visible manifestations of values. Artifacts may include signage, statues and other decorations, pictures, décor, dress code, traffic flow, medical equipment, and visible interactions. Values are explicitly stated norms and social principles and are manifestations of assumptions. Underlying assumptions are shared beliefs and expectations that influence perceptions, thoughts, and feelings about the organization; they are the core of the organization's culture. Assumptions define the culture of the organization, but because they are invisible, they may not be recognized. At times, the assumptions of an institution are

ambiguous and self-contradictory, especially when an institutional merger or acquisition has occurred.

A Framework for Describing Health Care Delivery Organizations

Pina et al. (2015) have developed a framework for describing health care delivery organizations. The framework includes six domains: capacity; organizational structure; finances; patients; care processes and infrastructure; and culture. The way in which they derived the domains and the contents of each domain are summarized in Evidence-Based Practice 9-1.

Organizational Culture, Employees, and the Community

Many organizations are aware of the impact of organizational culture on its employees. When filling positions, recruiters consider the "fit" between the organization and the potential employee, because a good "fit" results in better retention and satisfied employees. Nurses and other health care professionals also learn how to determine whether an organization will match their personal values. For example, a nurse who wants to provide care in a culturally competent manner to lesbian, gay, bisexual, and transgender (LGBT) individuals will not be happy in a critical care unit that restricts visitors to nuclear family members.

Humans need care to survive, thrive, and grow. According to Leininger (1996), organizations need to incorporate universal care constructs, including respect and genuine concern for clients and staff. These caring organizations are needed for nurses and other staff members. Historically, however, organizations have made few attempts to nurture and nourish the human spirit.

An inclusive workplace is characteristic of a caring organization. Such a workplace, however, is not satisfied simply by a diverse workforce.

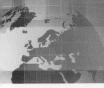

Health Care Delivery System Framework Domains and Elements

Pina et al. (2015) propose a framework for describing health care delivery systems that allows health care stakeholders to understand, evaluate, implement, and disseminate innovations to improve care and more easily compare health systems. For each step in the development of the framework, the researchers used two approaches: a review of the literature and the Delphi method with the Agency for Healthcare Research and Quality's Effective Health Care Stakeholders Group (SG). Nominations for the SG occurred via a public process. The group represented broad constituencies including patients, caregivers, and advocacy groups; clinicians and professional associations; hospital systems and medical clinics; government agencies; purchasers and payors; and health care industry representatives, policymakers and researchers. The Delphi method consisted of facilitated group discussions and interactive rounds of individual written feedback on each draft of the framework. The process yielded six domains with 26 elements as summarized below.

1. Capacity

Size—The system's productive capacity

Capital assets—The property, facilities, physical plant, and the property's ownership, equipment, and other infrastructure used to provide and manage health care services

Comprehensiveness of services—The scope and depth of services available in terms of setting, specialty, ancillary services, and acuity of care

2. Organizational structure

Configuration—The arrangement of the functional units in the system in terms of workflow, hierarchy of authority, patterns of communication, and resource flows among them

Leadership structure and governance—The level of formal decision-making authority for an office holder in terms of scope of decisions that can be made independently and with concurrence of others

Research and innovation—The extent to which participation in clinical and basic scientific research and health care innovation is a feature of the mission and activities of the organization

Professional education—The extent to which professional education and training is a feature of the mission and activities of the organization

3. Finances

Payment received for services—The categorical types of payment received, the approach to accountability for services provided, the proportion of each payment type, and the degree of financial risk held

Provider payment systems—The categorical types of payment to individual providers for their services and the proportion of each payment type

Ownership—The corporate status and health care industry affiliation of the owner of the health care system

Financial solvency—The extent to which the organization's financial resources exceed the organization's current liabilities and long-term expenses

4. Patients

Patient characteristics—Proportion of patients with different characteristics, health conditions, and coverage types

Geographic characteristics—Geographic location, type of community in which the health care delivery system functions, and size of the catchment area.

5. Care processes and infrastructure

Integration—The extent to which a network of organizations or units within one organization provides or arranges to provide a coordinated continuum of services to a population and is willing to be held clinically and fiscally accountable for the outcomes and health status of the population served

Standardization—The extent to which the health care delivery system reduces unnecessary

(continued)

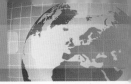

Health Care Delivery System Framework Domains and Elements (continued)

variation while encouraging differences dictated by diversity among patients in their conditions and preferences

Performance measurement, public reporting, and quality improvement—The extent to which the organization conducts regular measurement of performance with public reporting, feedback, and a systematic process for improvement

Health information system—The extent to which clinical and administrative information is organized and available to those who need it in a timely way and the extent to which they have electronic support for those functions

Patient care team—The extent to which patient care is delivered by clinicians and staff who regularly work together in an integrated way to serve patients and families

Clinical decision support—The extent to which clinical guideline-based reminders and decision aids are incorporated in the process of patient care

Care coordination—The deliberate organization of patient care activities between two or more participants involved in a patient's care to facilitate and maximize the appropriate delivery of health care services to achieve optimal patient experience and outcomes

6. Culture

Patient centeredness—The degree to which health care delivery is designed to serve the interests of patients rather than providers

Cultural competence—Ability of systems to provide care to patients with diverse values, beliefs, and behaviors, including tailoring delivery to meet patients' social, cultural, and linguistic needs

Competition–collaboration continuum—Where the organization falls on a scale from competitive to collaborative in relation to other organizations in its locale

Community benefit—The extent to which the organization is concerned about the health of the local community and takes advantage of community services for its patients through collaboration

Innovation diffusion—The degree to which the health care delivery organization or system is focused on creating and adopting new ways to provide care and accomplish its mission

Working climate—The degree to which the organization's employees perceive an environment of openness and fair process

Clinical Implications

During a clinical rotation, consider the following questions related to a domain and element.

Patients: Patient characteristics. What are the demographics of patients, such as age, gender, race, ethnicity, disability, education, income, and insurance coverage?

Culture: Patient centeredness. How are patients and family members involved in decision-making and the provision of care? How do clinicians adjust care based on the personal preferences of patients? How do they coordinate care for patients?

Culture: Cultural competence. What informational materials are available in which languages? How are professional interpreters arranged? What cultural competence goals are included in the organization's strategic plan? What strategies are in place to recruit, retain, and promote diverse leadership and staff?

Culture: Community benefit. How much uncompensated care is provided? How does the organization assess and prioritize local health care needs? What formal community partnerships are in place? What have the partnerships accomplished?

Reference: Pina, I. L., Cohen, P. D., Larson, D. B., Marion, L. N., Sills, M. R., Solberg, L. I., & Zerzan, J. (2015). A framework for describing health care delivery organizations and systems. *American Journal of Public Health, 105*(4), 670–679.

Instead, the organization focuses on capitalizing on the unique perspectives of a diverse workforce, in essence "managing for diversity" rather than "managing diversity" (Chavez & Weisinger, 2008). An inclusive workplace also reaches out beyond the organization by encouraging members of the workforce to become active in the community and participate in state and federal programs, working with the poor and with diverse cultural groups. Rather than espousing the golden rule (treat others as you wish to be treated), an inclusive workplace treats others as they wish to be treated, in what is sometimes called the platinum rule (Alessandra, 2010). Organizations with inclusive workplaces draw staff members who are committed to cultural competence and who value diversity and mutual respect for differences.

Although the impact of organizational culture on employees has been acknowledged, the impact of organizational culture on the community being served has received less attention. For years, hospitals and other health care organizations have espoused the view that "If we build it, they will come" (i.e., they need only offer the services). Now, there is a growing recognition that health care services should be structured in ways to appeal to and meet the needs of various members of the community. Health care leaders recognize that cultural competence in organizations is essential if organizations are to survive, grow, satisfy customers, and achieve their goals. Image is critically important for an organization's survival. A variety of factors are needed to move an organization toward cultural competence.

Assessment Tools

Organizational culture may be assessed in numerous ways. The Magnet Hospital Recognition Program for Excellence in Nursing Services evaluates organizational climate or culture (American Nurses Credentialing Center, 2017) and is used by many organizations as a blueprint for achieving excellence (Schaffner & Ludwig-Beymer, 2003). Evidence-Based Practice 9-2 outlines the

original research that resulted in the creation of **Magnet designation**. Evaluating the five key components of the Magnet model may be helpful in assessing the culture of an organization. These five key components are transformational leadership; structural empowerment; exemplary professional practice; new knowledge, innovations, and improvements; and empirical outcomes.

Leininger's (1991) theory of culture care diversity and universality is also helpful in assessing the culture of an institution. Leininger's culture care model may be used to conduct a cultural assessment of the organization, with dominant segments of the sunrise model identified. An example of such an assessment is provided in Box 9-6.

Other **cultural care assessment tools** are available to assess the culture of an institution. This assessment is then compared with the values and beliefs of the groups who use the health care organization. Andrews (1998) provides an assessment tool for cultural change that examines demographic/descriptive data; strengths; community resources; continued growth; perspectives of clients, families, and visitors; institutional perspective; and readiness for change. This tool allows organizational leaders to assess the needs of the community they serve and to use their findings to guide strategic planning for the future.

Building Culturally Competent Organizations

Cultural competence has been identified as a key strategy for eliminating racial and ethnic health disparities. However, the competence must extend beyond the provider, into the system of health care. It would be naive to assume that building culturally competent organizations will resolve all health disparities. However, when health care is delivered within a culturally competent organization, diverse health care consumers are more likely to access the services, return for services, adhere to the plan of care, and make necessary lifestyle changes.

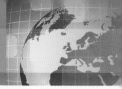

Magnet Research and the Magnet Model

The Magnet Recognition Program for Excellence in Nursing Services grew out of a 1982 descriptive study conducted by the American Academy of Nursing's Task Force on Nursing Practice (McClure, Poulin, Sovie, & Wandelt, 1983). The study began by asking Fellows from the American Academy of Nursing to identify hospitals that attracted and retained professional nurses who experienced professional and personal satisfaction in their practice. The Fellows nominated 165 institutions. These institutions were viewed as "Magnets." The task force then began narrowing the list based on specific criteria and the hospitals' willingness and availability to participate in the study.

Data were then collected from staff nurses and nursing directors in 41 hospitals. Nurses identified and described variables that created an environment that attracted and retained well-qualified nurses and promoted quality patient care. Nurses were asked nine questions, which remain valuable for structuring nursing input even today:

1. What makes your hospital a good place to work?
2. Can you describe particular programs that you see leading to professional/personal satisfaction?
3. How is nursing viewed in your hospital, and why?
4. Can you describe nurse involvement in various ongoing programs/projects whose goals are quality of patient care?
5. Can you identify activities and programs calculated to enhance, both directly and indirectly, recruitment/retention of professional nurses in your hospital?
6. Could you tell us about nurse–physician relationships in your hospital?
7. Describe staff nurse–supervisor relationships in your hospital.
8. Are some areas in your hospital more successful than others in recruitment/retention? Why?
9. What single piece of advice would you give to a director of nursing who wishes to do something about high RN vacancy and turnover rates in his or her hospital?

Staff nurses identified a variety of conditions that made a hospital a good place for nurses to work, specifically related to administration, professional practice, and professional development. Clustered together, a very clear culture of nursing emerged from this descriptive study.

Based on findings from the original Magnet study, the Magnet Recognition Program was developed in 1990. The program was created to advance three goals:

- Promote quality in a milieu that supports professional practice
- Identify excellence in the delivery of nursing services to patients/residents
- Provide a mechanism for the dissemination of "best practices" in nursing services

Clinical Implications

During clinical rotations to different facilities, nursing students are in an ideal position to evaluate organizational climate. Consider the following dimensions:

- Transformational leadership—How do the nursing leaders stimulate and inspire followers to achieve extraordinary outcomes? How do nursing leaders help others to develop their own leadership capacity?
- Structural empowerment—How are nurses involved in decision-making structures and processes to establish standards of practice and address opportunities for improvement? How does information flow between the chief nursing officer and all professional nurses? How do nurses partner with the community to improve patient outcomes and advance the health of the community? How do nurses enhance their professional development?
- Exemplary professional practice—What is the professional practice model? How do nurse partner with patients, families, and interprofessional team members to provide effective and efficient care? How do nurses enhance safety, quality,

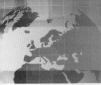

Magnet Research and the Magnet Model (continued)

and quality improvement? How is workplace advocacy supported within the organization?

- New knowledge, innovations, and improvements—How are evidence-based practice and research incorporated into clinical and operational processes? What infrastructure and resources are in place to support the advancement of evidence-based practices, research, and innovation in clinical settings?

- Empirical outcomes—What are the quantitative outcomes for the organization in terms of safety, quality, patient experience, and nurse satisfaction?

Nurses and nursing students are encouraged to use the Magnet framework to assess nursing subcultures and determine organizational fit.

References: McClure, M. L., Poulin, M. A., Sovie, M. D., & Wandelt, M. A.; for the American Academy Task Force on Nursing Practice in Hospitals. (1983). *Magnet hospitals. Attraction and retention of professional nurses.* Kansas City, MO: American Nurses Association.

American Nurses Credentialing Center. (2017). *2019 Magnet® application manual.* Silver Spring, MD: American Nurses Credentialing Center.

BOX 9-6	Example of Leininger's (1991) Culture Care Model Used to Conduct an Organizational Assessment

Factor: Environmental Context

Types of Questions: What is the general environment of the community that surrounds the organization? Socioeconomic status? Race/ethnicity? Emphasis on health? Living arrangements? Access to social services? Employment? Proximity to other health facilities?

Sample Findings: Hospital A is in a low-income urban setting. The neighborhood includes Blacks, Whites, and Hispanics. A public housing complex is located within a few blocks of the hospital. The economy is depressed, and many are out of jobs. Drug abuse and alcoholism are rampant. Families are challenged to survive, and they tend to view disease prevention as less important than their daily living. Health is defined as being able to participate in normal activities. Several social agencies nearby provide food pantries. There are no other hospitals within a 5-mile radius.

Factor: Language and Ethnohistory

Types of Questions: What languages are spoken within the institution? By employees? By patients and clients? How formal or informal are the lines of communication? How hierarchical?

What communication strategies are used within the institution? Written? Poster? Electronic? Oral? "Grapevine"? How did the institution come to be? What was the original mission? How has it changed over the years?

Sample Findings: Clients primarily speak English or Spanish. Employees typically speak English or Spanish, although Polish and Russian are heard, particularly among the housekeepers. The grapevine is alive and well at Hospital A. Although memos and e-mails are circulated, verbal communication is prized throughout the institution. The president/chief executive officer, chief nursing officer, and chief medical officer all maintain an open-door policy in their offices. Posters are also used to communicate, especially in the elevators. Electronic communication to direct care staff via e-mail has not been successful because computer workstations are in short supply throughout the institution. Hospital A was founded by a Roman Catholic religious order of nuns in 1885. The original mission was to provide care to immigrants and the poor. Immigrants from many nations, including Ireland, Poland, Hungary, and Russia originally inhabited the area.

(continued)

BOX 9-6	Example of Leininger's (1991) Culture Care Model Used to Conduct an Organizational Assessment (continued)

The mission is still to provide the highest quality of care to the poor and underserved, although that is becoming increasingly difficult financially.

Factor: Technology

Types of Questions: How is technology used in the institution? Who uses it? Is client documentation electronic? Is electronic order entry in place? Is cutting-edge technology in place in the emergency department (ED), critical care units, labor and delivery, radiology, surgical suites, and similar units? Are instant messaging, text messaging, and tweets used? Is Web-based technology embraced?

Sample Findings: There are a few computer workstations on each nursing unit. Nurses document electronically; physicians, Advanced Practice Registered Nurses (APRNs), and Physician Assistants (PAs) use computerized provider order entry (CPOE). Hospital A received external funding several years ago to renovate their old ED. The new ED has state-of-the art equipment, as do the critical care units. The labor and delivery unit is cramped and overcrowded. Equipment is well worn. Similarly, the surgical suites are dated. The radiology department is scheduled for a major capital investment next year.

Factor: Religious/Philosophical

Types of Questions: Does the institution have a religious affiliation? Are religious symbols displayed within the facility? By clients? By staff? Is the institution private or public? For-profit or not-for-profit?

Sample Findings: Founded by a religious order, Hospital A is very clearly viewed as Roman Catholic. Outside, the hospital is marked with a large cross on its roof. Inside, a crucifix hangs in each client room. A large chapel is used for daily mass. A chaplain distributes communion to clients and staff every evening. Nurses demonstrate a variety of religious symbols. One nurse is seen wearing a cross; another wears a Star of David. Clients adhere to a variety of faith traditions, including Roman Catholic, Southern Baptist, and Muslim. Chaplains come from a variety of faith traditions and attempt to meet the needs of diverse groups.

Factor: Kinship and Social Factors

Types of Questions: What are the working relationships within nursing? Between nursing and ancillary services? Between nursing and medicine? How closely are staff members aligned? Is the environment emotionally "warm" and close or "cold" and distant? How do employees relate to one another? Do they celebrate together? Rely on each other for support? Do employees get together outside of work?

Sample Findings: RNs at Hospital A tend to be White and are often the children of immigrants. They are most often educated in associate degree. Aides tend to be African American. There is tension between the two groups especially as the role of the aide has expanded. Nurses tend to be somewhat intimidated by physicians. Physicians' attitudes toward nurses range from respect to disrespect. Many physicians are angry about the erosion of their autonomy and economic security and the required use of CPOE. Most units tend to be tight knit, with celebrations of monthly birthdays and recognition provided when staff members "go the extra mile." Nurses rarely socialize with one another outside of work. Staff nurses have a mean age of 45. Most of them commute from the suburbs to the hospital and return home after their shift. In contrast, many of the aides are from the immediate community, know each other, and socialize outside of work.

Factor: Cultural Values

Types of Questions: Are values explicitly stated? What is valued within the institution? What is viewed as good? What is viewed as right? What is seen as truth?

Sample Findings: The institution clearly identifies its mission and strives to fulfill it in economically difficult times. Its stated values are collaboration and diversity. Although diversity training has been provided to managers, tensions still exist between work groups, particularly because the workforce tends to be racially divided.

BOX 9-6	Example of Leininger's (1991) Culture Care Model Used to Conduct an Organizational Assessment (continued)

Factor: Political/Legal

Types of Questions: How politically charged is the institution? Where does the power rest within the institution? With medicine? With finance? With nursing? With information technology? Is power shared? What types of legal actions have been taken against the institution? On behalf of the institution?

Sample Findings: Historically, Hospital A has been politically naive. It has gone about its mission without regard to the external environment. Recently, the hospital has begun to lobby for better reimbursement for care provided under Medicaid. Institutional power rests with the strong medical staff and department chairs.

Factor: Economic

Types of Questions: What is the financial viability of the institution? Who makes the financial decisions? How do the salaries and benefits compare with those of competitors in the immediate environment?

Sample Findings: Hospital A has a very low profit margin, 0.5%, compared with an industry standard of about 3%. This means that little money is available for capital improvements, which results in less technology and some units being cramped. Community needs are considered when making all financial decisions. People are valued, and efforts are made to keep salaries competitive. Starting salaries are increasing for new graduates, and experienced nurses are complaining of salary compression.

Factor: Educational

Types of Questions: How is education valued within the institution? What type of assistance (financial, scheduling, flexibility) is provided for staff seeking additional degrees? Does the institution provide education for medicine, nursing, and other professions? Are advanced practice nurses utilized? What is the educational background of staff nurses? Nurse managers? Nursing leaders? How does this compare with education of other professional groups? With competing organizations?

Sample Findings: Nurses are most often educated in associate degree programs. Although flexible scheduling and limited tuition reimbursement are provided, many nurses do not take advantage of the benefits because of the need to work extra shifts to ensure staffing and competing personal and family priorities. All nurse managers and directors are required to have a BSN. Some high-performing nurses are encouraged to return to school to become nurse practitioners, as the hospital plans to expand the use of that role. Nursing students from five different programs rotate through the institution, with priority given to students from the BSN programs. Medical education is provided at Hospital A, with 100 residents and many 3rd year and 4th year medical students rotating through the facility. The residents, while learning, also provide important service to the community, particularly through their clinic rotations. Students in respiratory, social work, dietitian, physical therapy, occupational therapy, speech therapy, and pastoral care also have clinical rotations at Hospital A.

Weech-Maldonado, Elliott, Pradhan, Schiller, Hall, et al. (2012) conducted research to examine the relationship between hospital cultural competence and satisfaction with inpatient care. They found that inpatients reported higher satisfaction with hospitals that had greater cultural competency. The findings were particularly striking among minority patients, who reported higher satisfaction with nurse communication, physician communication, staff responsiveness, pain control, and environmental factors in hospitals with greater cultural competency.

Guerrero (2012) examined the extent to which internal and external organizational pressures contributed to the degree of adoption of culturally and linguistically responsive practices in outpatient substance abuse treatment systems. Higher adoption of culturally competent practices was found in programs with more external funding and regulation and with managers who had higher levels of cultural sensitivity. Organizations with a large number of professional staff had lower adoption of culturally competent practices when compared to organizations with fewer professional staff members.

As with cultural competence in individuals, cultural competency in organizations develops over time as part of a journey. The process involves all aspects of the organization. Malone (1997) describes several strategies for improving organizational cultural competence. Strategies include training that helps the organization to value and manage cultural diversity; rewarding practice that values differences and is culturally appropriate and collaborative; recruiting nurses who are culturally competent; and hiring nurses who are culturally diverse. Castillo and Guo (2011) provide a framework for building cultural competence in health care organizations. They address governance,

vision, mission, and values; strategic planning; monitoring and evaluation; and communication. Purnell et al. (2011) provide a guide to developing culturally competent organizations that address four key areas: administration and governance, orientation and education, language, and staff competence. Marrone (2010) provides a comprehensive assessment of organizational cultural competency. Douglas et al. (2014) recommend 10 practices by leaders to build cultural competence in health care organizations, summarized in Box 9-7. Fung, Srivastava, and Andermann (2012) present a framework, consisting of eight domains, to plan for organizational cultural competence in mental health care service settings. Delphin-Rittmen (2013) describes seven essential strategies for promoting and sustaining cultural competence.

For the purpose of this chapter, the concepts identified above have been combined and consolidated. Seven specific areas critical to fostering culturally competent health care organizations are discussed in the sections below: governance and administration, internal evaluation of

---

BOX 9-7 | The Role of Health Care Organization Leaders in Developing Culturally Competent Health Care Systems and Organizations

1. Develop systems to promote culturally competent care delivery.
2. Ensure that mission and organizational policies reflect respect and values related to diversity and inclusivity.
3. Assign a managerial-level task force to oversee and take responsibility for diversity-related issues within the organization.
4. Establish an internal budget for the provision of culturally appropriate care, such as for the hiring of interpreters, producing multi-language client education materials, adding signage in different languages, and so on.
5. Include cultural competence requirements in job descriptions, performance measures, and promotion criteria.
6. Develop a data collection system to monitor demographic trends for the geographic area served by the agency.
7. Obtain patient satisfaction data to determine the appropriateness and effectiveness of services.
8. Collaborate with other health agencies to share ideas and resources for meeting the needs of culturally diverse populations.
9. Bring health care directly to the local ethnic populations.
10. Enlist community members to participate in the agency's program planning committees, for example, for smoking cessation or infant care programs.

Source: Douglas, M. K., Rosenkoetter, M., Pacquiao, D., Callister, L. C., Hattar-Pollara, M., Lauderdale, J., …, Purnell, L. (2014). Guidelines for implementing culturally competent nursing care. *Journal of Transcultural Nursing*, 25(2), 109–121.

adherence to cultural competence standards, staff competence, the physical environment of care, linguistic competence, community involvement, and culturally congruent services and programs.

Governance and Administration

For the purposes of this chapter, governance is defined as members of the board of directors and any sub-boards, such as Board Finance or Board Quality. Administration is defined as those individuals who serve as department heads. Together, governance and administration are responsible for ensuring that the organization is continually developing cultural competence. The Wellesley Institute in Ontario (Kouri, 2012) identifies key strategies and tools helpful for reducing health disparities; several strategies helpful for governance and administration to consider are summarized in Box 9-8.

Ideally, both board members and administrators reflect the ethnic and racial diversity of the community served. The board and administration set the strategic plan for the organization. The strategic plan sets the direction for an organization and is used to communicate organizational goals and the actions needed to achieve those goals. The strategic planning process should begin with an assessment of community strengths and needs. In a study designed to determine factors related to organizational cultural competence,

Guerrero (2013) found that leadership skills and strategic climate in addiction health service settings resulted in a better understanding and responsiveness to community needs.

Board members and administration also establish the mission, vision, and values for the organization. The mission statement describes the purpose of the organization, its reason for existing. The mission statement should be inclusive. The basic premises of an organization, reflected in its mission statement, provide insight into the presence or absence of a commitment to providing culturally competent care. Many organizations also establish a vision and values to guide their culture. The vision projects the future status of an organization and inspires and generates a shared purpose among organization members. Whether or not they are explicitly stated, all organizations have values. Values are sometimes called Pillars. Values are the standards that guide the perspective and action of the organization and help to define an organization's culture and beliefs. The strategic plan is based on the mission, vision, and values. The plan should include tactics for developing culturally congruent services and programs to meet community needs, partnering with key community organizations, and developing the organization's cultural competence. The mission, vision, and values may also include specific behaviors demonstrated toward both customers and colleagues.

BOX 9-8 | Strategies and Tools for Reducing Health Disparities

Conduct local research and analyze health disparities.

Provide primary health care practices and resources.
Offer convenient locations and hours.
Deliver appropriate care.

Form effective partnerships.
Collaborate to reduce poverty.

Provide opportunities for early childhood development.
Implement school-based strategies.

Advocate for public education and policy changes.

Participate in community development.

Source: Kouri, D. (2012, March). *Reducing health disparities: How can the structure of the health system contribute?* Wellesley Institute. Retrieved May 30, 2018 from http://www.wellesleyinstitute.com/wp-content/uploads/2012/09/Reducing-Health-Disparities-how-can-health-system-structure-contribute.pdf

Administration is responsible for developing the organization's budget, which is then approved by the board of directors. Financial resources, including funding for capital, staff, and programs for the delivery of care, must be allocated appropriately to foster organizational cultural competence. For example, the environment should be welcoming, with the space and décor appropriate for the cultural groups served. Funding for staff recruitment, orientation, and training is also essential. Funding for the delivery of care must always consider cultural components. For example, funding is needed to advertise new and existing programs, using the venues and languages appropriate to the community. Pictures on the advertising materials must reflect the client population.

Nurse executives can take the lead in developing culturally competent health care organizations. Leininger (1996) defined **transcultural nursing administration** as "a creative and knowledgeable process of assessing, planning, and making decisions and policies that will facilitate the provision of educational and clinical services that take into account the cultural caring values, beliefs, symbols, references and lifeways of people of diverse and similar cultures for beneficial or satisfying outcomes" (p. 30). Nurse administrators must ensure that organizational policies are culturally sensitive and appropriate and that

they recognize the rights of individuals and families. Such policies should incorporate Leininger's (1991) decisions and actions of culture care preservation/maintenance, culture care accommodation/negotiation, and culture care repatterning/restructuring.

Nurse leaders who recognize the importance of transculturally based administration are essential for culturally competent health care organizations. The American Organization of Nurse Executives (AONE, 2015) identifies five nurse executive competencies: communication, knowledge, leadership, professionalism, and business skills. Nurse executive competencies related to diversity are summarized in Box 9-9. Nurse administrators must foster a climate in which nurses and other health care providers realize that provider–client encounters include the interaction of three cultural systems: the organization, the providers, and the client.

In culturally competent health care organizations, nurse leaders also recognize the relationship between a culturally diverse nursing workforce and the ability to provide culturally competent patient care. The need to attract students from underrepresented groups is gaining importance (American Association of Colleges of Nursing, 2018) and calls for new partnerships between practice, community, and academic settings.

BOX 9-9	American Organization of Nurse Executives (AONE) Nurse Executive Communication and Relationship Building Competencies Related to Diversity

Diversity

- Establish an environment that values diversity (e.g., age, gender, race, religion, ethnicity, sexual orientation, culture).
- Establish cultural competency in the workforce.
- Incorporate cultural beliefs into care delivery.

- Provide an environment conducive to opinion sharing, exploration of ideas, and achievement of outcomes.

Community Involvement

- Represent the community perspective in the decision-making process within the organization/system

Source: American Organization of Nurse Executives. (2015). Nurse executive competencies. Retrieved May 16, 2016 from http://www.aone.org/resources/nec.pdf

Administration and the board of directors must work together to ensure that the health care organization continues the journey toward cultural competence. This includes setting strategic priorities and funding appropriate programs for staff and clients.

Internal Evaluation of Adherence to Cultural Competence Standards

In addition to recognizing and acknowledging the overall culture of a health care organization, organizations must also evaluate how they are adhering to cultural competence standards as an organization and determine how effectively the organization is meeting the needs of the populations they serve. The evaluation may be conducted in a variety of ways.

Roizner (1996) identifies a checklist for culturally responsive health care services. Health care services are evaluated based on their availability, accessibility, affordability, acceptability, and appropriateness. When the organization is evaluated by this model, it is important to consider these "five A's":

- Are the health services that are needed by the community readily available? In a community with rampant illicit drug use, for example, one should expect to find a variety of types of drug abuse prevention and treatment programs offered that are readily available to the local population.
- Are health care resources accessible? A pediatrician's office, for example, might need to expand its hours of operation to accommodate the schedules of working parents. Geographic location should be considered in terms of proximity to public transportation, traffic patterns, and available parking. Structural changes may also be needed to accommodate specific types of clients, such as those who use wheelchairs.
- Are the services affordable? Partnerships between public and private organizations may be needed to ensure that services are affordable. A sliding scale might be developed to accommodate the needs of people with limited financial resources.
- Are the services acceptable? Providers need to carefully consider this question. Do community members who use the services perceive the services to be of high quality? Do community members value the services? Are the waiting rooms stark, dimly lit, or untidy? Is the furniture worn or the reading material frayed and outdated? Providers need to understand what makes services acceptable to the community they seek to serve. Community members may avoid a particular agency or institution because services are delivered in a noncaring and patronizing fashion.
- Are the services appropriate? Community members may shun services if they do not perceive that these services meet their needs. For example, community members who struggle with day-to-day survival with limited financial and social resources may not use fitness classes. Programs that are disconnected from the daily life of community members constitute a recipe for failure.

Fung et al. (2012) present a methodology for evaluating cultural competence in health care organizations involving mixed qualitative and quantitative methods. An organization may also compare their performance to standards provided by regulatory bodies, government agencies, and professional organizations. Annually, members of the Language, Culture and Religion Committee at some organizations critically compare current practice with Joint Commission and CLAS standards. The committee members determine where there are gaps and develop a strategic plan to address the gaps.

The Cultural Competency Assessment Tool for Hospitals (CCATH) allows an organization to assess adherence to the CLAS standards (Weech-Maldonado et al., 2012). The instrument measures 12 composites: leadership and strategic planning, data collection on inpatient population, data collection on service area, performance management systems and quality improvement, HR practices, diversity training, community representation, availability of interpreter services, interpreter services policies, quality of interpreter services, translation of written materials, and clinical cultural competency practices. Weech-Maldonado, Elliott, Pradhan, Schiller, Dreachslin, et al. (2012) found that hospitals that were not-for-profit, served a more diverse inpatient population, and were located in more competitive and affluent markets exhibited a higher degree of cultural competency.

To evaluate how effectively the health care organization is meeting community needs, a variety of data elements may be considered, including clinical data and patient satisfaction. Health care organizations should assess their own practices to determine if there are unknown disparities in care. As an example, Figure 9-1 presents data for long

bone fracture pain management from the emergency department of a community hospital. The mean and median turnaround time for pain medication is shorter than the national average for all groups but is slightly longer for Asians compared to all other populations at the author's hospital. Examination of the data helps the organization to determine the causes of the variations.

Focused interventions can help administrators to improve their cultural competence. Weech-Maldonado et al. (2018) provided a systematic, multifaceted, and organizational-level cultural competency intervention to executive leadership at two hospitals within a system, with a third hospital in the system serving as a control. Overall performance improvement was greater in each of the two intervention hospitals than in the control

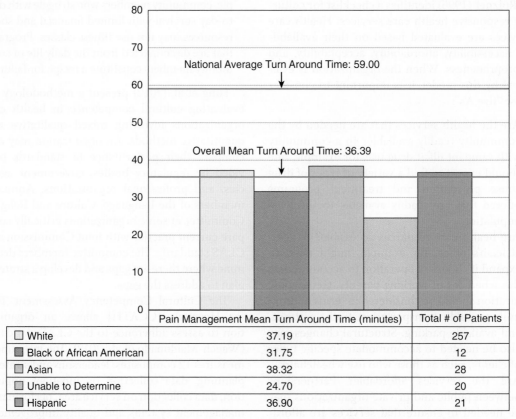

	Pain Management Mean Turn Around Time (minutes)	Total # of Patients
☐ White	37.19	257
■ Black or African American	31.75	12
☐ Asian	38.32	28
☐ Unable to Determine	24.70	20
■ Hispanic	36.90	21

Figure 9-1. Example of emergency department turnaround time for pain medication in clients with long bone fracture by race/ethnicity, FY2013. (Data from Edward Hospital at Edward-Elmhurst Health.)

hospital. Statistically significant improvements were noted in the organizational level of competencies of diversity leadership and strategic HR management; in individual-level competencies for diversity attitudes and implicit bias; and in overall diversity climate.

Staff Competence

Individual health care providers are essential for building culturally competent organizations. All staff members must be competent; this is especially critical for direct care nurses and other staff members. Many times, nurses and other care providers interact based on their own cultural values, experience, and preferences. They need to be taught how to interact with patients from various cultures to provide patient-centered care and serve as patient advocates (Sherrod, 2013). Key processes, including organizational support, orientation, and ongoing education, are needed to enhance staff competence.

The HR department typically provides organizational support for staff. The department plays a key role in ensuring that recruitment and hiring activities reflect the diversity of the community served by the health care organization. HR can also prioritize recruitment of bilingual staff members and ensure appropriate compensation. Policies, position descriptions, and performance reviews, typically overseen by HRs, must reflect cultural competence.

Orientation and ongoing education are needed for employees at all levels to develop and foster cultural sensitivity and competence. Diversity in its broadest terms should be discussed in orientation. This should include race, ethnicity, religion, age, gender, sexual orientation, sexual identity, socioeconomics, and educational backgrounds of both clients and staff members. Volunteers and medical staff members also need to be oriented to the organization's culture, strategy, and expectations.

Beyond orientation, ongoing education is needed to reinforce the learning. While staff cannot learn about all diversity, they should be equipped with a general cultural framework and have specific knowledge about the cultural groups for whom they most often provide care. A first step to learning about culture is to identify the values and worldview of one's own culture. This may be facilitated through reflection and discussion. By acknowledging one's own beliefs, staff members may be helped to avoid stereotyping and cultural imposition. A variety of formats may be used to educate staff, including live education sessions, electronic learning, journal clubs, and discussion groups. Inviting members of a particular culture or religion to discuss their beliefs and practices is often engaging for both the community and staff. To help hold staff members accountable for their actions, performance reviews must reflect the organization's commitment to cultural competence.

Nurses and other health care staff members need training on the importance of obtaining accurate patient data. According to a report from the Commonwealth Fund and the American Hospital Association's Health and Research Educational Trust (Hasnain-Wynia, Pierce, & Pittman, 2004), 80% of hospitals collect data on race and ethnicity. Data are collected primarily because of a law or regulatory requirement. However, the information may not be accurate or valid. The report recommends that hospitals standardize who provides the information, when it is collected, which racial and ethnic categories should be used, and how the data are stored.

Gomez, Le, West, Santariano, and O'Connor (2003) found that while 85% of hospitals reported collecting data on race, approximately half of them obtained the data by observing a client's physical appearance. In addition, only 12% of the hospitals reported having a procedure for recording the race and/or ethnicity of a client with mixed ancestry, and 55% reported never collecting ethnicity data. Regenstein and Sickler (2006) found that 78.4% of hospitals collect race information, 50.4% collect data on client ethnicity, and 50.2% collect data on language preference. However, only 20% have formal data collection policies, and fewer than 20% use the data to assess and compare care quality, health services utilization, health outcomes, or patient satisfaction.

The Institute of Medicine (2002) has standardized the collection of race, ethnicity, and language data. The Agency for Healthcare Research and Quality (2018b) has identified steps an organization can take to collect more accurate data. This includes how to ask patients and enrollees questions about race, ethnicity, and language and communication needs; how to train staff to elicit this information in a respectful and efficient manner; how to address the discomfort of registration/admission staff or call center staff about requesting this information; how to address potential patient or enrollee pushback respectfully; and how to address system-level issues, such as changes in patient registration screens and data flow.

In addition to understanding the need for accurate data, staff members must be culturally competent to help build culturally competent health care organizations. Staff members who lack competency may fail to take the client's culture seriously, misinterpret the client's value system, and elevate their own value systems. This posture is culturally destructive because it minimizes the other person's culture. Culturally competent staff members will take time to ask questions about what the client prefers and listen attentively. In the end, this will increase understanding, trust, collaboration, adherence, and satisfaction.

Nurses and other health care providers can help the organization grow in cultural understanding. If they listen and attend carefully, health care providers have a valuable window directly into the world of their clients. They can take what they learn and share it with the administration to improve the cultural responsiveness of their organization. Individuals and groups of clinicians can also develop special programs to meet the needs of the specific populations they serve. Speaking the language is a definite advantage.

The Physical Environment of Care

As part of building a culturally competent organization, the physical environment should always

be assessed. Approaching this assessment as a potential client is helpful, and a variety of factors should be considered. What message does the organization send through its physical surroundings? How is the facility organized physically? How does the entryway present the culture of the organization to the public? Is the entrance warm and inviting? Is the signage prominent? What languages are included on the signs? Is information presented clearly and unambiguously? Are amenities available to clients and their family members? Are the doors open or closed? Do people talk with one another, and what languages are spoken? What is the traffic pattern, and what is the general flow of traffic? Does the environment appear calm or turbulent? Are the staff members attentive and courteous?

A physical environment may send unintentional messages. For example, consider the birthing center at a city hospital. The hospital's service area is undergoing tremendous changes, with a large influx of African American, Hispanic, Indian, and Polish American populations. The birthing unit is beautifully and tastefully decorated with oak furniture and pastel prints. Every picture on the walls, however, shows a Caucasian family. This clearly sends a message of exclusivity rather than inclusiveness. When this is brought to the attention of the nurse manager, she is completely dumbfounded and quickly takes steps to rectify the situation. Ethnocentrism and stereotyping are in play here, and it takes a degree of cultural competence to identify this and bring it to recognition and resolution.

Organizational leaders must also assess the physical environment of care to identify potential barriers. A flow chart is a helpful tool for determining such barriers. For example, to provide comprehensive women's health programs in a caring fashion, organizational leaders may examine the steps for admission to the labor and delivery unit for the delivery of a baby. To determine this, staff members walk through the care process and create a flow chart that outlines the steps. Staff members must be alert for possible sources of confusion for parents at this highly stressful time. The flow chart can then be used to design changes in the environment that can be implemented to decrease barriers and improve services.

Linguistic Competence

Language is a major barrier to quality health care (Office of Minority Health, 2016b). The Institute of Medicine (2002) reports that 51% of providers believe that clients do not adhere to treatment because of culture or language. At the same time, nurses and other health care providers report having received no language or cultural competency training (Baldonado et al., 1998; Park et al., 2005). Twenty-two percent of medical residents feel unprepared to treat patients who have LEP (Weissman et al., 2005). Similarly, while both nurses and baccalaureate nursing students perceive an overwhelming need for transcultural nursing, only 61% report confidence in their ability to provide care to culturally diverse patients (Baldonado et al., 1998). Providing care to non–English-speaking patients presents a special challenge.

Addressing this challenge begins when the nurse determines the preferred language for health care discussions from the patient. This information must be recorded and shared with all health care providers. Patients must be informed that an interpreter will be provided for them at no cost. Interpreter services may be provided in person, by videoconferencing or by telephone.

Competent interpreter services are necessary when providing care and services. Because communication is a cornerstone of patient safety and quality care, every patient has the right to receive information in a manner he or she understands. Effective communication allows patients to participate more fully in their care, is critical to the informed consent process, and helps practitioners and health care organizations give the best possible care. For communication to be effective, the information provided must be complete, accurate, timely, unambiguous, and understood by the patient. Many patients of varying circumstances require alternative communication methods, including patients who speak and/or read languages other than English, patients who have limited literacy in any language, patients who have visual or hearing impairments, patients on ventilators, patients with cognitive impairments, and children.

Health care organizations have many options to assist in communication with these individuals, such as interpreters, translated written materials, pen and paper, and communication boards. It is up to the hospital to determine which method is the best for each patient. Various laws, regulations, and guidelines are relevant to the use of interpreters. These include Title VI of the Civil Rights Act, 1964; Executive Order 13166; policy guidance from the Office of Civil Rights regarding compliance with Title VI, 2004; Title III of the Americans with Disabilities Act, 1990; state laws; and the National Council on Interpreting in Health Care (2005).

Policies addressing interpreter services should be in place, and staff members should be educated on them. Signage, consent forms, patient education, and other written materials should be translated and available in the most commonly spoken languages. Written materials should augment, not substitute for, discussion in the patient's language. The organization should evaluate written documents for cultural sensitivity. When collecting data, such as patient satisfaction or quality of life surveys, the organization should provide the surveys in the patient's preferred language. The organization should also work with the community to address health literacy and provide and encourage attendance at English as a Second Language classes.

Large health care organizations may have resources to secure trained professional interpreters and bilingual providers. Regardless of setting, however, Youdelman and Perkins (2005) suggest the following eight-step process for developing appropriate language services:

1. Designate responsibility.
2. Conduct an analysis of language needs.

3. Identify resources in the community.
4. Determine what language services will be provided.
5. Determine how to respond to LEP patients.
6. Train staff.
7. Notify LEP patients of available language services.
8. Update activities after periodic review.

Community Involvement

Understanding what culturally competent health care means from the standpoint of patients is an important step in building culturally competent organizations. Napoles-Springer, Santoyo, Houston, Perez-Stable, and Stewart (2005) conducted 19 community focus groups to determine the meaning of culture and what cultural factors influenced the quality of their medical visits. Culture was defined in terms of value systems, customs, self-identified ethnicity, and nationality. African Americans, Latinos, and non-Latino Whites all agreed that the quality of health care encounters was influenced by clinicians' sensitivity to complementary/alternative medicine, health insurance discrimination, social class discrimination, ethnic concordance between patient and provider, and age-based discrimination. Ethnicity-based discrimination was identified as a factor for Latinos and African Americans. Latinos also described language issues and immigration status factors. Overall, participants indicated greater satisfaction with clinicians who demonstrated cultural flexibility, defined as the ability to elicit, adapt, and respond to patients' cultural characteristics.

Health care institutions exist to provide care. Many factors, such as tobacco, alcohol, and drug use; poor diet; and physical inactivity, contribute to mortality in the United States and Canada. Addressing these factors requires individual behavioral change, community change, social change, and economic change. Health care organizations cannot confront these complex factors in isolation; they must partner with their communities to build trust in their institutions and meet the needs of their local communities.

Community partnerships may be configured in a variety of ways. Hospitals and health care systems usually articulate their desire to improve the health of the communities they serve. Historically, hospitals have fulfilled this mission through charity care, health care provider education, health care research, community education programming, and community outreach (Pelfrey & Theisen, 1993). However, true improvements in the health of a community require the focused efforts of the entire community. Such improvements may occur only in partnerships with community members and community organizations.

An ethnographic study of community (Davis, 1997) revealed five themes related to the experience of community caring. Three of these themes are particularly significant to this discussion: (1) Reciprocal relationships and teams working together are central to building healthy communities, (2) education with a focus on prevention is key to enhancing health, and (3) understanding community needs is a primary catalyst for health care reform and change.

Health care professionals in culturally competent organizations collaborate with surrounding communities to conduct community health assessments. In community mapping, staff collect a variety of data, including demographics, health status, community resources, barriers, and enablers. Both strengths and needs are identified from the perspective of the community. Data are then used collaboratively with communities to set priorities. An example of such a community assessment is provided in Box 9-10. Data from these assessments are used to set priorities and guide the planning and implementation of key initiatives. These initiatives are most well accepted when they are sponsored by a variety of community organizations rather than by a single health care organization.

Focus groups may assist an organization in assessing how well they are meeting the needs of the populations they serve. For example, the Boston Pain Education Program worked collaboratively with community representatives to develop a culturally sensitive, linguistically appropriate cancer pain education booklet in 11 languages

BOX 9-10 | Community Assessment Example

As part of an assessment of the communities it serves, the hospital realized that Hispanics made up an increasing proportion of the population and were the most frequently underserved population. As a result, an interprofessional team led by a family practice physician proposed the idea of a community center for health and empowerment. A coalition composed of individuals from social services, health care agencies, schools, police, churches, businesses, city government, and other community services also identified the Hispanic community as underserved. This coalition provided an etic, or outsider, view of the Hispanic community.

To provide a local, or emic (insider) view, community members worked with health care personnel to design and conduct a door-to-door community assessment. Leininger's theory of cultural diversity and universality served to guide the assessment. The assessment process involved two focus groups, 15 community interviewers, and 220 door-to-door interviews. In addition, five meetings, attended by 180 community members, were held to report the findings to community members and solicit their input on how to maintain strengths and address needs. As a result, numerous task forces were formed to preserve strengths or mediate needs.

Major strengths identified were access to friends and families to socialize and get support;

prenatal and postnatal care; and pediatric care. Major needs identified were affordable housing; programs to help immigrants; Spanish-speaking dentists; and activities for youth.

The community was involved in key decisions from the beginning, including selecting the site for the center, choosing the name for the center, and establishing a sliding scale for fees. The bilingual center includes primary health care services, a Women–Infant–Children program run by the county health department, and a community empowerment program. A salaried community outreach worker coordinates the community empowerment program. In collaboration with businesses, churches, and city services, community members received training in group work and priority setting.

Because of the identified need for dental care, the center arranged for monthly dental services through a dental van. To address the concern about activities for youth, community members and center personnel actively partnered with the park district, schools, churches, and the police to provide recreational activities for the youth. The community uses this as an opportunity to celebrate their cultural heritage. Health promotion materials and activities are also provided through collaboration.

Source: Ludwig-Beymer, P., Blankemeier, J. R., Casas-Byots, C., & Suarez-Balcazar, Y. (1996). Community assessment in a suburban hispanic community: A description of methods. *Journal of Transcultural Nursing*, 8(1), 19–27.

and for 11 ethnic groups. Focus groups were used to develop materials that would empower patients and families to more effectively partner with health care professionals and manage pain in culturally competent ways (Lasch et al., 2000).

Community-based participatory research or **participatory action research** is helpful in understanding a community and developing health improvement initiatives with community members. The method uses collaborative, participatory approaches to develop sustainable services (Koch & Kralik, 2006). Reese (2011)

described a participatory action research project that addresses organizational barriers to cultural competence in hospice care through a university–community–hospice partnership. In addition, the National Center on Minority Health and Health Disparities (NCMHD), located within the National Institutes of Health, funds disease intervention research to reduce and eliminate health disparities using community-based participation research that is jointly conducted by health disparity communities and researchers (NCMHD, 2018).

Conducting community assessments requires cultural awareness and sensitivity. Interpreting the data requires knowledge of the cultural dimensions of health and illness. Using the data to develop and implement programs in conjunction with the community requires the ability to plan and implement culturally competent care. The skill of a transcultural nurse or other culturally competent health care professional is invaluable in these situations.

Culturally Congruent Services and Programs

Culturally competent nurses and other health care providers develop and evaluate culturally competent initiatives. Many important factors must be considered in planning programs across cultural groups. In many cases, cultural competence must be demonstrated with multiple cultures simultaneously. For example, one hospital

in the Chicago area provides care for individuals who speak 64 different languages. This calls for much effort and creativity on the part of patients, health care providers, and interpreters. Case Study 9-1 describes the development and implementation of a culturally competent initiative. This case study focuses on one culturally competent program provided to a community; however, additional programs, targeting the needs of other groups, may also be envisioned. For example, adult immunizations are a challenge for many communities, so a program might be developed that focuses specifically on older adults and their immunization needs. Similarly, programs might be instituted to deal with other health issues of concern to community members. The case study demonstrates the importance of incorporating an understanding of culture in every aspect of an initiative. To design and implement an effective program, the cultural values of patients must be understood and addressed.

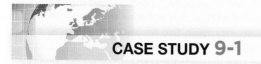

CASE STUDY 9-1

Caring Hospital, a not-for-profit hospital, serves clients who differ in multiple ways, including socioeconomic status, education, race, ethnicity, religion, language, sexual orientation, sexual identity, and culture. Organizational leaders embrace Leininger's theory of culture care. In particular, nursing leaders believe that nursing care must be congruent with the client's culture in order to promote the client's health and satisfaction.

Through a healthy community program, the hospital remains grounded in the reality of their clients. The healthy community program, developed and staffed by two nurses with community health backgrounds, is responsible for broadly defining community-based health promotion initiatives that address individual, social, and community factors. Their goal is to establish partnerships with commu-

nity members and governmental and community organizations to ensure that everyone has access to the basics needed for health; that the physical environment supports healthy living; and that communities control, define, and direct action for health.

The nurses in the healthy community program bring together resources from settings both within and outside their hospital. For example, they work closely with other community-focused staff members, such as home care and parish nurses. They also work with multiple external organizations, such as local health departments and other government agencies, religious institutions, community businesses, schools, and other health care entities. These nurses work specifically with the communities surrounding their facility. In this way, they acknowledge the specific needs of diverse groups.

The healthy community nurses use Leininger's culture care diversity and universality model in their practice. They use data gathered from cultural assessments to assist them in understanding the communities they serve. They consider environmental context, ethnohistory, language, kinship, cultural values and lifeways, the political and legal system, and technologic, economic, religious, philosophic, and educational factors. They understand the interactions among the folk system, nursing care, and the professional systems. They also understand the importance of using the three culture care modalities: preservation/maintenance, accommodation/negotiation, and repatterning/restructuring.

Because of their community health backgrounds, the nurses are knowledgeable about disparities in health. The nurses use data from a variety of sources, including hospital-specific data, census tract data, and health department data, to help them understand health and access disparities in their area. They also talk to community members and to health care providers to identify competing priorities. Using these processes, they discover that their communities have not achieved the Healthy People 2020 immunization goals for children by the age of 2 years.

To address the lack of immunizations, the nurses acknowledge that the issues that affect immunizations are multifaceted. The immunization schedule changes frequently and is quite complex. Even health care providers have difficulty interpreting it. Communication with parents has been sketchy and has been complicated by controversy. Immunizations are sometimes seen by parents as nonessential for young children until they enter elementary school. Immunizations may not be easily accessible, available, and affordable. Parents may make decisions based on misinformation, rumor, or hearsay. The nurses know, however, that community members want to keep their children healthy and that immunizations have contributed greatly to reducing illnesses in individuals and improving overall health for the community. They also know that community members prefer their children receive immunizations in a consistent place, as part of an overall medical home.

Because the childhood immunization levels are suboptimal in the communities served by the hospital, childhood immunization is selected as a quality initiative. A group of consumers and clinicians is convened to implement a program with the goal of increasing immunization to the Healthy People 2020 goals. There is much discussion on the best way for increasing immunization rates through a broad-based program. The group considers mailed, telephoned, e-mailed, and texted reminders and opts to combine texted reminders with follow-up mailed reminders.

Various materials are developed in both English and Spanish, and incentives are put into place to assist parents. Babies are automatically enrolled in the program when they are born in the hospital. Mailings occur at regular intervals and include a personalized letter indicating what vaccines are due, a vaccine record, vaccine information statements, and a growth and development newsletter. Additionally, incentives are mailed to help keep the parents motivated to use preventive services. Materials are written at a sixth-grade level. All materials are reviewed for cultural congruity, and the illustrations include babies from various ethnic groups.

New materials are developed as needed based on a continuous assessment of the needs of the parents. For example, reproducing all the materials in all the languages used by clients is found to be too expensive, so a multiple-language brochure is developed in the 11 most common languages spoken in the community. The brochure explains the program and asks that non–English-speaking and non–Spanish-speaking families obtain help in translating the materials. In addition, after families express a major concern about the multiple injections required to keep their babies fully immunized and their babies' resultant distress and crying, a "calming strategies" flyer is developed.

Because financial barriers still exist among parents seeking immunizations for their children, the healthy community nurses implement several additional strategies. First, they work with physicians and help them enroll in the Vaccines for Children program, making vaccines available at no cost. They also work with the staff in physicians' offices to enhance their role in fostering childhood immunizations. In addition, they work with the health department to provide monthly immunizations onsite at the hospital.

Overcoming the Barrier of Institutional Racism in Health Care

Prejudice, racism, stereotyping, and ethnocentrism are present in health care settings. **Institutional racism**, sometimes referred to as institutionalized racism, is defined as differential access to goods, services, and opportunities based on race (Peek et al., 2010); this includes differential access to health insurance. The dominant subgroup is often ignorant of its own privilege. For example, services may be organized for the convenience of providers, and providers may be unaware that inconvenient hours or locations are affecting the community members who seek services. In contrast to individual behaviors, institutional racism occurs when systematic policies and practices disadvantage certain racial or ethnic groups. Institutions may be overtly racist, as when they specifically exclude certain groups from service. More often, however, institutions are unintentionally racist. For example, a dress code that requires everyone to wear the same hat would institutionally discriminate against Sikh men, who are expected to wear turbans, and Muslim women, who wear the hijab or veil. Institutions do not necessarily adopt such policies with the intention of discriminating and often revise their practice once the discrimination is identified.

Institutional racism has been well documented in US health care (Clark, 2003; Feagin & Bennefield, 2014; Metzl & Hansen, 2014) and is a major contributor to the growing health inequities between the richest and poorest Americans (Krisberg, 2017). Institutional racism is also an international concern. In England, institutional racism is defined as "the collective failure of an organisation to provide an appropriate and professional service to people because of their colour, culture, or ethnic origin" (McKenzie & Bhui, 2007, p. 649). Differences in the treatment of mental illness have been documented in England and Wales (McKenzie & Bhui, 2007). Reports in Sweden and the United Kingdom suggest continued concerns about discrimination and inequity in services (Bhopal, 2007). Contributing factors include the actions of individual staff members and policies that are based on the needs of the ethnic majority population rather than considering the needs of minority populations (Bhopal, 2007). Henry, Houston, and Mooney (2004) suggest that health care in Australia is institutionally racist and that such racism represents one of the greatest barriers to improving the health of Aboriginal and Torres Strait Islander people. Examples include funding inequities, differences in performance criteria, and differences in treatment regimens.

Cultural differences and lack of knowledge create institutional racism, and indifference nurtures it. Cultural differences must be acknowledged and celebrated rather than denigrated (Henry et al., 2004). Metzl, Petty, and Olowojoba (2018) suggest using a structural competency framework to help health professionals understand how contextual factors such as racism shape health and illness. Health care organizations must be built upon the cultural values of the people they serve. The strategies outlined in this chapter and throughout this book are needed to overcome institutional racism and build culturally competent health care organizations.

Summary

As with individuals, the quest for organizational cultural competence is a continuous journey. There is always room for improvement. To be truly effective in improving patient care for all, health care services and social services must make an organizational commitment for cultural competence. Cultural competence cannot live in one or two nurses; it must be systemic. It must involve individuals at all levels of the organization: governance members, administrators, managers, providers, and support staff. In addition, an organization must have a mutually beneficial relationship with the community it serves to achieve cultural competence and must involve community members in its quest for cultural competence.

REVIEW QUESTIONS

1. What types of access, health care, and health outcome disparities exist nationally? In your community?
2. How does the culture of an organization affect the quality of care provided?
3. What tools or models are helpful for assessing organizational culture?
4. How does an organization's culture influence or affect its employees?
5. What specific areas must receive attention when building culturally competent health care organizations?

CRITICAL THINKING ACTIVITIES

1. An excellent way to understand a culturally competent organization is to assess the organizational culture using the "five A's" described in this chapter. With some of your classmates, evaluate the availability, accessibility, affordability, acceptability, and appropriateness of one health care organization. Discuss what actions could be taken by the organization to increase its cultural competency.

2. Use Leininger's (1991) theory of culture care diversity and universality to assess the culture of the same organization. Box 9-6 in this chapter provides an example of how Leininger's culture care model can be used. Compare and contrast the values and beliefs of the organization with the values and beliefs of the groups using the health care organization's services. What areas would be most problematic, and why?

3. Many individuals use the emergency departments (EDs) of city hospitals for episodic care. Visit a busy ED. What languages do you hear? Assess the physical environment to determine potential barriers to culturally competent care. Develop a flow chart that outlines the steps a client takes when he or she seeks care in an emergency room. Identify changes that would decrease barriers and improve services if they were implemented.

REFERENCES

Agency for Healthcare Research and Quality. (2016). National Healthcare Quality and Disparities Report. https://www.ahrq.gov/research/findings/nhqrdr/nhqdr16/index.html

Agency for Healthcare Research and Quality. (2018a). 2016 National Healthcare Disparities Report. Retrieved May 15, 2018 from https://www.ahrq.gov/research/findings/nhqrdr/nhqdr16/index.html

Agency for Healthcare Research and Quality. (2018b). Race, ethnicity, and language data: Standardization for health care quality improvement. Retrieved May 30, 2018 from http://www.ahrq.gov/research/findings/final-reports/iomracereport/index.html

Alessandra, T. (2010). The platinum rule. Retrieved May 30, 2018 from http://www.alessandra.com/abouttony/aboutpr.asp

Alter, D. A., Stukel, T., Chong, A., & Henry, D. (2011). Lessons from Canada's Universal Care: Socially disadvantaged patients use more health services, still have poorer health. *Health Affairs*, 30(2), 274–283.

American Association of Colleges of Nursing. (2018). Diversity and inclusion. Retrieved May 15, 2018 from http://www.aacnnursing.org/Diversity

American Nurses Association. (2016). The nurse's role in ethics and human rights: Protecting and promoting individual worth, dignity, and human rights in practice settings. Retrieved May 15, 2018 from https://www.nursingworld.org/globalassets/docs/ana/nursesrole-ethicshuman-rights-positionstatement.pdf

American Nurses Association. (2018). Diversity awareness. Retrieved May 15, 2018 from https://www.nursingworld.org/practice-policy/innovation-evidence/clinical-practice-material/diversity-awareness/

American Nurses Credentialing Center. (2017). *2019 Magnet® application manual.* Silver Spring, MD: American Nurses Credentialing Center.

American Organization of Nurse Executives. (2011). AONE guiding principles for diversity in healthcare organizations. Retrieved May 15, 2018 from http://www.aone.org/resources/diversity.pdf

American Organization of Nurse Executives. (2015). Nurse executive competencies. Retrieved May 16, 2016 from http://www.aone.org/resources/nec.pdf

Andrews, M. M. (1998). A model for cultural change. *Nursing Management, 66,* 62–64.

Baldonado, A., Ludwig-Beymer, P., Barnes, K., Starsiak, D., Nemivant, E. B., & Anonas-Ternate, A. (1998). Transcultural nursing practice described by registered nurses and baccalaureate nursing students. *Journal of Transcultural Nursing, 9*(2), 15–25.

Bhopal, R. S. (2007). Racism in health and health care in Europe: Reality of mirage? *European Journal of Public Health, 17*(3), 238–241.

Bolman, L. G., & Deal, T. E. (2017). *Reframing organizations: Artistry, choice, and leadership* (6th ed.). Hoboken, NJ: Jossey-Bass.

Castillo, R. J., & Guo, K. L. (2011). A framework for cultural competence in health care organizations. *The Health Care Manager, 30*(3), 205–214.

Centers for Medicare and Medicaid Services. (2012). Cultural competence: A national health concern. Retrieved May 15, 2018 from https://www.cms.gov/Outreach-and-Education/Medicare-Learning-Network-MLN/MLNMattersArticles/downloads/SE0621.pdf

Chavez, C. I., & Weisinger, J. Y. (2008). Beyond diversity training: A social infusion for cultural inclusion. *Human Resource Management, 47*(2), 331–350.

Clark, P. A. (2003). Prejudice and the medical profession: Racism, sometimes overt, sometimes subtle, continues to plague U.S. health care. *Health Progress, 84*(5), 12–23.

Davis, R. N. (1997). Community caring: An ethnographic study within an organizational culture. *Public Health Nursing, 14*(2), 92–100.

Delphin-Rittmen, M. E. (2013). Seven essential strategies for promoting and sustaining systemic cultural competence. *Psychiatric Quarterly, 84*(1), 53–64.

Douglas, M. K., Rosenkoetter, M., Pacquiao, D., Callister, L. C., Hattar-Pollara, M., Lauderdale, J., ..., Purnell, L. (2014). Guidelines for implementing culturally competent nursing care. *Journal of Transcultural Nursing, 25*(2), 109–121.

Feagin, J., & Bennefield, Z. (2014). Systemic racism and U.S. health care. *Social Science & Medicine, 103,* 7–14.

Flaskerud, J. H. (2007). Cultural competence: What effect on reducing health disparities? *Issues in Mental Health Nursing, 28,* 431–434.

Fung, K., Srivastava, R., & Andermann, L. (2012). Organizational cultural competence consultation to a mental health institution. *Transcultural Psychiatry, 49*(2), 165–184.

Gomez, S. L., Le, G. M., West, D. W., Santariano, W. A., & O'Connor, L. (2003). Hospital policy and practice regarding the collection of data on race, ethnicity, and birthplace. *Journal of Public Health, 93*(10), 1685–1688.

Greiner, A. C., & Knebel, E. (Eds.); Institute of Medicine. (2003). *Health professionals education: A bridge to quality.* Washington, DC: The National Academies Press.

Guerrero, E. (2012). Organizational characteristics that foster early adoption of cultural and linguistic competence in outpatient substance abuse treatment in the United States. *Evaluation and Program Planning, 35*(1), 9–15.

Guerrero, E. G. (2013). Organizational structure, leadership and readiness for change and the implementation of organizational cultural competence in addiction services. *Evaluation and Program Planning, 40,* 74–81.

Hasnain-Wynia, R., Pierce, D., & Pittman, M. A. (2004). *Who, when, and how: The current state of race, ethnicity, and primary language data collection in hospitals.* The Commonwealth Fund and the American Hospital Association's Health Research and Educational Trust. Retrieved May 30, 2018 from http://www.commonwealthfund.org/usr_doc/hasnain-wynia_whowhenhow_726.pdf

Henry, B. R., Houston, S., & Mooney, G. H. (2004). Institutional racism in Australian healthcare: A plea for decency. *Medical Journal of Australia, 180*(10), 517–520.

Institute of Medicine. (2002). *Unequal treatment: Confronting racial and ethnic disparities in health care.* Washington, DC: National Academies Press.

Joint Commission. (2018). Health equity. Retrieved May 15, 2018 from https://www.jointcommission.org/topics/health_equity.aspx

Joint Commission Resources. (2018). The Joint Commission Edition. Retrieved May 21, 2018 from https://e-dition.jcrinc.com/MainContent.aspx

Koch, T., & Kralik, D. (2006). *Participatory action research in health care.* Oxford: Wiley-Blackwell.

Kouri, D. (2012). *Reducing health disparities: How can the structure of the health system contribute?* Wellesley Institute. Retrieved May 30, 2018 from http://www.wellesleyinstitute.com/wp-content/uploads/2012/09/Reducing-Health-Disparities-how-can-health-system-structure-contribute.pdf

Krisberg, K. (2017). Economic, social inequities growing between richest, poorest Americans. *The Nation's Health, 47*(4), 6.

Lasch, K. E., Wilkes, G., Montuori, L. M., Chew, P., Leonard, C., & Hilton, S. (2000). Using focus group methods to develop multicultural cancer pain education materials. *Pain Management Nursing, 1*(4), 129–138.

Leininger, M. (1991). *Culture care diversity and universality: A theory of nursing care.* New York, NY: National League for Nursing Press.

Leininger, M. (1996). Founder's focus: Transcultural nursing administration: An imperative worldwide. *Journal of Transcultural Nursing, 8*(1), 28–33.

Ludwig-Beymer, P., Blankemeier, J.R., Casas-Byots, C., & Suarez-Balcazar, Y. (1996). Community assessment in a suburban hispanic community: A description of methods. *Journal of Transcultural Nursing, 8*(1), 19–27.

Malone, B. L. (1997). Improving organizational cultural competence. In J. A. Dienemann (Ed.), *Cultural diversity in nursing: Issues, strategies, and outcomes.* Washington, DC: American Academy of Nursing.

Marrone, S. R. (2010). Organizational cultural competency. In M. Douglas & D. Pacquiao (Eds.), *Core curriculum in transcultural nursing and health care*. Thousand Oaks, CA: Sage.

McClure, M. L., Poulin, M. A., Sovie, M. D., & Wandelt, M. A.; for the American Academy Task Force on Nursing Practice in Hospitals. (1983). *Magnet hospitals. Attraction and retention of professional nurses*. Kansas City, MO: American Nurses Association.

McKenzie, K., & Bhui, K. (2007). Institutional racism in mental health care. *BMJ, 334*(7595), 649–650.

Metzl, J. M. & Hansen, H. (2014). Structural competency: Theorizing a new medical engagement with stigma and inequality. *Social Science & Medicine, 103*, 126–133.

Metzl, J. M., Petty, J., & Olowojoba, O. V. (2018). Using a structural competency framework to teach structural racism in pre-health education. *Social Science & Medicine, 11*, 189–201.

Napoles-Springer, A. M., Santoyo, J., Houston, K., Perez-Stable, E. J., & Stewart, A. L. (2005). Patients' perceptions of cultural factors affecting the quality of their medical encounters. *Health Expectations, 8*, 4–17.

National Center on Minority Health and Disparities. (2018). Funding opportunities. Retrieved May 30, 2018 from https://www.nimhd.nih.gov/funding/

National Council on Interpreting in Health Care. (2005). National standards of practice for interpreters in health care. Retrieved May 30, 2018 from https://www.aamc.org/download/70338/data/interpreter-guidelines.pdf

Office of Disease Prevention and Health Promotion. (2018). Healthy people 2020. Retrieved May 15, 2018 from https://www.healthypeople.gov/

Office of Minority Health, Department of Health and Human Services. (2016a). The National CLAS standards. Retrieved May 15, 2018 from https://minorityhealth.hhs.gov/omh/browse.aspx?lvl=2&lvlid=53

Office of Minority Health, Department of Health and Human Services. (2016b). Retrieved May 15, 2018 from https://minorityhealth.hhs.gov/omh/browse.aspx?lvl=2&lvlid=53

Office of Minority Health, Department of Health and Human Services. (2017). Cultural and linguistic competency. Retrieved May 15, 2018 from https://minorityhealth.hhs.gov/omh/browse.aspx?lvl=1&lvlid=6

Park, E. R., Betancourts, J. R., Kim, M. K., Maina, A. W., Blumenthal, D., & Weissman, J. S. (2005). Mixed messages: Residents' experiences learning cross-cultural care. *Academic Medicine, 80*(9), 874–880.

Peek, M. S., Odoms-Young, A., Quinn, M. T., Gorawara-Bhat, R., Wilson, S. C., & Chin, M. H. (2010). Racism in healthcare: Its relationship to shared decision-making and health disparities. *Social Science & Medicine, 71*(1), 13–17.

Pelfrey, S., & Theisen, B. A. (1993). Valuing the community benefits provided by nonprofit hospitals. *Journal of Nursing Administration, 23*(6), 16–21.

Pina, I. L., Cohen, P. D., Larson, D. B., Marion, L. N., Sills, M. R., Solberg, L. I. & Zerzan, J. (2015). A framework for describing health care delivery organizations and systems. *American Journal of Public Health, 105*(4), 670–679.

Purnell, L., Davidhizar, R. E., Giger, J. N., Strickland, O. L., Fishman, D., & Allison, D. M. (2011). A guide to developing a culturally competent organization. *Journal of Transcultural Nursing, 22*(1), 7–14.

QSEN. (2018). Quality and safety education for nurses. Retrieved May 15, 2018 from http://qsen.org/

Reese, D. J. (2011). Proposal for a university-community-hospice partnership to address organizational barriers to cultural competence. *The American Journal of Hospital & Palliative Care, 28*(1), 22–26.

Regenstein, M., & Sickler, D. (2006). *Race, ethnicity, and language of patients*. National Public Health and Hospital Institute. Retrieved May 30, 2018 from https://publichealth.gwu.edu/departments/healthpolicy/DHP_Publications/pub_uploads/dhpPublication_3BD811C8-5056-9D20-3D8EFC1026A1B8A5.pdf

Roizner, M. (1996). *A practical guide for the assessment of cultural competence in children's mental health organizations*. Boston, MA: Judge Baker's Children's Center.

Schaffner, J. W., & Ludwig-Beymer, P. (2003). *Rx for the nursing shortage*. Chicago, IL: Health Administration Press.

Schein, E. H. (2016). *Organizational culture and leadership* (5th ed.). Hoboken, NJ: Jossey-Bass.

Sherrod, D. (2013). Ask, listen, respect. *Nursing Management, 44*(11), 6.

Statistics Canada. (2018). Life expectancy, 2017. Retrieved May 15, 2018 from www.statcan.gc.ca/pub/89-645-x/2010001/life-expectancy-esperance-vie-eng.htm

Strasser, D. C., Smits, S. J., Falconer, J. A., Herrin, J. S., & Bowen, S. E. (2002). The influence of hospital culture on rehabilitation team functioning in VA hospitals. *Journal of Rehabilitation Research and Development, 39*(1), 115–125.

Transcultural Nursing Society. (2018). Transcultural Nursing Society Mission. Retrieved May 15, 2018 from https://tcns.org/

U.S. Census. (2017). Income and poverty in the United States: 2016. Retrieved May 15, 2018 from https://www.census.gov/library/publications/2017/demo/p60-259.html

U.S. Department of Health and Human Services, Centers for Disease Control and Prevention, National Center for Health Statistics. (2017). Health, United States, 2016. Retrieved May 15, 2018 from https://www.cdc.gov/nchs/data/hus/hus16.pdf#015

Weech-Maldonado, R., Drecahskin, J.L., Epane, J.P., Gail, J., Gupta, S. & Wainio, J.A. (2018). Hospital cultural competency as a systematic organizational intervention: Key findings from the national center for healthcare leadership diversity demonstration project. *Health Care Management Review, 43*(1), 30–41.

Weech-Maldonado, R., Dreachslin, J. L., Brown, J., Pradhan, R., Rubin, K. L., Schiller, C., & Hays, R. D. (2012). Cultural competency assessment tool for hospitals: Evaluating hospitals' adherence to the culturally and linguistically appropriate services standards. *Health Care Management Review, 37*(1), 54–66.

Weech-Maldonado, R., Elliott, M. N., Pradhan, R., Schiller, C., Dreachslin, J., & Hays, R. D. (2012). Moving toward culturally competent health systems: Organizational and market factors. *Social Science & Medicine, 75*(5), 815–822.

Weech-Maldonado, R., Elliott, M., Pradhan, R., Schiller, C., Hall, A., & Hays, R. D. (2012). Can hospital cultural competency reduce disparities in patient experiences with care? *Medical Care, 50,* S48–S55.

Weissman, J. S., Betancourt, J. R., Campbell, E. G., Park, E. R., Kim, M., Clarridge, B., & Maina, A. W. (2005). Resident

physicians' preparedness to provide cross-cultural care. *Journal of the American Medical Association, 294*(9), 1058–1067.

Wilson, A. H., Sanner, S. J., & McAllister, L. E. (2003). The Honor Society of Nursing, Sigma Theta Tau International Diversity Paper. Retrieved May 15, 2018 from https://www.sigmanursing.org/docs/default-source/position-papers/diversity_paper.pdf?sfvrsn=4

Youdelman, M., & Perkins, J. (2005). *Providing language services in small health care provider settings: Examples from the field.* The Commonwealth Fund. Retrieved May 30, 2018 from http://www.commonwealthfund.org/usr_doc/810_Youdelman_providing_language_services.pdf

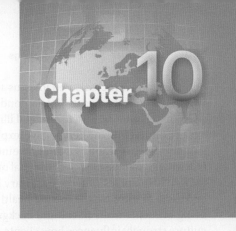

Chapter 10

Transcultural Perspectives in Mental Health Nursing

• Joanne T. Ehrmin

Key Terms

Cultural blindness
Cultural blind spot

Cultural norms
Cultural pain
Culture shock
Disenfranchised grieving

Historical trauma
Historical unresolved grief
Interpersonal communication
Mental health

Learning Objectives

1. Recognize the importance of cultural values, beliefs, and practices when planning and implementing mental health nursing care.
2. Examine best practice mental health treatment options in caring for clients from culturally diverse backgrounds.
3. Analyze the influence of culture on decisions about mental health care.
4. Evaluate strategies to provide competent transcultural mental health nursing care.
5. Recognize the importance of evidence-based transcultural mental health nursing research in caring for clients seeking mental health care in a culturally congruent and competent manner.

Mental health and mental illness are described as two extreme positions on a continuum, with many varying degrees between mental health and mental illness. For example, dealing with the loss of a job or the grief over losing a loved one versus having a severe mental illness, such as schizophrenia or depression, may all fall at varying degrees on the continuum. Mental health problems include emotional, psychological, and social well-being, affecting how individuals think, feel, and act. Mental health determines how we handle stress in our lives, how we interact with

others, and the choices we make. Mental health is important throughout our life span, from childhood through adulthood (Mental Health.gov, Retrieved May 5, 2018).

In 2016, the Surgeon General, Vivek Murthy, identified mental health as a "top priority." He identified nutrition and exercise as "critical pillars," to wellness, but further identified mental health as the third critical pillar. Murthy stated, "Emotional well-being is more than the absence of a mental illness, it's that resource within each of us that allows us to reach ever closer to our full potential, and which also enables us to be resilient in the face of adversity" (Diamond, 2016).

In this chapter, we discuss mental illness within a transcultural nursing perspective, exploring how culture influences the way in which we interpret and behave with mental illnesses. The goal of this chapter is to help nurses gain the necessary knowledge and skills to improve the mental health and well-being of clients from all cultural backgrounds. As culture strongly influences how clients experience illness, and culture is the framework for the interpretation of that experience, transcultural mental health nursing knowledge is integral for culturally competent mental health care. According to the American Psychiatric Association, Diagnostic & Statistical Manual of Mental Disorders-V (DSM-5) (2013), mental disorders are defined according to "cultural, social, and familial norms and values" (p. 14). Furthermore, culture provides the framework that is used to interpret "the experience and expression of the symptoms, signs, and behaviors that are criteria for diagnosis" (p. 14).

The concept of **cultural norms** is relevant to transcultural mental health nursing because the client's culture shapes what is considered normal and, by default, what is considered abnormal. Cultural norms are patterns, values, meanings, expressions, beliefs, practices, and experiences that are typical of specific cultural groups. Such norms are learned and passed down by family, friends, communities, and other members of the cultural group. Figure 10-1 is an American Indian "Feather Cleansing Ceremony" passed down from one generation to the next. Given the broad influence of culture, culture and mental health care are described as intricately related and dependent on one another. In fact, there is growing evidence that culture influences perceptions and attitudes with respect to mental illness (Heim, Wegmann, & Maercker, 2017).

Defining Mental Health Within a Transcultural Nursing Perspective

The World Health Organization (WHO) indicates that "over 450 million people suffer from mental disorders." WHO further postulates, "Mental

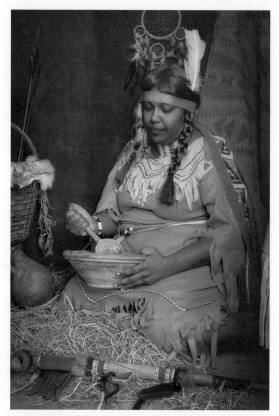

Figure 10-1. A ceremony is conducted to cleanse eagle feathers to honor the specific American Indian Tribe. The cleansing ceremony promotes cultural awareness and demonstrates honoring the life of the members of the Tribe and the spirit of the eagle. This is intended to provide blessings and strength for the people (Anneka/Shutterstock.com).

health is an integral and essential component of health." WHO includes mental well-being in their definition of health: "Health is a state of complete physical, mental, and social well-being and not merely the absence of disease or infirmity." Included in this definition is the implication that "mental health is more than the absence of mental disorders or disabilities" (Retrieved May 5, 2018). WHO further specifies that **mental health** is "a state of well-being in which the individual realizes his or her own abilities, can cope with the normal stresses of life, can work productively and fruitfully, and is able to make a contribution to his or her community" and that this understanding of mental health can be interpreted "across cultures" (p. 1). WHO further elaborates that "An environment that respects and protects basic civil, political, socioeconomic, and cultural rights is fundamental to mental health. Without the security and freedom provided by these rights, it is difficult to maintain a high level of mental health" (WHO, Retrieved May 5, 2018). Included in the WHO determinants of mental health are social, psychological, and biological factors. Some of the social/psychological factors include persistent poverty, risks of violence and human rights violations, gender discrimination, and social exclusion. Evidence indicates that the clearest evidence is associated with sexual violence (WHO, 2018a). There are also biological factors, including chemical imbalances.

The WHO (2018b) states, "Mental health is an integral part of health; indeed, there is no health without mental health." WHO's (2018a) work to improve the mental health of individuals and society at large involves improving psychological well-being, which may also involve facilitating an environment to support mental health. Some of the specific ways to promote mental health include: early childhood interventions, socio-economic support of women, programs targeting vulnerable populations, and mental health interventions in schools and work settings, reducing poverty and providing opportunities and care for individuals with mental disorders." (Retrieved May 5, 2018). WHO (2018a) developed a *Comprehensive Mental Health Action Plan for 2013–2020* to focus international attention on mental health as a neglected issue and as a human rights issue. The action plan calls for a change "in the attitudes that perpetuate stigma and discrimination that have isolated people since ancient times" (Retrieved May 5, 2018). It also calls for an increase in services to encourage efficient use of resources. The four major objectives of the action plan are to (1) strengthen effective leadership and governance for mental health; (2) provide comprehensive, integrated, and responsive mental health and social care services in community-based settings; (3)

implement strategies for promotion and prevention in mental health; and (4) strengthen information systems, evidence, and research for mental health.

According to the National Institute of Mental Health (NIMH) (2018), "depression is one of the most common mental disorders in the United States. Current research suggests that depression is caused by a combination of genetic, biological, environmental, and psychological factors" (see Evidence-Based Practice 10-1) (Retrieved March 12, 2018). According to the National Alliance on Mental Illness (NAMI) (2018), mental illness is a condition that "disrupts a person's thinking, feeling, mood, ability to relate to others, and daily functioning." NAMI identifies some of the most serious mental illnesses (SMIs). These include "major depression, schizophrenia, bipolar disorder, obsessive compulsive disorder (OCD), panic disorder, posttraumatic stress disorder (PTSD), and borderline personality disorder." NAMI further identifies that generally, a mental health condition is a result not of a single event but of multiple, linking causes. Genetics, environment, and lifestyle all play a role in an individual developing a mental health condition. Stress in a client's job or home life and traumatic life events, such as being a victim of a crime, can also play an influential role. Biochemical processes and circuits and basic brain structure may also play a role (Retrieved April 10, 2018).

Leininger (Leininger, 1991a; Leininger & McFarland, 2002; McFarland & Wehbe-Alamah, 2015) theorized the importance of identifying what is common and universal among cultures, while at the same time understanding there is individual diversity within cultures. Diversity for transcultural mental health nurses encompasses not only culture and ethnicity but also gender, sexual orientation, socioeconomic status, age, physical abilities or disabilities, religious beliefs, and political beliefs or other ideologies (see Figure 10-2).

Gaining a better understanding and more in-depth knowledge base of patterns of values, beliefs,

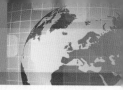

Depressive Disorders Interpreted Within a Cultural Context

According to the World Health Organization (WHO), depression is one of the most common mental disorders and the leading cause of disability worldwide. "Globally, more than 300 million people of all ages suffer from depression." Depression is not the same as usual mood fluctuations that are short in duration and in response to challenges of everyday life (Retrieved May 5, 2018). Similarly, the U.S. Office of Disease Prevention and Health Promotion, in the Healthy People 2020 report, identified that depressive disorders have been categorized as major, persistent, premenstrual, substance/medication-induced, depressive disorder R/T another health condition, other specified, and unspecified (Retrieved May 10, 2018). The American Psychiatric Association Common symptoms among the depressive disorders are "presence of sad, empty, or irritable mood, accompanied by somatic and cognitive changes" (DSM-5, 2013, p. 155) that significantly affect the individual's ability to carry out functions of daily living. What varies among the depressive disorders are "duration, timing, or presumed etiology" (DSM-5, 2013, p. 155).

Culture plays a central role in mental health care disparities among minority populations. Yet, cultural specific factors have not been a focus when assessing engagement in mental health services by diverse cultural groups. Yasui, Pottick, and Chen (2017) conducted a systematic review of the literature in order to develop the culturally infused engagement (CIE) model to focus on the role of cultural values, beliefs, and practices with engagement in mental health services by minority and immigrant children and families. This could help to identify diverse cultural groups' identification of somatic symptoms for mental health illnesses, such as depression. Somatic expressions of psychological symptoms are more common among Asian, Latino, and African Americans when compared to European Americans. The authors identified that the CIE model may help clinicians to consider that mainstream notions of depression may not

be understood by a minority client complaining of distress. This could help the clinician to better focus on the client's conceptualizations of distress rather than the DSM-5–specific criteria for diagnosing depression.

Abuelezam and Fontenot (2017) identified the current difficult political climate for Arab populations, which may be exacerbating mental health issues and decreasing the desire to seek mental health care. It is important for nurses to advocate for mental health screening, including screening for depression, intimate partner violence for Arab women, and other mental health needs of this "at-risk" population.

How depression is identified, treated, and talked about is frequently connected to one's cultural values, beliefs, and practices. For example, the cultural value of collectivism prioritizes cohesiveness of the cultural group over self. Xue-Ling Chang, Jetten, Cruwys, and Haslam (2017) identified Chinese individuals who strongly endorse that collectivism norms are more likely to somaticize depression more than in the West. For example, Chinese people may talk about having difficulty sleeping, feeling tired, and experiencing poor appetite rather than talk about feeling overwhelming sadness, low sense of self-worth, and feelings of depression.

Clinical Implications

It is important for nurses to understand that both past and present life experiences are interpreted through the lens of deeply held cultural, religious, and spiritual beliefs. Cultural beliefs, values, practices, and experiences grounded in one's culture need to be explored by practitioners in order to better understand a patient's symptoms, their perspective about their illness, and expected outcomes of treatment for depression. When health care providers lack an understanding of the diverse

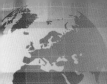

Depressive Disorders Interpreted Within a Cultural Context (continued)

cultural groups for whom they provide care, failure to accurately diagnose an individual with the correct diagnosis increases.

References: Abuelezam, N. N., & Fontenot, H. B. (2017). Depression among Arab American and Arab Immigrant women in the United States. *AWHONN, 21*(5), 395–399.

American Psychiatric Association. (2013). *Diagnostic and Statistical Manual of Mental Disorders, DSM-5* (5th ed.). Washington, DC: Author.

U.S. Office of Disease Prevention and Health Promotion, Healthy People 2020. (2015). Mental health and mental disorders. Retrieved May 10, 2018 from https://www.healthypeople.

gov/2020/topics-objectives/topic/mental-health-and-mental-disorders

World Health Organization. (2018a). Fact sheet N369. Retrieved April 4, 2018 from http://www.who.int/mediacentre/factsheets/fs369/en/

World Health Organization. (2018b). Retrieved May 5, 2018 from http://www.who.int/mediacentre/factsheets/fs220/en/

Xue-Ling Chang, M., Jetten, J., Cruwys, T., & Haslam, C. (2017). Cultural identity and the expression of depression: A social identity perspective. *Journal of Community & Applied Social Psychology, 27*, 16–34.

Yasui, M., Pottick, K. J., & Chen, Y. (2017). Conceptualizing culturally infused engagement and its measurement for ethnic minority and immigrant children and families. *Clinical Child Family Psychology Review, 20*, 250–332.

and practices for mental health care can be used as one "tool" in caring for clients, families, and communities from diverse cultural groups. This is different from simplistic overgeneralizations that can lead to stereotyping a particular culture. Cardwell, in 1996, identified stereotyping as a "fixed, overgeneralized belief about a particular group or class of people." Stereotypes can lead to

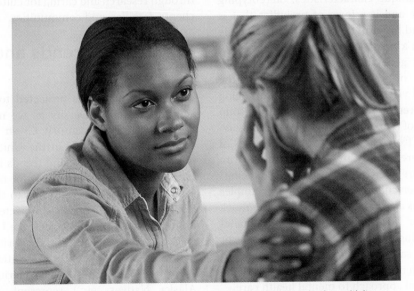

Figure 10-2. Transcultural nurses practice within a framework of sensitivity, knowledge, and skill to Promote health and care for individuals diagnosed with a mental illness in culturally congruent ways (Monkey Business Images/Shutterstock. com).

erroneous misrepresentations of diverse cultural groups, age groups, gender identity, etc.

Stereotypes can be used as an underlying rationale to distort mental illness symptoms and misdiagnose culturally diverse individuals, families, and communities. Stereotypes can also serve to exploit culturally diverse clients, particularly in the area of mental health care, where differences in group norms can sometimes be used to inappropriately label clients with a mental health diagnosis. According to a supplement by the Surgeon General, racism and discrimination are "umbrella terms referring to beliefs, attitudes, and practices that denigrate individuals or groups because of phenotypic characteristics (e.g., skin color and facial features) or ethnic group affiliation" (USDHHS, 1999, p. 38). It is important for mental health care providers to understand the impact minority clients may have experienced from prior stereotyping, racism, and discrimination when caring for their clients who seek mental health care services (Retrieved May 5, 2018).

Transcultural nurses do not promote stereotyping of clients, families, and communities because of unique characteristics. Stereotyping labels people and is a form of prejudice that is damaging and harmful to any recipient, let alone a client with a mental illness! Furthermore, stereotyping is generally inaccurate and is often based more on the individual expressing the stereotypical view than the cultural group being targeted. Stereotyping identifies a cultural group or members of that culture as identical and indistinguishable from each other. Some examples of common stereotyping are beliefs that African Americans are "better at sports" and "dancing" than are other cultural groups. Other examples of stereotypes are that Irish Americans are "quick tempered" or Turkish women are "belly dancers." Identifying people as all looking the same or thinking the same is stereotyping. Transcultural mental health nursing does not promote applying a stereotypical approach to mental health care.

Another concept that is important to consider in transcultural mental health nursing is ethnocentrism. "In its mildest form, ethnocentrism presents as subconscious disregard for cultural differences; in its most severe form, it presents as authoritarian" (Sutherland, 2002, p. 280). Ethnocentrism can manifest as feelings of superiority or discrimination with respect to one's own group or culture over another group or culture. For example, ethnocentrism can manifest as a belief that one's own religious beliefs are superior to another group or culture's religious beliefs and that one's own health care beliefs and practices are superior to another culture's health care beliefs and practices. US-educated health care professionals are frequently guilty of the latter ethnocentric assumption.

Many cultural groups have distinct patterns of values, beliefs, and practices that can be used as a basis for providing mental health care in a culturally congruent and competent manner. However, many individuals and families belonging to specific cultural groups may have more diverse mental health care needs than do those of the cultural group norm. The term "norm" is used to identify patterns of values, beliefs, and practices specific to mental health that have been identified through research and caring for culturally diverse clients, families, and communities.

Population Trends and Mental Health

The US population is projected to increase in age and cultural diversity as we move toward the middle of the century. Given the increasing numbers of elderly in the United States, it is important to understand trends in utilization of mental health care services for older populations of all cultures. According to the 2010 U.S. Census, the United States is projected to become a more diverse nation. In fact, the United States is expected to become a "majority–minority" nation by 2043. Currently, minorities (Hispanic, African American, Asian, American Indians, Alaska Natives, etc.) represent 37% of the US population and are expected to represent 57% of the population in the United States by 2060. The implications and need for educated transcultural mental health nurses are immense (Retrieved April 10, 2018).

According to NIMH, mental illnesses are identified as "common" in the United States. Approximately 44.7 million adults (approximately one in six of all adults in the United States), aged 18 or older, lives with a mental illness. In 2016, approximately 19.2 million adults received mental health treatment in that year. More women than men received treatment. Conditions vary in degree ranging from mild to moderate to severe. An SMI is defined as a "mental, behavioral, or emotional disorder resulting in serious functional impairment, which substantially interferes with or limits one or more major life activities." SMI is higher among women (5.3%) than men (3.0%), but young adults aged 18 to 25 years had the highest prevalence of SMI (5.9%) (NIMH, Retrieved March 12, 2018).

According to National Alliance on Mental Illness (NAMI) (2017) multicultural disparities in mental health is a continuing challenge in the United states. As the cultural demographics in the United States continues toward a more diverse, multicultural population, creating an equal, culturally competent mental health service for all remains a challenge. It was identified that European Americans see mental illness more in terms of biomedical basis, whereas Latino and African American cultures focus more on spirituality, moral character, and social rationale for mental illness. European Americans seek mental health care more frequently than do Latino or African American people. There is evidence of underutilization of mental health services by many minority groups. Minority populations tend to wait until symptoms are severe before seeking professional help (Retrieved March 12, 2018). Although mental health nurses care for clients of all age groups and all cultural groups, the current and future trends in population projections do have major implications for transcultural nursing and mental health services in the United States.

The institutionalized view of mental health care as portrayed in the movie "One Flew Over the Cuckoo's Nest" (1975) is no longer the norm for care today. Increasingly, mental health care is moving from state and general "mental" hospitals to community-based service centers. The U.S. Department of Health and Human Services' Center for Mental Health Services (CMHS) is the Federal agency within the U.S. Substance Abuse and Mental Health Services Administration (SAMHSA) charged with improving prevention and mental health treatment services in the United States. SAMHSA offers "Hotline" or "Lifeline" services for people in need to call in to professionals for help. According to SAMHSA's National Survey on Drug Use and Health (2014), approximately 43.6 million Americans 18 and older experienced some form of mental illness. In the past year (2017), 20.2 million adults had a substance use disorder. Of these, almost 8 million people had both a mental and substance use disorder, known as "co-occurring mental and substance use disorders" (SAMHSA, Retrieved May 14, 2018).

According to a television and radio series about "Recovery Among Diverse Populations," Limited English Proficiency (LEP), geographic location, and lack of health insurance are identified as reasons immigrants, cultural minorities, individuals of low socioeconomic status, and people living in rural communities frequently face problems accessing health care in general, and mental health care in particular. For the year 2015, Asians and Hispanics have significantly lower percentages of receiving mental health services (5.0% and 8.1%), respectively, compared to the national average of 14.2%. These statistics can help to guide the direction nursing will take in meeting the needs of mental health clients in the future (SAMHSA, 2017, Retrieved May 14, 2018).

Decision-Making and Mental Health Care

Consumers of mental health care (clients, families and significant others, and communities) are more knowledgeable now than they have ever been in the past. With the advent of the Internet, mental health care information is more widely available to those seeking knowledge. Continuous news broadcasts offer health care information to both consumers and professionals alike. National and international news and research breakthroughs are increasingly available to consumers, almost as soon as they are available to professionals. In addition, our society is more open to talking about mental health conditions, such as depression and bipolar disorder, in ways that would have been unthinkable just two decades ago.

Clients, families, and significant others want an active role in decision-making about their mental health care, and they use numerous resources to make those decisions. Mental health clients, particularly, can become agitated when their voice is not heard or taken into consideration with regard to treatment decisions. For culturally diverse clients with mental health care needs, and diverse values, beliefs, and practices that may not be understood by health care providers, this can be even more frustrating and can lead to misunderstandings on both sides. Clients may feel misunderstood and isolated in a health care system that can seem cold, frightening, rigid, and controlling.

Offering support and clear communication can be key to bringing about favorable outcomes for all clients, but it can be particularly challenging with clients, families, and significant others from diverse cultural groups seeking mental health care. In a study conducted by Eliacin, Slayers, Kukla, and Matthias (2015), shared decision-making (SDM) was found to be an important component of patient-centered care with positive outcomes. It was also identified that in addition to the collaboration between provider and patients in managing decisions, significant others need to be involved in the collaborative partnership in managing decisions. Challenges to the effectiveness of SDM included gender and culture. It was identified that it is crucial to focus on cultural competence in practice a gender and culture "are important building blocks for open communication, the development of meaningful patient–provider relationships, and person-centered care" (p. 676).

It has become important for mental health care professionals to attempt to include clients and family members in care decisions. At times, this can be problematic for mental health care providers, particularly if the mental health status of the client is considered to be questionable in making critical personal decisions regarding his or her own care. Consumer treatment input can also seem a daunting task for those care providers who have based practice decisions on a strictly authoritarian framework. Understanding and taking into account the client's values, beliefs, and practices is crucial to ensuring favorable outcomes. Evidence-based or "best" practice options can be discussed with clients and family members who are able to participate in care decisions. However, the ultimate decision lies with clients, their family, or significant others or relatives. It is important for nurses to assess the knowledge level of their clients, family members, and/or significant others regarding the client's status and care the client is receiving. Try to include the client in decisions affecting his or her care whenever possible.

Disparities in Mental Health Care

Reducing and eliminating disparities in health care has been a focus of numerous initiatives in recent years. The U.S. Office of Disease Prevention and Health Promotion, in the Healthy People 2010 report (Retrieved May 10, 2018), identified mental disorders as one of the most common causes of disability and further identified that one of the main goals was to "improve mental health through prevention and by ensuring access to appropriate, quality mental health services." The American Psychological Association (APA) called for reform in disparities in mental health status and care. APA identified that mental health is frequently lacking for diverse minority communities. The Council on Minority Mental Health and Health Disparities identified. "The Council on Minority Mental Health and Health Disparities identified the importance of reducing mental health disparities in clinical services and research, which disproportionately affect women and minority populations. The council aims to promote the recruitment and development of psychiatrists from minority and underrepresented groups both within the profession and in APA" (Retrieved May 1, 2018).

In addition, concerns were raised about mental health symptoms that are "undiagnosed, underdiagnosed, or misdiagnosed for cultural, linguistic, or historical reasons."

Disparities in mental health treatment have existed from the earliest historical recordings. Those with behavior that was considered to be "abnormal" were thought to be "deranged" or "mad," and in many cases, they were sent to asylums, under the harshest of conditions, to live out the remainder of their lives. Psychiatric mental health nurses have been at the forefront in paving the way for the humane care and treatment of mental health clients, and, yet, mental health still remains wrought with disparities and stigma that do not exist for many other health conditions (see Evidence-Based Practice 10-2). According to a study conducted by Wu et al. (2017) on a group of college students who participated across the United States and completed the Healthy Minds Study, "stigma functions as one of the major barriers that prevent college students in need of mental health services from seeking professional help" (p. 490). The fear of stigma generally does not result in specific changes in behavior but more often leads people to hide specific behaviors or actions (Bharadwaj, Pai, & Suziedelyte, 2017). In the case of mental illness, this can lead individuals to refrain from seeking much-needed mental health services. Immigrant populations have been found to have difficulties seeking help for mental health care. A decreased understanding of mental health services and stigma surrounding mental illness have been identified as barriers to seeking help among Latino immigrants (Dueweke & Bridges, 2017).

The first Surgeon General's report on mental health identified disparities among diverse cultural groups in seeking and being treated for mental illness: "Even more than other areas of health and medicine, the mental health field is plagued by disparities in the availability of and access to its services. These disparities are viewed readily through the lens of racial and cultural diversity, age, and gender" (USDHHS, 1999, p. iv, Retrieved May 5, 2018). A major factor in mental health disparities, particularly for underrepresented and underserved cultural groups, was the deinstitutionalization of mental health care in the mid 20th century. Moving mental health clients from psychiatric state hospitals to community-based settings never fully materialized. Instead, individuals with mental health problems frequently ended up in emergency rooms for short-term treatment. Eventually, jails and prisons became the long-term placement for many individuals with mental health diagnoses (Safran et al., 2009). Incarcerated minority populations, particularly youth, face noteworthy health disparities that may be exacerbated by the health consequences of incarceration (Barnert, Perry, & Morris, 2016). Through a concerted effort to improve the mental health of some of the most socially vulnerable individuals in our country remains a priority for mental health care providers.

Historically, racism in America has led to difficulties in acknowledging and/or discussing differences in cultural values and lifeways for diverse cultural groups. Bell and Peterson (1992) indicated that slavery, segregation, and institutionalized racism have resulted in numerous problems faced by African Americans, resulting in what the authors labeled as *cultural pain*. **Cultural pain** is defined as feeling "insecure, embarrassed, angry, confused, torn, apologetic, uncertain, or inadequate because of conflicting expectations of and pressures from being a minority" (p. 8). Leininger (1995) identified cultural pain as "the suffering, discomfort, or unfavorable responses of an individual group toward an individual who has different beliefs or lifeways, usually reflecting the insensitivity of those inflicting the discomfort" (p. 67).

A number of diverse cultural groups have experienced what is called **historical trauma** (also referred to as **historical unresolved grief**, **disenfranchised grieving or intergenerational transmission of trauma**). Historical trauma was first identified to explain clinical findings of

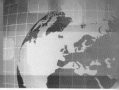

Overcoming Stigma for Those Seeking Mental Health Treatment

Unfortunately, mentally ill people have evoked adverse responses across various cultures, frequently leading to living with the mental illness, rather than seeking treatment, for fear of being labeled and rejected by society. Stigma is a word with Greek origins, which referred to a symbol cut or burnt into the body, and was used to signify something negative about the moral status of the individual. It was further identified that stigma could lead to a "spoiled identity" and "damaged sense of self" (Goffman, 1964, p. 116). Conner, Roker, McKinnon, Ward, and Brown (2018) identified that "stigma continues to be one of the most significant deterrents to professional mental health service utilization" (p. 2376).

Untoward consequences of mental illness, stigma, and discrimination can impact nearly every aspect of an individual's life, as well as the lives of their family and significant others. Bharadwaj et al. (2017) identified that the fear of stigma and social discrimination governs much of what we see in human behavior. This does not generally result in change in one's behavior but rather in simply hiding certain behaviors from others. The researchers found that patients diagnosed with a mental illness were significantly underreported when compared to physiological diagnoses. The researchers found that concerns about social discrimination may be related to intrinsic fears such as guilt, shame, self-image issues, etc. Furthermore, "in the absence of discrimination concerns, there is nothing to feel shameful/guilty about" (p. 60).

Given the importance of understanding stigma associated with mental illness, it is concerning that limited research has been conducted on this phenomenon. In a study by Han, Cha, Lee, and Lee, (2017) with Korean immigrant leaders living in the United states, primarily San Francisco for 11 to 49 years, the researchers wanted to understand different ways mental illness stigma was manifested in the Korean immigrant community in order to understand cultural norms and recommend educational prevention programs. Results found that Korean immigrants believed people with mental illness (PMI) were dangerous and abnormal. It was identified that "such a prevalent public stigma attached to mental illness may discourage sufferers from seeking help, to avoid being labeled a part of the stigmatized group" (p. 139). Fear of being stigmatized as a PMI can delay treatment until symptoms are more serious, such as developing psychotic symptoms that can lead to violent behaviors. This in turn reinforces the stigma associated with mental illness.

According to Tyson, Arriola, and Corvin (2016), Latino immigrants have a decreased rate of depression than do non-Latino Whites; however, they are also less likely to pursue professional mental health care. Interpersonal factors included a negative reaction with lack of support and understanding from family and friends including an unwillingness to help the individual seek mental health care. Intrapersonal factors included "not knowing where to go, fear, lack of acceptance, and stigma/shame" (p. 1294).

Haralambous et al. (2016) conducted a study on Chinese immigrants' experiences of depression and anxiety but chose to interview health professionals and community leaders rather than older Chinese immigrants directly, because there is such a strong stigma associated with mental health issues that older people would not feel comfortable discussing mental health issues. A major theme discovered in the study was stigma, which was related to the perception that mental illness was a result of character weakness. One participant stated, "Older Chinese people are reluctant/hesitate to admit that they suffer from depression or anxiety, because people with mental health problems are stigmatized. People would think them as crazy or mad persons and avoid contact with them" (p. 251). Older Chinese immigrants also suffered from feelings of shame, embarrassment, fear, and taboo. Again, fear of being stigmatized can result in individuals suffering with symptoms of depression and anxiety resulting in failure to seek help for treatable symptoms that could improve their quality of life.

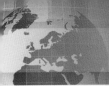

Overcoming Stigma for Those Seeking Mental Health Treatment (continued)

Clinical Implications

It is important for nurses and other health care providers caring for individuals, family members, and significant others to understand the impact of mental health stigma on the patient diagnosed with a mental illness. Understanding the stigma of mental illness can even influence the patient, family, and significant others' willingness to contact health care providers for treatment. If nurses are to help the patient deal with the untoward effects of stigma associated with mental illness, it is crucial that nurses get in touch with their own biases and negative attitudes about mental illness. It is also important for nurses to understand that the patient, family, and significant others may resist a mental illness diagnosis, based on the societal and specific cultural values, beliefs, and practices associated with mental illness. Peer discussions among nurses about personal and professional values, beliefs, and practices associated with mental illness could facilitate getting in touch with negative attitudes and beliefs about mental illness. Nurses can also participate in workshops and other educational experiences to improve their understanding of cultural values, beliefs, and practices related to mental illness in general and to specific mental illness diagnoses.

References: Bharadwaj, P., Pai, M. M., & Suziedelyte, A. (2017). Mental health stigma. *Economics Letters, 159,* 57–60.

Goffman, E. (1964). *Stigma.* London, UK: Penguin.

Han, M., Cha, R., Lee, H. A., & Lee, S. E. (2017). Mental-illness stigma among Korean Immigrants: Role of culture and destigmatization strategies. *Asian American Journal of Psychology, 8*(2), 134–141.

Haralambous, B., Dow, B., Goh, A., Pachana, N. A., Bryant, C., LoGiudice, D., & Lin, X. (2016). 'Depression is not an illness. It's up to you to make yourself happy': Perceptions of Chinese health professionals and community workers about older Chinese immigrants' experiences of depression and anxiety. *Australasian Journal on Ageing, 35*(4), 249–254.

Tyson, M. D., Arriola, N. B., & Corvin, J. (2016). Perceptions of depression and access to mental health care among Latino immigrants: Looking beyond one size fits all. *Qualitative Health Research, 26*(9), 1289–1302.

distress among Jewish Holocaust survivors and has since been used to explain suffering in various contexts in diverse cultural groups. Historical trauma is defined as mass trauma directed toward a group that shares an identity or affiliation and which has effects that transcend generational boundaries (Brave Heart, 1998; Brave Heart & DeBruyn, 1998). Evans-Campbell (2008) discussed historical trauma in Native American and Alaska Native communities and defined historical trauma as "a collective complex trauma inflicted on a group of people who share a specific group identity or affiliation—ethnicity, nationality, and religious affiliation. It is the legacy of numerous traumatic events a community experiences over generations" (p. 320). Cromer, Gray, Vasquez, and Freyd (2018) in a study with American Indians found "the more one identified with American Indian culture, the more he or she thought about historical losses, and the more one identified with White culture, the less he or she thought about historical losses" (2018).

Mental Health Care for Immigrants

Nurses have always cared for diverse populations of clients, and community-based nurses have focused in particular on newly arrived immigrant populations (see Figure 10-3). A century ago, nurses and other health professionals were concerned about contagious diseases and malnutrition in caring for immigrant populations. Currently, there is a great deal of research being conducted to better understand nursing care for culturally diverse immigrant clients and their

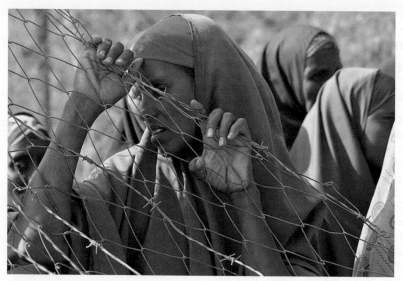

Figure 10-3. In addition to being uprooted or fleeing war-torn and impoverished living conditions in their home countries, many immigrants from diverse cultural groups suffer from mental health issues (hikrcn/Shutterstock.com).

family members who are seeking care. Many of these studies focus specifically on mental health care, particularly helping immigrant clients, families, and communities adjust to life in their new country. In addition, health care services for immigrant communities also place an emphasis on mental health, particularly since many recent immigrants have experienced war, displacement, and other associated traumas.

There has been extensive debate about immigration policy during the past several years in the United States as well as internationally. In the United States, the debate has become heated politically with political parties arguing the implications, from their standpoint, of immigration policies. Health care for those immigrants who are not in this country legally has also been extensively debated, again with both sides stating the merits of their views on whether such immigrants, or undocumented individuals, have a right to health care in this country. At the same time, however, there has been minimal understanding of these issues from the perspective of the undocumented immigrants and the impact immigration has on their mental health (see Evidence-Based Practice 10-3).

Use of the terms "illegal alien" and "illegal immigrant" is increasingly identified as "racially charged" and offensive terminology to describe "undocumented workers" or "undocumented immigrants." According to Dinan (2016), The Library of Congress Policy and Standards Division changed the term "Illegal Aliens" to "Noncitizen" and "Unauthorized Immigration" after thoroughly discussing the term "Alien." However, the House of Representatives in the U.S. Congress ordered The Library of Congress to continue using the term "illegal alien." Unfortunately, this seems to have turned into a legal debate (Retrieved May 12, 2018). According to the Central Broadcasting System (CBS) (2014), Supreme Court Justice Sonia Sotomayor, the first Hispanic Supreme Court Justice, uses the term "undocumented immigrants" rather than the term "illegal alien." Justice Sotomayor identified that "labeling immigrants criminals seemed insulting to her." She further stated, "I think people then paint those individuals as something less than worthy human beings and it changes the conversation." Illegal migration places immigrants in tenuous legal circumstances with limited rights and protections. In a study conducted on Deferred Action for

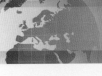

Mental Health Needs of the Immigrant Population

According to the U.S. Census Bureau (2018), "The foreign-born population includes anyone who was not a U.S. citizen or a U.S. national at birth. This includes respondents who indicated they were a U.S. citizen by naturalization or not a U.S. citizen." The percent of foreign-born persons for 2012 to 2016 was 13.2% (Retrieved April 5, 2018).

The immigrant population faces numerous challenges in seeking professional mental health care, including a lack of understanding of the mental health care, as well as access to care. Caballero et al. (2017) identified Latino children, either immigrants or the children of immigrants, are at high risk of developing mental health disorders related to increased poverty, exposure to trauma, assimilation stressors, and discrimination. In addition, Latino children are compromised by limited access to health care and failure to routinely screen the children for mental health disorders in primary care settings. Assimilation into the American culture may have a negative impact on mental health. The mental health needs of the immigrant population increase with the stresses encountered in learning the values, beliefs, and practices of a new culture. In addition, language and financial needs can limit the immigrant population from seeking adequate health care services, particularly mental health services.

According to Rojas-Flores, Clements, Koo, and London (2017), "The mental health impact of parental detention and deportation on citizen children is a topic of increasing concern. Forced parent–child separation and parental loss are potentially traumatic events (PTEs) with adverse effects on children's mental health" (p. 352). Given the current immigration climate in the United States, this is an area that mental health care providers will need to help parents and children work through for years to come. The researchers concluded, "These findings lend support to a reconsideration and revision of immigration enforcement practices to take into consideration the best interest of Latino citizen children. Trauma-informed assessments and interventions are recommended for this special population" (p. 352).

A major barrier that can impede an immigrant from seeking mental health care services is language. Immigrants may delay seeking mental health care based on fear of not being able to communicate or a fear of embarrassment about their language difficulties. Misdiagnoses may result from difficulties with communication and may impede appropriate mental health treatment. To help with the language barrier, Villalobos, Lynch, DeBlieck, and Summers (2017) proposed health care providers utilize a mobile technology app tool, such as the Canopy Translation App, to adequately assess the psychiatric symptoms of clients who spoke Spanish and had limited English proficiency. Participants identified the App as a resource that could help to decrease language barriers in health care. The App was able to translate questions into 15 languages. The Canopy Translation App did help to better interpret mental health symptoms described by Spanish-speaking participants. One drawback discovered in this study was that participants identified that using an App decreased the ability of health care professionals to have a very good therapeutic relationship with their patients.

Clinical Implications

Nurses and other health care providers caring for immigrant populations need to understand that the stress immigrants have undergone in moving to a new country. Given the numerous burdens to living in a foreign country and possibly having come from war-torn or other difficult situations in their own country, immigrants are at high risk for mental health disorders. Mental health care professionals need to empathize with the stressful experience immigrants have in reaching out to the health care system for themselves, their children, and/or significant others needing mental health care services. It is important to overcome the barrier language can have in accessing appropriate mental health treatments, based on accurate diagnoses. Villalobos et al. (2017) identified the importance of exploring new resources, including technologies, that can decrease language barriers and improve communication. Resources may

(continued)

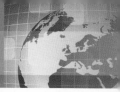

Mental Health Needs of the Immigrant Population (continued)

include tablets, computers and programs, interpreters, and professional translators. Adopting a lifelong learning philosophy for nurses and other mental health care providers, including continuing, to increase our professional cultural competence. Finally, it is important to understand the current political climate for immigrants in the United States today that places immigrants at higher risk for discrimination and could lead to deceased willingness or access to mental health care.

References: Caballero, T. M., DeCamp, L. R., Platt, R. E., Shah, H., Johnson, S. B., Sibinga, E. M., & Polk, S. (2017). Addressing the mental health needs of Latino children in immigrant families. *Clinical Pediatrics, 56*(7), 648–658.

Rojas-Flores, L., Clements, M. L., London, J., & Koo, J. H. (2017). Trauma and psychological distress in Latino citizen children following parental detention and deportation. *Psychological Trauma: Theory, Research, Practice, and Policy, 9*(3), 352–361.

U.S. Census Bureau. Foreign born persons, percent, 2012–2016. Retrieved April 5, 2018 from https://www.census.gov/quickfacts/fact/table/US/POP645216#viewtop

Villalobos, O., Lynch, S., DeBlieck, C., & Summers, L. (2017). Utilization of a mobile app to assess psychiatric patients with limited English proficiency. *Hispanic Journal of Behavioral Sciences, 39*(3), 369–380.

Childhood Arrivals (DACA) programs, despite an increase in sense of mental well-being when DACA participants felt less fear about their own temporary immigration status, mental health consequences persisted with increased concerns regarding fear of family member and significant others deportation risks (Siemons, Raymond-Flesh, Auerswald, & Brindis, 2017).

Setting aside the political debate, transcultural mental health nurses have cared for both documented and undocumented immigrants for many years and are increasingly caring for those immigrants who are feeling the emotional pressures of such a political climate. The term culture shock was coined by the anthropologist Kalervo Oberg (1960) to describe individuals, such as immigrants, who enter a new culture. Culture shock is "precipitated by the anxiety that results from losing all our familiar signs and symbols of social intercourse" (p. 177). Oberg suggested that the "signs" or "cues" that people use within a culture—such as the words people speak—customs people follow, and even nonverbal communication such as gestures and facial expressions are not recognized by those who are new to the culture. This leads to feelings of frustration and anxiety even in those persons who would be considered "mentally healthy." Imagine how these negative feelings would be confounded for an individual who has entered the country as an undocumented immigrant and fears arrest, detention, and deportation.

The concept of **acculturation** was initially defined by Redfield, Linton, and Herskovits (1936) as "those phenomena which result when groups of individuals having different cultures come into continuous first-hand contact, with subsequent changes in the original cultural patterns of either or both groups" (p. 149). Acculturation can be a stressful and complex process, particularly for immigrants who experience difficulty adjusting to the new culture.

In a study by Huq, Stein, and Gonzalez (2016), on Latino adolescents that differentiated general parent–child conflict as arguing in general and not specifically linked to culture; whereas, acculturation conflict was defined in the study as conflict specific to differences in cultural values between parents and their children. Latino cultural values were identified as placing a focus on strong family ties and harmonious relationships. Greater acculturation conflict with one's parents may lead to greater depressive symptoms as an adolescent may feel they are violating cultural norms and values, thereby, disappointing the family. Findings indicated that females experienced more general conflict with more depressive symptoms, whereas males reported experiencing more discrimination than females, such as how often they felt made fun of in school because of their race or ethnicity. The researchers identified the importance of working with Latino parents and adolescents regarding the acculturation process and conflict that may surround differences in cultural values between parents and their children. Some individuals may find themselves unable to work through the stress of acculturation and have great difficulty in modifying their **cultural values, beliefs, or practices** and feel isolated from their new culture or even from their culture of origin.

Depression (see Evidence-Based Practice 10-1) is the most common mental health problem in the United States (National Institute of Mental Health [NIMH], Retrieved March 12, 2018). One of the risk factors for depression is major life changes, trauma, or stress. Fox, Thayer, and Wadhwa (2017) identified that numerous academic disciplines question the postmigration and postcolonization impact cultural adjustment, or acculturation, has on minority migrant and indigenous populations' health. Since immigrants and refugees may be fleeing war and other traumatic political environments, symptoms of PTSD as well as depression are common mental health problems among immigrants in the United States.

Cultural Criteria Changes in Diagnostic Statistical Manual-5

In the most recent version DSM-5, the *culture-bound syndromes* that have routinely been used by mental health professionals have now been replaced with three cultural concepts. An overview of the three concepts follows, along with the reasons identified for the change in the DSM-5.

A Cultural Formulation Interview (CFI) has been identified in the DSM-5 and is a set of 16 questions clinicians can use in a mental health assessment. The questions are geared to the impact of culture on the individual's current clinical picture.

The three cultural concepts in the DSM-5 (American Psychiatric Association, 2013) are cultural syndrome, cultural idiom, and cultural explanation. Cultural syndrome is identified as a cluster or co-occurring group of symptoms found in a specific cultural group or community (e.g., *ataque de nervios*). The syndrome may not be identified as an illness by the cultural group yet would be identified as an illness by an outside observer. Cultural idiom of distress is a means of identifying suffering among a cultural group with shared ethnicity and religion (e.g., *kufungisisa*). Kufungisisa is associated with "a range of psychopathology," including "anxiety, excessive worry, panic attacks, depressive symptoms, and irritability" (p. 834). The cultural idioms of distress may not be associated with specific symptoms and may be used to demonstrate discomfort in a variety of situations, including social circumstances versus mental health issues, and cultural explanation or perceived cause is a label that provides a cultural etiology (e.g., *maladi moun*). "Interpersonal envy and malice cause people to harm their enemies by sending illnesses such as psychosis, depression. A related condition is the 'evil eye'" (p. 835). Explanations about the cause may be features or folk classifications used by cultural healers or lay individuals (see Table 10-1).

Culture-Bound Syndromes

Although culture-bound syndromes have been removed from the DSM-5 (American Psychiatric Association, 2013), they are presented here as still existent within the cultures identified and in the mental health system. Various mental health symptoms are experienced by people all over the world. Cultural meanings, beliefs, and practices regarding specific symptoms may vary depending on one's culture and socioeconomic status within

Table 10-1 | DSM-5 (2013) Cultural Concepts of Distress

Cultural Concept of Distress	Culture	Symptoms
Ataque de nervios	Latino	Intense emotional upset; acute anxiety, anger, or grief; screaming and shouting uncontrollably; attacks of crying; trembling; heat in the chest rising into the head; verbal and physical aggression Dissociative experiences; seizure-like and fainting; suicidal gestures
Dhat syndrome	India Pakistan	Associated with semen loss in young males Anxiety, fatigue, weight loss, impotence
Khyal cap	Cambodians in United States and Cambodia	Panic attacks; anxiety, tinnitus, and neck soreness
Kufungisisa	Shona of Zimbabwe	Anxiety, depression Somatic problems (Indicative of interpersonal and social difficulties)
Maladi moun Sent sickness	Haiti	Humanly caused illness (envy of other's success, hatred) Attractive, intelligent, and wealthy are at risk
Nervios	Latinos in the United States	Emotional distress Somatic disturbance Inability to function Headaches and brain aches
Shenjing shuairuo	Chinese	Weakness, emotions, excitement, nervous pain, sleep disturbances, 3:5 required
Susto	Some Latinos in United States, Central America, South America	Frightening event causing soul to leave body Unhappiness and sickness Difficulty in key social roles
Taijin kyofusho	Japanese	Interpersonal fear disorder Anxiety and avoidance of interpersonal situations Fear of inadequacy and offensiveness to others

From Cultural Concepts of Distress, American Psychiatric Association. (2013). *Diagnostic and Statistical Manual of Mental Disorders, DSM-5* (5th ed.). Washington, DC: Author.

the culture. Although specific identifying terms, manifestations, and meanings within different cultures may vary, a diagnosis such as depression is similar around the world. However, cultural values, beliefs, and practices shape how various groups interpret symptoms, identify causality, and determine appropriate treatment.

In contrast, **culture-bound syndromes**, also called folk illnesses, culture-specific illnesses, or culture-specific syndromes, often are localized to a particular cultural group. According to American Psychiatric Association (2000), culture-bound syndromes are described as recurrent, locality-specific patterns of aberrant behavior and troubling experiences that may or may not be linked to a particular DSM-IV diagnostic category. Many of these patterns are indigenously considered to be "illnesses," or at least afflictions, and most have local names. Culture-bound syndromes are generally limited to specific societies or culture areas and are localized, diagnostic categories that frame coherent meanings for certain repetitive, patterned, and troubling sets of experience and observations (p. 898).

As mental health care is changing to meet the increasing multicultural diversity of the client population, it is important for mental health nurses to recognize the culture-bound syndromes. Table 10-2 lists the most frequently cited culture-bound syndromes. Since values, beliefs, and practices of people are culturally constructed, the syndromes can only be interpreted within the context of the specific culture in which they exist.

Table 10-2 | Culture-Bound Syndromes

Syndrome	Culture	Symptoms
Amok Cafard, cathard Mal de pelea Iich'aa	Malaysia Polynesia Puerto Rico Navajo	Period of brooding with subsequent aggressive behavior followed by amnesia or exhaustion Typically occurs in young to middle-aged males who have experienced recent loss
Ataque de nervios	Latino Puerto Rico	Uncontrollable shouting, crying, trembling, and aggressive behavior Sensation of heat in the chest Possible fainting or seizure-like activity Triggered by stressful familial event and buildup of anger Typically occurs in women 45 years and older
Bilis, colera, muina	Latino	Acute nervous tension, trembling, screaming, gastrointestinal disturbances Cause is thought to be unexpressed anger or rage
Bouffee delirante	West Africa, Haiti	Abrupt outburst of agitation, aggression, and confusion May be associated with hallucinations (visual and auditory) and paranoia
Brain fag, brain fog	West Africa	Brain "fatigue," difficulty concentrating or sleeping, weakness Crawling sensation under skin Feelings of depression Most often afflicts high school or college students
Dhat, Jiryan Sukra Prameha Shen k'uei	India Sri Lanka China, Taiwan	Somatic complaints of dizziness, fatigue, weakness, loss of appetite, guilt, and sexual dysfunction associated with semen-loss anxiety
Falling out, blacking out	Southern United States, Caribbean	Spinning sensation and dizziness prior to collapse Visual impairment Difficulty interacting with environment
Ghost sickness	Navajo	Weakness, pending sense of "doom," loss of appetite, feeling of suffocation, fainting, dizziness, and hallucinations Preoccupation with death

(continued)

Table 10-2	Culture-Bound Syndromes (continued)	
Syndrome	**Culture**	**Symptoms**
Hwa-byung	Korea	Insomnia, chest discomfort, dizziness, headaches, fearful, sadness, suicidal ideation, and guilt Typically occurs in middle-aged or elderly women
Koro	Malaysia	Fear of penis in men and vulva and nipples in women retracting into the body and possibly causing death
Shuk yang, Shook yong, Suo yang	China	
Jinjinia bemar	Assam	
Rok joo	Thailand	
Latah	Malaysia	Exaggerated startle response, screaming, cursing, laughing, echopraxia, echolalia Typically occurs in women
Amurakh, irkunii, olan, myriachit, menkeiti	Siberia	
Bah tschi, bah tsi, baah ji	Thailand	
Imu	Ainu, Sakhalin, Japan	
Mali-mali, silok	Philippines	
Locura	Latin America and Latinos in United States	
Mal de ojo, evil eye	Mediterranean	Typically occurs with children and can also affect women Sleep disturbances, crying, diarrhea, vomiting, and fever
Nervios	Latino	Feeling of vulnerability and emotional distress to stressful life experiences Irritability, sleep disturbances, nervous, difficulty concentrating, tearfulness, and dizziness
Pibloktoq, Arctic hysteria	Inuit	Fatigue, depressive silences, confusion Typically follows a major loss
Qigong psychotic reaction	Chinese	Dissociation and paranoia Headache, dizziness, disorientation Can occur following Qigong meditation
Rootwork	Southern United States Caribbean	Witchcraft, voodoo, hexing, or evil influence are responsible for illnesses
Mal puesto, brujeria	Latino	GI disturbances, anxiety, fear of being poisoned or killed ("voodoo death")
Sangue dormido	Portuguese Cape Verde Islanders	Pain, numbness, paralysis, convulsions, stroke, heart attack, infection, and miscarriage
Shenjing	Chinese	Depression, anxiety, dizziness, headaches, GI and sleep disturbances, and sexual dysfunction
Shin-byung	Korean	Anxiety, weakness, dizziness, fear, sleep and GI disturbances Somatic complaints are followed by dissociation and feeling possessed by ancestral spirits

Table 10-2 | Culture-Bound Syndromes (continued)

Syndrome	Culture	Symptoms
Spell	Southern United States	Trancelike state, communication with deceased spirits May be misdiagnosed as psychosis
Susto, fright, soul loss (espantro, pasmo, perdida del alma chibi)	Latinos in United States Mexico Central America South America	Actual "fright" Sleep and appetite disturbances, tripa ida, sadness, lack of motivation, low self-esteem, muscle aches, headache, and GI disturbances Typically follows a frightening event resulting in the soul leaving the body Symptoms can occur immediately following event or years later
Taijin kyofusho	Japan	Intense fear that one's body (appearance, odor, nonverbal communication) embarrasses or offends others
Zar	North Africa Middle East	Feeling possessed by a spirit Dissociation (laughing, hurting self, singing, crying), withdrawal, difficulty caring for self May develop relationship with spirit

Sources: American Psychiatric Association. (2000). *Diagnostic and Statistical Manual of Mental Disorders* (4th ed.). Washington, DC: Author; Hales, Yudofsky, & Gabbard (Eds.). (2008). *The American Psychiatric Publishing Textbook of Psychiatry* (5th ed.), American Psychiatric Publishing, Inc.

Cultural Values, Beliefs, and Practices of Specific Cultural Groups as They Relate to Mental Health

Transcultural mental health nurses and other mental health care providers want to help clients of all cultures achieve their optimal level of human functioning. Modern medical care may not be viewed the same as traditional health care in many reservation or immigrant communities. Nurse researchers and other health-related disciplines have continued to explore the health beliefs and practices of culturally diverse clients specific to mental health. An overview of mental health beliefs and practices of selected cultural groups follows. The overviews are not intended to stereotype or generalize the specific cultures. They are only intended as a resource for transcultural nurses and others to increase the awareness of patterns of values, beliefs, and practices related to mental health of the selected cultural groups.

However, the transcultural nurse is also encouraged to understand the diversity within cultural groups with respect to mental health beliefs and practices. Many clients and families of specific cultural groups may not exhibit traditional patterns of values, beliefs, and practices of any specific cultural group. Transcultural nurses should conduct a thorough history and cultural assessment to ensure competent cultural care for each client.

African American Culture: An Overview of Mental Health Concerns

Individuals of African descent constitute approximately 13.5% of the total US population (United States Census Bureau, 2018). The concept of African Americans as a distinct group in the United States is grounded historically in their shared social and environmental contexts, historical events, as well as family and kin memories of those experiences. Bell and Peterson (1992) noted that slavery, segregation, and institutionalized racism created a climate that resulted in health disparities, structural inequalities, marginalization, and cultural pain for African Americans. Acknowledging and understanding this cultural context is an important first step prior to providing transcultural mental health care to African American individuals, families, and communities. Historically, African Americans were forced to deal with inequities with education, employment, and health care and thereby learned to turn to each other and community leaders for help. Currently, African Americans frequently turn to family, friends, neighbors, community, church, and religious leaders for help and to cope and deal with mental health issues.

African American men, as in other diverse cultural groups, often express their depression through bodily symptoms like headaches, stomach aches, pains, and so on. Within the African American community, there can be considerable stigma about mental illnesses. Prevention of depression and suicide is extremely important, and education is the key to early prevention. Although the African American church has traditionally viewed suicide as a sin, many religious organizations are now starting to create mental health programs. Conner et al. (2018) identified that the stigma of mental health for African Americans is a major barrier to seeking professional mental health services. The researchers identified "it is imperative for mental health professionals, interventionists, and researchers to make the effort to identify and examine novel ways to mitigate barriers to mental health service utilization among vulnerable populations who may be prone to experience more salient barriers to mental health service utilization, such as stigma" (p. 99).

In a study conducted by Mitchell, Watkins, Shires, Chapman, and Burnett (2017) studied self-reported responses of 1,666 African American men 60 years of age or older, mean age of 73.6 years. The researchers found that African American men may not identify with the term "depression," even though they exhibited the criteria of depression. Findings indicated that 74.8% of older African American men in the study reported feeling downhearted with only 18.5% identifying as depressed or anxious, thereby describing their emotional health state as downhearted rather than the clinical terminology of depression that may be more culturally stigmatized. The researchers suggested the importance of adding more culturally accepted terminology such as downhearted to the symptoms that are currently used to diagnose major depressive disorder (MDD). Since depression in African American individuals can be overlooked, it is imperative for professional mental health care providers to practice at a culturally competent level, to prevent overlooking symptoms of depression and other mental health needs of the African American community.

The "Black" church is a major institution in the African American community, and church leaders are frequently called upon for mental health issues in the African American community. Therefore, Bilkins, Allen, Davey, and Davey (2016) studied the leaders' attitudes in relation to seeking professional mental health services. The researchers found that church leaders tended to rely on church community and alternative health services, particularly for those leaders who frequently attended church. The closer the leaders felt to all "Black" people, the less satisfied they were with professional mental health services. Those leaders who had experienced more racial discrimination identified worse overall mental and physical health. The researchers identified that it would be important for clinical providers and Black churches to develop collaborative relationships in order to meet the needs of the communities they served. Once again, mental health stigma and fears of racial discrimination were reasons identified for African Americans to delay seeking professional mental health treatment.

There are other mental health issues within the African American community that lead to premature mortality or morbidity. The societal costs of substance abuse can be calculated in terms of violence, disease, and death. There is a close relationship between substance abuse and HIV/AIDS and other sexually transmitted diseases. Blake, Taylor, and Sowell (2017) identified that approximately 45% of new HIV cases in 2014 were diagnosed among African Americans. Poverty inadequate housing and access to health care, substance abuse, fear, and discrimination were identified as some of the reasons HIV rates are high among African Americans. The researchers conducted focus group research with 35 older African American men diagnosed with HIV. A number of participants also disclosed their personal history of drug and alcohol use and felt stigma associated with both HIV-positive status, in addition to their history of addiction. One man said, "It is almost easier to tell people you have HIV, uh, than the drug use." Another participant stated "I did not want to go to the clinic and let them find out about my HIV. I was ashamed" (p. 224).

There are several important factors to keep in mind when providing transcultural mental health care to African Americans. First, family and kin networks, while perhaps not as strong as in the past, are still extremely important in assisting the recovery process. Outreach and education to family members about depression, suicide, and substance abuse are extremely important. For many African Americans who have experienced difficulty with mental health issues of substance and drug abuse and serious and persistent mental illnesses, such as depression, family and community are very important components in the recovery process. As previously identified, the African American church is a key player in changing community perceptions about depression and suicide as well as a leading player in substance abuse programs. The Black church is a major institution and where many African Americans choose to go for help. Spirituality has been a traditional cultural norm in African cultures, and the modern African American church has incorporated the spiritual component into healing and care.

American Indian Culture: An Overview of Mental Health Concerns

According to the 2016 U.S. Census Bureau, Annual Estimates of the Resident Population, approximately 4 million individuals in the United States (of the 323 million people in United States) are American Indian and Alaska Native. In the United States, there are 573 federally recognized American Indian Tribes (Bureau of Indian Affairs, 2018, Retrieved May 27, 2018) and Nations. There is a need to improve mental health care for American Indians.

The Indian Health Service (IHS) (2018b), U.S. Department of Health and Human Services (Retrieved May 20, 2018) Mental Health Program, a part of the Federal Program for American Indians and Alaska Natives, offers culturally sensitive, comprehensive mental health services. For example, the Winnebago Counseling Center (WCC) in South Dakota offers counseling for "grief, anxiety, sleep problems, depression, anger management, stress, posttrauma reactions, family problems, interpersonal problems, and many other life situations." According to Walker (2014), the annual budget for IHS was $4.6 billion, of which only $266 million is allocated to mental health and substance abuse programs. Much work remains to be accomplished in overall mental health care for American Indians and Alaska Natives.

The Indian Health Services (IHS) (2018a) recognizes alcohol and drug abuse and the impact on the individual, family, community, and tribe as a major health problem. The American Indian Human Resource Center recognizes treatment and prevention are "through a coordinated multidisciplinary and intertribal effort" (Retrieved May 20, 2018). Alcohol abuse among the American Indian population continues to be a major concern. According to the National Institute of Drug Abuse (NIDA) (2014), Native American adolescents report initiating drug and alcohol use in 8th and 10th graders when compared to the national averages. For example, current marijuana use was 35%

for American Indian seniors versus the national average of 21.5% (Retrieved May 15, 2018).

In 2016, the National Tribal Behavioral Health Agenda (2016) (Retrieved March 15, 2018) was developed in collaboration with numerous American Indian and Alaska Native tribes, leaders, organizations, and federal agencies of the SAMHSA and the IHS as a result of the impact mental and substance use disorders impact tribal communities. Behavioral health, mental (including suicide), and substance use disorders have impacted tribal communities at disproportionately higher rates when compared to other communities in the United States. The goal of the agenda was to integrate authentic cultural traditional ways of knowing, being, and doing with current health care promotion to deliver culturally congruent care to the American Indian, Alaska Native tribes. In order to help preserve the family unit, interrelated behavioral health problems "that are often a result of child abuse and neglect, poverty, family violence, substance misuse, unemployment, and incarceration in American Indian and Alaska Native communities" (p. 40).

The Native American culture believes in holistic health care and generally has a holistic outlook in all aspects of their lives. Holism is a belief that the physical, mental, emotional, and spiritual dimensions of an individual are perceived as one. American Indians, as a cultural group, are also perceived as one, although each tribe may have unique characteristics. According to the National Tribal Behavioral Health Agenda (Retrieved March 15, 2018), "Our worldview on health and healing is holistic, encompassing the body, mind, spirit, nature, and our environment" (p. 5).

Native Americans frequently communicate through storytelling. So, allowing Native American clients to tell their story is an important and useful way to get information. Use of broad, open-ended questions facilitates obtaining a health history and other information in a culturally competent manner. It is important for nurses working with Native American clients to focus on such strengths as spirituality, resiliency, and positive identity to help clients in the healing process.

Asian/Pacific Islander Culture: An Overview of Mental Health Concerns

According to the United States Census Bureau (2012) for the United States 2010 to 2060 period, Asian Americans and Pacific Islanders are one of the fastest growing minority groups in the United States, second only to the Hispanic or Latino cultural groups. The Asian population is projected to more than double, from 15.9 million in 2012 to 34.4 million in 2060, with its share of nation's total population climbing from 5.1% to 8.2% in the same period. The Native Hawaiian and Other Pacific Islander population is expected to nearly double, from 706,000 to 1.4 million. Asian Americans and Pacific Islanders of Asian ancestry represent 43 diverse cultural groups from Korea, Japan, China, India, Cambodia, Vietnam, Indonesia, Philippines, and Papua New Guinea, to name only a few (Retrieved April 1, 2018).

For some Asian Americans, stigma related to mental health problems can be a stumbling block in their lives and in seeking services for their mental health. Millner and Kim (2017) conducted a study on challenges related to their psychiatric disabilities and their work life. The women had identified a history of psychiatric disability, received disability benefits because of their mental illness and had at least one hospitalization for mental health in the past year or psychiatric symptoms impaired major areas of their functioning (e.g., work, school). The women reported being ostracized by family and community members, because of their metal disability. One woman diagnosed with schizophrenia expressed that her father had disowned her, based on an inability to accept her mental illness. "Work-related failures deeply affected participants' perceptions of themselves (e.g., low self-esteem, feelings of worthlessness) and interactions with others (e.g., need to hide their mental health identity at work). Some individuals described self-blame and self-loathing for their poor work performance" (p. 184). The women identified an expectation to hide emotions, which delayed seeking appropriate care for their mental health disability. It was identified that culturally competent mental health services were important for Asian American women, particularly with the difficulties the women were experiencing with work, family, and community support. The researchers identified the importance of providing culturally congruent care for Asian Americans with mental health illness. Care providers need to explore the challenges faced by this population including the lack of family, peer, and community support, the impact of double discrimination of their minority status and mental illness. It was also suggested that it would be important to acknowledge the cultural strengths of a strong work ethic and cultural pride to help mitigate the negative impact of their mental illness.

Asian Americans' core cultural values of honor and pride and patriarchal obligations, particularly with elders, are important to understanding Asian American culture. Collective group harmony, including family and kin, rather than individual concerns, are significant cultural values (Leininger, 1995). Understanding core cultural values of the Asian American culture, particularly the importance of maintaining harmony, will help transcultural nurses plan care for clients with mental health problems in a culturally competent manner (see Figure 10-4).

Community agencies have often provided mental health services specifically to Asian Americans. According to the Cummings Institute (2016), recent budget cuts are impacting mental health care. Many community agencies have suffered a severe cutback in services and are unable to provide the level and kinds of care that they have provided in the past. Many individuals are seeking mental health care through hospital emergency departments, costing hospitals billions of dollars to care for those seeking mental health care services (Retrieved April 5, 2018). Recognition of cultural barriers, such as language, that have a direct effect on communication between nurses and other health care providers and clients and their family/significant other(s) can be preemptive and lead to more positive client outcomes.

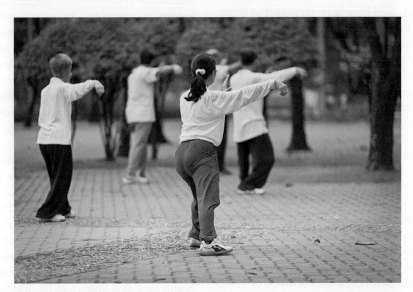

Figure 10-4. Tai chi, a low-impact Chinese martial art, is practiced to facilitate the relief of stress and a sense of mental well-being. Transcultural mental health nurses can explore the use of alternative techniques becoming more popular with diverse cultural groups (vanHurck/Shutterstock.com).

Hispanic/Latino Culture: An Overview of Mental Health Concerns

According to the United States Census Bureau (2012), individuals of Hispanic or Latino descent are the fastest growing cultural group in the United States. By 2060, approximately 128 million people, nearly one in three US residents, will self-identify as Hispanic Americans (Retrieved April 1, 2018). Hispanic countries include such diverse places as Mexico, Puerto Rico, Cuba, Spain, and the United States; there is tremendous cultural diversity among the Hispanic/Latino groups. According to the Pew Research Center (2016), the Hispanic population reached 55 million in the United States in 2015 (Retrieved May 5, 2018).

In general, Mexican Americans (American citizens identifying as having Mexican ancestry) tend to rely on their family and extended family networks. According to Hurwich-Reiss and Gudino (2016), traditional Latino cultural values of familism (familismo in Spanish) emphasize the central role the family plays, including feeling close, loyal, and obligated to the nuclear and extended family, and have been identified as being protective factors for Latino youth. Family and the extended family members are viewed as a whole and are highly valued. Nurses and other health care providers need to consider the importance of the family when making health care decisions for a client who has entered the mental health care system, where individuality is valued. Mexican Americans have a lower incidence of mental illness when compared to other diverse cultural groups, possibly due to strong extended family connections and the role family networks play in dealing with anxiety and stresses, as well as the role of religion.

Salinas, Heyman, and Brown (2017) conducted a study on financial barriers to health care with Mexican Americans with chronic disease and depression or anxiety in Texas. The researchers conducted a secondary data analysis of 1,002 Hispanics from El Paso, Texas. The average age for participants diagnosed with depression or anxiety was 51 years old. Participants with two or more chronic conditions were more likely to have been refused medical care because of financial barriers. Approximately 70% of participants had difficulty paying $100 for medical care, while 28% had postponed treatment because of cost. Those participants who had been diagnosed with depression or anxiety had been denied medical care more often than those without depression or anxiety. The authors identified the importance for nurses to provide culturally congruent care to those with depression or anxiety. "Nurses need to be particularly attuned to financial barriers to care and how to address them. Nurses can play an important role in addressing these disparities by identifying local resources that can help address financial barriers. Furthermore, nurses may also advocate for funding and policies that support access to care among Hispanics with depression and/or anxiety. Without such sensitivity, a substantial population of vulnerable persons with anxiety or depression will struggle to access lifesaving health care" (p. 493).

According to the Torres and Hicks (2018) for The American Counseling Association, the importance of understanding the cultural value of curanderismo many Mexican and Mexican American individuals rely on holistic traditional folk healers known as *curanderos*, *herbalists*, midwives, counselors, and spiritualists for help during a health crisis. The folk healers work with individuals on the physical, spiritual, and mental level in a holistic mind–body healing practices. Symbolism is also used by healers such as writing a letter of goodbye to loved ones, using a barrida, or broomlike object to sweep the top of individuals to symbolize removing the unwanted (Retrieved June 1, 2018). Many Hispanic individuals with mental illness often go without seeking professional help for mental health treatment in lieu of seeking traditional healing. Failure to seek professional mental health care services may be related to uninsured status. Cultural barriers, including language and fear of being stigmatized with a mental health illness, also serve to obstruct access to seeking professional mental health care. It is important for professional mental health care providers to understand the important meanings of techniques used by traditional healers, in order to appreciate and recognize important cultural values, beliefs, and practices of the culture.

Although intimate partner violence (IPV) and family violence associated with male dominance in the Mexican American culture may be prevalent, as in other cultural groups, it is frequently underreported (Kemp, 2005). It is important to talk to women about IPV when they come in for health care services. Mexican American women are generally open to disclosing and discussing their experiences of IPV if they believe the health care provider is willing to listen and facilitate breaking the silence surrounding the abuse; it is important to help the women find resources available to them in their respective communities. The Latino culture also holds strong expectations for women, with an emphasis on submissiveness and reverence toward men. The female role has its roots with the Virgin Mary and is referred to as *marianismo*, indicating women should be pure and self-sacrificing and devote their lives to their family. The traditional Hispanic cultural values for females may lead to a higher incidence of IPV, where women are encouraged to be submissive and "obey" their husbands. Nurses and other health care providers need to be aware of the importance of modesty for Hispanic women, particularly older women, and should try to keep them covered during physical exams (Galanti, 2003).

Religion is very influential in Hispanic communities and may play a major role in the mental health illnesses of Hispanic Americans. Many Hispanic Americans are Roman Catholics, and faith and church activities are an influential part of their daily life activities (Kemp, 2005). Some studies have identified religious and cultural barriers to professional mental health care as some Hispanic Americans report that they trust in God, and "if I am sick, it is his will" (Carter-Pokras et al., 2008). These attitudes often delay appropriate preventative care as well as treatment of mental health illnesses.

Arab Muslim Culture: An Overview of Mental Health Concerns

According to Harb (2018), it is difficult to get a census population number for the Arab culture in the United States, since there is no specific category for this population. The Arab cultural population remain "White" in the U.S. Census count and will remain so for the next 12 years, since there will be no Middle Eastern cultural category in the 2020 Census (Retrieved June 1, 2018).

Increasingly, Arab Americans are experiencing discrimination and marginalization and are at greater risk for mental health disorders. Samari (2016) conducted research on first-, second-, and third-generation Arab Americans, living in Detroit. Over 60% of 524 Arab Americans participating in the study were first generation, averaging 44 years old. First-generation Arab Americans were found to have more positive cross-border attitudes to countries of origin, consume more Arab media, and have more social ties compared to the other generations. It was also found that Arab Americans with more positive cross-border attitudes had a higher prevalence for psychological distress, which may indicate psychological distress associated with family and social support. If the participants were involved with cross-border Arab community organizations, the psychological distress was lower. Financial difficulties were associated with psychological distress. Respondents who were interviewed in Arabic versus English also demonstrated lower psychological distress. When working with Arab Americans in mental health clinical settings, it would be important to use interpreters when possible. It would also be important to help Arab Americans connect with Arab community organizations and connect with other Arab Americans. Helping Arab Americans who present with depression and other mental health disorders may need to work through feelings of isolation, discrimination, and an overall separation from Arab cultural norms.

Arab Americans have been described as "Invisible," based on past census results that historically and legally considered this cultural group "White." In a study conducted by Ajrouch and Antonucci (2018), Arab Americans were found to have more depressive symptoms than either Blacks or Whites. The Arab Americans identified as having more contact frequency; however, lower proportions of their network contacts were of the same culture. "With respect to Arab Americans, we live in a historical period marked by fast increasing marginalization" (p. 89).

Cultural beliefs about being possessed and sorcery or the "evil eye" affect interpretation of mental health symptoms. Prior to seeing health care professionals, Arab Muslims may seek traditional healers for mental health problems. Traditional healers hold special importance to Arab Muslim people because of their affiliation and connection to the community. Traditional healers also deal with mystical and unknown (Okasha, 2012). Little evidence exists that traditional healers have been effective in treating major mental health illnesses, such as schizophrenia or obsessive–compulsive disorder. However, for those individuals having cultural and spiritual beliefs different from conventional mental health, a more holistic care may be sought with traditional healers (Nortje, Oladeji, Gureje, & Seedat, 2016).

Jadalla and Lee (2012) conducted a study on the relationship between acculturation and health status for Arab Americans living in southern California to assess the physical and mental health of the participants. The researchers found that acculturation was an important factor when assessing the well-being of Arab Americans, particularly their mental health. The results indicated that the Arab American participants who had a higher assimilation into the American culture were associated with significantly better mental health. According to LeMaster et al. (2018) in research on acculturation psychological symptoms with Iraqi refugees, experiences of trauma prior to immigration was associated with PTSD and depressive symptoms and with decreased acculturation. "Interventions that aim to improve mental health and promote acculturation among refugees should assess their history of trauma, chronic disorders, and psychological symptoms soon after migration and promptly provide opportunities for social support" (p. 38).

Since acknowledging mental health issues, including sexual, physical, and substance abuse, is difficult for the Arab culture, mental health nurses need to have a good understanding of the cultural values, beliefs, and practices in dealing with such sensitive issues. The stigma of mental health in the Arabic culture is a challenge and can also be a barrier to mental health treatment. In recruiting Arabic participants for sensitive research, it was identified that some families will even go so far as to try to manage the mental health issue within the family rather than seek professional help, in order to avoid stigma and protect the secret (Timraz et al., 2017). Providing privacy, treating the client and family/significant others with respect, using an interpreter and care provider of the same culture, when possible, and understanding the role of stigma associated with seeking professional mental health care would be important for mental health nurses to understand in caring for the Arabic culture in a culturally congruent manner.

Culturally Competent Mental Health Care

The interpretation of behavior generally transpires within the context of the specific culture in which it occurs. However, when clients and families from diverse cultural groups come to institutions of the dominant culture, the behavior is identified and interpreted by the dominant culture. Frequently, behavior can be misinterpreted and/or distorted if health care providers are not knowledgeable about caring for clients from diverse cultural groups. Particularly with mental health, diagnoses applied to clients based on certain behaviors may be inaccurate; if the same behavior were understood and interpreted within the context of the client's culture, a different diagnosis might be made, with different treatment, or no diagnosis at all. Inaccurate mental health labels can have a negative impact on an individual and family for years. Communication and cultural knowledge, leading to cultural competency, can have a positive impact on the mental health care that is provided to clients of diverse cultural groups and lead to positive experiences for both clients and the nurses providing the care.

Developing Cultural Competence

Developing a mutually trusting relationship with clients improves plans of care and increases the likelihood of more optimal health outcomes; this is particularly important in mental health nursing care. Because of difficult experiences with past family and other relationships, it may be difficult for some clients with mental health needs to trust others, including mental health care providers. Early on, Leininger (1991b) recognized the importance of developing a trusting relationship with participants in a research study and developed "Leininger's Stranger to Trusted Friend Enabler Guide" (p. 82). Leininger also identified that the guide would be helpful for clinicians. The purpose of the enabler was to facilitate the researcher, or clinician, to "move from mainly a distrusted stranger to a trusted friend" (p. 82) in order to establish a trusting relationship as a clinician. According to Egan (2014), helpers need to have an understanding that some clients have a fear of betrayal and, therefore, have a more difficult time in developing trust with the helper. Even when caregivers make clear that they maintain confidentiality in their caring relationship, it is difficult for some clients to trust caregivers. Clients who have difficulty in trusting others may reveal themselves in a much more guarded manner, particularly in a mental health care setting. Patience and encouragement are needed when helping clients with a fear of trust. An understanding of the client's culture increases the likelihood of improved health outcomes.

Nurses are increasingly caring for clients from diverse cultures and are expected to have a broad understanding of culture in order to provide culturally competent mental health care. Culturally competent nursing care for clients from diverse cultures becomes crucial in caring for clients with mental health needs. Some questions that nurses may be asking are what exactly does *culturally congruent care* mean? How can a transcultural mental health nurse understand the cultural values, beliefs, and practices of all the culturally diverse clients a nurse will care for over the lifetime of his or her career? Well, one answer may be that, of course, you cannot understand the values, beliefs, and practices of all of the clients you will care for in your career. However, nurses can become familiar with the values, beliefs, and practices of the culturally diverse groups to whom they do provide care.

Buchwald et al. (1994) used the term "**cultural blind spot**," sometimes referred to as **cultural blindness**, to describe the assumption that if a person is similar in appearance and behaviors as the care provider, then there are no perceived cultural differences or potential barriers to giving appropriate care. The cultural blind spot supports people's beliefs that they understand the culture and have had similar cultural encounters. Thus, a person could conclude that he or she has culturally competent skills. However, it is this lack of awareness of differences that creates the cultural blind spot. Transcultural mental health nurses need to be aware of the phenomenon of cultural blind spot/cultural blindness because of the unintended influence it can have on care of diverse populations of mental health clients.

Intrapersonal Reflection

Leininger (2000) identified the importance of conducting a personal inventory of one's own cultural values, beliefs, and practices to begin to identify, understand, and remove personal cultural bias, ethnocentrism, and prejudice. It is important for nurses to explore and reflect on their own cultural values, beliefs, practices, expressions, meanings, and own cultural norms in order to identify and begin to understand personal biases, prejudices, and other barriers to caring for clients in a culturally congruent and competent manner. Although tolerance may be the opposite of prejudice, it is an inadequate benchmark in caring for clients in a culturally competent manner. It is important for nurses and other health care providers to celebrate diversity and recognize the challenge to continually explore areas within themselves or others that may block or serve as barriers to caring for clients in a culturally competent manner.

Each nurse needs to explore his or her own personal values, beliefs, and practices in order to recognize areas of prejudice, bias, stereotyping, and ethnocentrism of culturally diverse individuals, families, and communities. It is important for transcultural mental health nurses to explore their personal prejudices and biases toward people from diverse cultures and peel away and expose stereotypes that impede caring for culturally diverse clients. Learning about diverse cultural values, beliefs, and practices can help mental health nurses feel more competent in caring for clients from diverse cultural groups.

Important Factors to Consider in Transcultural Mental Health Nursing

Three important factors that need to be considered when discussing transcultural mental health nursing are communication and language, spirituality, and experiences of pain. Mental health care is dependent on initiating a dialogue with the client. It is even more important for transcultural mental health care providers to effectively communicate with clients who may have some difficulty with meanings and expressions of the dominant English language in the United States. Spirituality is an integral part of mental well-being and has become a focus for mental health care providers. Transcultural mental health care providers are increasingly exploring diverse cultural expressions, meanings, and practices of spirituality. Chronic pain is generally thought of as a physical, bodily pain; however, there is an emotional and mental health component to experiences of pain that may vary widely depending on one's cultural values, beliefs, and practices.

Communication

Communication, both verbal and nonverbal, is one of the most important skills for mental health nurses. Communication is even more important with culturally diverse mental health clients, where language may serve as a barrier and make the process of communication more difficult. **Interpersonal communication** helps mental health nurses assess each client's values, beliefs, and practices about their mental health care. Communicating with each client is important in caring for clients in a culturally congruent and competent manner.

Communication between the mental health nurse and the client and family generally brings together the exchange of two diverse cultures, that of the nurse and that of the client. Therefore, it is

also important for nurses to have an understanding of their own cultural values, beliefs, and practices, so they can better understand the diversity between their own cultural values, beliefs, and practices and those of the client and family, particularly as these phenomena relate to mental health care.

Culture influences each interaction nurses have with clients. Since an important part of mental health care is communicating and providing counseling for clients with mental health illnesses, if nurses are not knowledgeable about the cultural context in which their communication is being interpreted, there is a possibility that the message can be misunderstood.

Mental health nurses understand the importance of developing trust with clients and their family/kin networks. Taking time to develop trust with clients who do not speak English or speak minimal English can be very challenging, particularly given the increasingly culturally diverse population seeking mental health care. Sometimes, health care providers can become irritated that clients and family members do not speak the dominant English language. When there is a possibility to have a certified translator/interpreter serve as an interpreter, that is the ideal choice rather than using family members or other staff who may not understand complex health situations. Family members should be encouraged to offer family support rather than serve as an interpreter.

Empathy is one of the most important communication skills that transcultural mental health nurses and other health care providers can use with clients from diverse cultural backgrounds. In using empathy in communicating with clients, health care providers are attempting to understand what a client is experiencing or has experienced—trying to put themselves in the client's place and feel and experience what the client is feeling and experiencing—and then communicating that understanding back to the individual client (Egan, 2014). Empathic communication helps the health care provider to better understand the situation or context of the client as well as the cultural norms and values that structure that context and influence the client. It is important to communicate back to the client and family your understanding of their experience so they may clarify whether you have accurately identified the client's perception of a particular experience (Egan, 2014).

Empathy becomes very important in trying to understand the experience and feelings of mental health clients and their families. Attempting to understand the experience of abuse, schizophrenia, depression, bipolar disorders, and other mental health issues is crucial to understand the perspectives of the client and family (see Figure 10-5). For transcultural mental health care providers, empathy needs to be communicated, taking into consideration the beliefs, values, and practices, or in other words the "norms" of a culture. When communicating with clients from other cultures, particularly for those who do not speak English or for whom English is a second language, there is an increased risk of miscommunication.

Mental health nurses need to practice culturally competent communication skills to improve care for an ever-increasing population of culturally diverse mental health clients. Becoming aware of the importance of communication is key to providing culturally competent mental health care.

Taking into account the cultural values, beliefs, meanings, practices, expressions, and cultural norms of specific cultures takes knowledge, experience, and patience in acquiring these skills. In addition, basic verbal and nonverbal communication skills such as tone of voice, use of probes and clarification, listening, empathy, facial expressions, and body gestures, for both the nurses themselves and for the clients and family members, will help to improve overall communication and culturally competent mental health care.

Spirituality

Because spirituality is a central theme that governs Nigerian's lives, counselling interventions should attempt to include aspects of spirituality in the assessment and treatment processes to help develop engagement, promote empathy, reduce other stigma, and limit counselling attrition rates (Meniru & Schwartz, 2018).

Although the terms spirituality and religion are sometimes used interchangeably, *spirituality* refers to a broad sense of the inner experience of the self and a search for meaning while *religion*

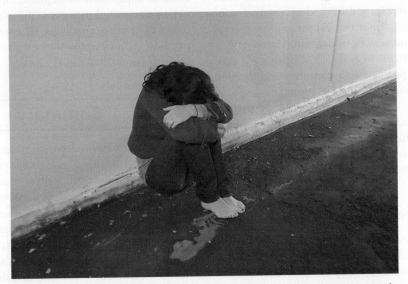

Figure 10-5. A rape victim covers her face. Numerous feelings haunt rape survivors for years. Fear, shame, humiliation, and emotional pain are areas transcultural mental health nurses can facilitate healing through therapeutic empathy and counseling (ChameleonsEye/Shutterstock.com).

generally involves an institution with a given set of rules and observances involving devotion and ritual. There are many spiritual and religious themes to mental health disorders such as schizophrenia, bipolar disorder, psychosis, hallucinations, and delusions. Transcultural mental health nurses care for clients who have diverse cultural values, beliefs, meanings, and practices, many of which are grounded in spiritual and religious beliefs. This applies to clients and families from all of the world's major religious systems, Jewish, Christian, Islamic, and others.

Spirituality and religious practices can play an influential role in enhancing mental health and emotional stability. For example, many African Americans view their church as the focal point of their lives. Within the African American church, emotions can be released that cannot be expressed in many other social situations and friendships. The African American church functions in promoting a high level of self-esteem, particularly for those individuals and communities in poverty-stricken environments. Given the important role the African American church plays in the lives of parishioners, the churches may be uniquely positioned to overcome barriers such as stigma, distrust, and limited access that contribute to racial disparities in professional mental health care and service utilization (Hankerson & Weissman, 2012). In addition, health care providers could partner with churches and develop culturally congruent interventions to improve care African Americans connected to various churches. Church leaders could also begin to develop relationships with professional mental health care providers to refer parishioners needing more acute mental health care services.

Experiences of Pain

In mental health nursing, the client's experience of pain can be manifested in many different ways. Unlike other somatic symptoms frequently associated with mental health issues, pain has a component that includes emotional elements. Psychosocial factors have been found to influence pain. There is increasing evidence to suggest that pain can be a physical symptom of depression and that pain and depression are common comorbidities. According to Hall-Flavin (2013), depression can lead to pain and vice versa. In fact, pain and depression may create a "vicious cycle in which pain worsens symptoms of depression, and then the resulting depression worsens feelings of pain." It seems to be extremely difficult to separate the somatic, physical component of pain from the psychological component of pain.

There is the concept of psychosomatic pain, or pain with psychological components, and this pain is expressed differently by cultural groups. One of the distinct types of depression with Haitian women is "douleur de corps (pain in the body)" (Nicholas et al., 2007, p. 87). Barkwell (2005) studied Native Americans (Ojibwa) with cancer pain. They described their pain as "all that was most painful in life" and included the following properties in their description of cancer pain: "physical sensation, threatening cognitions, emotional, social and spiritual anguish, and intuitive sensing" (p. 454). In a study to differentiate somatic versus psychological symptoms as a cultural expression of depression, Chinese outpatients reported more somatic symptoms compared to Euro-Canadians, who reported more psychological symptoms specific to the diagnosis of depression (Ryder et al., 2008).

Summary

This chapter explored perspectives on transcultural mental health nursing care. The goal is to help nurses provide culturally competent care that improves the health and well-being of culturally diverse mental health clients. Nurses can increase their competency by understanding cultural values, beliefs, practices, meanings, expressions, and cultural norms of diverse cultures specific to the mental health and well-being of individuals, families/kin, and communities. Competency-based transcultural knowledge is essential in today's complex mental health environment.

REVIEW QUESTIONS

1. Describe the influence of culture on mental health care values, beliefs, and practices.
2. Identify specific cultural values, beliefs, and practices of three diverse cultural groups and how transcultural mental health nurses might facilitate culturally congruent care in a mental health care system.
3. Compare and contrast your cultural values, beliefs, and practices about mental health care with that of another cultural group.
4. Critically explore and reflect on any personal or familial biases, prejudices, and other culturally specific barriers that would impact your ability to provide culturally congruent care.
5. Identify five communication skills that facilitate culturally competent mental health care.

CRITICAL THINKING ACTIVITIES

1. Describe a personal clinical experience you have had or observed where a cultural misunderstanding occurred. How did you feel either as a participant or as an observer? How do you believe the other individual(s) involved in the situation felt? How might the situation have been resolved in a culturally congruent manner?

2. Role-play several clinical situations in which cultural misunderstandings occurred. Then, role-play how you would resolve the cultural misunderstandings in a culturally congruent manner.

3. Discuss the impact an incorrect mental health diagnosis and label might have on individuals' lives.

4. Collect data on knowledge and skills for culturally congruent transcultural mental health nursing by interviewing someone from a culture that is very different from your own. Practice some basic interpersonal communication skills to get to know the person and establish some basic trust; ask the individual about their values, beliefs, and practices related to mental health and mental illness. Then, search the literature for information to read about that individual's cultural group. Regardless of whether your interviewee is from Haiti, Japan, or another cultural group and is gay, young, or elderly, consider if what you have read either represents or does not represent the individual you have interviewed.

5. Think about various times in your life that you have been involved with a group of people with whom you have felt comfortable, connected to, and shared similar values, beliefs, and practices. Think about the times in your life that you have been involved with a group of people with whom you did not feel comfortable and connected to and did not share similar values, beliefs, and practices. Compare and contrast those different experiences in your life. How might it feel for an individual from a different culture to come into the group you felt comfortable with, connected to, and shared similar values, beliefs, and practices?

6. Imagine you are working with several nurses who imitate clients and their families who have difficulty speaking English and make fun of some of the cultural values, beliefs, and practices of culturally diverse individuals and families who are different from their own. How might you deal with this situation? Try role-playing the situation from different perspectives and using different communication skills not only to challenge the actions of your coworkers but also to help them begin to understand the impact of their behavior on others.

7. Imagine you are working with a client and his or her extended family who do not speak English. What are some ways you might communicate with your client and the family? Role-play some options you might try to communicate with your client and family.

8. You are caring for a patient from an Arab Muslim culture in a clinical setting, and the patient is exhibiting behaviors that you believe may be signs and symptoms of mental illness. Describe some of the signs and symptoms you might be observing. Describe some of the techniques you might use to differentiate whether the behavior is a manifestation of cultural values, beliefs, and practices you are not familiar with or are a result of a mental illness?

REFERENCES

Abuelezam, N. N., & Fontenot, H. B. (2017). Depression among Arab American and Arab Immigrant Women in the United States. *AWHONN, 21*(5), 395–399.

Ajrouch, K. J., & Antonucci, T. C. (2018). Social relations and health: Comparing "invisible" Arab Americans to blacks and whites. *Society and Mental Health, 8*(1), 84–92.

Barkwell, D. (2005). Cancer pain: Voices of the Ojibway people. *Journal of Pain and Symptom Management, 30*(5), 454–464.

Barnert, E. S., Perry, R., & Morris, R. E. (2016). Juvenile incarceration and health. *Academic Pediatrics, 16*(2), 99–109.

Bell, P., & Peterson, D. (1992). *Cultural pain and African Americans: Unspoken issues in early recovery.* Hazelden Publishing Center City, MN.

Bharadwaj, P., Pai, M. M., & Suziedelyte, A. (2017). Mental health stigma. *Economics Letters, 159*, 57–60.

Bilkins, B., Allen, A., Davey, M. P., & Davey, A. (2016). Black church leaders' attitudes about mental health services: Role of racial discrimination. *Contemporary Family Therapy, 38*, 184–197.

Blake, B. J., Taylor, G. A., & Sowell, R. L. (2017). Exploring experiences and perceptions of older African American males aging with HIV in the rural Southern United States. *American Journal of Men's Health, 11*(2), 221–232.

Brave Heart, M. Y. H. (1998). The return to the sacred path: Healing the historical trauma and historical unresolved grief response among the Lakota through a psychoeducational group intervention. *Smith College Studies in Social Work, 68*, 288–305.

Brave Heart, M. Y. H., & DeBruyn, L. M. (1998). The American Indian holocaust: Healing historical unresolved grief. *American Indian & Alaska Native Mental Health Research, 8*, 60–82.

Buchwald, D., Caralis, P. V., Gany, F., Hardt, E. J., Johnson, T. M., Muecke, M. A., & Putsch, R. W. (1994). Caring for patients in a multicultural society. *Patient Care, 28*, 105–123.

Bureau of Indian Affairs. (2018). About us. Retrieved May 27, 2018 from https://www.bia.gov/about-us

Caballero, T. M., DeCamp, L. R., Platt, R. E., Shah, H., Johnson, S. B., Sibinga, E. M., & Polk, S. (2017). Addressing the mental health needs of Latino children in immigrant families. *Clinical Pediatrics, 56*(7), 648–658.

Carter-Pokras, O., Brown, P., Martinez, I., Solano, H., Rivera, M., & Pierpont, Y. (2008). Latin American–trained nurse perspective on Latino health disparities. *Journal of Transcultural Nursing, 19*(2), 161–166.

Central Broadcasting System. (2014). Sotomayor: Labeling illegal immigrants criminals is insulting. Retrieved May 12, 2018 from http://washington.cbslocal.com/2014/02/04/sotomayor-labeling-illegal-immigrants-criminals-is-insulting

Conner, K. O., Roker, R., McKinnon, S. A., Ward, C. J., & Brown, C. (2018). Mitigating the stigma of mental illness among older adults living with depression: The benefit of contact with a peer educator. *Stigma and Health, 3*(2), 93–101.

Cromer, L. D., Gray, M. E., Vasquez, L., & Freyd, J. J. (2018). The relationship of acculturation to historical loss awareness, institutional betrayal, and the intergenerational transmission of trauma in the American Indian experience. *Journal of Cross-Cultural Psychology, 49*(1), 99–114.

Cummings Institute. (2016). How budget cuts are affecting mental health care. Retrieved April 5, 2018 from https://cummingsinstitute.com/resources/infographics/budget-cuts-affect-mental-health-care/

Diamond, M. (2016). Retrieved from https://www.huffingtonpost.com/entry/why-emotional-well-being-is-a-top-priority-for-the-us-surgeon-general_us_57866486e4b08608d3327828

Dinan, S. (2016). House orders Library of Congress to maintain 'illegal alien'. *The Washington Times*. Retrieved March 10, 2018 from https://www.washingtontimes.com/news/2016/jun/10/house-orders-library-congress-keep-illegal-alien/

Dueweke, A. R., & Bridges, A. J. (2017). The effects of brief, passive psychoeducation on suicide literacy, stigma, and attitudes toward help-seeking among Latino immigrants living in the United States. *Stigma and Health, 2*(1), 28–42.

Evans-Campbell, T. (2008). Historical trauma in American Indian/Native Alaska communities: A multilevel framework for exploring impacts on individuals, families, and communities. *Journal of Interpersonal Violence, 23*(3), 316–38.

Egan, G. (2014). The skilled helper: A problem management and opportunity development approach to helping (10th ed.), Belmont, CA: Thomson Brooks/Cole.

Eliacin, J., Slayers, M. P., Kukla, M., & Matthias, M. S. (2015). Patients' understanding of shared decision making in a mental health setting. *Qualitative Health Research, 25*(5), 668–678.

Fox, M., Thayer, Z., & Wadhwa P. D. (2017). Assessment of acculturation in minority health research. *Social Science & Medicine, 176*, 123–132.

Galanti, G. A. (2003). The Hispanic family and male-female relationships: An overview. *Journal of Transcultural Nursing, 14*(3), 180–185.

Goffman, E. (1964). *Stigma.* London, UK: Penguin.

Hall-Flavin, D. K. (2013). Is there a link between pain and depression? Can depression cause physical pain? Disease and Conditions (Major Depressive Disorder). Retrieved January10, 2015 from http://www.mayoclinic.org/diseases-conditions/depression/expert-answers/pain-and-depression/faq-20057823

Han, M., Cha, R., Lee, H. A., & Lee, S. E. (2017). Mental-illness stigma among Korean immigrants: Role of culture and destigmatization strategies. *Asian American Journal of Psychology, 8*(2), 134–141.

Hankerson, S. H., & Weissman, M. M. (2012). Church-based health programs for mental disorders among African Americans: A review, *Psychiatric Services, 63*(3), 243–249.

Haralambous B., Dow, B., Goh, A., Pachana, N. A., Bryant, C., LoGiudice, D., & Lin, X. (2016). 'Depression is not an illness. It's up to you to make yourself happy': Perceptions of Chinese health professionals and community workers about older Chinese immigrants' experiences of depression and anxiety. *Australasian Journal on Ageing, 35*(4), 249–254.

Harb, A. (2018). US Census fails to add MENA category: Arabs to remain 'white' in count. *The Middle East Eye*. Retrieved June 1, 2018 from http://www.middleeasteye.net/news/us-census-continue-count-arabs-white-1206288795

Heim, E., Wegmann, I., & Maercker, A. (2017). Cultural values and the prevalence of mental disorders in 25 countries: A secondary data analysis. *Social Science & Medicine, 189*, 96–104.

Huq, N., Stein, G. L., & Gonzalez, L. M. (2016). Acculturation conflict among Latino youth: Discrimination, ethnic identity, and depressive symptoms. *Cultural Diversity and Ethnic Minority Psycholog, 22*(3), 377–385.

Hurwich-Reiss, E., & Gudino, O. G. (2016). Acculturation stress and conduct problems among Latino adolescents: The impact of family factors. *Journal of Latina/o Psychology, 4*(4), 218–231.

Indian Health Service. (May 20, 2018a). Alcohol counseling. Retrieved May 20, 2018 from https://www.ihs.gov/winnebago/services/alcoholcounseling/

Indian Health Service. (May 20, 2018b). Mental health. Retrieved May 20, 2018 from https://www.ihs.gov/winnebago/services/mentalhealth/

Jadalla, A., & Lee, J. (2012). The relationship between acculturation and general health of Arab Americans. *Journal of Transcultural Nursing, 23*(2), 159–165.

Kemp, C. (2005). Mexican and Mexican-Americans: Health beliefs & practices. Retrieved from http://bearspace.baylor.edu/Charles_Kemp/www/hispanic_health.htm

Leininger, M. M. (1991a). The theory of culture care diversity and universality. In M. M. Leininger (Ed.). *Culture care diversity and universality: A theory of nursing* (pp. 5–68). New York, NY: National League for Nursing Press.

Leininger, M. M. (1991b). Ethnonursing: A research method with enablers to study the theory of culture care. In M. M. Leininger (Ed.) *Culture care diversity and universality: A theory of nursing* (pp. 73–117). New York, NY: National League for Nursing Press.

Leininger, M. M. (1995). *Transcultural nursing: concepts, theories, research and practice.* New York, NY: McGraw-Hill.

Leininger, M. M. (2000). Founders focus: Transcultural nursing is discovery of self and the world of others. *Journal of Transcultural Nursing, 11*, 312–313.

Leininger, M. M., & McFarland, M. R. (2002). *Transcultural nursing: Concepts, theories, research and practice* (3rd ed.), New York: McGraw Hill.

McFarland, M. R., & Wehbe-Alamah, H. B. (2015). *Leininger's culture care diversity and universality : A worldwide nursing theory* (3rd. ed.), Jones and Bartlett Learning: MA.

LeMaster, J. W., Lumley, M. A., Arnetz, J. E., Arfken, C., Jamil, H., Broadbridge, C. L., ..., Arnetz, B. B. (2018). Acculturation and post-migration psychological symptoms among Iraqi refugees: A path analysis. *American Journal of Orthopsychiatry, 88*(1), 38–47.

Meniru, M. O., & Schwartz, R. C. (2018). The influence of Afrocentric spirituality on counselling stigma and help-seeking perceptions among Nigerian Americans. *International Journal of Advanced Counseling, 40*, 26–38.

Mental Health.gov. (May 5, 2018). Retrieved May 5, 2018 from https://www.mentalhealth.gov/basics/what-is-mental-health

Millner, U. C., & Kim, M. (2017). Perspectives on work and work-related challenges among Asian Americans with psychiatric disabilities. *Asian American Journal of Psychology, 8*(3), 177–189.

Mitchell, J. A., Watkins, D. C., Shires, D., Chapman, R. A., & Burnett, J. (2017). Clues to the blues: Predictors of self-reported mental and emotional health among older African American Men. *American Journal of Men's Health, 11*(5), 1366–1375.

National Alliance on Mental Health. (2017). Retrieved March 12, 2018 from https://namitexas.org/challenging-multicultural-disparities-mental-health/

National Alliance on Mental Health. (April 10, 2018). Mental health conditions. Retrieved April 10, 2018 from https://www.nami.org/Learn-More/Mental-Health-Conditions

National Institute of Mental Health. (March 12, 2018). Retrieved March 12, 2018 from https://www.nimh.nih.gov/health/topics/depression/index.shtml

National Institute on Drug Abuse. (2014). Substance use in American Indian youth is worse than we thought. Retrieved May 15, 2018 from https://www.drugabuse.gov/about-nida/noras-blog/2014/09/substance-use-in-american-indian-youth-worse-than-we-thought

National Tribal Behavioral Health Agenda. (2016). Retrieved March 15, 2018 from https://store.samhsa.gov/shin/content/PEP16-NTBH-AGENDA/PEP16-NTBH-AGENDA.pdf

Nicholas, G., Desilva, A. M., Subrebost, K., Breland-Noble, A., Gonzalez-Eastep, D., Manning, N., ... Prater, K. (2007). Expression and treatment of depression among Haitian immigrant women in the United States: Clinical observations. *American Journal of Psychotherapy, 61*(1), 83–98.

Nortje, G., Oladeji, B., Gureje, O., & Seedat, S. (2016). Effectiveness of traditional healers in treating mental disorders: A systematic review. *Lancet Psychiatry, 3*, 154–170.

Oberg, K. (1960). Cultural shock: Adjustment to new cultural environments. *Practical Anthropology*, 177–182.

Okasha, A. (2012). Mental health services in the Arab world. *World Psychiatry, 11*(1), 52–54.

Pew Research Center. (2016). Key facts about how the U.S. Hispanic population is changing. Retrieved May 5, 2018 from http://www.pewresearch.org/fact-tank/2016/09/08/key-facts-about-how-the-u-s-hispanic-population-is-changing/

Redfield, R., Linton, R., & Herskovits, M. (1936). Memorandum on the study of acculturation. *American Anthropologist, 38*, 149–152.

Rojas-Flores, L., Clements, M. L., London, J., & Koo, J. H. (2017). Trauma and psychological distress in Latino citizen children following parental detention and deportation. *Psychological Trauma: Theory, Research, Practice, and Policy, 9*(3), 352–361.

Ryder, G., Yang, J., Zhu, X., Yao, S., Yi, J., Heine, S. J., & Bagby, M. R. (2008). The Cultural shaping of depression: Somatic symptoms in china, psychological symptoms in North America? *Journal of Abnormal Psychology, 117*(2), 300–313.

Safran, M. A., Mays, R. A., Huang, N. L., McCuan, R., Pham, P. K., Fisher, S. K., ..., Trachtenberg, A. (2009). Mental Health Disparities. *American Journal of Public Health, 99*(11), 1962–1966.

Salinas, J. J., Heyman, J. M., & Brown, L. D. (2017). Financial barriers to health care among Mexican Americans with chronic disease and depression or anxiety in El Paso, Texas. *Journal of Transcultural Nursing, 28*(5), 488–495.

Samari, G. (2016). Cross-border ties and Arab American mental health. *Social Science and Medicine, 155*, 93–101.

Siemons, R., Raymond-Flesh, M., Auerswald, C. L., & Brindis, C. D. (2017). Coming of age on the margins: Mental health and wellbeing among Latino Immigrant Young Adults Eligible for Deferred Action for Childhood Arrivals (DACA). *Journal of Immigrant Minority Health, 19*, 543–551.

Substance Abuse and Mental Health Services Administration. (2017). Recovery among diverse populations discussion guide. Retrieved May 14, 2018 from https://www.recoverymonth.gov/sites/default/files/roadtorecovery/r2r-september-2017-discussion-guide.pdf

Sutherland, L. L. (2002). Ethnocentrism in a pluralistic society: A concept analysis, *Journal of Transcultural Nursing, 13*(4), 274-281.

Timraz, S. M., Alhasanat, D. I., Albdour, M. M., Lewin, L., Giurgescu, C., & Kavanaugh, K. (2017). Challenges and strategies for conducting sensitive research with an Arab American population. *Applied Nursing Research, 33*, 1–4.

Torres, N., & Hicks, J. F. (2018). Cultural awareness: Understanding Curanderismo. Retrieved June 1, 2018 from https://www.counseling.org/docs/default-source/vistas/article_396cfd25f16116603abcacff0000bee5e7.pdf?sfvrsn=4

Tyson, M. D., Arriola, N. B., & Corvin, J. (2016). Perceptions of depression and access to mental health care among Latino immigrants: Looking beyond one size fits all. *Qualitative Health Research, 26*(9), 1289–1302.

U.S. Census Bureau. (2012). U.S. Census Bureau projections show a slower growing, older, more diverse nation a half century from now. Retrieved April 1, 2018 from https://www.census.gov/newsroom/releases/archives/population/cb12-243.html

U.S. Census Bureau. (2018). Foreign born persons, percent, 2012–2016. Retrieved 5, 2018 from https://www.census.gov/quickfacts/fact/table/US/POP645216#viewtop

U.S. Department of Health and Human Services. (1999). *Mental health: A report of the surgeon general.* Rockville, MD. Retrieved May 5, 2018 from https://profiles.nlm.nih.gov/ps/access/NNBBHT.pdf

U.S. Department of Health and Human Services, Substance Abuse and Mental Health Services Administration, Center for Mental Health Services, National Institutes of Health, National Institute of Mental Health. What is mental health? Available online at: U.S. Department of Health and Human Services. Retrieved May 14, 2018 from http://www.mentalhealth.gov

U.S. Office of Disease Prevention and Health Promotion, Healthy People 2020. 2015. Mental health and mental disorders. Retrieved May 10, 2018 from https://www.healthypeople.gov/2020/topics-objectives/topic/mental-health-and-mental-disorders

Villalobos, O., Lynch, S., DeBlieck, C., & Summers, L. (2017). Utilization of a mobile app to assess psychiatric patients with limited English proficiency. *Hispanic Journal of Behavioral Sciences, 39*(3) 369–380.

The World Health Organization. (2018a). Retrieved May 5, 2018 from http://www.who.int/mental_health/action_plan_2013/en/

The World Health Organization. (2018b). Retrieved May 5, 2018 from http://www.who.int/mediacentre/factsheets/fs220/en/

Walker, D. (2014). Detecting the True "Culture" of Indian Health Service Mental Health Programs, Mad in America, science, *Psychiatry and community.* Retrieved January 5, 2015 from http://www.madinamerica.com/2014/09/detecting-true-culture-indian-health-service-mental-health-programs-counting-words/

Wu, I. H. C., Kalibatseva, Z., Leong, F. T. L., Bathje, G. J., Sung, D., & Collins-Eaglin, J. (2017). Stigma, mental health, and counseling service use: A person-centered approach to mental health stigma profiles. *Psychological Services of the American Psychological Association, 14*(4), 490–501.

Xue-Ling Chang, M., Jetten, J, Cruwys, T., & Haslam, C. (2017). Cultural identity and the expression of depression: A social identity perspective. *Journal of Community & Applied Social Psychology, 27*, 16–34.

Yasui, M., Pottick, K. J., & Chen, Y. (2017). Conceptualizing culturally infused engagement and its measurement for ethnic minority and immigrant children and families. *Clinical Child Family Psychology Review, 20*, 250–332.

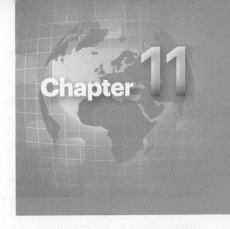

Chapter 11

Culture, Family, and Community

- Joyceen S. Boyle, Martha B. Baird, and John W. Collins

Key Terms

Acculturation
Aggregates
Assimilation
Asylees
Community-based collaborative action research (CBCAR)
Community-based nursing
Community-based setting

Community health nursing
Community nursing
Community settings
Cultural assessment
Cultural knowledge
Cultural sensitivity
Culturally competent care
Immigrants
Integration
Levels of prevention

Medically underserved
Primary prevention
Public health nursing
Refugees
Secondary prevention
Specialized community interventions
Subcultures
Tertiary prevention
Traditional health beliefs and practices

Learning Objectives

1. Use cultural concepts to provide nursing care to families, communities, and aggregates.
2. Understand the necessary components of a cultural assessment of an aggregate group.
3. Explore interactions of community and culture as they relate to concepts of community-based nursing practice and specialized community interventions.
4. Analyze how cultural factors influence health and illness of groups.
5. Assess factors that influence the health of diverse groups within the community.
6. Evaluate potential health problems and solutions in refugee and immigrant populations.
7. Identify interventions that are culturally sensitive and relevant to address health concerns of a refugee population.

An understanding of culture and cultural concepts contributes to the nurse's knowledge and facilitates culturally competent nursing care in **community-based settings**. Currently, many nurses practice in community settings with clients from a wide variety of cultural backgrounds; this trend is expected to increase with more nurses moving from acute care institutions to community settings. The care of clients in the community can be extremely complex, calling for a high level of nursing skill. Cultural diversity is also expected to increase in the United States as reported; "by 2050 nearly one-half of the U.S. population will be composed of racial minorities" (McKenzie, Pinger, & Seabert, 2017, p. 256). Significant changes in the health care system, including an increased emphasis on health promotion and disease prevention, have influenced nurses to make changes in their practice and the setting in which care is delivered. Concepts such as health equality, diversity, partnership, empowerment, and facilitation now form the basis for community-based nursing practice with individuals, families, and **aggregates** in the community. An aggregate is a collection of people who can be thought of as a whole simply because they happen to be in the same place at the same time. For some time, national nursing associations, including the National Institute of Nursing Research (NINR), have urged an aggregated community and population focus in both nursing research and practice. Involving clients in planning for and providing community nursing services is the foundation of culturally competent care and involves learning individual and community perspectives to plan and provide community-aggregated services.

Specialized community interventions that are culturally relevant to the people served are built on collaboration and partnerships between community leaders, health consumers, and health care providers. When community residents or health consumers are involved as partners, community-based services are more likely to be responsive to locally defined needs, are better used, and are sustained through local actions. **Community-based collaborative action research (CBCAR)** is an approach for nurses to partner with communities to address health issues (Pavlish & Pharris, 2012). Specialized community interventions are complex and often very time consuming. They require a high level of nursing knowledge and skill in working with and relating to different individuals and groups. In many instances, the complexity is increased when clients and their families come from diverse cultures. Nurses must understand how to help persons from various cultures work with community leaders and health care providers to form partnerships that are responsive and can structure nursing and health care in ways that are culturally sensitive and appropriate. It is often the cultural factors that determine whether a particular population or group will choose to participate in community-based health services. There is always a need for continuing communication among health care providers and community residents, which is characterized by mutual understanding and respect. It is this understanding and respect that forms the basis for culturally relevant and competent nursing care.

In this chapter, the terms **community nursing**, **community-based nursing**, **community health nursing**, and **public health nursing** are used interchangeably, even though they have different meanings in some settings and in different contexts (Canales & Drevdahl, 2014; Williams, 2012). Whether the nurse is employed as a public health nurse or a community health nurse in a health department or practices in a community-based setting, he or she needs the knowledge and skills to provide **culturally competent care**. The practice of nursing in a community setting requires that nurses be comfortable with clients from diverse cultures and the broader socioeconomic context in which nurses personally live. As the population continues to grow in diversity, health disparities have become more apparent in diverse populations and are now a vital area of focus for researchers and practitioners. Care that is not congruent with the client's value system is likely to increase the cost of care because it compromises quality and inhibits access to services (Gainsbury, 2017). Furthermore, members of diverse cultural groups, such as the officially designated minority groups in the United States, tend to experience greater

BOX 11-1	What's New in Healthy People 2020?

- Emphasizing ideas of health equity that address social determinants of health and promote health across all stages of life
- Replacing the traditional print publication with an interactive Web site as the main vehicle for dissemination

- Maintaining a Web site that allows users to tailor information to their needs and explore evidence-based resources for implementation

Source: https://www.healthypeople.gov/

health inequalities than do members of the general population. This was the impetus for targeting the four ethnic minority groups in *Healthy People 2000* (National Health Promotion and Disease Prevention Objectives, 1991 and Human Services, 1990) and *Healthy People 2010* (National Health Promotion and Disease Prevention Objectives, 2000) because cultural diversity must be respected and taken into account by health care professionals. Equally important, we must address the stark inequalities that exist in health status between minority groups and the wider American society. *Healthy People 2020* (Healthy People 2030 goals are being determined at time of press, for updates visit the Healthy People 2030 website) is a set of goals and objectives with 10-year targets designed to guide national health promotion and disease prevention efforts to improve the health of all people in the United States (HealthyPeople 2020, 2018). Box 11-1 shows what is new in *Healthy People 2020*.

Overview of Culturally Competent Nursing Care in Community Settings

Nurses practice in many settings within the community, including worksites, schools, physicians' offices, health care program sites, clinics, churches, and public health departments. The use of cultural knowledge in community-based nursing practice begins with a careful assessment of clients and families in their own environments. Cultural data that have implications for nursing care are selected from clients, families, and the environment during the

assessment phase and are discussed with the client and family to develop mutually shared goals. The Andrews/Boyle Transcultural Nursing Assessment Guide for Individuals and Families (Appendix A) and the Andrews/Boyle Transcultural Nursing Assessment Guide for Groups and Communities (Appendix B) are helpful when assessing clients, families, groups, and communities.

Cultural data are important in the care of all clients; however, in community nursing, they are a prerequisite to successful nursing interventions. Community nursing is practiced in a community setting, often in the home of the client, and frequently requires more active participation by the client and family. Frequently, the client and family must consider making basic changes in lifestyle, such as changes in diet and exercise patterns. Cultural competence requires that the nurse understand the family lifestyle and value system, as well as those cultural forces that are powerful determinants of health-related behaviors. Nurses often work closely with clients with chronic diseases or those who have other health problems, and nursing interventions must include aspects of counseling and education as well as anticipatory guidance directed toward helping clients and families adjust to what may be lifelong conditions. Nurses must take into account the diverse cultural factors that will motivate clients to make successful changes in behavior because improvement in health status requires lifestyle and behavioral modifications.

Transcultural nursing practice has the potential to improve the health of the community as well as the health of individual clients and families. An additional consideration of the nurse who is involved in community-focused planning is the health needs of populations at risk. Special at-risk groups can be found in all communities: the homeless, the poor, persons with HIV/AIDS and/or tuberculosis, **refugees**, prison populations, and the elderly are groups at risk for decreased health status.

Consider the difficulty of designing a health program for a community composed primarily of refugees who recently arrived in the United States. By definition, refugees are individuals who have been forced to leave their home country due to war, violence, or persecution. They may have spent years in refugee camps in other countries, may have lost family members, and may have family members still living in their home country, and yet the refugees are now making a life for themselves in a strange country. While refugees may come from all levels of the socioeconomic status in their homeland, many refugees will have not had access to medical, dental, and other health care services while in refugee status, regardless if they may have had health care access prior to fleeing their native country. Certainly, language would be a major problem, but so could many other cultural differences, from nuances in communication to differences in beliefs of what constitutes health and illness as well as treatment and cure. A failure to understand and deal with these differences would have serious implications for the success of any health or nursing intervention. Nurses who have knowledge of, and an ability to work with, diverse cultures are able to devise effective community interventions to reduce risks in a manner that is consistent with the community and group, as well as individual values and beliefs of community members.

A Transcultural Framework

A distinguishing and important aspect of community-based nursing practice is the nursing focus on the community as the client (Stanhope & Lancaster, 2016). Effective community nursing practice must reflect accurate knowledge of the causes and distribution of health problems and of effective interventions that are congruent with the values and goals of the community. A social–ecological approach can be used by the community nurse to collect, organize, and analyze information about high-risk groups that are encountered in community practice. The underlying foundation of the social–ecological approach is that behavior has multiple levels of influences. This approach focuses on the interaction between and the interdependence of factors within and across all levels of a health problem (McKenzie et al., 2017). Using a cultural overlay with a social–ecological approach enhances nurse–community interactions in numerous ways.

Identifying Subcultures and Devising Specialized Community-Based Interventions

A transcultural framework for nursing care helps the nurse to identify subcultures within the larger community and to devise community-based interventions that are specific to community health and nursing goals. For example, in the multicultural society of the United States, it is common to speak of "the Black community," "the Hispanic community," or "the Francophone community." We might also speak more broadly of "the immigrant community," or the "refugee community," or of other unique groups within or near a local community. A cultural focus allows this variety and facilitates data collection about specific groups based on their health risks. A cultural/social/ecological framework facilitates a view of the community as a complex collective yet allows for diversity within the whole. Interventions that are successful in one subgroup may fail with another subgroup of the same community, and often, the failure can be attributed to cultural differences or barriers that arise because of these differences. Often, the community location of a diverse subculture reflects distinctive aspects of the cultural group. Figure 11-1 shows murals on the wall of a library in El Rio, a Mexican American barrio in Tucson, AZ.

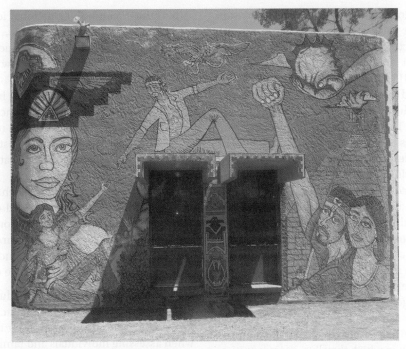

Figure 11-1. These murals reflect the Mexican American culture of the El Rio barrio. They were painted by community residents.

Identifying the Values and Cultural Norms of a Community

A transcultural framework is essential for the community health nurse to identify the values and cultural norms of a community. Although values are universal features of all cultures, their types and expressions vary widely, even within the same community. Values often serve as the foundation for a community's acceptance and use of health resources or a group's participation in community-based intervention programs to promote health and wellness. Just as nurses share data and collaborate with clients and families to establish mutually acceptable goals for nursing care, the community-based nurse works with the community or aggregates within the community to plan community-focused health programs. Correctly identifying values and cultural norms within a community or aggregate often requires community nurses to spend time interacting with and learning from members of those

populations. In addition to forming partnerships with communities, the community nurse considers the influences of social, economic, ecological, and political issues. Larger policy issues directly and profoundly affect many, if not all, community health issues. These larger policy issues are, in turn, influenced by the wider national and/or international culture.

Cultural Issues in Community Nursing Practice

The need for nurses to be sensitive to clients who are culturally different is increasing as we become more aware of the complex interactions between health care providers and clients and how these interactions might affect the client's health. Diverse client groups who have limited access to health services, along with barriers resulting from language and cultural differences, often suffer from a variety of health inequalities

(Weech-Maldonado et al., 2018). The information in this chapter will assist nurses to become aware of cultural factors that affect health, illness, and the practice of nursing in community settings.

Purnell (2013) and Andrews and Boyle (2016) have provided models or frameworks to guide the nurse in the assessment of cultural factors in patient care. The Andrews/Boyle Transcultural Nursing Assessment Guide (see Appendices A and B) provides outlines for the nurse to collect and assess cultural data relevant to individuals, families, and communities. Most cultural assessment guides are oriented to individual clients and occasionally to families. The Andrews/Boyle assessment guides have the comprehensive view necessary for assessing cultural factors for intervention at the individual, family, and community levels. Because individual clients and their families constitute larger communities, nurses who work in community settings must understand cultural issues as they relate to individuals and families and the context in which they live—communities.

Cultural Influences on Individuals and Families

Cultural influences—values, norms, beliefs, and behaviors—have a profound effect on health. When assessing individuals and families, the community health nurse should carefully examine the following:

1. Family structure and makeup (multigenerational, nuclear, extended family, significant others, etc.), individual roles and responsibilities, and dynamics in the family, particularly communication patterns and decision-making
2. Health beliefs and practices related to disease causation, treatment of illness, and the use of indigenous healers or folk practitioners and other alternative/complementary therapies
3. Patterns of daily living, including work, school, and leisure activities
4. Social networks, including friends, neighbors, kin, and significant others, and how they influence health and illness
5. Ethnic, cultural, or national identity of client and family, for example, identification with a particular group, including language
6. Nutritional practices and how they relate to cultural factors and health
7. Religious preferences and influences on well-being, health maintenance, and illness, as well as the impact religion might have on daily living and taboos or restrictions arising from religious beliefs that might influence health status or care
8. Culturally appropriate behavior styles, including what is manifested during anger, competition, and cooperation, as well as relationships with health care professionals, relationships between genders, and relations with other groups in the community

A cultural assessment of individuals and families includes all of the preceding factors. This list is a starting point for community nurses to use when assessing individuals and families in everyday practice. Cultural values shape human health behaviors and determine what individuals and families will do to maintain their health status, how they will care for themselves and others who become ill, and where and from whom they will seek health care. Most importantly, family members are often the ones who decide on the course of treatment. Families have an important role in the transmission of cultural values and learned behaviors that relate to both health and illness. It is within the family context that individuals learn basic ways to stay healthy and to ensure their own well-being and that of their family members.

One commonality shared by members of well-functioning families is a concern for the health and wellness of each individual within the family by taking responsibility for and providing for the health needs of its members. The nurse must not only assess the health of each family member but also determine how well the family can meet family health needs. Just how well families can meet the needs of each family member will determine how, when, and where interventions will take place. A cultural orientation assists the nurse in understanding cultural values and interactions, the roles that family members assume, and the support system available to the family to help them when health problems are identified.

The family is usually an individual's most important social unit and provides the social context within which illness occurs and is resolved. Health promotion and maintenance also occur within the family group. Most **traditional health beliefs and practices** promote the health of the family because they are generally family and socially oriented. Frequently, traditional beliefs and practices reinforce family cohesion. Some values are more central and influential than others; given a competing set of demands, these central values will typically determine a family's priorities. In families that adhere to traditional cultural values, the families' (or tribe's and/or community's) needs and goals often will take precedence over an individual's needs and goals. The culturally competent nurse can recognize and use the family's role in promoting and maintaining health. This requires an appreciation of the family context in health and illness and how this varies among diverse cultures.

Cultural Factors Within Communities

In addition to identifying and meeting the cultural needs of clients and families, the community health nurse must consider social and cultural factors on a community level to understand and respect cultural values, mobilize local resources, and develop culturally appropriate health programs and services. Important factors to consider include the influence of demographics on health care, subcultures within refugee and immigrant populations, degree of acculturation and/or maintenance of traditional values and practices, and access to health and nursing care for these population groups.

Demographics and Health Care

During the 21st century, the United States and many other countries will face enormous demographic, social, and cultural changes. The United States is becoming more diverse, and it is incumbent on nurses to be prepared to respond appropriately as the health status of individuals differs dramatically across cultural/ethnic groups and social classes. Certain groups in the United States face greater challenges than does the general population in accessing timely and needed health care services. Major indicators such as morbidity and mortality rates for adults and infants show that the health status of minority Americans in the United States is substantially worse than that of White Americans. Health status is worse among those who are **medically underserved**—populations who have inadequate access to quality health care. Community nurses must assess groups within the community in a very sensitive manner; often those characteristics that we assume are related to the group's culture may be influenced by other factors instead.

Subcultures or Diversity Within Communities

Caring for diverse groups within the community has been a focus of public health nursing since the days of Lillian Wald, an early nurse leader. Home care was provided to inner city residents, particularly recently arrived immigrants. Because nurses were not from the same cultural background as their clients, they had to deal with cultural differences between themselves and the persons in their care. The need for nurses to provide culturally relevant care is greater than ever. Currently, the focus of community nursing is on diversity in the United States across and within **subcultures** (Phillips & Malone, 2014). Subcultures are aggregates of people who establish certain rules of behavior, values, and living patterns that are different from mainstream culture. Leininger described subcultures as having "distinctive patterns of living with sets of rules, special values and practices that are different from the dominant culture" (Leininger, 1995, p. 60). There can also be diversity within each subculture. Hispanic culture as a group is very broad and includes Mexican

Americans, Puerto Ricans, Dominicans, Cubans, and Central and South Americans. There is diversity within each of these groups as well.

Certain geographic areas of the country, such as Appalachia, can be singled out as containing subcultures. Persons born and reared in the southern states or in New York City can often be identified by their dialect and mannerisms as members of a distinct subculture. The United States used to be described as a "melting pot" culture, indicating that new arrivals gave up their former languages, customs, and values to become Americans. This concept may not be appropriate, however. A more accurate metaphor for the American population is a rich and complex tapestry of colors, backgrounds, and interests. One subculture that has retained many aspects of their traditional culture is the Hmong people from Southeast Asia. They came to the United States in the 1970s as refugees after the Vietnam War. The large Hmong community in Fresno, CA, sponsors a New Year's Day Celebration that is attended by as many as 100,000 Hmong from all over the United States (Figure 11-2).

Refugee and Immigrant Populations

Immigrants are persons who voluntarily and legally immigrate to the United States to live.

Immigrants come of their own choice, and most hope to eventually become citizens of their new host country. Persons coming to the United States, Canada, and Western Europe without the proper documentation may be referred to as "undocumented" migrants, "illegal immigrants," or "illegal aliens." The terms **illegal** and **alien** should be avoided in nursing discourse and the professional literature to show respect for the undocumented immigrant as a human being (McGuire, 2014). Currently, immigration of undocumented individuals, or those who do not have the appropriate documentation to immigrate, can be a contentious issue in the industrialized nations of the world. Many of the key issues in the debate about immigration policies in the United States are based on economic and political issues (Ayón, 2018).

Under international law, **refugee** is a special term that describes a person who is outside of his or her country of nationality or habitual residence and who has a well-founded fear of persecution if he or she returns to his or her own country. By definition, refugees are persons escaping persecution based on race, religion, nationality, or political stance (Convention and protocol relating to the status of refugees, 2010). Evidence-Based Practice 11-1 presents a study about the barriers

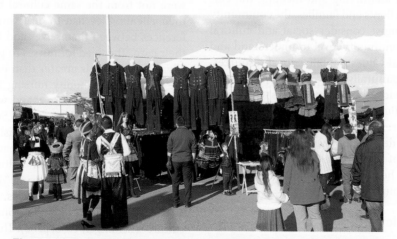

Figure 11-2. The Hmong New Year's Celebration in Fresno, CA, is attended by 100,000 Hmong. In this photo, several Hmong admire the merchandise in a booth selling traditional clothes.

Human Rights Barriers for Displaced Persons in Southern Sudan

This is a community-based research study that explores community perspectives on barriers to human rights that women encounter in a postconflict setting of southern Sudan. Violence against women is considered the most pervasive human rights violation in the world and is exacerbated in war-torn countries with high incidence of rape and other physical/sexual abuse during armed conflicts; women and girls are at particularly high risk. Violence against women is often rooted in social values and mores and potential success of change depends on learning more about local priorities regarding gender relationships, practices, and rights.

The region of southern Sudan is the site of a 40-year civil war that has had a horrific effect on the population as well as the social, economic, and physical infrastructures and health care services. Focus groups and key informant interviews provided the data for this ethnographic study. Themes found in human rights structures and subsequent barriers to human rights are described. Most human rights situations are dealt with by the traditional clan system and then go on to the more formal court and police system. Customary behavior often prevails and often women are disadvantaged because of their social positions and power differentials. Although some police officials receive procedural training in law enforcement and occasionally informal training in human rights, key informants reported that the police might actually perpetuate human rights abuses. The formal court system is still "developing" and does not always offer protection to women. Numerous barriers exist to extending human rights and protection to women. These barriers include (1) shifting legal frameworks that create a lack of knowledge about what constitutes a human rights violation, (2) mistrust and doubt about human rights, (3) weak government infrastructure, and (4) poverty.

Clinical Implications

- Nurses should be aware of the everyday struggle for justice and human dignity that refugees from the Sudan have experienced. Similarly, nurses must consider the broader historical and cultural factors that contribute to human rights abuses when working with displaced or refugee communities.
- Given their advocacy role and direct contact with communities, nurses can help educate community members regarding the health effects of human rights violations. Furthermore, by questioning social practices that violate women's rights (e.g., domestic violence), nurses can create opportunities for social change.
- Research results also indicated that enacting human rights was frequently associated with a sense of connectedness and community responsibility, suggesting that nurses can work with local residents and service providers in addressing violence against women and promoting human rights.
- Nurses are in a key position to help refugee communities analyze and address human rights barriers, thus advancing women's health and well-being.

Reference: Pavlish, C., & Ho, A. (2009). Human rights barriers for displaced persons in southern Sudan. *Journal of Nursing Scholarship*, *41*(3), 284–292. doi: 10.1111/j.1547-5069.2009.01281.x

to human rights that women encountered in southern Sudan. Violence against women is considered the most pervasive human rights violation in the world. Violence against women is exacerbated in war-torn countries, with a high incidence of rape and other physical/sexual abuse during armed conflicts. Women and girls, often unaccompanied by family members, are particularly at high risk. Many refugee women who come to the United States have experienced these human rights violations (Meffert et al., 2016; Musalo & Lee, 2017).

Studies have suggested that there is a need for research about refugees who are distinct from other categories of immigrants (Betancourt et al., 2017; Golub et al., 2018). The circumstances that lead to forced migration of refugees are very different from those that influence an immigrant to relocate, and these differences can have distinct health implications. In recent times, refugees fleeing war, famine, and other social upheavals have come to the United States from the Democratic Republic of the Congo, the Middle Eastern countries of Afghanistan, Iraq, and Syria, as well as Myanmar (Burma), African nations Sudan and Somalia, and other countries undergoing violent conflicts (Igielnik & Krogstad, 2017; Krogstad, 2017). Refugees flee for their lives and safety rather than personally choosing to leave their homeland and thus may experience very different circumstances, health care needs, and acculturation challenges differing from those of immigrants.

Another classification of newcomers is **asylees**—persons who come to a particular country seeking political asylum from some sort of persecution in their home country. These various types of classification—immigrant, undocumented immigrant, refugee, and asylee—often

determine the rights of individuals. The individual's status will determine eligibility for work permits, residency status, and the types of social and health services he or she may be entitled to. In addition, those who are undocumented, or without appropriate residency status, may face arrest and deportation to their country of origin. Table 11-1 shows terms used for individuals residing in a country who are not citizens.

Many recent immigrants and refugees are not acculturated to prevailing Western norms related to health beliefs or behaviors. Furthermore, they do not understand the complex US health care system. Many arrive with scant economic resources and must learn English and become economically self-sufficient as quickly as possible. Certain factors, such as settlement patterns, that is, living near family, friends, or others from their home region, communication networks, social class, and education, have helped many immigrants maintain their cultural traditions. Immigrant or refugee communities provide support for newcomers and opportunities for cultural continuity because these ethnic communities reflect the identities of the home countries. At the same time, belonging to such a community tends

Table 11-1	Terms Used for Individuals Residing in a Country Who Are Not Citizens	
Term	**Description**	
Illegal immigrant	A person who is in a country without the appropriate documentation and permission	
Immigrant	A person who comes to a country to take up permanent residence	
Refugee	A person who is escaping persecution based on race, religion, nationality, or political persuasion	
Emigrant	A person departing from a country to settle elsewhere	
Émigré	A person forced to emigrate for political reasons	
Asylee	A person seeking political asylum from persecution in his or her home country	
Temporary stay migrant	A person who moves to another country with the intention of staying there for only a limited time, usually for occupational reasons	
Undocumented	A person without the required documents that provide evidence of status or qualification, such as nationality or specified length of time a person may legally reside within a country	

to set immigrants and refugees apart and isolate them from the larger community. For example, newcomers from Mexico realize that they need to learn English to get better jobs, but they often join expanding Latino communities where most residents speak Spanish. Learning English well enough to obtain employment in the English-speaking world is difficult and takes time. It is to their credit that most immigrants and refugees do learn English and make significant contributions to their new country.

In addition to the legal entrance of immigrants and refugees, other persons seeking political asylum have entered the United States from all over the world. Regardless, those seeking asylum or those who enter the country legally or illegally are at considerable risk for health and social problems. In particular, health care along the US–Mexico border, where many individuals are undocumented, poses special problems and challenges for health care providers (Ayón, 2018; McEwen, Boyle, & Hilfinger Messias, 2015). Immigrants, refugees, and asylees face language and employment barriers often with little or no economic reserve to draw from. Some have experienced rapid change and traumatic life events with few resources available to assist them. Refugees, asylees, and immigrants in general have special health risks that health care clinicians must be aware of and sensitive to.

Planning Nursing Care for Refugee Families and Communities

Careful assessment of cultural backgrounds and individual factors can help nurses anticipate and work with challenges experienced by refugees and immigrants seeking health care. The Boyle/Baird Assessment Guide for Refugees (Appendix D) is recommended for use with refugee clients and their families. In response to the large numbers of refugees admitted to the United States after the Vietnam War, the early work of Lipson and Meleis identified important factors to assess when working with refugees (Lipson & Meleis, 1983). This outline provides minimum information for the nurse to plan culturally competent care:

- Length of time since the client and family left the country of origin.
- The different locations (countries or refugee camps) and number of years spent prior to resettlement. Not only is the country important but rural and urban differentiation may also be important, as well as social, political, and economic levels.
- Language spoken in the home and language skill in English.
- Nonverbal communication style.
- Religious practices.
- Ethnic affiliation or identity.
- Family roles and how they are influenced by the resettlement experience.
- Social support or networks, especially relatives or family members in the new country.

Assessment of these factors will assist the nurse in planning health care for refugee and/or immigrant families. Health services, preventive care, and health education have repeatedly been identified as important needs in health surveys that have been conducted in refugee communities. Conflicts worldwide continue to generate refugees fleeing violence and war.

The stress of resettlement is often a significant problem of refugees. Stress is related to the refugee experience and also to inadequate income, work-related problems, and loss of culture and traditions. The lack of mental health services is a real concern in refugee and immigrant communities and requires creative and innovative solutions. In refugee communities, a church, synagogue, or mosque can play a positive and important role—religion is often identified as a protective factor by refugees in facilitating wellness and increasing quality of life. Refugee men and women may be reluctant to seek mental health services because of the stigma of mental illness. Postmigration stress may be exacerbated by unemployment or underemployment and may contribute to depression, posttraumatic stress disorder (PTSD), alcohol abuse, and poor general health status.

Many refugees come from underdeveloped countries with limited availability of health care services, and the idea of preventive care is foreign to them. Preventive health practices such as dental care, breast self-examination, mammography, and Papanicolaou (Pap) smears are important for refugee women (see Evidence-Based Practice 11-2). Refugee men need preventive health care as well as including regular prostate and testicular examinations. Many barriers to good preventive care for newcomers to the United States are environmental and social rather than cultural. Constraints are based on the refugee's individual situations as well as language, economic, occupational, and transportation problems. Cultural groups differ in regard to the priority given to individual goals versus those of the larger group. For example, many refugee communities are collectivist societies that value the good of the group, traditional values, and group loyalty. This often conflicts with the individualistic American society. Many African refugees may suffer from racism and discrimination when they resettle in the United States, and this too impacts mental health and successful resettlement.

Health education, including information about access to care, is always important in planning services for refugee and immigrant communities. Many refugees and immigrants do not use health education services, not necessarily because of cultural barriers but because of difficulties with language and access, the need for translation and transportation, the desire for women health care providers, and other barriers such as child care.

Health care institutions and agencies serving refugee and immigrant communities should include bicultural health care providers on their staff. Further, community health workers should be trained to serve as interpreters and translators, as it is often problematic for health care providers to use family members as interpreters because of divisions along age and gender lines. Children learn English more quickly than do their parents and could conceivably serve as interpreters, but it would be inappropriate to expect a young boy to interpret a conversation about his mother's Pap smear. The health care provider's gender is also important, as many refugee women are not comfortable with male doctors or nurses and might avoid health care altogether if female care providers are not available. Health care providers must be knowledgeable about the refugees' or immigrants' experiences and background, cultural and social factors, and other unique aspects of the population they serve. Refugees and new immigrants need access to language-appropriate and culturally relevant health care. Many refugees from community-oriented societies prefer to receive such information in a group or social setting rather than a one-to-one basis that is common in many US health care settings. For many refugee and/or immigrant communities, churches, mosques, and synagogues are appropriate settings for health education. Health fairs sponsored by community nurses and held within the refugee or immigrant communities have been very successful. Often, health fairs have been cosponsored by churches that serve immigrant or refugee communities.

Many refugee women may have experienced gender-based violence (GBV) including torture, rape, and human rights abuses. Nurses and other health professionals especially women physicians and nurses, must learn sensitive ways of broaching these subjects and helping refugee women access culturally appropriate care. Clinicians must be cognizant to design programs that address challenges in health care access, and delivery of services in appropriate dialect as well as provision of culturally sensitive health care for women who have experienced GBV.

The classic definition of community uses a geographic boundary such as a village, town, or urban settlement/city to provide parameters for and context of the population being described. This sense may be conveyed somewhat in terms such as Little Havana, Little Kabul, and Little Saigon, but such designations do not really convey the nature or quality of the refugee or

A Community-Based Collaborative Action Research (CBCAR) Intervention with Sudanese Refugee Women

This project was a partnership between students and faculty from a Midwestern school of nursing and a group of refugee women from South Sudan to address some of the health concerns in their community. This CBCAR intervention provided informational support, social support, and job skills to empower the women to help themselves, their families, and their community.

The intervention was a series of five educational seminars held at the Sudanese Community Church on a Saturday to accommodate the women's work schedules. Transportation and child care were provided. The students and faculty presented information to the women on the following topics:

- Well-woman health
- Parenting children in the United States
- Prevention of sexually transmitted diseases (STDs)
- Managing childhood illnesses
- Women's stress (depression, anxiety, and PTSD)

After each seminar, the students, faculty, and women shared social time and ate lunch together. Then a focus group was held to get the women's perspectives about the information presented in the seminars. A final focus group was held at the end of the project, so participants could evaluate the project and discuss plans for future partnerships. A young refugee woman from South Sudan, who was trained as a professional interpreter, interpreted for each of the seminars and focus groups in both Dinka and Arabic, the primary languages spoken by the Sudanese women, and back into English.

The women responded very positively to the health information. Five of the thirteen women who attended the seminar on well-woman health followed up and scheduled their first mammogram. The students and faculty reported that they learned as much from the experience as the refugee women. For instance, the women explained that the concept of preventive health care did not exist in South Sudan and people only went to clinics or hospitals when they were seriously ill. Some of the refugee women experienced discrimination during their visits with US health providers in settings such as the emergency department and health clinics. The women explained that it was difficult to communicate their concerns to health providers using an interpreter in the brief, 15-minute time-limited visits typical in these settings. Overall, the faculty, students, and refugee women learned valuable lessons about the differences in cultural perspectives that will influence future health encounters.

Clinical Implications

- Involve clients in a partnership to address health concerns that are important to them.
- Use trained, professional interpreters.
- Understand that many clients are most comfortable in a place that is familiar to them, such as a community church.
- Encourage clients/participants to discuss traditional health care behaviors and to describe their encounters with the US health care system.

Reference: Baird, M. B., Domian, E. W., Mulcahy, E. R., Mabior, R., Jemutai-Tanui, G., & Filippi, M. K. (2015). Creating a bridge of understanding between two worlds: Community-based collaborative-action research with Sudanese refugee women. *Public Health Nursing, 32*(5), 388–396. doi: 10.1111/phn.12172

immigrant experience, which tends to cross geographic boundaries. Although refugees from certain geographical areas such as Sudan tend to be resettled in common locations when they arrive in the United States, they may later move to be closer to relatives or families who came from the same village or region of their homeland. The sense of shared displacement or "uprootedness" that serves to unite and distinguish immigrant or refugee communities from other groups or communities is quite profound and cannot be ignored when planning for community-based health services.

Immigrants and refugees are often seen by health professionals as dominated by psychoemotional experiences and consequences of relocation. In other words, we focus on the effects of stress, relocation, and human rights violations. Indeed, much of the literature on immigrants and refugees focuses on PTSD. Although many immigrants and refugees have endured horrific experiences, this focus alone is not holistic. This view, according to DeSantis' early work (1997) and McEwen et al. (2015), focuses on the primacy of the individual (an American value) rather than the community and thus prescribes psychiatric treatment instead of addressing the sociocultural and economic barriers at the macro level. It is at the macro level that transcultural health care providers must be engaged if they are to be effective participants in building healthy refugee and immigrant communities. This does not mean that individual health concerns should be ignored; it simply acknowledges that health care can be more effective when incorporated within a community focus, especially when dealing with immigrant or refugee communities.

Maintenance of Traditional Cultural Values and Practices

An important aspect of transcultural nursing is the collection of cultural data and the assessment of traditional values and practices and how they are maintained over time. The terms **assimilation** and **acculturation** are often used to describe how immigrants and refugees adapt and change over time in a new country. Both of these terms imply that newcomers modify their traditional cultural traditions to adapt to the dominant culture. **Integration** may be a better term to describe the experience: it implies that an immigrant or refugee incorporates certain aspects of the new culture into his or her lifestyle, such as language

and food, while still maintaining his or her cultural traditions and values. Both individuals and groups may be resistant to some changes and retain many traditional cultural traits. Hispanics are the largest cultural/ethnic group in the United States, and in several large American cities, they constitute large percentages of the population. In these ethnic communities, it is easier to speak Spanish and to maintain traditional cultural practices of their native land. Because traditional health beliefs and practices influence health and wellness, it is important for the nurse to understand the degree to which clients, families, and communities adhere to traditional health values and how nursing practice should reflect those values. Spector (2013) suggests that a person's health care and behavior during illness may well have roots in that person's traditional belief system. Unless community health nurses understand the traditional health beliefs and practices of their clients and communities, they may intervene at the wrong time or in an inappropriate way. Evidence-Based Practice 11-3 describes the hypertension prevention beliefs of a group of Hispanics and how they might influence barriers to preventive behaviors.

Many factors influence the likelihood that clients, families, and communities will maintain traditional health beliefs and practices. For example, the length of time a person lives in the new host country will influence factors such as language and the use of media (e.g., radio, television, and computers). Teenagers may quickly adjust to American culture and use a smartphone or an iPad. The ability to understand and speak English to communicate with members of the majority culture is crucial to learning about American culture and beginning to feel comfortable. The size of the ethnic or cultural group is also important; if the group is small, individuals from that group are more likely to be exposed to outsiders and will not spend all their time within their own group or community. Although this may hasten integration in the new culture, not being around individuals from their own cultural group may deprive

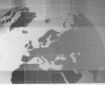
Hypertension Prevention Beliefs of Hispanics

This qualitative study used focus group methodology to explore attitudes and beliefs of Hispanics regarding hypertension prevention behaviors. The investigators found that participants were knowledgeable about hypertension and had a positive attitude about prevention. However, they identified numerous barriers to preventive behaviors.

The participants believed that hypertension is strongly influenced by unhealthy diets, lack of exercise, and being overweight. Certain emotions such as "worry" and "upset" were also identified as causes of hypertension. Participants agreed that the consequences of hypertension were serious, such as stroke or kidney disease. They believed that lifestyle modification (diet and managing stress) would be best to control hypertension, although medication was helpful too.

The participants described three subcategories of limitations—health insurance for hypertension screening, money for purchasing healthy food, and lack of time. Lack of time was the greatest barrier to preventing hypertension as time constraints interfered with a healthy lifestyle and engaging in activities to reduce stress.

Every participant described Hispanic food as "a link to the past" and saw Hispanic food as a symbol of love, affection, and hospitality. Hispanic food was generally described as "unhealthy" because it was fried, salty, and contained large portions of lard, meat, and carbohydrates. While healthy adaptations of Hispanic food were acknowledged, traditional foods were the choice for social occasions as they are symbolic of hospitality and affection.

The participants described cultural norms that valued spending time with family and friends rather than regularly scheduled exercise or "working out." Dancing (with Latin music) was suggested as more appropriate than going to a yoga class. Another deterrent to hypertension prevention was not seeking health care unless symptomatic—"I'd better be pretty darn sick before I step into a doctor's office." Participants described a cultural norm that defined overweight as normative. Many Hispanics think being a little heavy is healthy; one explained, "Culturally, we don't look like little toothpicks." Being overweight may also be more acceptable to older Hispanics.

Clinical Implications

- Younger and more highly educated Hispanics may be more knowledgeable about and open to lifestyle changes than are older adults.
- Assess cultural norms when prescribing lifestyle changes for adult Hispanics who have hypertension. For example, exercise, stress reduction, and diet modification strategies may have significant cultural barriers.
- Social interactions are highly valued. Exercise and stress reduction can capitalize on this cultural value by building on another cultural value—dancing.
- Public health campaigns should emphasize that modifying traditional foods to make them healthy is appropriate, not only for regular meals but also for parties and social events.

Reference: Aroian, K. J., Peters, R. M., Rudner, N., & Waser, L. (2012). Hypertension prevention beliefs of Hispanics. *Journal of Transcultural Nursing, 23*(2), 134–142. doi: 10.1177/1043659611433871

members of an immigrant or refugee community of the social support and presence of a large ethnic community.

Generally, children acculturate more quickly because they are exposed to their peer group through schooling and they learn cultural characteristics through that association. The need to work outside the household often exposes women from traditional cultures to others of the majority culture; thus, they learn English more quickly than if they remain isolated at home. When individuals from other cultures seek health

BOX 11-2 | Factors Influencing Traditional Beliefs and Practices

1. Length of time in the new host country.
2. Size of the ethnic or cultural group with which an individual identifies and interacts.
3. Age of the individual. As a general rule, children acculturate more rapidly than do adults or seniors.
4. Ability to speak English and communicate with members of the majority culture. Language spoken in the home among family members.
5. Economic status. For example, if the family economic situation necessitates that a Salvadoran woman work outside the home, she may learn English more quickly than if she remains within the household and speaks only Spanish with her family members.
6. Educational status. In general, higher levels of education lead to faster acculturation.
7. Health status of family members. If individuals and their families seek health care

in their host country, they begin to "learn the system." This does not mean that they comply with all of the health advice, but contacts with the system should decrease anxiety and confusion.

8. Distinguishing ethnic characteristics, such as skin color. These individuals may be more isolated because of discrimination and thus may retain traditional values related to health beliefs and behavior.
9. Intermarriage. Ethnic intermarriage is associated with a greater loss of traditional ethnic identity.
10. Rigidity or flexibility of the host society. This refers to the extent to which the host society is willing to allow members of different ethnic groups, along with their traditions, beliefs, and practices, into their structure, culture, and identity.

care in their host country, they become familiar with its health care system. This does not necessarily mean that they comply with all health advice, but contact with the system decreases anxiety and confusion, and individuals are more likely to seek care again. In addition, if individuals or groups have distinguishing ethnic characteristics, such as skin color, they may be more isolated because of discrimination and thus retain traditional values, beliefs, and practices over a longer time. Some factors that influence the likelihood that clients, families, and communities will maintain traditional health beliefs and practices are shown in Box 11-2.

Access to Health and Nursing Care for Diverse Cultural Groups

Members of diverse cultural groups, especially those who are poor and without health insur-

ance, face special problems in accessing health and nursing care. Access to care is often determined by economic and geographic factors. Certain cultural groups have faced discrimination and poverty, and their ability to access care has been compromised. Sensitivity to cultural factors has often been lacking in the health care of traditional communities and identified minority groups.

In addition to economic status and discriminatory factors that limit access to care, geographic location plays an important role in health care. Many **medically underserved areas** lack medical personnel and the variety of health facilities and services that are available to urban populations. For example, Native Americans living in sparsely settled and isolated reservations in the western part of the United States must travel long distances, sometimes over primitive roads, to obtain health care services. Individuals who

BOX 11-3	Factors to Consider in the Nursing Care of Culturally Diverse Groups

1. Employment opportunities and insurance coverage or the financial ability to pay for health care services
2. Different traditional belief systems as well as different norms and values
3. Lack of cultural sensitivity on the part of social service and health care workers
4. Lack of bilingual personnel or staff members or the lack of interpreters to assist clients and care providers

5. Rapid changes in the US health care system, where clients are "lost" in the gaps between agencies and services
6. Inconvenient locations or hours of health and social services that preclude clients from accessing care
7. Lack of understanding, trust, and commitment on the part of health care providers

live on the Navajo or Hopi reservations in northern Arizona and have type 2 diabetes or kidney failure requiring dialysis must travel long distances for care. They may be picked up as early as 4 AM by a shuttle van that takes them into Tuba City, AZ for renal dialysis; the van takes them home later in the afternoon. Depending on the route and weather conditions, some individuals may arrive home as late as 5 or 6 PM having spent up to 8 hours per day in travel time plus the time required for dialysis. This arduous routine may take place as often as 3 days each week.

Other factors that may also limit access and use of health care services include the following:

- Reluctance of clients from culturally diverse backgrounds to seek the services of health care professionals who do not speak their language.
- Undocumented persons may be reluctant to seek health care because they are afraid of revealing their immigration status.
- Women from traditional Muslim cultures will be reluctant to seek care from male health care providers.
- Lack of understanding by clients of how to use health resources.

Nurses can develop sensitivity to diverse groups within communities and reach out to them with culturally specific health programs.

Box 11-3 lists some important factors that nurses must take into account for culturally appropriate community-based care.

Assessment of Culturally Diverse Communities

A **cultural assessment** is the process used by nurses to assess cultural needs of individual clients (Leininger, 1991, 1995) (see Appendix A). In general, the purpose of all successful cultural assessments is to collect information that helps health professionals better understand and address the specific health needs and interests of their target populations. Individual cultural assessments are accomplished through the use of a systematic process. In community health nursing, the community is considered the client, and several models have been proposed to help nurses assess the community (Stanhope & Lancaster, 2016), including the Andrews/Boyle Transcultural Nursing Assessment Guide for Groups and Communities (Appendix B). A community nursing assessment requires gathering relevant data, interpreting the data (including problem analysis and prioritization), and identifying and implementing intervention activities for community health (Stanhope & Lancaster, 2016). The community nursing assessment often focuses on a broad goal, such as improvement in the health status of a group of people. It is often the characteristics of people that give each community its uniqueness, and these common characteristics, which influence norms, values, religious practices, educational aspirations, and health and illness behaviors, are frequently determined by shared cultural experiences. Thus, including the cultural component to a community nursing assessment strengthens the assessment base. Box 11-4 provides basic principles underlying all cultural assessments.

Cultural Competence in Health Maintenance and Health Promotion

Leininger (1978, 1995) suggested that cultural groups have their own culturally defined ways of maintaining and promoting health (McFarland & Wehbe-Alamah, 2015). Nursing interventions to improve the health of individuals, groups, and communities can best be planned and

implemented by considering persons within their social, cultural, and environmental contexts.

Community nurses, who have direct access to clients in the context of their daily lives, should be especially aware of the importance of cultural knowledge in promoting and maintaining health, because the promotion and maintenance of health occurs in the context of everyday lives rather than in the doctor's office or in a hospital. The range of cultural influences on health maintenance and promotion is considerable. Major cultural issues and considerations must be addressed before health maintenance and promotion programs are implemented for culturally diverse groups. Evidence-Based Practice 11-4 describes a study that sought to understand parental perceptions of rural African American parents about the human papillomavirus (HPV) vaccine and how HPV vaccination rates among children in rural minority communities might be increased.

Cultural competence in community settings begins with anticipatory planning. In addressing

---

BOX 11-4 | **Basic Principles of Cultural Assessments**

1. **All cultures must be viewed in the context in which they have developed.** Cultural practices develop as a "logical" or understandable response to a particular human problem, and the setting as well as the problem must be considered. This is one reason why environmental and/or contextual data are so important.

2. **The meaning and purpose of the behavior must be interpreted within the context of the specific culture.** For example, the Hispanic client's refusal to take a "hot" medication with a cold liquid is understandable if the nurse is aware that many Hispanic patients adhere to hot/cold theories of illness causation. There is often a range or spectrum of illness beliefs, with one end encompassing illnesses defined within the biomedical model and the other

end firmly anchored within the individual culture (Huff, Kline, Peterson, & Green, 2015). The more widely disparate the differences between the biomedical model and the beliefs within the cultural group, the greater the potential for encountering resistance to biomedical interventions.

3. **There is such a phenomenon as intracultural variation.** Not every member of a cultural group displays all the behaviors that are associated with that group. For instance, not every Hispanic client will adhere to hot/cold theories of illness, and not every Hispanic mother will have a close personal relationship with her son. It is only by careful appraisal of the assessment data, and validation of the nurse's assessment with the client and family, that culturally competent care can be provided.

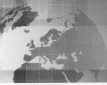

Rural African American Parents' Knowledge and Decisions About Human Papillomavirus Vaccination

Identifying those cultural factors or predictors of preventive health behaviors is an important activity in community health. The National Cancer Institute advises that certain strands of the human papillomavirus (HPV) are responsible for nearly 99% of cervical cancer cases and at least 20% of cancers of the head, neck, and anogenital areas (HPV and Cancer, 2015). The HPV vaccine can prevent many of these cancers if given to children (both girls and boys) at the age of 11 to 12 years. Previous research has shown that African American women are often skeptical about the HPV vaccine and that African American men are not knowledgeable about HPV or the HPV vaccine.

Understanding parental perceptions about the HPV vaccine is key to increasing vaccine rates, which are significantly lower for children from minority groups living in rural areas. The study sought to find culturally specific points of intervention that would increase HPV vaccination rates among children in rural African American communities. The researchers used a descriptive cross-sectional design and quantitative methods to collect data in three rural communities in Georgia. Four hundred parents participated in the study. Findings imply three major points of intervention: culture, religious affiliation, and parent education.

- *Culture:* Findings describe rural communities with low income, geographic challenges to access care, and large numbers of self-reported religious affiliation (Baptist). Local culture shapes people's perceptions of risk or perceived vulnerability. People assign value (either positive or negative) to an issue on the basis of their experience, and they trust experts who have a similar background to their own.
- *Religious affiliation:* Among participants in this study, religious affiliation had a correlation with vaccinating or planning to vaccinate a child. This is a significant finding since religion and spirituality are integral components of sociodemographics (rural culture) and influence perceived vulnerability to HPV infection and perceived severity of HPV infection and subsequent HPV-related cancer. The study found a "disconnect"

between people's attitudes about faith and healing and their actual choice to vaccinate their children. In other words, those that designated themselves as "Baptist," a reportedly "conservative" religion, reported high rates of HPV vaccination and intent to vaccinate.
- *Parent education:* The findings suggest that in this population of rural African American parents, both low knowledge of HPV vaccination and low level of perceived barriers could be attributed to the lack of knowledge about the connection between persistent HPV infection and HPV-related cancer.

This study reveals several intervention points: educating parents or caregivers about HPV-related cancers, HPV transmission, and HPV vaccination. Other possible interventions include increasing access to health care, reducing the cost of vaccination, and implementing school-based vaccine programs.

Clinical Implications

- Use culturally relevant interventions to educate both parents and youth about HPV. For rural African Americans, sensitivity and respect for the tenets of their faith are important. These tenets include but are not limited to belonging to the church family, giving problems over to God, and recognizing the human body as a temple of God.
- Access to care, cost, and availability of the vaccine influence HPV vaccination rates.
- Advocate for access to health care for rural residents and their children.
- Parental perceptions about the HPV vaccine are key to increasing vaccine rates among African American children in rural communities.
- Direct community interventions to minority families, communities, and the larger systems in which social injustice and racial discrimination have occurred.

Reference: Thomas, T. L., Strickland, O. L., DiClemente, R., Higgins, M., & Haber, M. (2012). Rural African American parents' knowledge and decisions about human papillomavirus vaccination. *Journal of Nursing Scholarship*, 44(4), 358–367. doi: 10.1111/j.1547-5069.2012.01479.x

cultural issues, it is important to involve local community leaders or "elders" who are members of the cultural group being targeted to promote the acceptance of health promotion programs. Such a leader, for example, might be the pastor of an African American church in the rural south or a member of the tribal council for a Native American tribe. The nurse must also be sensitive to cultural differences in leadership styles. For example, the African American pastor may not speak in favor of the health education program from his or her pulpit, choosing instead to work through more informal networks. Numerous nurse researchers (Abrums, 2004; Shambley-Ebron & Boyle, 2006; Zuniga, Wright, Fordyce, West Ohueri, & Garcia, 2018) over many years have found that many African Americans rely on spirituality and/or religious practices when they are ill, and in general, a health program that has the support of the church pastor would be viewed favorably by the church community. In addition to local community and religious leaders, it is important to involve those who are most affected by the health-related problems in the planning process. Those involved in planning and participating in the program's activities should likewise participate in its evaluation. Collaboration between the planner and the participants is often the key to success in community-based health programs (Stanhope & Lancaster, 2016).

Second, family members, churches, employers, and community worksites need to be involved in supporting health promotion/education programs through the use of networks that already exist. For example, a health education program about the importance of having a routine screening such as a mammography can be established at a worksite that employs mostly women. A display could be set up in the cafeteria, dining room, or other accessible site. Women could view the educational material during breaks or after lunch. Providing information about sites where women could obtain a mammography would be an important component of such a program.

Third, health messages are more readily accepted if they do not conflict with existing cultural beliefs. If the nurse plans to talk about prevention of teenage pregnancy to mothers and daughters at a local church, he or she should be sensitive to the group's religious values and norms. The nurse could discuss these plans in advance with some of the mothers and the pastor and ask for ways to strengthen the church's position, such as the support of abstinence programs. This is the time to be sensitive to the group's religious values.

Fourth, language barriers and cultural differences are very real problems in many large cities as well as rural areas. For example, in the US–Mexico border areas, *promotoras* (community health workers) are used to disseminate messages in Spanish and to help organize and present information that is culturally appropriate and understood by community members. Many Native American tribes make use of community health representatives (CHRs) to assist individuals to improve their health and/or access care. The health care professional should not be afraid to ask for help and suggestions in finding suitable educational material such as brochures or videos in the appropriate language and with a culturally acceptable message.

Last, **cultural sensitivity**, the ability to be aware of the needs and emotions of others, is essential to meeting health needs that exist within diverse cultural groups. For example, HIV/AIDS is spreading rapidly in some Hispanic and African American populations and is associated with intravenous drug use, violence, and the use of crack cocaine (Shambley-Ebron, Dole, & Karikari, 2016). Culturally relevant drug treatment programs should be implemented, thereby addressing both the drug abuse problem and the spreading HIV/AIDS epidemic. However, minority women seeking treatment programs for cocaine addiction may encounter barriers that seem insurmountable. Treatment programs may not be available in many areas, and child care facilities may not be provided, even in day-treatment programs. Thus, a young mother living in a rural area with children may not be able to find a treatment center that meets her needs. If she seeks admittance to a residential treatment program, she might have to agree to place her children in foster care.

Cultural competence to promote and maintain health in families requires knowledge about family systems, including relationships between family members, and how family members individually and collectively cope with health issues and challenges. Promoting and maintaining health also requires that the nurse understand cultural lifeways or practices within the family. Culturally competent nursing care in health maintenance and promotion is guided by four principles (Davis et al., 1992).

1. Care is designed for the specific client.
2. Care is based on the uniqueness of the client's culture and includes cultural norms and values.
3. Care includes self-empowered strategies to facilitate client decision-making in health behavior.
4. Care is provided with sensitivity and is based on the cultural uniqueness of the client.

Family Systems

Because the family is the basic social unit, it provides the context in which health promotion and maintenance are defined and carried out. The nurse can recognize and use the family's role in altering the health status of a family member and in supporting lifestyle changes. This requires an appreciation of the role of the family in diverse cultural groups. African American families, for example, may demonstrate interchangeable roles for their male and female members, extended ties across generations, and strong social support systems for the family such as the African American church, all of which can be tapped by a community health nurse to activate health and wellness in families (Campinha-Bacote, 2013; Chatters, Taylor, Woodward, & Nicklett, 2015). Immigrant and refugee families also tend to have strong extended ties with their kin, and changes in lifestyle, diet, and other established patterns of daily life that influence health status

will need the understanding and support of all family members.

Coping Behaviors

Clients often have distinct, culturally based behaviors to cope with illness as well as to maintain and promote health. These behaviors may be traced to the health–illness paradigms discussed in Chapter 4. Beliefs about hot and cold, yin and yang, and harmony and balance may underlie actions to prevent disease and maintain health. Community nurses must understand their clients' cultural values and beliefs to correctly assess clients understanding of health and illness. These assessment data serve as the basis for planning health guidance and teaching strategies that incorporate cultural beliefs and practices in the nursing care plan. It seems likely that clients in the process of coping with illness and seeking help may involve a network of persons, ranging from family members and select laypersons, as well as health care professionals.

Seeking social support is often a means of coping. Social support varies widely across people, cultural groups, and circumstances. An individual's coping behaviors during a personal or family member illness may differ remarkably over the course of time from diagnosis until resolution depending on intrapersonal, interpersonal, and environmental factors. Nurses working with diverse cultural populations understand how coping styles are used by individuals and family members, and how they are often influenced by culture.

Lifestyle Practices

Lifestyle is the typical way of life of an individual, group, or culture. Cultural influences that shape lifestyles have a significant impact on such health-promoting practices as diet, exercise, and stress management. Community health nurses should assess the implications of diet planning and teaching to clients and family members who adhere to culturally prescribed practices concerning foods. Some cultural groups believe that certain foods maintain or promote health. Specific foods often are restricted or promoted during illness, for example, the proverbial chicken soup. Cultural preferences determine the style of food preparation and consumption, the frequency of eating, the time of eating, and the eating utensils. Milk is not always considered a suitable source of protein for Native Americans, Hispanics, African Americans, and some Asians because of their relatively high incidence of lactose intolerance.

Nurses who work with culturally diverse clients must evaluate patterns of daily living as well as culturally prescribed activities before they suggest forms of physical activity or exercise to clients. Not everyone has access to a tennis court or a gym, and many individuals would not feel comfortable in such surroundings, or in aerobics classes regardless of the setting. Helping clients plan physical activities that are culturally acceptable is an important first step in implementing a program of physical activity for clients in diverse cultures. For example, traditional tribal dancing has become popular on some reservations for Native Americans. Running remains popular for members of the Hopi tribe. Running is deeply rooted in Hopi traditions as a way to carry messages from village to village and is also prominent in Hopi ceremonies. In the past, men of the Hopi tribe were superb distance runners, and the tribe still sponsors running events for its members. Hopi High School in Arizona has earned 23 state cross-country titles in a row and is well known throughout the state for its excellent track teams (Fonseca, 2013).

Another aspect of lifestyle that must be understood for the successful promotion of health and wellness is the manner in which culturally different clients manage stress. Stress management is learned from childhood through our parents, our social group, and our cultural group. Smoking and chewing tobacco, although not healthy habits, are often used to manage stress. Although these practices are not associated with a group's culture per se, they are often found in groups whose members feel that they do not have other options or alternatives based on economic or access challenges.

Evidence-Based Practice 11-5 describes how cardiovascular disease is defined and how Canadian Aboriginal women in tribal communities deal with such a diagnosis. Aboriginal women believed that they had taken on additional responsibilities including care of grandchildren, foster children and adopted children within their families and communities and that they could not manage any more lifestyle changes, not even to improve cardiac health. Providing culturally competent nursing care to heal their "broken hearts" requires an understanding of Aboriginal history in Canada and cultural knowledge about how the women made meaning out of their diagnosis and treatment programs.

The presence of large numbers of families with altered family processes and unhealthy lifestyles within any community may create problems for all members of the larger community or society. The nurse who works in **community settings** will frequently encounter these families and is in an ideal position to act as their advocate, to refer them to appropriate care, and, in effect, to improve the health of the community at large. This often requires understanding the individual's or family's lifestyle.

The nurse may find that in some cultural groups, such as Mexican Americans, traditional healers, such as *curanderos*, can be helpful for persons with some emotional or psychological disorders. It has been a tradition for many Mexican Americans to seek care from traditional healers. This lifestyle practice or health-seeking behavior seems "appropriate" and the right thing to do, whereas seeking care from a psychiatrist for this particular occasion or situation would be highly unlikely behavior. In some aggregate ethnic settings, such as the Chinatown area in San Francisco, there are practitioners of traditional Chinese medicine as well as Western medicine, acupuncturists, neighborhood pharmacies, and herbalists, all of which are available to meet the diverse needs of that particular neighborhood. Lifestyle is about the parts of our lives that make us feel comfortable and "right with the world." It's how we make our homes, relate to our loved

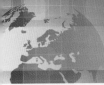
Broken Heart Stories: Understanding Aboriginal* Women's Cardiac Problems

The morbidity associated with heart disease is significantly higher in Aboriginal than non-Aboriginal Canadians with Aboriginal women showing the highest rate. Cardiovascular disease is commonly viewed as "White man's sickness." It is important to understand how individuals attribute meaning to cardiac health, healing, and overall life under complex social and cultural conditions. The role of colonialism is not only a historical fact but also a reality of today that serves to maintain health inequalities. Colonialism served to destroy traditional community structures that supported the role of the grandmother and that of women in general. Along with Aboriginal communities becoming more patriarchal, colonialism has altered the responsibilities and identities of women with particular consequences for women's health and also for that of their families and communities.

Cardiovascular disease is highly defined by biomedical terms; thus, the diagnosis of such a disease means introducing a highly medicalized "Western" sickness into a new cultural setting where there are few traditional healing options. The authors used a narrative–discursive approach in their study to capture subtle meaning-making processes that reflected the interplay between the individual and the culture. Sixteen women, all with various heart problems, volunteered for the study. Three major narratives were identified in the findings: problems of the heart, healing, and sociocultural context.

- *Problems of the heart:* While the participants described an illness genealogy of cancer, stroke, and diabetes, they reported that they were shocked to learn that they had heart problems. The women tried to downplay their symptoms and worries while struggling with fear and anxiety, afraid that a racing heart might be the precursor of another cardiac episode. Many of the participants were unaware that there are unique heart symptoms for women and for Aboriginal people.
- *Healing:* Many of the women relied on their Christian beliefs and turned to prayers and

reading the Bible. Only one woman practiced traditional alternatives to Western medicine. All were willing to take pharmaceutical medications, believing that taking pills required very little effort on their part. There was great ambivalence and even hostility toward the typically recommended heart-healthy lifestyle changes such as diet management, increasing exercise, and quitting smoking. Generations of White people had told Aboriginal people how to live in the name of "civilization," now health care providers are telling them how to live, this time in the name of "health."

- *Sociocultural context:* The mainstay of the women's narratives focused on the care and attention they gave to others, providing a backdrop to understand why living a heart-healthy lifestyle was so difficult for them. Aboriginal women take care of children and grandchildren, as well as foster and/or adopted children, many of whom had developmental difficulties due to fetal alcohol syndrome. The women made it clear that they often took on extra responsibilities in their families and communities with little or no support from men. Heart problems were not positioned as major concerns. It seemed the women intended to not burden others with what they called their "broken hearts."

Clinical Implications

- Aboriginal women need additional information about the unique symptoms of cardiovascular problems in women and in Aboriginal people. They also need information about the dangers of high blood pressure and the close relationship between anxiety and heart disease; panic attacks can be heart problems in disguise in postmenopausal women.

---

*Aboriginal or First Nations are the terms used by Canadians to refer to Native Peoples of Canada.

(continued)

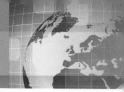

Broken Heart Stories: Understanding Aboriginal* Women's Cardiac Problems (continued)

- Health messages need to focus on positive and achievable goals. Taking prescribed medications can be an achievable goal that has positive results for women's health. Downplay the diet and exercise regimens. Talk about healthy eating and enjoyable activities.
- Traditional healing practices, such as sharing circles, sweat lodges, smudging, and artwork, include family and community and have repeatedly been associated with positive health outcomes. Health promotion activities that are less "top-down" would create more interest and support and less negativity.

- Consider how heart-healthy messages could be tied into the rich storytelling traditions of First Nations or Native Americans.
- Become knowledgeable and sensitive to First Nation/Native American cultures, belief systems, lifeways, and traditions as a first step in developing culturally competent care.

Reference: Medved, M. I., Brockmeier, J., Morach, J., & Chartier-Courchene, L. (2013). Broken heart stories: Understanding aboriginal women's cardiac problems. *Qualitative Health Research*, 23(12), 1613–1625. doi: 10.1177/1049732313509407

ones, raise our children, and manage our health and the well-being of those around us. Feeling comfortable with a health care provider's office may depend on the health care provider sharing the same ethnic heritage or at least speaking the language of the client.

Cultural Competence in Primary, Secondary, and Tertiary Preventive Programs

Nurses working in community settings use health-related concepts that are identified with the practice of community health nursing. Concepts such as "community as client" and "population-focused practice" were discussed briefly in the first sections of this chapter. Another important concept for community nurses is levels of prevention. Preventive care, consisting of primary, secondary, and tertiary activities, is directed toward high-risk groups or aggregates within a community setting. Primary prevention is composed of activities that prevent the occurrence of an illness, disease, or health risk. The preventive actions take place before the disease or illness

occurs. Secondary prevention involves the early diagnosis and appropriate treatment of a condition or disease. Tertiary prevention focuses on rehabilitation and the prevention of recurrences or complications.

The major aim of community-based preventive programs is to reduce the risk for the population at large, rather than to prevent illnesses in specific individuals. As long as preventive actions are directed toward a given population rather than toward individuals, there is a chance of altering the general balance of forces so that even if not all individuals benefit, many will have a chance to avoid illness. Evidence-Based Practice 11-6 *Yellow Dirt* documents the impact of uranium mining on the Navajo reservation and is an account of the tragic failure of preventive programs at all levels.

Primary Prevention

In their daily practice, community nurses are often involved in activities related to all three levels of prevention. Primary prevention is aimed at individuals and groups who are susceptible to disease or injury but have no discernible pathology or illness. The example of primary prevention

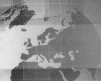

Yellow Dirt by Judy Pasternak

Yellow Dirt is a book that documents the impact of uranium mining on the land and the people of the Navajo Nation. During World War II, the Navajo Nation, wanting to support America's role in the war, permitted uranium mining on reservation land. The project was originally kept secret under the guise of national security. As early as 1952, the Public Health Service warned of cancer risks associated with uranium exposure. The Navajo cancer rate doubled between the 1970s and 1990s.

The initial case of *Navajo Neuropathy* was diagnosed in 1959; but it was only a matter of time before other Navajo children were diagnosed with the same syndrome. Scarce research monies were focused solely on genetics as the probable cause, ignoring the role of uranium exposure.

Hodgins and Hodgins (2013) describe the high incidence of severe combined immunodeficiency syndrome (SCIDS) among the Navajo, which results in a failure of the antibody response and cell-mediated immunity. In 2006, SCIDS was "discovered" to be the result of a mutation of the MPV17 gene.

Pasternak describes corporate and government actions, as well as the portrayal of the personal anguish experienced by many Navajo. *Yellow Dirt* is a compelling account that demonstrates the socio-economic, political, cultural, and policy factors that facilitated the exploitation of the Navajo Nation.

Clinical Implications

- Advocacy and education are important roles in community health nursing.
- Nurses can also play a role in community empowerment.
- Become knowledgeable about environmental concerns and their impact on health.
- Become familiar with local, state, and national agencies that are responsible for protecting the environment.
- Identify environmental concerns in your own community. How are they being dealt with?

References: Hodgins, O., & Hodgins, D. (2013). American Indians and Alaskan Natives. In L. D. Purnell (Ed.), *Transcultural health care: A culturally competent approach* (4th ed.). Philadelphia, PA: F. A. Davis Company.

Pasternak, J. (2010). *Yellow dirt*. New York, NY: Free Press, A Division of Simon & Schuster, Inc.

Prengaman, M. V. (2013). Review of yellow dirt by Judy Pasternak. *Journal of Transcultural Nursing, 24*(4), 417. doi: 10.1177/1043659613493442

---

used here is prenatal health services in Mexican American communities. Prenatal services serve as primary preventive measures for both the mother and her infant.

Overview of the Health Concern

When viewed as a group, racial and ethnic minorities suffer from worse health compared to White counterparts. Differences in the incidence, prevalence, mortality, and burden of diseases and other adverse health conditions exist among ethnic population groups in the United States (2016 National Healthcare Quality and Disparities Report, 2017). For many years, public health agencies have tried to improve maternal and infant services to high-risk populations.

In 1985, a special government seminal report on minority health reported that many minority women do not begin prenatal care during the first trimester (Heckler, 1985) and that this has serious consequences for mothers and infants. In response to this report, there was a considerable national effort to provide prenatal services to all pregnant women, but especially minority women and teenagers, and to reach them early in their pregnancy. Many communities now have broad-based coalitions that facilitate a comprehensive approach, especially for pregnant teenagers.

The risk factors of pregnancy include age (both extremes), parity, low socioeconomic status, and other factors such as diabetes and substance abuse. Additionally, other children within the family (need for child care), transportation problems, and other health care access issues negatively influence use of prenatal care and other health services. Many Mexican American women regularly face these challenges. Obtaining early and regular prenatal care greatly enhances a young woman's chance of delivering a healthy, full-term baby.

A program of primary prevention would focus on preventing infant morbidity and mortality and other health problems in Mexican American mothers and their infants. Early prenatal care may enhance pregnancy outcome and maternal health by assessing risk, providing health advice, and managing chronic and pregnancy-related health conditions (McKenzie et al., 2017). Nurses are in a unique position to advocate for policies that increase women's access to services for prenatal care. Nursing care must be broadly focused, not only providing some specific services but also helping clients access other resources in the community.

Access to Care. There are various reasons why Mexican American women might not seek care during pregnancy. Cost is often a factor, and in many areas of the country, Mexican Americans have tended to belong to poorer socioeconomic groups. Twenty-one percent of Mexican American families in the United States live below the poverty level, and many are headed by a single female parent (US Census Bureau Facts for Features: Hispanic Heritage Month, 2016). Mexican Americans are concentrated in blue-collar jobs, farm work, domestic work, and service occupations; lower status jobs translate into lower income and higher poverty rates (Ayón, 2018).

The value of routine prenatal visits to a health care provider should be repeatedly emphasized by nurses; some Mexican American women may stop regular visits if they are feeling well, because they are not accustomed to seeing a health care provider unless they are ill. The community health nurse can provide information about community resources and help clients access care early in pregnancy by referral to appropriate

agencies. Nearly all states offer programs that provide funds and services for low-income pregnant women. Although not a health program specifically, the Women, Infants, and Children (WIC) Program provides nutritious food and nutrition education to low-income pregnant and breast-feeding mothers, their infants, and their children under age 5 who are found at nutritional risk. WIC also provides health care referrals (U.S. Department of Agriculture, Food, and Nutrition Service, Women, Infants, and Children (WIC), 2018). The rate of low-birth-weight babies among infants born to women on WIC is 25% lower than for infants born to similarly situated women not receiving WIC benefits. WIC is an example of one of the most popular, successful, and cost-effective public health programs. Referring pregnant women to WIC services is a strong primary prevention intervention by community nurses.

Many Mexican Americans are more comfortable accessing health educational services in a setting that is known to them and where they feel comfortable. Neighborhood churches or neighborhood centers are excellent settings for health education; women know where they are located and are familiar with them in contrast to a hospital or clinic setting away from their neighborhood. Also, churches can provide child care so that mothers can leave their children in a safe place while they are attending prenatal classes.

Cultural Views About Modesty. Prenatal programs that serve Mexican American women may be underused unless consideration is given regarding some Mexican American women's reluctance to be examined by male health care providers. Female nurse practitioners and midwives are preferred for this population. Further, consideration should be given to incorporating the traditional *parteras* (lay midwives) or female *promotoras* (community health workers) in preventive educational services to increase use of prenatal services. *Promotoras* who speak Spanish are especially effective in delivering primary health care services to expectant mothers both in community settings and in clients' homes.

Language Barriers. Nurses working in community settings must always be aware of language barriers and plan accordingly. In some border communities, such as Nogales, Arizona, the Hispanic population is predominant (95.0%), and most residents speak Spanish in their homes (Nogales primary care area statistical profile—2017, 2017). It is absolutely essential in prenatal programs for Mexican American populations that the majority of health care professionals be bilingual. If that is not possible, interpreters must be employed to facilitate professional services. All prenatal classes should be offered in Spanish and English. This sometimes means that two classes must be offered concurrently; Mexican American women speak predominantly either Spanish or English and choose the class with the language they understand best. The availability of health education material in Spanish is critical to reinforce teaching and anticipatory guidance. Further, videos may be more effective than written material.

Cultural Views of Motherhood and Pregnancy. Some evidence indicates that women of Mexican American heritage may adhere to slightly different value orientations and cultural views of motherhood and pregnancy than do those found in mainstream American culture (Zoucha & Zamarripa, 2013). The Mexican American culture traditionally places high value on motherhood, and young women are encouraged to prepare themselves for this role. Community health nurses, nurse practitioners, and professional midwives are in important positions to help pregnant women prepare for motherhood and its associated responsibilities. Understanding of and reinforcing cultural views of pregnancy are helpful for clients, because trust and mutual goal setting can develop more rapidly. All nursing interventions should incorporate family members, especially mothers and sisters, for support of the pregnant woman. Emphasizing the responsibility for the mother to be healthy for her baby's health and welfare is appropriate for this cultural group.

Traditional Pregnancy-Related Folk Beliefs. Many Mexican Americans adhere to some traditional beliefs and practices related to pregnancy and childbirth. Traditionally, children are greatly valued and are desired soon after marriage. Census data from the 2000 and 2010 census indicate that Mexican Americans tend to marry and have children at earlier ages (Orengo-Aguayo, 2015; Zoucha & Zamarripa, 2013). As in many other cultures, Mexican Americans consider pregnancy, birth, and the immediate postpartum period as a time of great vulnerability for women and their newborns. Box 11-5 shows selected beliefs and practices of pregnancy and childbirth in traditional Mexican American culture. Each generation of childbearing women perceives pregnancy and birth differently. It is important for the nurse to assess the views of members of the pregnant mother's support system, especially her mother, who typically would adhere to more traditional values. It is always necessary to assess intracultural variation; not every member of any given culture adheres to the same beliefs and behaviors typical of that culture.

Mexican American Cultural Networks. Family is very important social structural factor in traditional Mexican American culture; nursing care should be patient and family focused, including those kinship ties including fictive kin, such as godparents. If nursing care is to be effective, nurses must tap these kinds of cultural networks to ensure the support of family members, neighbors, or friends.

Using Cultural Competence at the Primary Level of Prevention

The community health nurse should target certain high-risk behaviors for change during pregnancy, such as smoking, using drugs, consuming alcohol, and poor nutritional habits. A Mexican American mother-to-be may respond well to suggestions for change if she is convinced that her current behavior will cause harm to her baby. Family and social support groups in Mexican American culture can also be helpful and

---

BOX 11-5 | **Selected Beliefs and Practices of Pregnancy and Childbirth in Traditional Mexican American Culture**

- Avoid strong emotions such as anger and fear during pregnancy.
- Cool air is dangerous during pregnancy and should be avoided.
- Bathe often during pregnancy; be active so that the baby will not grow too big and hinder delivery.
- Eat a nutritious diet; "give in" to food cravings.
- Massage is helpful to place the baby in the right position for birth.
- Don't raise your arms above your head or sit with your legs crossed during pregnancy

because these actions will cause knots in the umbilical cord.
- Moonlight should be avoided during pregnancy, especially during an eclipse, because it will cause a birth defect.
- After delivery, a 40-day period known as *la diet* or *la cuarentena* is observed. Certain activities and foods are restricted during this time.
- Chamomile tea will relieve nausea and vomiting in pregnancy.
- Heartburn can be treated with baking soda.
- Laxatives and purges may be used to "clean" the intestinal tract.

---

supportive to expectant mothers wishing to make lifestyle changes. Hispanic women in general have low rates of smoking, about 7% compared with the general population at 15.5% (Hispanics/Latinos and Tobacco Use, 2017).

Prenatal services should include information about breast-feeding and family planning and reproductive health services. Traditionally, some health care professionals have assumed that family planning services will not be accepted in a Mexican American population because of religious opposition and *machismo*—the need of the man to prove his manhood by having children or to believe in the biologic superiority of men. However, Mexican American men and women may indeed be interested in family planning, particularly if they are concerned about the number of children they can support. This issue should be validated with individual clients and their spouses. During *la cuarentena*, the 40 days after the birth of the baby, women kin of the new mother often help with infant care, household tasks, and preparation of special foods for the mother (Zoucha & Zamarripa, 2013). Many Hispanic families believe that chili and other spicy foods should be avoided during and immediately after pregnancy.

Strategies for promoting breast-feeding should be identified and encouraged. Educational levels, family experiences with breast-feeding, the husband's attitude, the need to return to work, and feelings of embarrassment are all associated with infant-feeding choices among Mexican American women as well as other groups. These factors need to be explored with individual women to help them make the best choices for themselves and their babies. Breast-feeding is becoming more common in the United States as mothers become more educated about the advantages that breast-feeding can provide for a new baby.

Traditionally, Hispanic mothers may bind their own abdomen and also may place a cotton band around the baby's umbilicus (*ombligero*) to prevent the navel from protruding when the baby cries. The nurse can show the mother how to remove the *ombligero*, clean the umbilicus, and put on a clean *ombligero*. Many traditional customs should be supported by nurses who work with postpartum Mexican American women and their babies.

Secondary Level of Prevention

Secondary prevention involves interventions designed to diagnose a disease at a stage when treatment is likely to result in a cure. Nurses often use health education interventions when caring for individuals with a diagnosed health problem with the aim of preventing further complications or exacerbations. For example, at the individual and family level, teaching a patient with diabetes and his or her family members about eating healthy foods and incorporating physical activities into daily activities could be considered secondary prevention.

Overview of the Health Concern

Type 2 diabetes is seen commonly among many Native Americans, and certain tribes have extremely high rates of the disease. The American Diabetes Association recently indicated that American Indians and Alaska Natives are 2.2 times more likely to have diabetes compared with non-Hispanic Whites. In addition, there has been a 110% increase in diabetes from 1990 to 2009 in American Indian and Alaska Native youth aged 15 to 19 years (Diabetes in American Indians and Alaska Natives Facts At-a-Glance, 2014). By all accounts, the high rate of diabetes in Native Americans is a leading health concern; diabetes is a leading cause of outpatient visits at Indian Health Service facilities. Although Native Americans make up just 1.5% of the US population, they have the highest rate of diabetes in the world and one of the highest rates of end-stage renal disease (Native Americans and Chronic Kidney Disease, n.d.). Type 2 diabetes has become an epidemic and a national tragedy among many Native peoples.

The reasons for the epidemic of type 2 diabetes among some Native Americans are not clear. It has long been believed that some Native North American tribes have an underlying genetic propensity for the disease that is triggered by major changes in dietary practices, a sedentary lifestyle, and increasing obesity (Ratner, Davis, Lhotka, Wille, & Walls, 2017). These factors have been complicated by social conditions, such as poverty and inadequate access to health care, as well as by problems of compliance or lack of adherence to medical regimens. Because of the high rate of diabetes on some reservations, numerous secondary preventive services that focus on early diagnosis and treatment have been initiated. Box 11-6 shows beliefs and practices about diabetes of some Native Americans that could influence the success of secondary preventive programs for diabetes. Validation of beliefs and practices should always take place with individual clients and families, and stereotyping (thinking that all Native Americans are the same) should be avoided.

Using Cultural Competence at the Secondary Level of Prevention

Nursing interventions at the secondary level of prevention should focus on the implementation of healthful lifestyle changes that will ultimately decrease the complications of diabetes. Most of these are related to what health professionals call diet and exercise, but what is appropriate for Native North American culture is an emphasis on health and a healthy lifestyle. Nurses should emphasize health and a healthy lifestyle rather than negative factors such as control of diabetes, prevention of complications, weight reduction, and exercise. The choice of words, as well as the emphasis, is important.

For example, when teaching the client and family about diabetic diets, the nurse can substitute the word "nutrition" for "diet," removing the negative perceptions and leading to a nursing plan that emphasizes substitution of healthy foods rather than deprivation of unhealthy foods. Substituting fruits for candy bars and packaged pastries; whole grains for French fries, potato chips, or doughnuts; and vegetables for sugared snacks will improve the client's nutritional status and lead to a healthier lifestyle. Special traditional foods, even fried bread, can be eaten on special occasions, and other types of bread can be substituted during regular meals. Some reservations have restaurants or cafes that serve traditional foods such as tepary beans, squash, and Indian corn (Figure 11-3). Many Native Americans are interested in eating traditional foods that are more beneficial for a healthy lifestyle.

BOX 11-6	Beliefs and Practices Related to Diabetes of Some Native Americans

Nutritional Practices

- Diets are high in calories, carbohydrates, and fats.
- Sharing communal meals is a common and valued cultural practice.
- Some tribes have a high incidence of obesity and type 2 diabetes.
- Food preparation often adds fats and calories.
- Snack foods (potato chips, carbonated beverages, prepackaged pastries) are common.
- Alcohol abuse is often a concern. High intake of alcohol seriously compromises the treatment of diabetes.

Activity Levels/Fitness Practices

- Sedentary lifestyles have become common.
- Many reservations lack recreational facilities.
- Sometimes, formal exercise activities are associated with the White man's culture and are thought to be inappropriate for Native Americans. This is changing as Native youth excel at sports, and more tribes use "casino" money (funds generated from casinos) to build recreational and exercise facilities on tribal lands.

Beliefs and Values Related to Diabetes

- Ideal body image favors a heavier physique, and weight gain is considered normal; thinness is a cause for worry and concern.
- Concept of "control of one's body," that is, weight, glucose levels, blood pressure, may conflict with values and norms of Native American culture. For example, Native American clients may be uncomfortable with comparison of individual performance against others or against the norms and standards of biomedical care.
- Many Native Americans are uncomfortable with discussing or exposing private body functions, such as providing urine samples or participating in blood testing in a public situation.
- Illness is a personal and unpleasant topic, and Native American clients may be uncomfortable when asked to talk about it.
- Diabetes is a "White man's disease"; Native Americans did not have diabetes until Whites came to this continent.
- The term "diabetic" may be offensive to some, and the label "diabetic clinic" may discourage clients from seeking health care services.
- White health professionals may be viewed with some suspicion and distrust, given the history of cultural contact between Whites and Native Americans.
- Because diabetes is so common in some tribal groups, there is a fatalism about the disease, especially if a family member already has diabetes.
- Beliefs and health practices surrounding diabetes may vary according to the Native American tribe.

Health education should be oriented toward the individual client and his or her family as well. Often health education is more effective in a home situation rather than an impersonal clinic. Physical activities that are culturally relevant, such as traditional dancing or even basketball, can be encouraged. Many Native American high schools now have basketball teams for boys and girls, and the competition is significant; games are avidly watched by the entire community. The value of health and a healthy lifestyle should be stressed over exercise and weight reduction. Physical activities that are congruent with overall lifestyle and cultural context will be easier to incorporate into daily living situations.

The Native American family system is typically an extended family that includes several

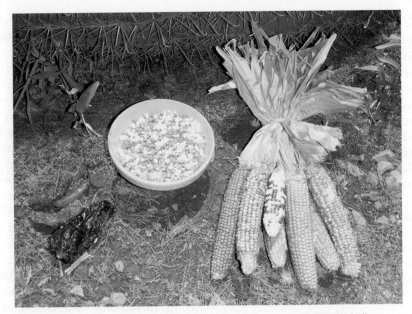

Figure 11-3. These colorful ears of Indian corn were named after the indigenous people of North America who had been cultivating corn for years when they introduced it to the Europeans who arrived in the New World in the 15th century. Unlike the typical niblets of corn on the cob, Indian corn is not sweet. It also has a starchy texture when cooked. The tepary beans are the preferred beans of the Tohono O'odham (the people of the desert). They have a slightly sweet flavor and a firm texture.

households of closely related kin. Family members become exceedingly important during times of crisis because they are a source of support, comfort, assistance, and strength. The importance of cultural ties with kin and other members of the reservation community must always be considered in planning for early diagnosis and treatment programs. It is in this context (family and community) that clients are encouraged and supported, not only to seek care but also to institute lifestyle changes that are congruent with cultural practices and that will enhance the health status of all members of the family and, ultimately, the tribal community.

The increasing rates of type 2 diabetes are of great concern to Native American communities. Introducing preventive health programs requires great sensitivity to cultural traditions and to the past experiences that native communities

have had with health care and health research. Understanding the needs of community members is essential for the development of culturally appropriate programs, and each Native American community has its own cultural traditions and beliefs that make up the details of daily life. Understanding the needs of Native communities begins by asking them what they want and need from preventive programs, rather than imposing ideas upon them. The best way to find out what matters to people is to get out into the community and talk to them. In Native American communities, it is wise to begin with respected and esteemed members of the tribal council.

Appendix D, Components of a Cultural Assessment: Traditional Native American Healing provides a framework that can be used to assess traditional healing beliefs and practices in Native communities.

Tertiary Level of Prevention

Tertiary prevention includes interventions aimed at limiting disability and rehabilitation from disease, injury, or disability. Sometimes, the distinction between primary, secondary, and tertiary levels of prevention can blur; tertiary prevention usually includes compliance with long-term treatment and provision of aftercare services. The following example focuses on African Americans who have high rates of hypertension, often leading to heart disease and stroke. African Americans are a highly heterogeneous group and display considerable variation in health beliefs and behaviors. For the most part, this section discusses a more traditional, rural African American culture; always validate beliefs and behaviors with individual clients and communities.

Overview of the Health Concern

Hypertension is a major risk factor for heart disease and stroke. Mean blood pressure levels are higher in African Americans than in White Americans, with a marked excess in African Americans. Further, the prevalence of hypertension in African Americans in the United States is still among the highest in the world (Musemwa & Gadegbeku, 2017). It is critical that efforts to treat hypertension in African American populations be continued, because hypertension affects African Americans in unique ways. African Americans develop high blood pressure at younger ages than other groups in the United States. In addition, they are more likely to develop complications associated with high blood pressure. These problems include stroke, kidney disease, blindness, dementia, and health disease (Beckerman, 2017).

Unfortunately, appropriate care often has been complicated by discrimination, poverty, and limited access to care. Poverty is often a problem in rural African American communities, and African Americans often experience severe economic deprivation. In 2016, 22% of all African Americans were living below the national poverty level (Poverty Rate by Race/Ethnicity, 2016). Some researchers believe that high blood pressure in African Americans may be due to factors that are unique to the experiences of African Americans in the United States. To date, researchers do not know exactly why high blood pressure is more common in African Americans. However, we do know that increased age, excessive weight, diabetes, inactivity, diet, and smoking are some risk factors for developing high blood pressure.

The goal of tertiary prevention is to reduce disability and prevent complications from developing further. Weight management; increased physical activities; appropriate diet, such as decreasing dietary salt and fat; and smoking cessation are all amenable to tertiary preventive measures. A major aim of nursing care in the implementation of tertiary activities is to help clients adjust to limitations or changes in daily living, to increase their coping skills, to control symptoms, and in general to minimize the complications of disease by reducing the rate of residual damage in a given population. Cultural factors that should be considered in tertiary prevention programs for African Americans are shown in Box 11-7.

Using Cultural Competence at the Tertiary Level of Prevention

Community nurses have demonstrated competence in the management of community hypertension programs. Although these programs are vital to the early diagnosis and management of hypertension, they also include a component that focuses on helping clients manage a chronic disease—an aspect of tertiary prevention. Numerous studies have shown that African American churches are excellent sites for community-based health programs such as hypertension clinics. The African American community should be involved in every aspect of community-based programs. The goals, objectives, and interventions of the services should reflect the expressed needs of the community target group, as well as their values, beliefs, and interests.

Community health nurses are in the advantageous position of assessing clients and families

BOX 11-7	Cultural Factors to Consider in Planning Tertiary Prevention for a Traditional African American Population

Language

African American communication concepts and patterns can be identified and used in community education programs.

Cultural Health Beliefs

Good health comes from good luck.

Health is related to harmony in nature. Illnesses are classified as "natural" or "unnatural."

Illness may be God's punishment.

Maintenance of health is associated with "reading the signs," for example, phase of the moon, season of the year, position of the planets.

Cultural Health Practices

The use of herbs, oils, powders, roots, and other home remedies may be common.

Prayers, reading the Bible, and attending church services will promote health and help cure diseases.

Cultural Healers

Older woman ("old lady") in the community who has knowledge of herbs and healing

Spiritualist who is called by God to heal disease or solve emotional or personal problems

Voodoo priest/priestess who is a powerful cultural healer who uses voodoo, bone reading, and so on to heal or to bring about desired events

Root doctor who uses roots, herbs, oils, candles, and ointments in healing rituals

Time Orientation

May be present-time oriented, which makes preventive care more difficult to implement and maintain

Nutritional Practices

Soul food takes its name from a feeling of kinship among African Americans and may be served at home, provided at church dinners, or served at home-style restaurants.

Diets may reflect traditional rural Southern foods such as fried chicken, collard greens cooked with bacon or ham, grits with butter, corn bread, and chickpeas. Dessert may be peach cobbler.

With the exception of chickpeas, the other foods have a high caloric and fat content.

Economic Status

In 2014, 35% of African Americans were living below the national poverty level (Poverty Rate by Race/Ethnicity, 2014). This has a very negative impact on health status.

Educational Status

High aspirations for education but socioeconomic status and other complex factors limit educational opportunities

Family and Social Networks

Often strong extended family networks with a sense of obligation to relatives

Self-concept

The importance of race has been a continual issue for the self-identity of African Americans.

Impact of Racism

Unfortunately, racism is still present, and a negative perception of the African American's skin color by health professionals will seriously interfere with efficacious health care.

Religion

African American churches have tremendous influence on the daily lives of their members because they serve as a source of spiritual and social support.

The African American church acts as a caretaker for the cultural characteristics of Black culture.

| **BOX 11-7** | Cultural Factors to Consider in Planning Tertiary Prevention for a Traditional African American Population |

Biologic Variations

There is a high incidence of lactose intolerance and lactase deficiency; this has implications for diet planning if African American clients cannot tolerate milk or milk products.

There is a higher prevalence of hypertension among African Americans than among Americans of European heritage. Sickle cell anemia is more common among African Americans.

References: Andrews, M. M., & Bolin, L. (1993). The African American community. In J. M. Swanson, & M. Albrecht (Eds.), *Community health nursing: Promoting the health of aggregates* (pp. 443–458). Philadelphia, PA: W. B. Saunders; Campinha-Bacote, J. (2013). People of African American heritage. In L. D. Purnell (Ed.), *Transcultural health care: A culturally competent approach* (4th ed.). Philadelphia, PA: F. A. Davis Company.

---

in their own homes and neighborhoods. This provides an understanding of the daily life situation faced by clients that other health care professionals often lack. Community health nurses can bring this understanding to bear on helping clients with tertiary preventive activities. African American clients who have been diagnosed with hypertension can be encouraged to lose weight by eating healthier foods, eliminating dietary salt and fat from their diets, and increasing their intake of potassium. If an African American client has diabetes, the nurse can encourage him or her to incorporate healthy eating habits and increase physical activities in their lifestyle as appropriate. Clients who smoke can be encouraged to join smoking cessation programs; nurses can work with family members to encourage and support healthy activities that will keep high blood pressure from further damaging the health of African Americans. Tertiary preventive measures often involve long-time lifestyle changes, and clients can become discouraged when they see no immediate signs of improvement. Encouraging clients and families to continue with tertiary preventive measures requires the nurse to establish rapport by listening and attending to what the client is saying and doing. Mutual goal setting is important, and support for the individual client and family, although change provides support and motivation to continue with the tertiary preventive activities.

Summary

Cultural concepts related to community health nursing practice serve as a guide or framework for nurses who work with diverse populations. A guide or framework for providing culturally competent nursing care helps nurses and other health professionals provide care to individuals and groups with diverse cultural backgrounds. Nurses use cultural knowledge in assessing, planning, implementing, and evaluating nursing care. This chapter addressed cultural diversity of clients, families, and communities. Various subcultures, including refugees, asylees, and immigrants, were described to help nurses understand and become comfortable working with these groups in community settings.

Cultural concepts as they relate to the community at large will help nurses plan care for diverse individuals, families, and communities. A cultural assessment is as an integral component of a community nursing assessment. Culturally competent nursing interventions are an integral part of the nurse's role and ensure health maintenance and health promotion at a community level. Preventive care in the community is of particular importance to community health nursing. The use of cultural knowledge will help nurses in primary, secondary, and tertiary levels of prevention. Examples of cultural diversity and levels of prevention illustrate how cultural knowledge can be used in community health nursing practice.

REVIEW QUESTIONS

1. Describe four cultural concepts, and discuss how they can be used to provide transcultural nursing care to families and community aggregates.
2. Describe an example of how cultural factors influence the health of an aggregate group within the community.
3. List the major cultural considerations in implementing preventive programs for culturally diverse groups. How can cultural considerations be used to identify barriers and facilitators for preventive programs?
4. Identify special health considerations in immigrant groups within the community.
5. Describe secondary and tertiary programs targeting hypertension for elderly Chinese Americans living in San Francisco's Chinatown.
6. Describe similarities and differences between folk and scientific health care systems. Give an example of each.

CRITICAL THINKING ACTIVITIES

Describe sociocultural factors and their impact on health care for a cultural group within your community. Evaluate the access to, availability of, and acceptability of various health care services. Is this cultural group at risk? Why?

1. Conduct a community cultural assessment of a group within your community. Critically analyze the cultural knowledge and/or information that should be considered when planning care for the group. Use Appendix B to identify and collect cultural assessment data—family and kinship, social life, political systems, language, worldview, religious behaviors, health

beliefs and practices, and health concerns. Compare and contrast the assessment of other groups in your community.

2. For a cultural group in your community, develop a program plan or intervention that has components of primary, secondary, and tertiary prevention.

3. Attend religious services at a church, temple, mosque, synagogue, or place of worship to learn about a religion different from your own. How does the church meet the unique needs of its congregation?

4. Identify alternative health care practitioners within your community. Which subcultures do they serve? Describe the kinds of care that they offer to residents.

REFERENCES

2016 National Healthcare Quality and Disparities Report. (2017). Rockville, MD: Agency for Healthcare Research and Quality. Retrieved from https://www.ahrq.gov/workingforquality/about/nqs-fact-sheets/fact-sheet.html

Abrums, M. (2004). Faith and feminism: How African American women from a storefront church resist oppression in healthcare. *ANS. Advances in Nursing Science*, *27*(3), 187–201. Retrieved from https://www.ncbi.nlm.nih.gov/pubmed/15455581

Andrews, M. M., & Bolin, L. (1993). The African American community. In J. M. Swanson, & M. Albrecht (Eds.), *Community health nursing: Promoting the health of aggregates* (pp. 443–458). Philadelphia, PA: W. B. Saunders.

Andrews, M. M., & Boyle, J. (Eds.). (2016). *Transcultural concepts in nursing care* (7th ed.). Philadelphia, PA: Wolters Kluwer.

Aroian, K. J., Peters, R. M., Rudner, N., & Waser, L. (2012). Hypertension prevention beliefs of Hispanics. *Journal of Transcultural Nursing*, *23*(2), 134–142. doi: 10.1177/1043659611433871

Ayón, C. (2018). "Vivimos en Jaula de Oro": The impact of state-level legislation on immigrant latino families. *Journal of Immigrant & Refugee Studies*, *16*(4), 351–371. doi: 10.1080/15562948.2017.1306151

Baird, M. B., Domian, E. W., Mulcahy, E. R., Mabior, R., Jemutai-Tanui, G., & Filippi, M. K. (2015). Creating a bridge of understanding between two worlds: Community-based collaborative-action research with Sudanese refugee women. *Public Health Nursing*, *32*(5), 388–396. doi: 10.1111/phn.12172

Beckerman, J. (2017). High blood pressure in African-Americans. Retrieved from https://www.webmd.com/hypertension-high-blood-pressure/guide/hypertension-in-african-americans#1

Betancourt, T. S., Newnham, E. A., Birman, D., Lee, R., Ellis, B. H., & Layne, C. M. (2017). Comparing trauma exposure, mental health needs, and service utilization across clinical samples of refugee, immigrant, and U.S.-origin children. *Journal of Traumatic Stress*, *30*(3), 209–218. doi: 10.1002/jts.22186

Campinha-Bacote, J. (2013). People of African American heritage. In L. D. Purnell (Ed.), *Transcultural health care: A culturally competent approach* (4th ed.). Philadelphia, PA: F. A. Davis Company.

Canales, M. K., & Drevdahl, D. J. (2014). Community/public health nursing: Is there a future for the specialty? *Nursing Outlook*, *62*(6), 448–458. doi: 10.1016/j.outlook.2014.06.007

Chatters, L. M., Taylor, R. J., Woodward, A. T., & Nicklett, E. J. (2015). Social support from church and family members and depressive symptoms among older African Americans. *The American Journal of Geriatric Psychiatry*, *23*(6), 559–567. doi: https://doi.org/10.1016/j.jagp.2014.04.008

Convention and protocol relating to the status of refugees. (2010). Geneva, Switzerland: Retrieved from https://www.unhcr.org

Davis, L. H., Dumas, R., Ferketich, S., Flaherty, M. J., Isenberg, M., Koerner, J. E., . . . Meleis, A. I. (1992). American Academy of Nursing expert panel report: Culturally competent health care. *Nurs Outlook*, *40*(6), 277–283.

DeSantis, L. (1997). Building healthy communities with immigrants and refugees. *Journal of Transcultural Nursing*, *9*(1), 20–31. doi: 10.1177/104365969700900104

Diabetes in American Indians and Alaska Natives Facts At-a-Glance. (2014). Indian Health Service. Retrieved from https://www.ihs.gov/sdpi/includes/themes/responsive2017/display_objects/documents/factsheets/Fact_sheet_AIAN_508c.pdf

Fonseca, F. (November 2, 2013). Championships run deep at Hopi high school, News. *Arizona Daily Star*.

Gainsbury, S. M. (2017). Cultural competence in the treatment of addictions: Theory, practice and evidence. *Clinical Psychology & Psychotherapy*, *24*(4), 987–1001. doi: 10.1002/cpp.2062

Golub, N., Seplaki, C., Stockman, D., Thevenet-Morrison, K., Fernandez, D., & Fisher, S. (2018). Impact of length of residence in the united states on risk of diabetes and hypertension in resettled refugees. *Journal of Immigrant and Minority Health*, *20*(2), 296–306. doi: 10.1007/s10903-017-0636-y

HealthyPeople 2000. *National health promotion and disease prevention objectives*. (1991). Rockville, MD: U.S. Department of Health & Human Services.

HealthyPeople 2010. *National health promotion and disease prevention objectives*. (2000). Rockville, MD: Centers for Disease Control and Prevention.

HealthyPeople 2020. (November 9, 2018). Retrieved from https://www.healthypeople.gov/

Heckler, M. M. (1985). *Report of the secretary's task force on black & minority health*. Retrieved from https://www.nal.usda.gov/

Hispanics/Latinos and Tobacco Use. (2017). Retrieved from https://www.cdc.gov/tobacco/disparities/hispanics-latinos/index.htm

Hodgins, O., & Hodgins, D. (2013). American Indians and Alaskan Natives. In L. D. Purnell (Ed.), *Transcultural health care: A culturally competent approach* (4th ed.). Philadelphia, PA: F. A. Davis Company.

HPV and Cancer. (2015). About cancer. Retrieved from https://www.cancer.gov/about-cancer/causes-prevention/risk/infectious-agents/hpv-fact-sheet

Huff, R. M., Kline, M. V., Peterson, D. V., & Green, L. W. (2015). *Health promotion in multicultural populations: A handbook for practitioners and students* (3rd ed.). Los Angeles, CA: Sage.

Igielnik, R., & Krogstad, J. (February 3, 2017). Where refugees to the U.S. come from. *Factank News in the Numbers*. Retrieved from http://www.pewresearch.org/fact-tank/2017/02/03/where-refugees-to-the-u-s-come-from/

Krogstad, J. (2017). Key facts about refugees to the U.S. Retrieved from http://www.pewresearch.org/AUTHOR/JRADFORD/)

Leininger, M. (1978). *Transcultural nursing: Concepts, theories and practice*. New York, NY: John Wiley & Sons.

Leininger, M. (1991). Leininger's acculturation health care assessment tool for cultural patterns in traditional and non-traditional lifeways. *Journal of Transcultural Nursing*, *2*(2), 40–42. Retrieved from https://www.ncbi.nlm.nih.gov/pubmed/2043295

Leininger, M. (1995). *Transcultural nursing: Concepts, theories, research and practice*. New York, NY: McGraw-Hill.

Lipson, J. G., & Meleis, A. I. (1983). Issues in health care of Middle Eastern patients. *Western Journal of Medicine*, *139*(6), 854–861. Retrieved from http://www.ncbi.nlm.nih.gov/pmc/articles/PMC1011016/

McEwen, M., Boyle, J., & Hilfinger Messias, D. (2015). Undocumentedness and public policy: The impact on communities, individuals, and families along the Arizona/Sonora border. *Nursing Outlook*, *63*(1), 77–85. doi: 10.1016/j.outlook.2014.10.009

McFarland, M. R., & Wehbe-Alamah, H. B. (2015). *Leininger's culture care diversity and universality: A worldwide nursing theory* (3rd ed.). Burlington, MA: Jones & Bartlett Learning.

McGuire, S. (2014). Borders, centers, and margins: Critical landscapes for migrant health. *Advances in Nursing Science*, *37*(3), 197–212.

McKenzie, J. F., Pinger, R. R., & Seabert, D. (2017). *An introduction to community & public health* (9th ed.). Burlington, MA: Jones & Bartlett Learning.

Medved, M. I., Brockmeier, J., Morach, J., & Chartier-Courchene, L. (2013). Broken heart stories: Understanding aboriginal women's cardiac problems. *Qualitative Health Research, 23*(12), 1613–1625. doi: 10.1177/1049732313509407

Meffert, S. M., Shome, S., Neylan, T. C., Musalo, K., Fineberg, H. V., Cooke, M. M., ... Goosby, E. P. (2016). Health impact of human rights testimony: Harming the most vulnerable? *BMJ Global Health, 1*(1), e000001. doi: 10.1136/bmjgh-2015-000001

Musalo, K., & Lee, E. (2017). Seeking a rational approach to a regional refugee crisis: Lessons from the summer 2014 "Surge" of Central American women and children at the US-Mexico border. *Journal on Migration and Human Security, 5*(1), 137–179. doi: 10.14240/jmhs.v5i1.78

Musemwa, N., & Gadegbeku, C. A. (2017). Hypertension in African Americans. *Current Cardiology Reports, 19*(12), 129. doi: 10.1007/s11886-017-0933-z

Native Americans and Chronic Kidney Disease. (n.d.). DaVita kidney care: Education. Retrieved from https://www.davita.com/education/kidney-disease/risk-factors/native-americans-and-chronic-kidney-disease-ckd

Nogales primary care area statistical profile—2017. (2017). Retrieved from https://www.azdhs.gov/documents/prevention/health-systems-development/data-reports-maps/primary-care/santa-cruz/126.pdf

Orengo-Aguayo, R. E. (2015). Mexican American and other Hispanic couples' relationship dynamics: A review to inform interventions aimed at promoting healthy relationships. *Marriage & Family Review, 51*(7), 633–667. doi: 10.1080/01494929.2015.1068253

Pasternak, J. (2010). *Yellow dirt.* New York, NY: Free Press, A Division of Simon & Schuster, Inc.

Pavlish, C., & Ho, A. (2009). Human rights barriers for displaced persons in southern Sudan. *Journal of Nursing Scholarship, 41*(3), 284–292. doi: 10.1111/j.1547-5069.2009.01281.x

Pavlish, C. P., & Pharris, M. D. (2012). *Community-based collaborative action research: A nursing approach.* Sudbury, MA: Jones & Bartlett Learning.

Phillips, J. M., & Malone, B. (2014). Increasing racial/ethnic diversity in nursing to reduce health disparities and achieve health equity. *Public Health Reports, 129*(1 suppl. 2), 45–50. doi: 10.1177/00333549141291s209

Poverty Rate by Race/Ethnicity. (2014). State health facts. Retrieved from https://www.kff.org/other/state-indicator/poverty-rate-by-raceethnicity/

Poverty Rate by Race/Ethnicity. (2016). State health facts. Retrieved from https://www.kff.org/other/state-indicator/poverty-rate-by-raceethnicity/

Prengaman, M. V. (2013). Review of yellow dirt by Judy Pasternak. *Journal of Transcultural Nursing, 24*(4), 417. doi: 10.1177/1043659613493442

Purnell, L. D. (Ed.) (2013). *Transcultural health care: A culturally competent approach* (4th ed.). Philadelphia, PA: F. A. Davis Company.

Ratner, N. L., Davis, E. B., Lhotka, L. L., Wille, S. M., & Walls, M. L. (2017). Patient-centered care, diabetes empowerment, and type 2 diabetes medication adherence among American Indian patients. *Clinical Diabetes, 35*(5), 281. Retrieved from http://clinical.diabetesjournals.org/content/35/5/281.abstract

Shambley-Ebron, D. Z., & Boyle, J. S. (2006). Self-care and mothering in African American women with HIV/AIDS. *Western Journal of Nursing Research, 28*(1), 42–60; discussion 61–49. doi: 10.1177/0193945905282317

Shambley-Ebron, D., Dole, D., & Karikari, A. (2016). Cultural preparation for womanhood in Urban African American girls: Growing strong women. *Journal of Transcultural Nursing, 27*(1), 25–32. doi: 10.1177/1043659614531792

Spector, R. E. (2013). *Cultural diversity in health and illness* (8th ed.). Boston, MA: Pearson.

Stanhope, M., & Lancaster, J. (2016). *Public health nursing: Population-centered health care in the community* (9th ed.). St. Louis, MO: Elsevier.

Thomas, T. L., Strickland, O. L., DiClemente, R., Higgins, M., & Haber, M. (2012). Rural African American parents' knowledge and decisions about human papillomavirus vaccination. *Journal of Nursing Scholarship, 44*(4), 358–367. doi: 10.1111/j.1547-5069.2012.01479.x

U.S. Department of Agriculture, Food, and Nutrition Service, Women, Infants, and Children (WIC). (2018). Retrieved from https://www.fns.usda.gov/wic/women-infants-and-children-wic

U.S. Census Bureau Facts for Features: Hispanic Heritage Month (CB16-FF.16). (2016). Suitland, MD: United States Census Bureau.

Weech-Maldonado, R., Dreachslin, J. L., Epane, J. P., Gail, J., Gupta, S., & Wainio, J. A. (2018). Hospital cultural competency as a systematic organizational intervention: Key findings from the national center for healthcare leadership diversity demonstration project. *Health Care Management Review, 43*(1), 30–41. doi: 10.1097/HMR.0000000000000128

Williams, C. (2012). Population-focused practice: The foundation of specialization in public health nursing. In M. Stanhope, & J. Lancaster (Eds.), *Public health nursing: Population-centered health care in the community* (pp. 3–21). Maryland Heights, MO: Elsevier/Mosby.

Zoucha, R., & Zamarripa, C. (2013). People of Mexican heritage. *Transcultural health care: A culturally competent approach* (2013 ed., pp. 374–390). Philadelphia, PA: F. A. Davis Company.

Zuniga, J. A., Wright, C., Fordyce, J., West Ohueri, C., & Garcia, A. A. (2018). Self-management of HIV and diabetes in African American women: A systematic review of qualitative literature. *The Diabetes Educator, 44*(5):419–434. doi: 10.1177/0145721718794879

Other Considerations in Culturally Competent Care

PART

FOUR

Other Considerations in Culturally Competent Care

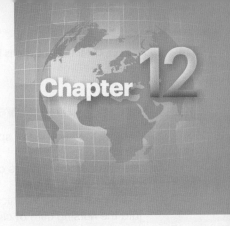

Chapter 12

Religion, Culture, and Nursing

- Patricia A. Hanson and Margaret M. Andrews

Key Terms

Allah
Amish
Anointing of the Sick
Bad death
Bereavement
Brahman
Brit milah
Buddha
Buddhism
Caste system
Catholic
Catholic Charities USA
Christian Science
Church of Jesus Christ of
    Latter-Day Saints
Consequential dimension
Enlightenment
Ethnoreligion
Experiential dimension
Faith healing
Fasting
Four Noble Truths

Friendscraft
Funeral
Garment
Good death
Grief
Hadith
Halal
Health Ministries
Hindu
Home going
Ideologic dimension
Intellectual dimension
Islam
Jehovah
Jehovah's Witnesses
Judaism
Karma
Kosher
Mennonites
Mohel
Moslem/Muslim
Mourning
Native American Church
    (Peyote Religion)

Nirvana
Noble Eightfold Way
Ordinances
Pillars of Faith
Principle of totality
Protestantism
Qur'an (Koran)
Reincarnation
Religion
Ritualistic dimension
Seventh-Day Adventists
Shema
Spiritual assessment
Spiritual distress
Spiritual health
Spirituality
Spiritual nursing care
Talmud
Torah
The Relief Society
Vedas
Wake
Word of Wisdom

Learning Objectives

1. Explore the meaning of spirituality and religion in the lives of clients across the life span.
2. Identify the components of a spiritual needs assessment for clients from diverse cultural backgrounds.
3. Examine the ways in which spiritual and religious beliefs can be incorporated into the nursing care of clients from diverse cultures.
4. Discuss cultural considerations in the nursing care of dying or bereaved clients and families.
5. Describe the health-related beliefs and practices of selected religious groups in North America.

As an integral component of culture, religious and spiritual beliefs may influence a client's explanation of the cause(s) of illness, perception of its severity, decisions about healing intervention(s), and choice of healer(s). In times of crisis, such as serious illness and impending death, religion and spirituality are often a source of consolation for the client and family and may influence the course of action believed to be appropriate by the nurse involved in the person's care and the care of their family.

The first half of this chapter discusses dimensions of religion, religion and spiritual nursing care, religious trends in the United States and Canada, and contributions of religious groups to the health care delivery system. The second half highlights the health-related beliefs and practices of selected religions, which are presented in alphabetical order.

Dimensions of Religion

Religion is complex and multifaceted in both form and function. Religious faith and the institutions derived from that faith become a central focus in meeting the human needs of those who believe. The majority of faith traditions address the issues of illness and wellness, disease and healing, and caring and curing (Sorajjakool, Carr, & Bursey, 2017).

Religious Factors Influencing Human Behavior

First, it is necessary to identify specific religious factors that may influence human behavior. No single religious factor operates in isolation, but rather exists in combination with other religious factors and the person's ethnic, racial, and cultural background. When religion and ethnicity combine to influence a person, the term **ethnoreligion** is sometimes used. Examples of ethnoreligious groups include the Amish; Russian Jewish; Lebanese Muslims; Italian, Irish, and Polish Catholics; Tibetan Buddhists; and so forth.

In their classic work, Faulkner and DeJong (1966) proposed five major dimensions of religion: experiential, ritualistic, ideologic, intellectual, and consequential. The **experiential dimension** recognizes that every religious person will experience religious emotion and/or feeling about their purpose in life and their connection with a higher power. The **ritualistic dimension** refers to religious practices, such as prayer, attending worship services, participating in sacraments, and reading religious literature. The **ideologic dimension** consists of the shared beliefs that members of a religion must adhere to in order to be considered members. The **intellectual dimension**, which is closely related to the ideologic dimension, consists of the cognitive understanding of the basic tenets or beliefs of the religion and its sacred writing or scriptures. Finally, the **consequential dimension** consists of how closely members adhere to the prescribed standards of conduct and/or attitudes as a consequence of belonging to a religion, such as political beliefs, attitudes about sex, and observing holy days.

Religious Dimensions in Relation to Health and Illness

Each religious dimension has a different significance when related to matters of health and illness. Different religious cultures may emphasize one of the five dimensions to the relative exclusion of the others. Similarly, individuals may develop their own priorities related to the dimensions of religion. This affects the nurse providing care to clients with different religious beliefs in several ways.

First, it is the nurse's role to determine from the client, or from significant others, the dimension or combinations of dimensions that are important so that the client and nurse can have mutual goals and priorities. Second, it is important to determine what a given member of a specific religious affiliation believes to be important by asking the client or, if the client is unable to communicate this information personally, a close family member. Third, the nurse's information must be accurate. Making assumptions about clients' religious belief systems on the basis of their cultural, racial, ethnic, or even religious affiliation is imprudent and may lead to erroneous inferences. Our Lady of Lourdes is a Catholic shrine, yet people from many different Christian and non-Christian faiths visit Lourdes each year seeking peace and healing from illnesses and injuries. Figure 12-1 shows people entering the shrine seeking peace and healing.

Fourth, even when individuals identify with a particular religion, they may accept the "official" beliefs and practices in varying degrees. It is not the nurse's role to judge the religious virtues of clients, but rather to understand those aspects related to religion that are important to the client

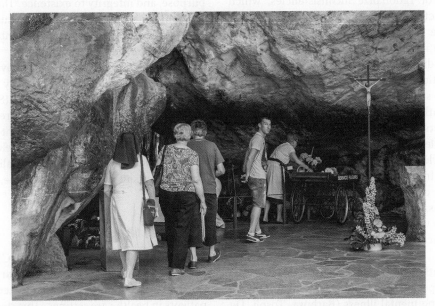

Figure 12-1. Our Lady of Lourdes shrine is in Lourdes, France, and commemorates the site of a Marian apparition in 1858. Four to six million people visit the shrine each year, seeking peace and healing from physical and mental afflictions. (Pierre-Olivier/ Shutterstock.com.)

and family members. When religious beliefs are translated into practice, they may be manipulated by individuals in certain situations to serve particular ends; that is, traditional beliefs and practices are altered. Thus, it is possible for a Jewish person to eat pork or for a Catholic to take contraceptives to prevent pregnancy. Homogeneity among members of any religion cannot be assumed. The nurse should be open to variations in religious beliefs and practices and allow for the possibility of change in an individual's views. Individual choices frequently arise from new situations, changing values and mores, and exposure to new ideas and beliefs. Few people live in total social isolation surrounded by only those with similar religious backgrounds.

Fifth, ideal norms of conduct and actual behavior are not necessarily the same. The nurse is frequently faced with the challenge of understanding and helping clients cope with internal conflict, which can occur when the patient faces differences between their own behaviors and the norms of their religion. Sometimes, conflicting norms are manifested by guilt or by efforts to minimize or rationalize inconsistencies, which may impact their health and desires regarding health care.

Sometimes, norms are vaguely formulated and filled with discrepancies that allow for a variety of interpretations. In religions having a lay organization and structure, moral decision-making may be left to the individual without the assistance of members of a church hierarchy. In religions having a clerical hierarchy, moral positions may be more clearly formulated and articulated for members. Individuals retain their right to choose, regardless of official church-related guidelines, suggestions, or laws; however, the individual who chooses to violate the norms may experience the consequences of that violation, including social ostracism, public removal from membership rolls, or other forms of censure. Social ostracism is especially problematic for those clients experiencing mental illness (Barbosa, Tosoli, De Oliveira Fleury, Dib, De Oliveira Fleury, & da Silva, 2018).

Religion and Spiritual Nursing Care

For many years, nursing has emphasized a holistic approach to care in which the needs of the total person are recognized. Most nursing textbooks emphasize the physical and psychosocial needs of clients rather than ways to address spiritual needs (Scammell, 2017). Recently, more has been written about guidelines for providing spiritual care to clients from diverse cultural backgrounds (Cates, 2014; Friedman, 2013; Jeffers, Nelson, Barnet, & Brannigan, 2013). Because nurses endeavor to provide holistic health care, addressing spiritual needs becomes essential.

Religious concerns evolve from and respond to the mysteries of life and death, good and evil, and pain and suffering. Although the religions of the world offer various interpretations of these phenomena, most people seek a personal understanding and interpretation at some time in their lives. Ultimately, this personal search becomes a pursuit to discover a Supreme Being, God, gods, or some unifying truth that will give meaning, purpose, and integrity to existence. The concerns related to life and death, pain and suffering are often present in the lives of the patients and their families under the care of nurses.

While religion and spirituality have similarities and overlapping concepts, they are separate and distinct from one another (Sorajjakool et al., 2017). In general, religion addresses questions related to what is true and right and helps individuals determine where they belong in the scheme of their life's journey. Spirituality emphasizes the pursuit of meaning, purpose, direction, and values.

Spiritual Nursing Care

In 2001, The Joint Commission (TJC) included an accreditation standard that required a brief spiritual assessment to be conducted with all patients in health care settings. This standard was revised in November 2008. It is nonprescriptive but states that each organization will define what spiritual assessment means for them and how it will be evaluated. Suggestions include such items as "who or what provides the patient/client with strength and hope, how does the patient express their spirituality, what kind of religious/spiritual support does the patient desire, etc." (Standard FAQ details, 2008). Given that pastoral services may be limited, the responsibility of obtaining this brief spiritual assessment may fall to the nurse. This assessment is the beginning of providing **spiritual nursing care**.

Spiritual nursing care promotes clients' physical and emotional health as well as their spiritual health. When providing care, the nurse must remember that the goal of spiritual intervention is not, and should not be, to impose his or her own religious beliefs and convictions on the client (Scammell, 2017).

Although spiritual needs are recognized by many nurses, spiritual care is often neglected. There are many reasons why nurses fail to provide spiritual care, including the following:

1. They view religious and spiritual needs as a private matter concerning only an individual and his or her Creator.
2. They are uncomfortable about their own religious beliefs or deny having spiritual needs.
3. They lack knowledge about spirituality and the religious beliefs of others.
4. They mistake spiritual needs for psychosocial needs.
5. They view meeting the spiritual needs of clients as a family or pastoral responsibility, not a nursing responsibility.

Spiritual intervention is as appropriate as any other form of nursing intervention and recognizes that the balance of physical, psychosocial, and spiritual aspects of life is essential to overall good health. Nursing is an intimate profession, and nurses routinely inquire without hesitation about very personal matters such as hygiene and sexual habits. The spiritual realm also requires a personal, intimate type of nursing intervention

(Bone, Swinton, Toledo & Cook, 2018; Rahmwati, Wihatstuti, Rachmawatic, & Kumboyono, 2018).

In 1978, the Third National Conference on the Classification of Nursing Diagnoses recognized the importance of spirituality by including "spiritual concerns," "spiritual distress," and "spiritual despair" in the list of approved diagnoses. Because of practical difficulties, these three categories were combined at the 1980 National Conference into one category, **spiritual distress**, which is defined as disruption in the life principle that pervades a person's entire being and that integrates and transcends the person's biologic and psychosocial nature. Pattison (2013) acknowledges the multidimensional nature of spiritual concerns and defines them as the human need to deal with sociocultural deprivations, anxieties and fears, death and dying, personality integration, self-image, personal dignity, social alienation, and philosophy of life.

Assessment of Ethnoreligious and Spiritual Issues

As discussed in Chapters 3 and 11, cultural assessment includes assessment of religious and spiritual issues as they relate to the health care status of clients. In the integration of health care and religious/spiritual beliefs, the focus of nursing intervention is to help the client maintain his or her own beliefs in the face of a serious health challenge or crisis and to use those beliefs to strengthen the client's coping patterns. Box 12-1 includes guidelines for assessing spiritual needs in clients from diverse cultural backgrounds.

Spiritual Nursing Care for Ill Children and Their Families

Any hospitalization or serious illness can be viewed as stressful and, therefore, has the potential to develop into a crisis. Religion may play an especially significant role when a child is seriously ill and in circumstances that include dying, death, or bereavement.

BOX 12-1	Assessing Spiritual Needs in Clients from Various Ethnoreligious Backgrounds

What Do You Notice About the Client's Surroundings?

- Does the client have religious objects, such as the Qur'an (Koran), Bible, prayer book, devotional literature, religious medals, rosary or other type of beads, photographs of historic religious persons or contemporary religious leaders (e.g., Catholic Pope, Dalai Lama, or image of another religious figure), paintings of religious events or persons, religious sculptures, crucifixes, objects of religious significance at entrances to rooms (e.g., holy water founts, a mezuzah, or small parchment scroll inscribed with an excerpt from scripture), candles of religious significance (e.g., Paschal candle, menorah), shrine, or other items?
- Does the client wear clothing that has religious significance (e.g., head covering, undergarment, uniform)? Does the hairstyle connote affiliation with a certain ethnoreligious group, for example, earlocks worn by Hasidic Jewish men?
- Are get well greeting cards religious in nature or from a representative of the client's church, mosque, temple, synagogue, or other religious congregations?

How Does the Client Act?

- Does the client appear to pray at certain times of the day or before meals?

- Does the client make special dietary requests (e.g., kosher diet, vegetarian diet, or refrain from caffeine, pork or pork derivatives such as gelatin or marshmallows, shellfish, or other specific food items)?
- Does the client read religious magazines or books?

What Does the Client Say?

- Does the client talk about God, Allah, Buddha, Yahweh, Jehovah, prayer, faith, or other religious topics?
- Does the client ask for a visit by a clergy member or other religious representatives?
- Does the client express anxiety or fear about pain, suffering, dying, or death?

How Does the Client Relate to Others?

- Who visits? How does the client respond to visitors?
- Does a priest, rabbi, minister, elder, or other religious representatives visit?
- Does the client ask the nursing staff to pray for or with him/her?
- Does the client prefer to interact with others or to remain alone?

Illness during childhood may be an especially difficult clinical situation. Children have spiritual needs that vary according to their developmental level and the relative importance of religion and spirituality in the lives of their primary providers of care. Parental perceptions about the illness of their child may be partially influenced by religious beliefs. For example, some parents may believe that a transgression against a religious law has caused a congenital anomaly in their offspring. Other parents may delay seeking medical care because they believe that prayer should be tried first.

The nurse should be respectful of parents' preferences regarding the care of their child. If the nurse determines that parental beliefs or practices threaten the child's well-being and health, he or she is obligated to discuss the matter with the parents. It may be possible to reach a compromise in which parental beliefs are respected and necessary care is provided. On rare occasions, it may become a legal matter. Religion may be a source of consolation and support to parents, especially those facing the unanswerable questions associated with life-threatening illness in their children.

Spiritual Nursing Care for the Dying or Bereaved Client and Family

While all people mourn, all people do not mourn alike. Mourning is a form of cultural behavior, and it is manifest in a multicultural society. Mourning customs help people cope with the loss of loved ones. Nurses inevitably focus on restoring health or on fostering environments in which the client returns to a previous state of health or adapts to physical, psychological, or emotional changes. However, one aspect of care that is often avoided or ignored, although it is every bit as crucial to clients and their families, is death and the accompanying dying and grieving processes.

Death is indeed a universal experience, but one that is highly individual and personal. Although each person must ultimately face death alone, rarely does a person's death fail to affect others. There are many rituals serving many purposes that people use to help them cope with death. These rituals are often determined by cultural and religious orientation. Situational factors, competing demands, and individual differences are also important in determining the dying, bereavement, and grieving behaviors that are considered socially acceptable.

The role of the nurse in dealing with dying clients and their families varies according to the needs and preferences of both the nurse and client as well as the clinical setting in which the interaction occurs. By understanding some of the cultural and religious variations related to death, dying, and bereavement, the nurse can individualize the care given to clients and their families (Ohr, Jeong, & Saul, 2017).

Nurses are often with the client through various stages of the dying process and at the actual moment of death, particularly when death occurs in a hospital, nursing home, extended care facility, or hospice. The nurse often determines when and whom to call as the impending death draws near. Knowing the religious, cultural, and familial heritage of a particular client, as well as his or her devotion to the associated traditions and practices, may help the nurse determine whom to call when the need arises.

Death Practices

Universally, people want to die with dignity. Historically, this was not a problem when individuals died at home in the presence of their friends and families. Now, when more and more people are dying in institutions (hospitals, hospices, and extended care facilities), with a variety of technological advances available that may prolong life but decrease dignity, ensuring dignity throughout the dying process is more complex. When death is seen as a problem requiring professional management, instead of a natural process, the hospital displaces the home, and specialists with different kinds and degrees of expertise take over for the family (Sherwen, 2014).

Preparation of the Body

A nurse may or may not actually participate in the rituals following death. When people die in the United States and Canada, they are usually transported to a mortuary, where the preparation for burial occurs.

In many cultural groups, preparation of the body has traditionally been very important. Whereas members of many cultural groups have now adopted the practice of letting the mortician prepare the body, there are some who want to retain their native and/or religious customs. For example, for immigrants of certain Asian religions, it remains an important ritual for families and friends of the same sex to wash and prepare the body for burial or cremation. In other situations, the family or religious representatives may go to the funeral home to prepare the body for burial by dressing the person in special religious clothing.

If a person dies in an institution, it is common for the nursing staff to "prepare" the body according to standard policy and procedure. Depending on the ethnoreligious practices of the family, this may be objectionable—the family members may view this washing as an infringement on a special task that belongs to them alone. If the family is present, it is important to ask family members about their preference. If ritual washings will eventually take place at the mortuary, it may be necessary to carry out the routine procedures of the institution and reassure the family that the mortician will comply with their requests, if that has in fact been verified.

The initial preparation of the body, as commonly practiced in the United States and Canada, has been described in a classic work by Kalish and Reynolds (1981) in the following way:

> *"After delivery to the undertaker, the corpse is in short order sprayed, sliced, pierced, pickled, trussed, trimmed, creamed, waxed, painted, rouged and neatly dressed...transformed from a common corpse into a beautiful memory picture. This process is known in the trades as embalming and restorative art, and is so universally employed in North America [the United States and Canada] that the funeral director does it routinely without consulting the corpse's family. He regards as eccentric those few who are hardy enough to suggest it might be dispensed with. Yet no law requires it, no religious doctrine commends it, nor is it dictated by considerations of health, sanitation or even personal daintiness. In no part of the world but in North America is it widely used. The purpose of embalming is to make the corpse presentable for viewing in a suitably costly container, and here too the funeral director routinely without first consulting the family prepares the body for public display" (Kalish & Reynolds, 1981, p. 65).*

This extensive preparation and attempt to make the body look "alive," "just as he used to," or "just as if she were asleep" may reflect the fact that people from the United States and Canada have come into contact with death and dying less than other cultural groups.

Funeral Practices

By their very nature, people are social beings who need to develop social attachments. When these social attachments are broken by death, people need to bring closure to the relationships. The **funeral**, a formal commemoration of the person's life, and the wake/viewing are an appropriate and socially acceptable time for the expression of sorrow and grief. Whether it is called a wake, viewing, or **home going**, it serves the same function: allowing the survivors to mourn together, comfort each other, and say a last goodbye.

Customs for disposal of the body after death vary widely. Muslims have specific rituals for washing, dressing, and positioning the body as well as time constraints regarding how soon the person is to be buried. In traditional Judaism, cosmetic restoration is discouraged, as is any attempt to hasten or retard decomposition by artificial means. As part of their lifelong preparation for death, Amish women sew white burial garments for themselves and for their family members (Amish Customs and Culture for Funerals and Burials, Death and Dying, 2015). For the viewing and burial, faithful Mormons are dressed in white temple garments. Burial clothes and other religious or cultural symbols may be important items for the funeral ritual. If such items are present in the hospital or long-term care facility, ensure that they are taken by the family or sent to the funeral home.

Believing that the spirit or ghost of the deceased person is contaminated, some Navajos are afraid to touch the body after death. In preparation for burial, the body is dressed in fine apparel, adorned with expensive jewelry and money, and wrapped in new blankets. After death, some Navajos believe that the structure in which the person died must be burned. There are specific members of the culture whose role is to prepare the body and who must be ritually cleansed after contact with the dead.

Funeral arrangements vary from short, simple rituals to long, elaborate displays. Among the Amish, family members, neighbors, and friends are relied on for a short, quiet ceremony. Many Jewish families use unadorned coffins and stress simplicity in burial services. Some Jews fly the body to Jerusalem for burial in ground considered to be holy. Regardless of economic considerations, some groups believe in lavish and costly funerals.

Taboos

In some cultures, people believe that particular omens, such as the appearance of an owl or a message in a dream, warn of approaching death. Breaking a taboo, for example, removing an object believed to have healing powers, is also believed by some to cause death. Nurses should take care to avoid moving or removing any objects of religious or spiritual significance without first consulting the client or family members.

Voodoo beliefs and practices are present in the United States and Canada. Incidents of sudden death or minor injuries after hexing have been attributed to the power of suggestion and to total social isolation, which have been thought to trigger fatal physiologic responses and sensitization of the autonomic nervous system.

Unexpected and Violent Death

Acceptance of sudden, violent death is difficult for family members in most societies. For example, suicide is strictly forbidden under Islamic law. In the Filipino culture, suicide brings shame to the individual and to the entire family. Many Christian religions prohibit suicide and may impose sanctions even after death for the "sin." For example, a Roman Catholic who commits suicide may be denied burial in blessed ground or in a Catholic cemetery. In some religions, a church funeral is not permitted for a suicide victim, requiring the family to make alternative arrangements. This imposition of religious law can further add to the grief of surviving family members and friends.

The Northern Cheyenne believe that suicide, or any death resulting from a violent accident, disturbs the individual's spiritual balance. This disharmony is termed **bad death** and is believed to render the spirit earthbound in its wanderings, thus preventing it from entering the spirit world. A **good death** among the Tohono O'odham comes at the end of a full life, when a person is prepared for death. A bad death, by contrast, occurs unexpectedly and violently, leaving the victim without a chance to settle affairs or to say goodbye. "A 'bad death' is 'bad' because evil caused it, which leaves the soul of the dead unrestful, unfulfilled, and desirous of returning to the living out of a longing for what has been taken away. The soul returns to the living, although not out of malevolence, to visit loved ones. It is on these visits, that the dead can bring a form of *ka:cim mumkidag* (staying–Indian–sickness), to the living—hence their dangerousness" (McIntyre, 2008).

The categories of "good" and "bad" deaths among the Tohono O'odham have implications for research on excess deaths. Accidents, homicide, and suicide produce bad deaths; in Tohono O'odham view, these are deaths that should not occur, deaths that should be avoided if possible. "Bad" deaths are excess deaths. If the medical community's concern is with eliminating excess deaths, it must also be concerned with the larger cultural, social, and economic context in which these deaths occur. Other causes of death, while still important, may affect a people to a much lesser degree. Diabetes mellitus, for example, most often affects people of more advanced years and, because of its slow progress, allows them to prepare for death. This is still an excess death by Western medical standards, but it is not a "bad" death (Anderson, n.d.).

Death memorials provide a place for the dead to go without bringing harm to the living and a place for the living to go to help the dead to a proper afterlife. Among the Tohono O'odham, there has been a notable increase in violent deaths, particularly for young males. The majority of these violent deaths are the result of motor vehicle accidents and are marked by roadside death memorials or shrines. Suicides and homicides are also sometimes commemorated with death memorials.

Deaths resulting from nonviolent but untimely causes can be equally difficult for the client, family, and friends. Cancers and chronic diseases may give the client and family time to "prepare" for the death, but the death still occurs and must receive attention. A good death to the elderly Japanese American often means to not have been a burden to others (Mori, Kuwama, Ashikaga, Henrique & Miyashita, 2018).

The Death of a Child

Although a great deal has been written about children's conceptions of death, cross-cultural studies have not yet been reported. Children develop a concept of death through innate cognitive development, which has significant cultural variations, and through acquired notions conveyed by the family, which vary according to the family's cultural beliefs. Thus, it is unsafe to assume that all children, regardless of family culture, will develop parallel concepts of and reactions to death.

Most children's initial experiences with death occur with the loss of a pet rather than a person. Because of reduced childhood mortality and delayed adult mortality, children in the United States and Canada are now much less exposed to death in family than they used to be, and they tend to be sheltered from the experience. The current lack of direct exposure of children to death is both a class phenomenon and a cultural phenomenon.

In many Western societies, children are considered precious, valued, and vulnerable; they are protected and often the first to be saved in emergencies. In less developed societies, by contrast, parents are less likely to see most of their children grow into adulthood because of a high infant mortality rates. As a result, a child's life may be viewed as less valued and precious than an adult's, although the child is still viewed as valuable to the parents and other loved ones. Regardless of the sociocultural situation, each society has a special view of the significance of children and their death as it affects the bereaved family.

Bereavement, Grief, and Mourning

Bereavement is a sociologic term indicating the status and role of the survivors of a death. **Grief** is an affective response to a loss, whereas **mourning** is the culturally patterned behavioral response to a death. What differs between cultural groups is

not so much the feelings of grief but their forms of expression or mourning.

Different family systems may alleviate or intensify the pain experienced by bereaved persons. In the typical nuclear American family, the death of a member leaves a great void because the same few individuals fill most of the roles. By contrast, cultural groups in which several generations and extended family members commonly reside within a household may find that the acute trauma of bereavement is softened by the fact that the familial role of the deceased is easily filled by other relatives. It should be noted, however, that the loss is experienced and mourned irrespective of the person's cultural background.

Although nurses frequently encourage clients and their families to express their grief openly, many people are reluctant to do so in the institutional setting. The nurse often sees family members when they are still in shock over the death and are responding to the situation as a crisis rather than expressing their grief. When asked who would be sought for comfort and support in a time of bereavement, most frequently named were a family member or a member of the clergy. In an institutional setting, a nurse who has been with the patient and family throughout the dying process may be surprised at the time of death when the grieving persons turn to other family, and the nurse is "left out."

Contemporary bereavement practices of various cultural and religious groups demonstrate the wide range of expressions of bereavement. Each group reflects practices that best meet its members' needs. The nurse can help promote a culturally appropriate grieving process; hindering or interfering with practices that the client and family find meaningful can disrupt the grieving process. Bereaved people can experience physical and psychological symptoms, and they may succumb to serious physical illnesses, leading even to death. Although bereavement is regarded as a universal stressor, the magnitude of the stress and its meaning to the individual vary significantly cross-culturally. For example, one Western misconception is that it is more stressful to mourn the death of a child than the death of an older or more distant relative. Yet, cross-cultural studies show that emotional attachments to relatives vary significantly and are not based on Western concepts of kinship.

Although traditional funeral and postfuneral rituals have benefited both bereaved persons and their social groups in their original settings, the influence of the contemporary Western urban setting is unknown. It is likely that in North America, most individuals have assimilated US and Canadian practices in varying degrees. The role of the nurse is to obtain information from individual clients in a caring manner, explaining that you wish to provide culturally appropriate nursing care.

Religious Trends in the United States and Canada

The United States and Canada are cosmopolitan nations to which all of the major and many of the minor faiths of Europe and other parts of the globe have been transplanted. Figure 12-2 illustrates the diversity of religions present in the world. Religious identification among people from different racial and ethnic groups is important because religion and culture are interwoven. Table 12-1 details the statistical breakdown of major religious affiliations of the United States and Canada.

As discussed, a wide range of beliefs frequently exists within religions—a factor that adds complexity. Some religions have a designated spokesperson or leader who articulates, interprets, and applies theological tenets to daily life experiences, including those of health and illness. These leaders include, but are not limited to, Jewish rabbis, Catholic priests, Lutheran ministers, and Muslim imams. Some religions rely more heavily on individual conscience, whereas others entrust decisions to a group of individuals or to a single person vested with ultimate authority within their religious tradition.

Contributions of Religious Groups to the Health Care Delivery System

In the United States and Canada, many denominations own and operate health care institutions and make significant fiscal contributions that help

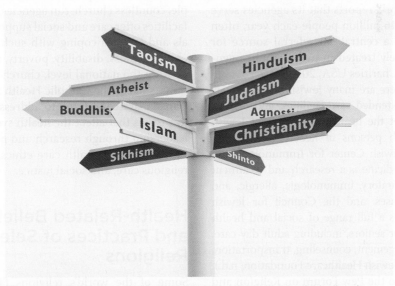

Figure 12-2. Multiple religions are present in all societies, and this diversity enhances opportunities for nurses to encounter multiple belief systems and to adjust their care accordingly. (Ryan DeBerardinis/Shutterstock.com.)

Table 12-1 | Major Religious Affiliations of the United States and Canada (%)

	United States	Canada	World
Christianity	69.7	67.3	31.2
Atheism, Agnosticism, no affiliation	29.9	23.9	16
Judaism	1.9	1.0	0.22
Islam	0.9	3.2	24.1
Buddhism	0.7	1.1	6.9
Hinduism	0.7	1.5	15.1
Major Christian Faith Groups			
Roman Catholic	20.8	38.7	32.3
Protestant	46.6	19.2	9.2

Source: Religious Landscape Study. (2017). Retrieved from http://www.pewforum.org/religious-landscape-study/.

control health care costs. For example, the Roman Catholic Church, the largest single denomination in the United States, is also a major stakeholder in the health care field. In the United States, there are more than 600 Catholic hospitals, 1,600 long-term care facilities treat 5.4 million people annually, meaning that 1 out of every 6 patients is cared for in a Catholic hospital (Catholic Health Care in the United States, 2018). **Catholic Charities USA**, an umbrella agency that oversees nonhospital work, reports that its agencies serve more than 1,046 million people each year, often functioning as a centralized referral source for clients ultimately treated in non-Catholic agencies (Catholic Charities USA, 2018).

Similarly, there are many Jewish hospitals, day care centers, extended care facilities, and organizations to meet the health care needs of Jewish and non-Jewish persons in need. For example, the National Jewish Center for Immunology and Respiratory Medicine is a research and treatment center for respiratory, immunologic, allergic, and infectious diseases, and the Council for Jewish Elderly provides a full range of social and health care services for seniors, including adult day care, care/case management, counseling, transportation, and advocacy (Jewish Healthcare Foundation, n.d.).

According to the Pew Forum on Religion and Public Policy, many other denominations, including the Lutheran, Mennonite, Methodist, Muslim, and Seventh-Day Adventist groups, also own and operate hospitals and health care organizations.

In Canada, hospital care, outpatient care, extended care, and medical services have been publicly funded and administered since the Medical Care Act of 1966. However, before the Medical Care Act and into the present, religious organizations have made important contributions to the health and well-being of Canadians at individual, community, and societal levels. For example, countless church-run agencies, charities, and facilities offer care and social support to individuals and families coping with such conditions as chronic illness, disability, poverty, and homelessness. At the national level, church-run organizations, such as the Catholic Health Association of Canada, are committed to addressing social justice issues that affect the health system and offer leadership through research and policy development regarding health care ethics, spiritual and religious care, and social justice.

Health-Related Beliefs and Practices of Selected Religions

Some of the world's religions fall into major branches or divisions, such as Vaishnavite and Shaivite Hinduism; Theravada and Mahayana

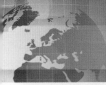
Two Studies on Religion and Health Care Practices

The Adventist Health Study-2 studied the relationship of vegan, lacto-ovo vegetarian, pesco-vegetarian, semivegetarian, and nonvegetarian dietary patterns of 97,000 members of the Seventh-Day Adventist church exploring the relationship of those dietary patterns to health outcomes, specifically obesity, metabolic syndrome, hypertension, type 2 diabetes mellitus, osteoporosis, cancer, and mortality. While the data regarding cancer have yet to be analyzed in depth, the data showed that "vegetarian diets in the AHS-2 population studied are associated with lower BMI values, lower prevalence of hypertension & metabolic syndrome and lower prevalence and incidence of type 2 diabetes as well as lower all-cause mortality" (p. 357S). While there has long been a concern that vegetarian diets put the person at risk for osteoporosis, it appears from this study that when plant sources of protein are consumed, the risk is decreased.

Reference: Orlich, M. J., & Fraser, G. E. (2014). Vegetarian diets in the Adventist health study 2: A review of initial published findings. *American Journal of Clinical Nutrition, 100*(Suppl 1), 353S–358S.

In this study, the researchers explored whether Hispanics, in general, and Catholic Hispanics, in particular, follow a "cultural belief" called "fatalism," which precludes the person from participating in cancer screening practices. Sixty-seven participants (33 men, 34 women) attended one of eight focus groups with 8 to 10 participants per group. Men and women attended separate groups. The intent was to explore the "participants' cultural explanatory models of cancer, including their cultural beliefs, attitudes, personal life experiences and their understanding of both biomedical and population explanations of health and illness" (p. 841). Contrary to the stereotype of "fatalism," this group "expressed few fatalistic beliefs with regard to cancer" and instead indicated a general belief that cancer was preventable if caught early. This group reported that their religion supported them in their search for health, including cancer screening. They also indicated that there is a role for faith and calling upon God and saints in the face of illness.

Reference: Leyvam, B., Allen, J. D., Tom, L. S., Ospino, H., Torres, M. I., & Abraido-Laza, A. F. (2014). Religion, fatalism and cancer control: A qualitative study among Hispanic Catholics. *American Journal of Health Behavior, 38*(6), 839–849.

Clinical Implications

- What questions might you consider after thinking about the evidence provided in these studies?
- How might this information impact your care of patients who are not from any of the ethnic backgrounds found in these studies?
- What other evidence might you want to explore to seek answers to clinical questions that you have faced?

Buddhism; Orthodox, Reform, and Conservative Judaism; Roman Catholic, Orthodox, and Protestant Christianity; and Sunnite and Shi'ite Islam. There also are subdivisions into what are often called denominations, sects, or schools of thought and practice.

Health-related beliefs and practices of select religions are important to understand, especially considering the diverse religious groups in the United States and Canada. Evidence-Based Practice 12-1 provides information regarding other research done on this topic. Box 12-2 summarizes some of the religious and nonreligious holidays covered in this chapter. A brief overview of selected religious groups and their health-related beliefs and practices follows.

Amish

The term **Amish** refers to members of several ethnoreligious Christian groups who choose to live separately from the modern world through

BOX 12-2	Religious and Nonreligious Holidays in the United States and Canada

This calendar is a guide to religious and nonreligious holidays that are celebrated in the United States and Canada. This not an exhaustive list, but instead reflects major holidays and festivals for religious and ethnic groups in the United States and Canada.

B = Buddhist
Ba = Baha'i
C = Christian (general)
Ci = Civic holiday
H = Hindu

I = Islam
J = Jewish
Ja = Jain
M = Mormon

O = Eastern Orthodox
   Christian
P = Protestant
RC = Roman Catholic
S = Sikh

January
1 New Year's Day (Ci)
1 Feast of St. Basil (O)
6 Epiphany (C)
7 Nativity of Jesus Christ (O)
3rd Monday Martin Luther King, Jr. Birthday Observance (Ci)

February
Black History Month (United States)
8 Scout Day (Ci)
14 Valentine's Day (Ci)
Midmonth President's Day (United States; Ci)
Other holidays that often fall in February according to the lunar calendar:
Chinese New Year
Ramadan (30 days; I)
Nehan-e (Death of Buddha; B)
Vasant Panchami (Advent of Spring; H, Ja)
Ash Wednesday (RC, P)
Purim (J)

March
Women's History Month (United States)
17 St. Patrick's Day (C)
25 Annunciation (C)
Other holidays that often occur in March according to the lunar calendar:
Eastern Orthodox Lent begins (O)
Higan-e (First Day of Spring; B)
Naw-Ruz (Baha'i and Iranian New Year)
Palm Sunday (RC, P)
First Day of Passover (8 days; J)
Holi (Spring Festival; H, Ja)

Maundy Thursday (The Thursday prior to Easter; RC, P)
Good Friday (The Friday prior to Easter; RC, P)
Easter (C, RC, P, M)
Mahavir Jayanti (Birth of Mahavir; Ja)

April
16 Yom Ha'atzmaut (Israel Independence Day; J)
Holidays that often occur in April according to the lunar calendar:
Hana-Matsuri (Birth of Buddha; B)
Yom HaShoah (Holocaust Remembrance Day; J, Ci)
Baisakhi (Brotherhood; S)
Huguenot Day (P)
Ramavani (Birth of Rama; H)
Palm Sunday (O)
Holy Friday (O)
Easter (O)

May
5 Cinco de Mayo (Ci)
23 Victoria Day (Canada)
30 Memorial Day (Ci)
Holidays that often occur in May according to the lunar calendar:
Shavuot (J)
Idul-Adha (Day of Sacrifice; I)
Ascension Day (RC, P)
Pentecost (RC, P)

June
12 Anne Frank Day
14 Flag Day (United States; Ci)
24 Nativity of St. John the Baptist (RC, P, O)

| BOX 12-2 | Religious and Nonreligious Holidays in the United States and Canada (continued) |

Holidays that often occur in June according to the lunar calendar:
Ratha-Yatra (H)
Ascension Day (O)
Muharram (I)
Pentecost (O)
Islamic New Year (I)
Hindu New Year (H)

July
1 Canada Day (Canada; Ci)
4 Independence Day (United States; Ci)
24 Pioneer Day (M)
Holidays that often occur in July according to the lunar calendar:
Obon-e (B)

August
6 Transfiguration (C)
15 Feast of the Blessed Virgin Mary (RC, O)

September
First Monday Labor Day (United States; Ci)
15 National Hispanic Heritage Month (30 days; Ci)
17 Citizenship (US Constitution; Ci)
19 San Gennaro Day (RC)
25 Native American Day (Ci)
Holidays that often occur in September according to the lunar calendar:
Higan-e (First Day of Fall; B)
Rosh Hashanah (Jewish New Year, 2 days; J)

October
12 Columbus Day (United States, Ci)
Thanksgiving Day (Canada, Ci)
24 United Nations Day (Ci)

31 Reformation Day (P)
31 Halloween (RC, P, Ci)
Holidays that often occur in October according to the lunar calendar:
Dussehra (Good over Evil; H, JA)
Yom Kippur (Atonement; J)
Sukkot (Tabernacles; J)
Shemini Atzeret (End of Sukkot; J)
Diwali or Deepavali (Festival of Lights; H, Ja)

November
1 All Saints Day (RC, P)
11 Veterans Day (Ci)
25 Religious Liberty Day (Ci)
First Tuesday Election Day (United States; Ci)
4th Thursday Thanksgiving Day (United States; Ci)
Holidays that often occur in November according to the lunar calendar:
Baha'u'llah Birthday (Ba)
Guru Nanak Birthday (S)

December
6 St. Nicholas Day (C)
8 Feast of the Immaculate Conception (RC)
10 Human Rights Day (Ci)
12 Festival of Our Lady of Guadalupe (Mexico–Hispanic)
25 Christmas (C, RC, P, M, Ci)
Holidays that often occur in December according to the lunar calendar:
Bodhi Day (Enlightenment; B)
Hanukkah (8 days; J)
Kwanzaa (7 days)

manner of dress, language, family life, and selective use of technology. There are four major orders or affiliating groups of Amish:

1. *Old Order Amish*, the largest group, whose name is often used synonymously with "the Amish"

2. The ultraconservative *Swartzentruber* and *Andy Weaver Amish*, both more conservative than the Old Order Amish in their restrictive use of technology and shunning of members who have dropped out or committed serious violations of the faith

3. The less conservative *New Order Amish*, which emerged in the 1960s with more liberal views of technology but with an emphasis on high moral standards in restricting alcohol and tobacco use and in courtship practices
4. The *Liberal Beachy Amish*, more commonly known as **Mennonites**, who maintain many of the same features as the more conservative Amish, but allow electricity and use of automobiles

The total population of Amish is estimated at 300,000 spread throughout more than 500 settlements in 31 states and two Canadian provinces (Farrar, Kulig, & Sullivan-Wilson, 2018).

Substance Use

Once baptized, alcoholic beverages and drugs are forbidden unless prescribed by a physician. Teenagers and unmarried young adults may experiment with cigarettes, alcohol, and sometimes other chemical substances. It is important to assess persons in this age group for substance abuse.

Health Care Practices

Illness is seen as the inability to perform daily chores; physical and mental illness are equally accepted. Health care practices within the Amish culture are varied and include folk, herbal, homeopathic, and biomedicine. Unlike the use of episodic biomedicine, however, preventive medicine may be seen as against God's will. The use of the biomedical health care system is largely episodic and crisis oriented. If biomedicine fails, there is no hesitancy in visiting an herb doctor, pow-wow doctor (a practitioner of a folk healing art, known as *brauche*, in which touch is used to heal), or a chiropractor. Folk, professional, and alternative care are often used simultaneously. Cost, access, transportation, and advice from family and friends are the major factors that influence healing choices. The Amish are at risk for a variety of genetic diseases due to frequent intermarriage among close relatives.

Farming accidents are also a common reason for seeking health care service.

Medical and Surgical Interventions

The use of narcotic drugs is prohibited. There are no restrictions against the use of blood or blood products, if advised by health care providers. Vaccinations are acceptable, especially for children, but may not be accepted for adults or elderly individuals.

Practices Related to Reproduction

The Amish believe that the fundamental purpose of marriage is procreation, and couples are encouraged to have large families. Children are an economic asset to the family because they assist their parents with housework, farm chores, gardening, and family business. Women are expected to have children until menopause. If situations arise that justify sterilization (e.g., removal of cancerous reproductive organs), those called upon to make the decisions would rely on the best medical advice available and the council of the church leaders. Although the Amish family structure is patriarchal, the grandmother is often a key decision-maker concerning reproductive and other health-related issues.

Abortion is inconsistent with Amish values and beliefs. Artificial insemination, genetics, eugenics, stem cell research, and in vitro fertilization are also inconsistent with Amish values and beliefs.

Religious Support System for the Sick

Individual members of local and surrounding communities assist and support one another in times of need. From birth to death, each person knows that he or she will be cared for by those in the community. **Friendscraft** is a unique three-generational extended family support network inherent in the Amish community that provides informal support, emotional and financial assistance, and advice. The extended family consists of aunts, uncles, cousins, and grandparents, who usually live only a few miles away and can be counted on to assist in times of illness.

The Amish do not use religious titles. So, a nurse may call any visitor by typical titles of Mr. or Mrs. There are approximately 300,000 Amish in the United States and Canada living in 31 states and 2 Canadian provinces, each representing about 20 to 35 families (approximately 500 settlements) and a minimal hierarchy of church leaders (a bishop, deacon, and two ministers). The bishop is the spiritual head; the deacon assists the bishop and is responsible for donations to help members with medical bills and other expenses; and the ministers help the bishop with preaching at church services and providing spiritual direction for the church district and its members. Although bishops meet periodically, there is no church hierarchy above the level of the church district. Because the Amish are surrounded by US and Canadian societies, which continuously exert strong economic and cultural pressures that are incompatible with Amish values, the Amish represent a subculture that is among the most "self-consciously engineered of all societies"(Farrar et al., 2018).

Individual members of local church districts look after the needs of the sick person and his or her family. When an Amish person is hospitalized, there will likely be a large number of visitors. Since they will not want to be in the way, asking them to step out when necessary is acceptable. Physical touch should be limited except for direct care. Parents will likely stay with children. Home health care is acceptable and often welcomed. While most will speak both English and Pennsylvania Dutch, in times of stress, they may revert to their Pennsylvania Dutch dialect and interpreters may be necessary.

Practices Related to Death and Dying

Advanced directives are uncommon. With a fatalistic view of life (God's will), there may be resistance to extensive procedures, tests, and life-prolonging interventions. Decisions are made on a family-by-family basis. When death is imminent, the bishop may perform an anointing, which is usually silent. Space and privacy need to be provided. Prolongation of life (right to die) and euthanasia are personal matters that may be discussed with the bishop, ministers, and/or family members. Autopsy is acceptable in the case of medical necessity or legal requirement but is seldom performed on the Amish. Although there is no specific prohibition, the Amish usually prefer to bury the intact body and generally do not donate body parts for medical research. Organ and tissue donation will require consultation with church leaders. While not expressly forbidden, it is a matter that is determined on an individual basis. Bodies are buried in small cemeteries in Amish communities on private property. Cremation is not acceptable.

Additional Considerations

The Amish beliefs of self-sufficiency, separation from the world, and mutual aid have resulted in their rejection of formal assistance from outside the Amish community. For example, the Amish obtained exemption for self-employed workers from Social Security, including Medicare, in 1965 on religious grounds and received exemption for all Amish workers from these programs in 1988. The Amish have also been exempted from the stipulations of the Affordable Care Act (Kelley, October 5, 2013). Amish seldom purchase commercial health insurance; instead, they have traditionally relied on personal savings and various methods of mutual assistance within the immediate and larger Amish community to meet their medical expenses. It is expected that each family has planned for future health care needs (e.g., childbirth and minor illness), but it is recognized that catastrophic illnesses resulting in extensive medical expenses do sometimes occur. In these instances, the Amish community provides assistance, usually through participation in one of the Amish Hospital Aid plans.

Changing occupational patterns among the Amish have resulted in shifting views toward commercial health insurance. Data on the Amish are limited. A recent study on the Amish use of commercial health insurance was conducted in the late 1990s in Holmes County, Ohio, where only 32.9% of Amish breadwinners earn their living as farmers: 24.5% are active farmers, 4% are retired farmers, and 3.4% hold dual occupations (both farm and nonfarm). Similar trends have been reported among other Amish settlements, where 30% to 80% of adult men work in nonfarm wage labor jobs in construction, factories, and home-based shops (e.g., cabinetmaking, harness making, blacksmithing, and so forth). The underlying reasons for the change are attributed to two factors: population growth and difficulty finding sufficient farmland for the growing numbers of Amish (Farrar et al., 2018).

Buddhist Churches of America

Buddhism is a general term that indicates a belief in Buddha and encompasses many individual churches. There are approximately 2.7 million Buddhists in the United States and Canada (Buddhism Canada on-the-move, n.d.; Buddhist Churches of America, 2018), and the worldwide membership is greater than 488 million (Religious Landscape Study, 2017).

The Buddhist Churches of America is the largest Buddhist organization in mainland United States. There are numerous Buddhist sects in the United States and Canada, including Indian, Sri Lankan, Vietnamese, Thai, Chinese, Japanese, and Tibetan.

General Beliefs and Religious Practices

Buddha's original teachings included Four Noble Truths and the Noble Eightfold Way, the philosophies of which affect Buddhist responses to health and illness. The **Four Noble Truths** expound on suffering and constitute the foundation of Buddhism:

1. The truth of dissatisfaction and suffering
2. The truth of the origin of dissatisfaction and suffering
3. The truth that dissatisfaction and suffering can be destroyed
4. The way that leads to the cessation of pain

The **Noble Eightfold Way** gives the rule of practical Buddhism, which consists of:

1. Right views
2. Right intention
3. Right speech
4. Right action
5. Right livelihood
6. Right effort
7. Right mindfulness
8. Right concentration

Nirvana or **Enlightenment**, a state of greater inner freedom and spontaneity, is the goal of all existence. When one achieves Nirvana, the mind has supreme tranquility, purity, and stability. Although the ultimate goals of Buddhism are clear, the means of obtaining those goals are not religiously prescribed. Buddhism is not a dogmatic religion, nor does it dictate any specific practices. Individual differences are expected, acknowledged, and respected. Each individual is responsible for finding his or her own answers through awareness of the total situation.

Religious Objects

Prayer beads and images of Shakyamuni Buddha and other Buddhist deities may be utilized for specific prayer or meditation practices (Sorajjakookl, Carr & Bursey, 2017). Figure 12-3 shows Buddhist monks creating a sand mandala a spiritual and ritual symbol representing the universe.

Holy Days

The major Buddhist holy day is Saga Dawa (or Vesak), which is the observance of Shakyamuni Buddha's birth, Enlightenment, and parinirvana. This holiday falls during the months of May or June. It is based on a lunar calendar, and therefore, the actual date varies from year to year. Although there is no religious restriction for therapy on this day, it can be highly emotional, and a Buddhist client should be consulted about his or her desires for medical or surgical intervention. Some Buddhists may fast for all or part of this day.

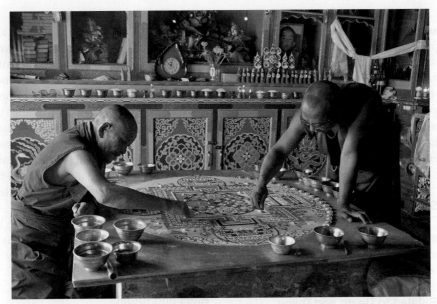

Figure 12-3. Buddhist monks making a sand mandala. The mandala is a spiritual and ritual symbol in both Hinduism and Buddhism, representing the universe. (Vladimir Melnik/ Shutterstock.com.)

Rites and Rituals

Buddhism does not have any sacraments that need to be taken into consideration for a hospitalized member of the Buddhist faith. A ritual that symbolizes one's entry into the Buddhist faith is the expression of faith in the Three Treasures (Buddha, Dharma, and Sangha).

Diet

Moderation in diet is encouraged. Specific dietary practices are usually interconnected with ethnic practices. Some branches of Buddhism have strict dietary regulations, for example, vegetarianism, while others do not. It is important to inquire about the client's preferences.

Health Care Practices

Buddhists do not believe in healing through a faith or through faith itself. However, Buddhists do believe that spiritual peace and liberation from anxiety by adherence to and achievement of awakening to Buddha's wisdom can be important factors in promoting healing and recovery.

Medical and Surgical Interventions

There are no restrictions in Buddhism for nutritional therapies, medications, vaccines, and other therapeutic interventions, but some individuals may refrain from alcohol, stimulants, and other drugs that adversely affect mental clarity. Buddha's teaching on the Middle Path may apply here: He taught that extremes should be avoided. What may be medicine to one may be poison to another, so generalizations are to be avoided. Medications should be used in accordance with the nature of the illness and the capacity of the individual. Whatever will contribute to the attainment of Enlightenment is encouraged. Treatments such as amputations, organ transplants, biopsies, and other procedures that may prolong life and allow the individual to attain Enlightenment are encouraged.

Practices Related to Reproduction

The immediate emphasis is on the person living now and the attainment of Enlightenment. If practicing birth control or having an amniocentesis or sterility test will help the individual attain Enlightenment, it is acceptable.

Buddhism does not condone the taking of a life. The first of Buddha's Five Precepts is abstention from taking lives. Life in all forms is to be respected. Existence by itself often contradicts this principle (e.g., drugs that kill bacteria are given to spare a patient's life). With this in mind, it is the conditions and circumstances surrounding the client that determine whether abortion, therapeutic or on demand, may be undertaken.

Religious Support System for the Sick
Support of the sick is an individual practice in keeping with the philosophy of Buddhism, but Buddhist priests often render assistance to those who become ill.

Practices Related to Death and Dying
If there is hope for recovery and continuation of the pursuit of Enlightenment, all available means of support are encouraged. If life cannot be prolonged so that the person can continue to search for Enlightenment, conditions might permit euthanasia. If the donation of a body part will help another continue the quest for Enlightenment, it might be an act of mercy and is encouraged. The body is considered a shell; therefore, autopsy and disposal of the body are matters of individual practice rather than of religious prescription. Burials are usually a brief graveside service after a funeral at the temple. Cremations are common.

Catholicism According to the Roman Rite

Roman Catholic membership in the United States and Canada includes approximately 89 million people; worldwide membership is more than 1.1 billion (Pew Research Center for Religion and Public Life, 2017).

General Beliefs and Religious Practices

The Roman Catholic Church traces its beginnings to about 30 AD, when Jesus Christ is believed to have founded the church.

Holy Days
Catholics are expected to observe all Sundays as holy days. Sunday or holy day worship services may be conducted any time from 4:00 PM on Saturday (a vigil mass celebrated on Saturday evening) until Sunday evening. Other days set aside for special liturgical observance include the Solemnity of Mary, Mother of God (January 1st), Ascension Thursday (the Lord's ascension bodily into Heaven, observed 40 days after Easter), Feast of the Assumption (August 15th), All Saints' Day (November 1st), the Feast of the Immaculate Conception (December 8th), and Christmas (December 25th). Other days that may be particularly important to the observant Roman Catholic include the Easter Triduum (Holy Thursday, Good Friday, and Easter Sunday).

Rites and Rituals
The Roman Catholic Church recognizes seven sacraments: Baptism, Reconciliation (or Penance or Confession), Holy Communion (or the Eucharist) (Figure 12-4), Confirmation, Matrimony, Holy Orders, and Anointing of the Sick (or Extreme Unction).

Religious Objects
Rosaries, prayer books, and holy cards are often present and may be of great comfort to the client and their family. They should be left in place and within the reach of the client whenever possible.

Diet
The goods of the world have been given for use and benefit. The primary obligation people have toward food and beverages is to use them in moderation and in such a way that they are not injurious to health. Fasting in moderation is recommended as a valued discipline. Additionally, Catholics have an obligation to fast on Ash Wednesday and Good Friday. When fasting, a person is permitted to eat one full meal. Two smaller meals may also be taken, but not to equal a full meal. Abstinence from meat is also required on these days and on all of the Fridays of Lent. The sick are never bound by this prescription of the law. Healthy persons between the ages of

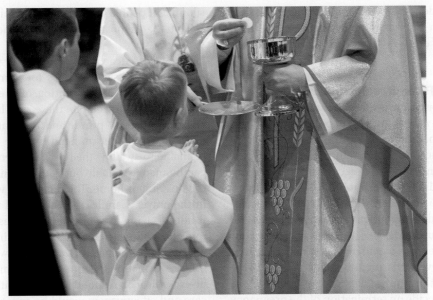

Figure 12-4. In the Roman Catholic tradition, when children reach the age of reason (7 years), they continue the ongoing initiation into their religion by making their First Communion, usually during 2nd grade. In addition to the religious ritual, there are sometimes cultural traditions surrounding this event, many of which involve a family celebration after the religious services have concluded. (Wideonet/Shutterstock.com.)

18 and 59 are encouraged to engage in fasting as described; abstinence applies to those over the age of 14.

Social Activities

The major principle is that Sunday is a day of rest; therefore, unnecessary servile work is prohibited. The holy days of obligation are also considered days of rest, although many persons must engage in routine work-related activities on some of these days.

Substance Use

Alcohol and tobacco are not evil per se. They are to be used in moderation and not in a way that would be injurious to one's health or that of another party. The misuse of any substance is not only harmful to the body but also sinful.

Health Care Practices

In time of illness, the basic rite is the sacrament of **Anointing of the Sick**, which is performed by a priest and includes reading of scriptures, prayers, communion if possible, and anointing with oil. Prayers are frequently offered for the sick person and for members of the family. The Eucharistic wafer (a small unleavened wafer made of flour and water) is often given to the sick as the food of healing and health. Other family members may participate if they wish to do so.

Medical and Surgical Interventions

As long as the benefits outweigh the risk to the individuals, judicious use of medications is permissible and morally acceptable. A major concern is the risk of mutilation. The Church has traditionally cited the **principle of totality**, which states that medications are allowed as long as they are used for the good of the whole person. Blood, blood products, and amputations are acceptable if consistent with the principle of totality. Biopsies and circumcision are also permissible.

The transplantation of organs from living donors is morally permissible when the anticipated benefit to the recipient is proportionate to the harm done to the donor, provided that the loss of such an organ does not deprive the donor of life itself or of the functional integrity of his or her body.

Practices Related to Reproduction

The basic principle is that the conjugal act should be one that is love-giving and potentially life-giving. Only natural means of contraception, such as abstinence, the temperature method, and the ovulation method, are acceptable. Ordinarily, artificial aids and procedures for permanent sterilization are forbidden. Birth control (anovulants) may be used therapeutically to assist in regulating the menstrual cycle.

Amniocentesis in and of itself is not objectionable. However, it is morally objectionable if the findings of the amniocentesis are used to lead the couple to decide on termination of the pregnancy or if the procedure injures the fetus.

Direct abortion is always morally wrong. Indirect abortion may be morally justified by some circumstances (e.g., treatment of a cancerous uterus in a pregnant woman). Abortion on demand is prohibited. The Roman Catholic Church teaches the sanctity of all human life from the time of conception.

The use of sterility tests for the purpose of promoting conception, not misusing sexuality, is permitted. Although artificial insemination has been debated heavily, traditionally, it has been looked on as illicit, even between husband and wife.

Research in the fields of eugenics and genetics is objectionable. This violates the moral right of the individual to be free from experimentation and also interferes with God's right as the master of life and human beings' stewardship of their lives. Some genetic investigations to help determine genetic diseases may be used, depending on their ends and means. There is support for research using adult stem cells, but opposition to the use of embryonic stem cells.

Religious Support System for the Sick

Although a priest, deacon, or lay minister usually visits a sick person alone, the family or other significant people may be invited to join in prayer. In fact, that is most desirable, since they too need support.

The priest, deacon, or lay minister will usually bring the necessary supplies for administration of the Eucharist or Anointing of the Sick. The nursing staff can facilitate these rites by ensuring an atmosphere of prayer and quiet and by having a glass of water on hand (in case the patient is unable to swallow the host). Consecrated wine can be made available but is usually not given in the hospital or home. The nurse may wish to join in the prayer. Candles may be used if the patient is not receiving oxygen. The priest, deacon, or lay minister will usually appreciate any information pertaining to the patient's ability to swallow. Any other information the nurse believes may help the priest or deacon respond to the patient with more care and effectiveness would be appreciated, but HIPAA laws must be remembered and information that violates privacy must not be divulged.

Catholic lay persons of either gender may visit hospitalized or homebound elderly or sick persons. Although they may not administer the sacraments of Anointing of the Sick or Reconciliation, they may bring Holy Communion (the Eucharist).

The titles of religious representatives include Father (priest), Mr. or Deacon (deacon), Sister (Catholic woman who has taken religious vows), and Brother (Catholic man who has taken religious vows).

Privacy is most conducive to prayer and the administration of the sacraments. In emergencies, such as cardiac or respiratory arrest, medical personnel will need to be present. The priest will use an abbreviated form of the rite and will not interfere with the activities of the health care team.

Most major cities have outreach programs for the sick, handicapped, and elderly. More serious needs are usually handled by Catholic Charities and other agencies in the community or at the local parish level. Organizations such as the St. Vincent de Paul Society may provide material support for the poor and needy as well as some counseling services, depending on the location.

In the United States, the Catholic Church owns and operates hospitals, extended care facilities, orphanages, maternity homes, hospices, and other health care facilities. Although the majority of tertiary care facilities in Canada are publicly owned, many such institutions are strongly influenced by the leadership of the Catholic Church and its members. It is usually best to consult the pastor or chaplain in specific cases for local resources.

Practices Related to Death and Dying

The Catholic Church endorses the use of advanced directives and recommends that its members prepare these documents and review them periodically.

Members are obligated to take ordinary means of preserving life (e.g., intravenous medication) but are not obligated to take extraordinary means. What constitutes as extraordinary means may vary with biomedical and technological advances and with the availability of these advances to the average citizen. Other factors that must be considered include the degree of pain associated with the procedure, the potential outcome, the condition of the patient, the economic factors, and the patient's or family's preferences.

Direct action to end the life of patients is not permitted. Extraordinary means may be withheld, allowing the patient to die of natural causes. There are sentiments regarding organ donation, as well: "when an indisputable pronouncement of death has been made donation of organs can commence" (What is the position of the Catholic Church on Organ Donation, 2016).

Autopsy is permissible as long as the corpse is shown proper respect and there is sufficient reason for doing the autopsy. The principle of totality suggests that organ donation is justifiable, being for the betterment of the person who does the giving.

Ordinarily, bodies are buried. Cremation is acceptable in certain circumstances, such as to avoid spreading a contagious disease. Because life is considered sacred, the body should be treated with respect. Any disposal of the body should be done in a respectful and honorable way.

Christian Science

Christian Science accepts physical and moral healing as a natural part of the Christian experience. Members believe that God acts through universal, immutable, spiritual law. They hold that genuine spiritual or Christian healing through prayer differs radically from the use of suggestion, willpower, and all forms of psychotherapy, which are based on the use of the human mind as a curative agent. In emphasizing the practical importance of a fuller understanding of Jesus' works and teachings, Christian Science believes healing to be a natural result of drawing closer to God in one's thinking and living. The church does not keep specific membership data; however, they report that there are approximately 400,000 adherents and approximately 3,000 congregations worldwide (Christian Science, 2017).

General Beliefs and Religious Practices

Christian Science beliefs and practices rely on the individual's faith and a reliance on prayer to achieve health when disease is present. Christian Science is based on the teachings of Christ Jesus, who said, "He that believeth on me, the works that I do shall he do also..." (John 14:12). Mary Baker Eddy, the founder of Christian Science, said, "these mighty works are not supernatural, but supremely natural..." (*Science and Health*, p. xi:14). This can mean resolving difficult challenges with health, relationships, employment, and other personal and global issues through prayer. People who practice Christian Science are free to make their own choices about what to think and do in each situation, including health care. But Christian Science is more than a system of self-help or health care. Ultimately, it is a way to draw closer to our loving Father–Mother, God, as well as all of humanity.

Holy Days

Besides the usual weekly day of worship (Sunday), other traditional Christian holidays are observed on an individual basis. Worldwide, Wednesday evenings are observed as times for members to gather for testimony meetings.

Rites and Rituals

Although sacraments in a strictly spiritual sense have deep meaning for Christian Scientists, there are no outward observances or ceremonies. Baptism and Holy Communion are not outward observances but deeply meaningful inner experiences. Baptism is the daily purification and spiritualization of thought, and communion is finding one's conscious unity with God through prayer.

Social Activities and Substance Use

Members are encouraged to be honest, truthful, and moral in their behavior. Although every effort is made to preserve marriages, divorce is recognized. The Christian Science Sunday School teaches young people how to make their religion practical in daily life as related to school studies, social life, sports, and family relationships. Members abstain from alcohol and tobacco; some abstain from tea and coffee.

Health Care Practices

Viewed as a by-product of drawing closer to God, healing is considered proof of God's care and one element in the full salvation at which Christianity aims. Christian Science teaches that faith must rest not on blind belief but on an understanding of the present perfection of God's spiritual creation. This is one of the crucial differences between Christian Science and **faith healing**. The practice of Christian Science healing starts from the Biblical basis that God created the universe and human beings "and made them perfect." Christian Science holds that human imperfection, including physical illness and sin, reflects a fundamental misunderstanding of creation and is therefore subject to healing through prayer and spiritual regeneration.

An individual who is seeking healing may turn to Christian Science practitioners, members of the denomination who devote their full time to the healing ministry in the broadest sense. In cases requiring continued care, nurses grounded in the Christian Science faith provide care in facilities accredited by the mother church, the First Church of Christ, Scientist, in Boston, Massachusetts. Individuals may also receive such care in their own homes. Christian Science nurses are trained to perform the practical duties a patient may need while also providing an atmosphere of warmth and love that supports the healing process. No medication is given, and physical application is limited to the normal measures associated with hygiene. The *Christian Science Journal*, a monthly publication, contains a directory of qualified Christian Science practitioners and nurses throughout the world.

Before they can be recognized and advertised in *The Christian Science Journal*, practitioners must have instruction from an authorized teacher of Christian Science and provide substantial evidence of their experience in healing. There are approximately 942 Christian Science practitioners throughout the world. Practitioners who speak other languages may also be listed in appropriate editions of *The Herald of Christian Science*, which is published in 12 languages.

The denomination has no clergy. Practitioners are thus lay members of the Church of Christ, Scientist, and do not conduct public worship services or rituals. Their ministry is not an office within the church structure but is carried out on an individual basis with those who seek their help through prayer. Both members and nonmembers are welcome to contact practitioners by telephone, by letter, or in person for help or for information.

Christian Science practitioners are supported not by the church but by payments from their patients. Their ministry is not restricted to local congregations but extends worldwide. Many insurance companies include coverage of payments to practitioners and Christian Science nursing facilities in their policies. In spite of such superficial resemblances to the health care professions, the work of Christian Science practitioners involves a deeply religious vocation, not simply alternative health care. Practitioners do not use medical or psychological techniques.

The term *healing* applies to the entire spectrum of human fears, grief, wants, and sin as well as to physical ills. Practitioners are called upon to give Christian Science treatment not only in cases of physical disease and emotional disturbance but also in family and financial difficulties, business problems, questions of employment, schooling problems, theological confusion, and so forth. The purpose of prayer, or Christian Science treatment, is to deal with these interrelated and complex problems of establishing God's law of harmony in every aspect of life. When healings are accomplished through perception and living of spiritual truth, they are effective and permanent. Physical healing is often the manifestation of a moral and spiritual change.

Ordinarily, a Christian Science practitioner and a physician are not employed in the same case, because the two approaches to healing differ so radically. During childbirth, however, an obstetrician or qualified midwife is involved. Since bone setting may be accomplished without medication, a physician is also employed for repair of fractures if the patient requests this medical intervention. In cases of contagious or infectious disease, Christian Scientists observe the legal requirements for reporting and quarantining affected individuals. The denomination recognizes public health concerns and has a long history of responsible cooperation with public health officials.

Christian Scientists are not necessarily opposed to doctors. They are always free to make their own decisions regarding treatment in any given situation. They generally choose to rely on spiritual healing because they have seen its effectiveness in the experience of their own families and fellow church members—experience that goes back over 100 years and in many families for three or four generations. Where medical treatment for minor children is required by law, Christian Scientists strictly adhere to the requirement. At the same time, they maintain that their substantial healing record needs to be seriously considered in determining the rights of Christian Scientists to rely on spiritual healing for themselves and their children. They do not ignore or neglect disease, but they seek to heal it by the means they believe to be most effective.

Medical and Surgical Interventions

Christian Scientists ordinarily do not use medications. Immunizations and vaccines are acceptable only when required by law. Ordinarily, members do not use blood or blood products. A Christian Scientist who has lost a limb might seek to have it replaced with a prosthesis. Christian Scientists are unlikely to seek transplants and are unlikely to act as donors. Christian Scientists do not normally seek biopsies or any sort of physical examination. Circumcision is considered an individual matter.

Practices Related to Reproduction

Matters of family planning (i.e., birth control) are left to individual judgment. Because abortion involves medication and surgical intervention, it is normally considered incompatible with Christian Science. Artificial insemination is unusual among Christian Scientists. Christian Scientists are opposed to programs in the field of eugenics and genetics.

Religious Support System for the Sick

Christian Scientists have their own nurses and practitioners. No special religious titles are used. Organizations to assist the sick include Benevolent Homes, staffed by Christian Science nurses, and visiting home nurse services.

Practices Related to Death and Dying

A Christian Science family is unlikely to seek medical means to prolong life indefinitely. Family members pray earnestly for the recovery of a person as long as the person remains alive. Euthanasia is contrary to the teachings of Christian Science. Most Christian Scientists believe that they can make their particular contribution to the health of society and of their loved ones in ways other than donation of the body. Disposal of the body is left to the individual family to decide. The individual family decides the form of burial and burial service (Christian Science fast facts, 2017).

Additional Considerations

A wide variety of books and journals are published by the Christian Science Publishing

Society, Boston, Massachusetts. Most major cities have Christian Science Reading Rooms, which carry these publications and are staffed by church members, who are available to provide additional information (Christian Science, 2017).

The Church of Jesus Christ of Latter-day Saints

The Church of Jesus Christ of Latter-day Saints is a Christian religion established in the United States in the early 1800s. The title of "Church of Jesus Christ of Latter-Day Saints" and "Members" are preferred over the more commonly known name of Mormonism. Worldwide membership in the United States and Canada is approximately 16.1 million (Toone, 2018).

General Beliefs and Religious Practices

Members of the Church of Jesus Christ of Latter-day Saints believe in Christianity as preached by Jesus Christ. They believe that the church was lost shortly after the death of Christ and was restored in the early 1800s by Joseph Smith. As a consequence, Latter-day Saints hold that God the Father is an embodied being, yet the roles Latter-day Saints ascribe to members of the Godhead largely correspond with the views of others in the Christian world. Latter-day Saints believe that God is omnipotent, omniscient, and all-loving, and they pray to Him in the name of Jesus Christ. They acknowledge the Father as the ultimate object of their worship, the Son as Lord and Redeemer, and the Holy Spirit as the messenger and revealer of the Father and the Son.

Religious Objects

Copies of scriptures are often found at the bedside of members of this church. Reading these scriptures often brings comfort during times of illness. Scriptures sacred to members of the Church of Jesus Christ of Latter-day Saints include the Bible (Old and New Testament), the Book of Mormon, Doctrine and Covenants, and Pearl of Great Price.

Holy Days

For members, Sunday is the day observed as the Sabbath in the United States. In other parts of the world, the Sabbath may be observed on a different day; in Israel, for example, members observe the Sabbath on Saturday.

Rites and Rituals

Within the Church of Jesus Christ of Latter-day Saints, an **ordinance** is a formal, sacred act representing a commitment of the person to the beliefs of the church.

An adult member of the Church of Jesus Christ of Latter-day Saints may wear a special type of underclothing, called a garment. In a health care setting, the garment may be removed to facilitate care. As soon as the individual is well, he or she is likely to want to wear the garment again. The garment has special significance to the person, symbolizing covenants or promises the person has made to God.

Diet

Members have a strict dietary code called the Word of Wisdom. This code prohibits all alcoholic beverages (including beer and wine), hot drinks (e.g., tea and coffee, although not herbal tea), tobacco in any form, and any illegal or recreational drugs.

Fasting to a member means no food or drink (including water), usually for 24 hours. Fasting is required once a month on the designated fast Sunday. Pregnant women, the very young, the very old, and the ill are not required to fast. The purpose of fasting is to bring oneself closer to God by controlling physical needs. The person is expected to donate the price of what has not been eaten to the church to be used to care for the poor.

Social Activities

The Church of Jesus Christ of Latter-day Saints has a wide variety of activities for its youth and encourages group activities until young people are at least 16. Young men are highly encouraged to perform missions for the church for 2 years at their own expense, beginning at the age of 18.

Women may go on missions when they are 19, but marriage is more strongly emphasized for them.

Substance Use

Alcohol, caffeinated beverages (such as tea, coffee, and soda), and tobacco are forbidden. In recent years, "recreational drugs" and non–medically indicated sedatives and narcotics have also been considered forbidden substances.

Health Care Practices

The members of the Church of Jesus Christ of Latter-day Saints believe that the power of God can be exercised on their behalf to bring about healing at the time of illness. The ritual of blessing the sick consists of one member (Elder) of the priesthood (male) anointing the ill person with oil and a second Elder "sealing the anointing with a prayer and a blessing." Commonly, both Elders place their hands on the individual's head. Faith in Jesus Christ and in the power of the priesthood to heal, requisite to the healing use of priesthood, does not preclude medical intervention but is seen as an adjunct to it. Members believe that medical intervention is one of God's ways of using humans in the healing process.

Medical and Surgical Interventions

There is no restriction on the use of medications or vaccines. It is not uncommon to find many members using herbal folk remedies, and it is wise to explore in detail what an individual may already have done or taken. There is no restriction on the use of blood or blood components.

Surgical intervention is a matter of individual decision in cases of amputations, transplants, and organ donations (both donor and recipient). Biopsies and resultant surgical procedures are also a matter of individual choice. The circumcision of infants is viewed as a medical health promotion measure and is not a religious ritual.

Practices Related to Reproduction

According to church doctrine, one of the major purposes of life is procreation; therefore, any form of prevention of the birth of children is contrary to church teachings. Exceptions to this policy include ill health of the mother or father and genetic defects that could be passed on to offspring. The decision of how many children to have and when to have them is extremely intimate and private, and the position of the church is that it should be left between the couple and the Lord.

Amniocentesis is a matter of individual choice. However, even if the fetus is found to be deformed, abortion is not an option unless the mother's life is in danger.

Abortion is forbidden in all cases except when the mother's life is in danger or when a competent physician determines that the fetus has severe defects that will not allow the baby to survive birth. Even in these circumstances, abortion is looked upon favorably only if the local priesthood authorities, after fasting and prayer, receive divine confirmation that the abortion is acceptable. In the event of pregnancy resulting from rape or incest, the church encourages that the child should be born and put up for adoption if necessary, rather than be aborted. The final decision rests with the mother. No official church sanction is used if she chooses to abort the child. Abortion on demand is strictly forbidden.

Because bearing children is so important, all measures that can be taken to promote having children are acceptable. Artificial insemination is acceptable if the semen is from the husband.

Religious Support System for the Sick

The Church of Jesus Christ of Latter-day Saints has a highly organized network, and many church representatives are likely to visit a hospitalized member, including the bishop and two counselors (leaders of the local congregation), Members are assigned to minister to each other. Two men are usually assigned to men and two women to other women. Sometimes, married couples minister together to other members and families. Friends within the local congregation can also be expected to visit.

Various titles are used for members of this church's hierarchy. For men, the term *Elder* is generally acceptable, regardless of the man's position; the term Sister is acceptable for women. (No one will object if they are simply addressed as Mr., Mrs., or Ms.)

To perform a blessing of the sick, the Elders performing the blessing need privacy and, if possible, silence. They generally bring a vial of consecrated oil with which to anoint the person. If they plan to perform a Sacrament of the Lord's Supper, they usually bring what they need with them. Bread and water are used for this ordinance.

The Relief Society is the organization for helping members. It is organized by the women of the church, who work closely with priesthood leaders to determine the general needs of members, including use of the church-run welfare organization. Church members who are in need may receive local help, such as child care when parents are ill or hospitalized and money for medical expenses or food when the family is in need.

Practices Related to Death and Dying

Whenever possible, medical science and faith healing are used to reverse conditions that threaten life. When death is inevitable, the effort is to promote a peaceful and dignified death. The church teaches that life continues beyond death and that the dead are reunited with loved ones; death is another step in eternal progression.

Euthanasia is not acceptable because the church teaches that life and death are in the hands of God, and humans must not interfere in any way. Autopsy is permitted with the consent of the next of kin and within local laws. Organ donation is permitted; it is an individual decision. Cremation is discouraged but not forbidden; burial is customary. A local priesthood member dedicates the graves.

Hinduism

The **Hindu** religion may be the oldest religion in the world. There are approximately 950 million Hindus worldwide, with approximately 2.23 million members in the United States and 157,015 members in Canada.

General Beliefs and Religious Practices

Hindus may be monotheistic, polytheistic, or atheistic; the basis of Hindu belief is the unity of everything. The major distinguishing characteristic is the social caste system.

Hinduism is founded on sacred, written scripture called the **Vedas**. **Brahman** is the principle and source of the universe and the center from which all things proceed and to which all things return. **Reincarnation** is a central belief in Hinduism. The law of **karma** determines life. According to karma, rebirth is dependent on moral behavior in a previous stage of existence. Life on earth is transient and a burden. The goal of existence is liberation from the cycle of rebirth and redeath and entrance into what in Buddhism is called Nirvana (a state of extinction of passion).

The practice of Hinduism consists of roles and ceremonies performed within the framework of the **caste system**, a social order determined by birth. These rituals focus on the main ethnoreligious events of birth, marriage, and death. Hindu temples are dwelling places for deities to which people bring offerings. There are numerous places for religious pilgrimage.

Social Activities, Diet, and Substance Use

Social activities are strictly limited by the caste system.

The eating of meat is forbidden because it involves harming a living creature. Most will not eat beef and many are vegetarian. At different stages of one's life, one may change one's dietary habits. For instance, in old age, a person who has been vegetarian may begin to eat fish or chicken.

Substance use is not restricted.

Religious Objects

A small picture of a deity may be found at the bedside. Prayer is often accompanied by the use of a "mala" (prayer beads) and a mantram (a sound representing an aspect of the divine). Facing North or East during prayer is preferable, but not required.

Health Care Practices

Some Hindus believe in faith healing; others believe illness is God's way of punishing people for their sins.

Medical and Surgical Interventions

The use of medications, blood, and blood components is acceptable. Persons who lose a limb are not outcasts from society. Loss of a limb is considered to be caused by "sins of a previous life." Organ transplantations are acceptable for both donors and recipients. Women may prefer to be examined by a female health care practitioner. Both men and women may retain their own clothes underneath a hospital gown.

Practices Related to Reproduction

All types of birth control are acceptable. Amniocentesis is acceptable, although not often available. Abortion, except for medical reasons, is discouraged. Artificial insemination is not restricted, but it is not often practiced because the technology to perform artificial insemination is not readily available, especially in rural areas.

Noting the exact time of a baby's birth is very important because it is used to determine the baby's horoscope. Males are not circumcised. Breast-feeding is expected. The infant is traditionally given a name on the 10th day following the birth, although in American hospitals, the child is sometimes named at birth.

Religious Support System for the Sick

Religious representatives use the title of priest. Church organizations to assist the sick do not exist; family and friends within the caste provide help.

Practices Related to Death and Dying

No religious customs or restrictions related to the prolongation of life exist. Life is seen as a perpetual cycle, and death is considered as just one more step toward Nirvana. Euthanasia is not practiced. Autopsy is acceptable. The donation of body or parts is also acceptable.

Cremation is the most common form of body disposal. Ashes are collected and disposed of in holy rivers. The fetus or newborn is sometimes buried (Hindu funeral customs and rituals, n.d.).

Islam

Islam is a monotheistic religion founded between 610 and 632 AD by the prophet Muhammad. Derived from an Arabic word meaning "submission," Islam literally translated means "submission to the will of God." A follower of Islam is called Moslem or Muslim, which means "one who submits." The current United States and Canadian membership is approximately 3,480,000 million, with a worldwide membership of between 1.7 billion (Desilver & Masci, 2017).

Muhammad, revered as the prophet of **Allah** (God), is seen as succeeding and completing both Judaism and Christianity. Good deeds will be rewarded at the last judgment, whereas evil deeds will be punished in hell.

General Beliefs and Religious Practices

Islam has five essential practices, or **Pillars of Faith** (Religious Literacy Project: Islam, n.d.). These are:

1. The profession of faith (*Shahada*), which requires bearing witness to one true God and acknowledging Muhammad as his messenger
2. Ritual prayer five times daily—at dawn, noon, afternoon, sunset, and night—facing Mecca, Saudi Arabia, Islam's holiest city (*salat*)
3. Almsgiving (*zakat*) to the needy, reflecting the Koran's admonition to share what one has with those less fortunate, including widows, orphans, homeless persons, and the poor
4. Fasting (*sawm*) from dawn until sunset throughout Ramadan during the 9th month of the Islamic lunar calendar
5. Making a pilgrimage to Mecca at least once during one's lifetime (*Hajj*) (Figure 12-5)

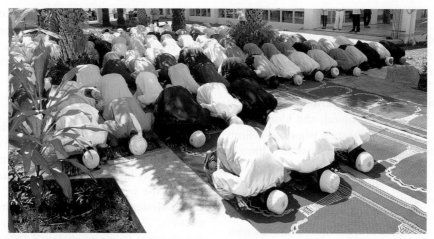

Figure 12-5. Pilgrims praying in the historic Pattani Masjid Mosque. (Titima Ongkantong/Shutterstock.com.)

The sources of the Islamic faith are the **Qur'an (Koran)**, which is regarded as the uncreated and eternal Word of God, and **Hadith** (tradition), regarded as sayings and deeds of the prophet Muhammad. All Muslims recognize the existence of the sharia and the five categories into which it divides human conduct: required, encouraged, permissible, discouraged, and prohibited.

Various sects of Islam have developed. When Muhammad died, a dispute arose over the leadership of the Muslim community. One faction, the *Sunni*, derived from the Arabic word for "tradition," felt that the caliph, or successor of Muhammad, should be chosen as Arab chiefs customarily are by election. Therefore, they supported the succession of the first four (the "rightly guided") caliphs who had been Muhammad's companions. The other group maintained that Muhammad chose his cousin and son-in-law, Ali, as his spiritual and secular heir and that succession should be through his bloodline. In 680 AD, one of Ali's sons, Hussein, led a band of rebels against the ruling caliph. In the course of the battle, Hussein was killed, and with his death began the *Shi'a* (sometimes called the *Shi'ite*) movement, whose name comes from the word meaning "partisans of Ali." The Shi'a and the Sunni are the two major branches of Muslims; the Sunni constitute about 85% of the total. The Sunni are found in Lebanon, the West Bank, Jordan, and throughout Africa; the Shi'a are in Iran, Iraq, Yemen, Afghanistan, and Pakistan. The Shi'a and the Sunni also have different rituals, practices, and structural and political orientations.

Holy Days

Days of observance in Islam are not "holy" days but days of celebration or observance. The Muslims follow a lunar calendar, so the days of observance change yearly.

Diet and Substance Use

Eating pork and drinking alcoholic or other intoxicating beverages are strictly prohibited. In all cases, moderation in one's life is expected. Some Muslims consume meat that has been ritually slaughtered by the process called **halal**, which means "the lawful or that which is permitted by Allah." A patient may inquire if the food received is "halal." If it is not, the client may request that food be brought from home by family or friends.

Fasting during the month of Ramadan is one of the pillars of Islam. Children (boys 7 years old, girls 9 years old) and adults are required to fast. Fasting means to abstain from food from dawn until dusk. Pregnant women, nursing mothers, the elderly, and anyone whose physical condition is so fragile that a physician recommends not fasting are exempt from fasting but are expected to fast later in the year or to feed a poor person to make up for the unfasted Ramadan days (Religious Literacy Project: Islam, n.d.).

Religious Objects

A prayer rug and the Koran are often present with a Muslim patient and should not be handled or touched by anyone who is ritually unclean. Nothing should be placed on top of these items. Some Muslims may wear an amulet, which is a black string or a silver or gold chain, on which sections of the Koran are attached. If worn by the patient, it should not be removed and should remain dry.

Health Care Practices

Muslim women typically prefer to have female physicians and health care providers, while men prefer male physicians and health care providers (Attun & Shamoon, 2018). Faith healing is not acceptable unless the psychological health and morale of the patient are deteriorating. At that time, faith healing may be used to supplement the physician's efforts. Vaccinations are encouraged. Touching between men and women is discouraged, another reason why health care providers of the same sex are preferred (Attun & Shamoon, 2018).

Medical and Surgical Interventions

There are no restrictions on medications. Even items normally forbidden (e.g., pork derivatives) are permitted if prescribed as medicine, although some Muslims will request medications that don't have a pork derivative, such as insulin. The use of blood and blood components is not restricted. Amputations are not restricted. Organ transplantations are acceptable for both donor and recipient. Biopsies are acceptable. No age limit is fixed, but circumcision is practiced on boys at an early age. For adult converts, circumcision is not obligatory, although it is sometimes practiced.

Practices Related to Reproduction

All types of birth control are generally acceptable in accordance with the law of "what is harmful to the body is prohibited." The family physician's advice on method of contraception is required. The husband and wife should agree on the method.

Amniocentesis is available in many Islamic countries. "Progressive" doctors and expectant parents use amniocentesis only to determine the status of the fetus, not the sex of the child; this is left in the hands of God.

There is a strong religious objection to abortion, which is based on Muhammad's condemnation of the ancient Arabian practice of burying unwanted newborn girls alive. If in vitro fertilization takes place, the destruction of fertilized eggs would be considered an abortion and not allowed (Attun & Shamoon, 2018).

Artificial insemination is permitted only if from the husband to his own wife. No official policy exists on practices in the fields of eugenics and genetics. Different Islamic schools of thought accept differing opinions.

Religious Support System for the Sick

In Islam, care of the physical body is not regarded highly. In many wealthy, oil-rich Middle Eastern nations, expatriates are hired to staff hospitals and provide for health care. Islamic clerics, called imams, may provide guidance that could be helpful for emotional and psychological disorders. Formal, organized support systems to assist the sick do not exist; family and friends provide emotional and financial support.

Practices Related to Death and Dying

The right to die is not recognized in Islam. Any attempt to shorten one's life or terminate it (suicide or otherwise) is prohibited. Euthanasia is not acceptable. Autopsy is permitted only for medical and legal purposes. The donation of body parts or body is acceptable, without restrictions.

Withholding of life-sustaining care is acceptable to both Sunni and Shi'a Muslims; however, withdrawal of care is not acceptable from the

Shi'a perspective. Maintaining a terminal patient on artificial life support is not encouraged in the Sunni tradition, but is encouraged in the Shi'a tradition.

Burial of the dead, including fetuses, is compulsory. It is important in Islam to follow prescribed burial procedures. Under conditions that cause fragmentation of the body, sections of the burial ritual may be omitted. The burial procedure consists of five steps:

1. *Ghasl El Mayyet*: Rinsing and washing of the dead body according to Muslim tradition. Muslim women cleanse a woman's body and Muslim men a man's body. At the time of death, the person's eyes are closed, the limbs straightened, and the entire body is covered with a sheet of cloth (Attun & Shamoon, 2018).

2. *Muslin*: After being washed three times, the body is wrapped in three pieces of clean white cloth. The Muslim word for "coffin" is the same as that for "muslin."

3. *Salat El Mayyet*: Special prayers for the dead are required. They are performed by those in attendance for the ritual washing, which prepares the body for burial (Attun & Shamoon, 2018).

4. The body should be prepared and buried as soon as possible. This must occur within 24 hours of the death. Cremation and embalming are prohibited. The body should always be buried so that the head faces toward Mecca.

5. Burial of a fetus: Before a gestational age of 130 days, a fetus is treated like any other discarded tissue. After 130 days, the fetus is considered a fully developed human being and must be treated as such.

Jehovah's Witnesses

Membership of the **Jehovah's Witnesses** is 1.2 million United States and 112,705 in Canada for a total of about 1.3 million. Worldwide membership is approximately 8.4 million (Jehovah's Witnesses Around the World: USA, 2018).

General Beliefs and Religious Practices

Jehovah's Witnesses are Christians and derived their name from the Hebrew name for God (**Jehovah**), according to the King James Bible. Thus, Jehovah's Witness is a descriptive name, indicating that members profess to bear witness concerning Jehovah, his Godship, and his purposes. Every Bible student devotes approximately 10 hours or more each month to proselytizing activities (Jehovah's Witnesses Official Website, n.d.).

Jehovah's Witnesses are opposed to saluting the flag, serving in the armed forces, voting in civil elections, and holding public office. These prohibitions are related to belief in a theocracy that is in harmony with their understanding of New Testament Christianity. Governed by a body of individuals, members united with the theocracy are to dissociate themselves from all activities of the political state and give full allegiance to "Jehovah's organization." This practice is related to the belief that Jesus Christ is King and Priest and that there is no need to hold citizenship in more than one kingdom. Members also refrain from gambling (Interesting Jehovah's Witness Statistics).

Membership in the Jehovah's Witness faith is difficult to ascertain. A member who fulfills their monthly obligation in proselytizing is known as a "publisher," while those who attend the yearly Memorial service are counted as members only and membership data are reported differently according to whether a person is a "publisher" or a "member," which confounds the statistics.

Holy Days

Although Witnesses do not celebrate Christmas, Easter, or other traditional Christian holy days, a special annual observance of the Lord's Supper is held. Witnesses and others may attend this important meeting, but only those numbered among the 144,000 chosen members (Revelation 7:4) may partake of the bread and wine as a symbol of the death of Christ and the dedication to God. This memorial of Christ's death takes place on the day corresponding to Nisa 14 of the Jewish calendar, which occurs sometime in March or

April. These elite members will be raised with spiritual bodies (without flesh, bones, or blood) and will assist Christ in ruling the universe. Others who benefit from Christ's ransom will be resurrected with healthy, perfected physical bodies (bodies of flesh, bones, and blood) and will inhabit this earth after the world has been restored to a paradisiacal state.

Social Activities and Substance Use

Youth are encouraged to socialize with members of their own religious background. Members abstain from the use of tobacco and hold that drunkenness is a serious sin. Alcohol used in moderation is acceptable.

Health Care Practices

The practice of faith healing is forbidden. However, it is believed that reading the scriptures can comfort the individual and lead to mental and spiritual healing.

Medical and Surgical Interventions

Vaccinations are encouraged. Use of vaccinations is an individual's choice, even those made from a small fraction of blood (Jehovah's Witnesses Official Website, n.d.). To the extent that they are necessary, medications are acceptable.

Blood in any form and agents in which blood is an ingredient are not acceptable. Blood volume expanders are acceptable if they are not derivatives of blood. Mechanical devices for circulating the blood are acceptable as long as they are not primed with blood initially. The determination of Jehovah's Witnesses to abstain from blood is based on scriptural references and precedents in the history of Christianity. Courts of law have often upheld the principle that each individual has a right to bodily integrity, yet some physicians and hospital administrators have turned to the courts for legal authorization to force blood to be used as a medical treatment for an individual whose religious convictions prohibit the use of blood. In some cases, children have been made wards of the court so that they could receive blood when a medical condition mandating blood transfusion was life-threatening. This can threaten the standing of the child in the community and must be approached with great care.

Although surgical procedures are not in and of themselves opposed, the administration of blood during surgery is strictly prohibited. There is no church rule pertaining to the loss of limbs or the amputation of body parts. If they are a violation of the principle of bodily mutilation, transplants are forbidden. However, this is usually an individual decision. Biopsies are acceptable. Circumcision is an individual decision.

Practices Related to Reproduction

Sterilization is prohibited because it is viewed as a form of bodily mutilation. Other forms of birth control are left to the individual. Amniocentesis is acceptable. Both therapeutic and on-demand abortions are forbidden. Sterility testing is an individual decision. Artificial insemination is forbidden both for donors and for recipients. Jehovah's Witnesses do not condone any activities in the areas of eugenics and genetics; they are considered to interfere with nature and therefore are unacceptable.

Religious Support System for the Sick

Individual members of a congregation, including elders, visit the ill. Visitors pray with the sick person and read scriptures. Male religious representatives are referred to as "Mr." or "Elder" and females as "Ms." or "Mrs." Religious titles are not generally used. Individuals and members of the congregation look after the needs of the sick.

Practices Related to Death and Dying

The right to die or the use of extraordinary methods to prolong life is a matter of individual conscience. Euthanasia is forbidden. An autopsy is acceptable only if it is required by law. No parts are to be removed from the body. The human spirit and the body are never separated. The donation of a body is forbidden. Disposal of the body is a matter of individual preference. Burial practices are determined by local custom. Cremation is permitted if the individual chooses it.

Judaism

Judaism is an Old Testament religion that dates back to the time of the prophet Abraham. Worldwide, there are approximately 14.5 million Jewish people. Membership includes approximately 5.7 million members in the United States and 390,000 members in Canada (American Jewish Yearbook, 2017).

General Beliefs and Religious Practices

Judaism is a monotheistic religion. Jewish life historically has been based on interpretation of the laws of God as contained in the **Torah** and explained in the **Talmud** and in oral tradition. Ancient Jewish law prescribed most of the daily actions of the people. Diet, clothing, activities, occupation, and ceremonial activities throughout the life cycle are all part of Jewish daily life.

Today, there are at least three schools of theological thought and social practice in Judaism. The three main divisions include Orthodox, Conservative, and Reform. There is also a fundamentalist sect called Hasidism. Hasidic Jewish communities cluster in metropolitan areas and live and work only within their Jewish communities.

Any person born of a Jewish mother or anyone converted to Judaism are considered Jewish. All Jewish people are united by the core theme of Judaism, which is expressed in the **Shema**, a prayer that professes a single God.

Holy Days

The Sabbath is the holiest of all holy days. The Sabbath begins each Friday 18 minutes before sunset and ends on Saturday, 42 minutes after sunset, or when three stars can be seen in the sky with the naked eye.

Other Holy Days include:

1. Rosh Hashanah (Jewish New Year)
2. Yom Kippur (Day of Atonement, a fast day)
3. Sukkot (Feast of Tabernacles)
4. Shemini Atzeret (8th Day of Assembly)
5. Simchat Torah
6. Chanukah (Festival of Lights, or Rededication of the Temple in Jerusalem)
7. Asara B'Tevet (Fast of the 10th of Tevet; not observed by liberal or Reform Jews)
8. Fast of Esther
9. Purim
10. Passover
11. Shavuot (Festival of the Giving of the Torah)
12. Fast of the 17th of Tammuz
13. Fast of the 9th of Ave (Commemoration of the Destruction of the Temple)

Holy days are very special to practicing Jewish people. If a condition is not life-threatening, medical and surgical procedures should not be performed on the Sabbath or on holy days. Preservation of life is of greatest priority and is the major criterion for determining activity on holy days and the Sabbath. If a Jewish patient is hesitant to receive urgent and necessary treatment because of religious restrictions, a rabbi should be consulted.

Rites and Rituals

Brit milah, the covenant of circumcision, is performed on all Jewish male children on the 8th day after birth. Although circumcision is a surgical procedure, for members of the Jewish faith, it is a fundamental religious obligation. Circumcision is usually performed by a **mohel**, usually a pious Jewish person with special training or by the child's father. Because the severing of the foreskin constitutes the essence of the ritual, the practice of having a non-Jewish or non-Observant physician perform the circumcision (even in the presence of a rabbi or other person who pronounces the blessing) is not acceptable according to Jewish law. Circumcision may be delayed if medically contraindicated. For example, if the child has hypospadias, a congenital defect of the urethral wall for which surgical repair usually occurs at age 3 years and requires the use of the foreskin in reconstructive plastic surgery, the circumcision may be delayed. At times, Jewish law requires postponement of circumcision, though contemporary medical science recognizes no potential threat to the health of the baby (e.g., for physiologic jaundice). As soon as the jaundice disappears, the brit milah may be performed. In Reform and Conservative traditions, girls mark the 8th day of life with a dedication ceremony in which prayers and blessings are invoked on her behalf.

The *bar mitzvah* (meaning "son of the commandment") is a confirmation ceremony for boys at age 13 that has been preceded by extensive religious study, including mastery of key Torah passages in Hebrew (Figure 12-6). In Reform and Conservative traditions, the *bas* (or *bat*) *mitzvah* (meaning "daughter of the commandment") is the equivalent ceremony for girls.

Diet

The dietary laws of Judaism are very strict; the degree to which they are observed varies

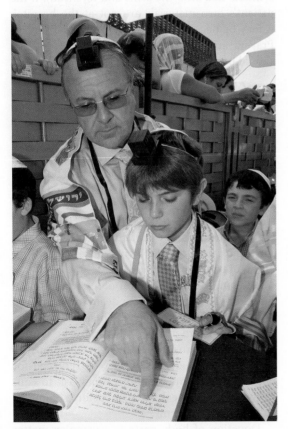

Figure 12-6. Bar Mitzvah ritual at the Wailing Wall in Jerusalem. When a boy becomes bar mitzvah at around the age of 13, he is morally and ethically responsible for his decisions and actions. (Chameleons Eye/Shutterstock.com.)

according to the individual. Strictly Observant Jewish people never eat pork or predatory fowl and never mix milk dishes and meat dishes. Only fish with fins and scales are permissible; shellfish and other water creatures are prohibited.

The word kosher comes from a Hebrew word *kashrut* that means "proper." All animals must be ritually slaughtered to be kosher. This means that the animal is to be killed by a specially qualified person, quickly, with the least possible pain. More colloquially, many people think that "kosher" refers to a type of food. If a patient asks for kosher food, it is important to determine what he or she means.

Religious Objects

On the Sabbath and on holidays, it is customary to light two candles in candleholders. Many Jewish men and some women wear *kippot* or *yarmulkes* (small head coverings) and *tallit* (prayer shawls) when praying. A *siddur* (prayer book) may also be present.

Social Activities

Like all ethnic groups, Jewish people tend toward socializing among themselves. Social activities that might lead to marriage outside the faith are discouraged. However, it is recognized that a significant number of individuals in Jewish society will seek partners outside of the Jewish faith. When this occurs, every effort is made to bring the non-Jewish partner into Judaism and to keep the Jewish partner a member and part of Jewish society.

Substance Use

The guideline is moderation. Wine is a part of religious observance and used as such. Historically, Jewish people are well connected with their faith and have a low incidence of alcoholism.

Health Care Practices

Medical care from a physician in the case of illness is expected according to Jewish law. There are many prayers for the sick in Jewish liturgy. Such prayers and hope for recovery are encouraged.

Medical and Surgical Interventions

There are no restrictions when medications are used as part of a therapeutic process. There is a prohibition in Judaism against ingesting blood (e.g., blood sausage, raw meat). This does not apply to receiving blood transfusions. Beliefs and practices related to body mutilation (e.g., organ transplantation, amputations) vary widely in Judaism. Individual beliefs should be explored with the client before any procedure that involves body mutilation.

Practices Related to Reproduction

It is said in the Torah that the Jewish people should be fruitful and multiply; therefore, it is a *mitzvah* (a good deed) to have at least two children. Since the Holocaust of World War II, it has been increasingly acceptable to have more children to replace those who were lost. It is permissible to practice birth control in traditional and liberal homes. In the past, contraception was limited to the woman; vasectomy was prohibited. Currently, Judaism permits contraception by either partner, although Hasidic and Orthodox Jewish people rarely use vasectomy.

Although therapeutic abortion is always permitted if the health of the mother is jeopardized, traditional Judaism regards the killing of an unborn child to be a serious moral offense; liberal Judaism permits it with strong moral admonitions (i.e., it is not to be used as a means of birth control). The fetus, although not imbued with the full sanctity of life, is a potential human being and is acknowledged as such.

Sterility testing is permissible when the goal is to enable the couple to have children. Artificial insemination is permitted under certain circumstances. A rabbi should be consulted in each individual case.

Members of the Jewish faith have an understandable aversion to genetic engineering because of the experimentation carried on during the Nazi era. At the same time, eugenic practices are permitted under a limited range of circumstances. The Jewish belief in the sanctity of life is a guiding factor in rabbinical counseling.

Religious Support System for the Sick

The most likely visitors will be family and friends from the synagogue. To visit the sick is a mitzvah of service (an obligation, a responsibility, and a blessing). There are often many Jewish social service agencies to help those in need. The Jewish Federation and Jewish Community Service are two large organizations that provide services to fulfill a variety of needs.

The formal religious representative from a synagogue is the rabbi. A visit from the rabbi may be spent talking, or the rabbi may pray with the person alone or in a minyan, a group of 10 adults (aged 13 years or older). If the patient is male and strictly observant, he may wish to have a prayer shawl (*tallit*), a cap (*kippah*), and *tefillin* (special symbols tied onto the arms and forehead). If the patient's own materials are not at the hospital, it may be necessary to ask that they be brought. Prayers are often chanted. If possible, privacy should be provided.

Practices Related to Death and Dying

A person has the right to die with dignity. If a physician sees that death is inevitable, no new therapeutic measures that would artificially extend life need to be initiated. It is important to know the precise time of death for the purpose of honoring the deceased after the first year has passed.

Euthanasia is prohibited under any circumstances. It is regarded as murder. However, in the administration of palliative medications that carry the calculated risk of overdose, the amelioration of pain is paramount.

Any unjustified alteration of a corpse is considered a desecration of the dead, to be avoided in normal circumstances. When postmortem examinations are justified, they must be limited to essential organs or systems. Needle biopsy is preferred. All body parts must be returned for burial. Jewish family members may ask to consult with a rabbinical authority before signing an autopsy consent form.

Donation of body parts is a complex matter according to Jewish law. If it seems necessary, consultation with a rabbi should be encouraged.

The body is ritually washed at a funeral home after death, if possible by members of the Chevra Kadisha (Ritual Burial Society). The body is then clothed in a simple white burial shroud. Embalming and cosmetic treatment of the body are forbidden. Public viewing of the body is considered a humiliation of the dead. Relatives are forbidden to touch or embrace the deceased, except when involved in preparation for interment. The exact time of burial is significant for *sitting Shiva*, the mourning period. After death in an institution, a nurse may wash the body for transport to the funeral home. Ritual washing then occurs later. Human remains, including a fetus at any stage of gestation, are to be buried as soon as possible. Cremation is not in keeping with Jewish law (Klug, n.d.).

Native American and Indigenous People's Churches

There are 6.6 million **Native Americans** in the United States, who comprise approximately 573 Native American tribes legally recognized by the Bureau of Indian Affairs (2018). **First Nations** is a term used to describe the 3.1 million *Aboriginal people* in Canada who are not *Métis* or *Inuit* and self-identify as being of First Nations heritage. There are 634 First Nations in Canada (Statistics Canada, 2018). Native American and First Nations people have a wide range of group-specific, health-related spiritual and religious beliefs and practices. Healers are known by a wide array of names, and their scope of practice varies widely from group to group, often encompassing herbal remedies and traditional healing rituals. Traditional healing practices may be used concurrently with contemporary biomedical interventions. General beliefs and practices are discussed in the remainder of this section. In Canada, similar native people are referred to as Indigenous people.

General Beliefs and Religious Practices

In both the United States and Canada, Native Americans and Indigenous Canadians may adopt both a Christian tradition with its accompanying health beliefs and practices as well as traditional healing practices. The **Oklevueha Native American Church** or **Peyote Religion** encompasses members of many tribes. Its focus is on the revival of Native American culture, beliefs, and spirituality.

When trying to support a Native American in physical or psychological crisis, the nurse needs to remember several important items:

1. The Native North American belief about disease is not necessarily based on symptoms. Disease may be attributed to intrusive objects, soul loss, spirit intrusion, breach of taboo, or sorcery. Disease may also be attributed to natural or supernatural causes.
2. The Native North American may embrace an organized (usually Christian) religion and still be a member of their tribe and its religion.
3. Native North Americans also balance "modern theories of disease" with long-standing tribal beliefs or customs. Therefore, during illness and particularly hospitalization, Native Americans may ask to see a priest or minister in addition to their tribe's healer. Visits from these people will likely be spiritually supportive, although the form of the support may vary greatly.

Health Care Practices

The spiritual basis for much of Native North American belief and action is symbolized by the number four. This number is seen in the extended hand, which means life, unity, equality, and eternity. The clasped hand symbolizes unity, the spiritual law that binds the universe.

It is this unity on which decisions should be made. Questions about abortion, the use of drugs, giving and receiving blood, the right to life, euthanasia, and so on do not have dogmatic "yes" or "no" answers; rather, answers are based on the situation and the ultimate unity or disunity that a decision would produce.

To the Native American, everything is cyclical: Communication is the key to learning and understanding, understanding brings peace of mind, peace of mind leads to happiness, and happiness is communicating. Other guidelines also function in groups of four.

Four guidelines toward self-development:

1. Am I happy with what I am doing?
2. What am I doing to add to the confusion?
3. What am I doing to bring about peace and contentment?
4. How will I be remembered when I am gone, in absence, and in death?

Four requirements of good health:

1. Food
2. Sleep
3. Cleanliness
4. Good thoughts

Four divisions of nature:

1. Spirit
2. Mind
3. Body
4. Life

Four divisions of goals:

1. Faith
2. Love
3. Work
4. Pleasure

Four ages of development:

1. Learning age
2. Age of adoption
3. Age of improvement
4. Age of wisdom

Four expressions of sharing:

1. Making others feel you care
2. An expression of interest
3. An expression of friendship
4. An expression of belonging

Unity, the great spiritual law, also can be expressed in four parts:

1. Going into the silence in spirit, mind, and body

2. The union through which all spirituality flows
3. A goal toward communicating with all things in nature
4. Recognized through sense, emotions, and impressions

In concert with the belief in the interconnectedness of all things, natural remedies in the form of herbal medicine are often used. Native American folk medicine and herbal remedies provided the forerunners of many of today's pharmaceutical remedies. Herbal treatments are still used today and may be requested by Native North American patients. A nurse caring for a Native American client should obtain a careful and complete history, including a list of whatever folk remedies have been tried. The patient may not know the names of herbs used in the treatment, and the tribal medicine man or woman may need to be consulted.

Respecting the concept that religion, medicine, and healing are inseparable to the Native American, one must be sensitive to the fact that asking for the names of native medicines or descriptions of healing practices tried in an attempt to cure the person is not just simply obtaining a history but also entering into the realm of what is not only private but also very sacred. The nurse must use care and sensitivity and show deep respect for the information received (Oklevueha: Native American Church, n.d.).

Protestantism

General Beliefs and Religious Practices

In its broadest meaning, **Protestantism** denotes the whole movement within Christianity that originated in the 16th century with Martin Luther and the Protestant Reformation. Historically and traditionally, the chief characteristics of Protestantism are the acceptance of the Bible as the only source of infallible revealed truth, the belief in the universal priesthood of believers, and the doctrine that Christians are justified in their relationship to God by faith alone, not by good works or dispensations of the church.

It is difficult to accurately categorize Protestant churches and impossible to mention them all; there are more than 30,000 different denominations. Protestantism can be divided into four major forms: Lutheran, Anglican, Reformed, and the free (or independent) church.

The oldest and second largest Protestant religion, *Lutheranism*, began in 1517 with Martin Luther's split from the Roman Catholic Church. Lutherans emphasize theological doctrine and spirituality. Many Lutherans in the United States and Canada are of German or Scandinavian heritage. There are approximately 64 million Lutherans worldwide ("Major Branches of Religions Ranked", 2005).

Anglicanism is represented by the established Church of England and similar churches. Unlike most other Protestant churches, they have an episcopal system of government in which each church or parish is served by a priest who is supervised by a bishop. A bishop supervises a group of churches called a diocese. A bishop, in turn, is responsible to a council of bishops. Anglican churches allow their clergy to marry. The Methodist church was established by followers of John Wesley, an 18th-century Anglican who sought to bring reform to the Church of England. Wesley's movement spread to the United States and Canada in the 18th century. There are approximately 73 million Anglicans worldwide ("Major Branches of Religions Ranked", 2005).

The *Reformed denominations* include Presbyterianism and are based on the teachings of John Calvin and his followers. These churches are distinguished from Lutheranism and Anglicanism, which maintain symbolic and sacramental traditions that originated before the Protestant Reformation. There are approximately 75 million people who practice one of the reformed denominations ("Major Branches of Religions Ranked", 2005).

Free or *independent churches*, including Baptists, Congregationalists, Adventists, and Churches of Christ, exercise congregational government. Each local denomination is an independent autonomous unit, and there is no official doctrine. With 27 million members of the Baptist faith in the United States and more than 70 million worldwide, the Baptist church makes up more than 10% of the population of the United States. Black and White Baptist church denominations exist separately. The largely White Southern Baptist Convention has about 12 million members, whereas 9 million Black people (30% of all Black people in the United States) are members of the National Baptist Conventions.

Health Care Practices

Given the wide diversity that exists within Protestant denominations, it is beyond the scope of this text to identify health-related beliefs and practices for each group.

Seventh-Day Adventists

Membership of **Seventh-Day Adventists** in United States and Canada is approaching 1 million, with worldwide membership now (Seventh Day Adventist Statistics, 2018). Doctrinally, Seventh-Day Adventists are heirs of the interfaith Millerite movement of the late 1840s, although the movement officially adopted the name Seventh-Day Adventist in 1863.

General Beliefs and Religious Practices

Seventh-Day Adventists accept the Bible as their only creed and hold certain fundamental beliefs to be the teaching of the Holy Scriptures. There are official statements by the General Conference of the Seventh-Day Adventists concerning the scriptures, the trinity, creation, nature of man, the great controversy (Christ vs. Satan), life, death, resurrection, and other topics.

Holy Days

The seventh day (Saturday) is observed as the Sabbath—from Friday sundown to Saturday sundown. The Sabbath is the day that God blessed and sanctified. It is a sacred day of worship and rest. Worship services are held on Saturday; weekly evening prayer meetings are usually held midweek.

Rites and Rituals

There are three church **ordinances**: (1) baptism by immersion, (2) the Ordinance of Humility, and (3) the Lord's Supper or Communion. There are no rituals at the time of birth. There is no requirement for a final sacrament at death. If requested by the individual or family member, the dying person might be anointed with oil.

Diet and Substance Use

Seventh-Day Adventists believe that because the body is the temple of God, it is appropriate to abstain from any food or beverage that could prove harmful to the body. Because the first human diet consisted of fruits and grains, the Church encourages a vegetarian diet. Nevertheless, some members choose to eat beef and poultry. Based on a passage in Leviticus 11:3, nonvegetarian members refrain from eating foods derived from any animal having a cloven hoof that chews its cud (e.g., meat derived from pigs, rabbits, or similar animals). Although fish with fins and scales are acceptable (e.g., salmon), shellfish are prohibited. Consumption of some birds is prohibited, but common poultry such as chicken and turkey are acceptable. Fasting is practiced, but only when members of a specific church elect to do so. Practiced in degrees, fasting may involve abstention from food or liquids. Fasting is not encouraged if it is likely to have adverse effects on the individual. Fermented beverages are prohibited. Members should abstain from the use of tobacco products.

Social Activities

Dancing is not encouraged as a form of recreation or social activity. Members are encouraged to date other members or persons holding similar beliefs and values.

Health Care Practices

The church believes in divine healing and practices anointing with oil and prayer. This is in addition to healing brought about by medical intervention. Since 1865, the church has maintained chaplains and physicians as inseparable in its institutions. There are eight principles that guide decisions/actions related to health: nutrition, divine power, exercise, rest, abstemiousness, fresh air, water, and sunlight (Health Principles, n.d.).

Surgical Interventions

Adventists operate one of the world's largest religiously operated health systems, including a medical school. The **Health Ministries** include 142 hospitals and sanitariums worldwide, with 68 in the United States. Worldwide, there are also 16 nursing home/rehabilitation sites and 27 senior living centers. Worldwide, there are many clinics and dispensaries, orphanages, and children's homes, as well as a number of airplanes and medical launches. Physical medicine and rehabilitation are emphasized and recommended, along with therapeutic diets. There are no restrictions on the use of vaccines. Similarly, there are no restrictions on the use of blood and blood products, amputations, organ transplants, donation of organs, biopsies, and circumcisions.

The Seventh-Day Adventist church is opposed to the use of hypnotism in the practice of medicine or under any other circumstance. Clinical implications for psychotherapy from the Seventh-Day Adventist tradition have been addressed by faculty from Loma Linda University School of Medicine (Mental Health and Wellness, n.d.).

Practices Related to Reproduction

The use of birth control is an individual decision; the church prohibits cohabitation except between husband and wife. There are no restrictions on amniocentesis. Therapeutic abortion is acceptable if the mother's life is in danger and in cases of rape and incest. On-demand abortion is unacceptable because Adventists believe in the sanctity of life. Artificial insemination between husband and wife is acceptable. Although the church views practices in the fields of eugenics and genetics as an individual decision, it upholds the principle of responsibility in dealing with children.

Religious Support System for the Sick

At the request of the sick person or the family, the pastor and elders of the church will come together to pray and anoint the sick person with oil. The religious representative is referred to as Doctor, Pastor, or Elder.

Practices Related to Death and Dying

Although there is no official position, the church has traditionally followed the medical ethics of prolonging life and prohibiting euthanasia. Autopsy and the donation of the entire body or parts are acceptable. No directives or recommendations exist regarding disposal of the body. No specific directives concerning burial exist; this is an individual decision (Markey, 2017).

Summary

Religious and cultural beliefs are interwoven and influence a client's understanding of illness and health care practices. In times of serious illness and death, religion may be a source of consolation for the client. Five dimensions of religion influence human behavior, including health-related practices. The goal of spiritual nursing care is to assist clients in integrating their own religious and spiritual beliefs into an ultimate reality that gives meaning to their lives. For the nurse providing spiritual nursing care, issues related to death and dying are of particular importance. Health-related beliefs and practices of select religions are important to understand, especially considering the diverse religious groups in the United States and Canada.

REVIEW QUESTIONS

1. When assessing the spiritual needs of clients from diverse cultural backgrounds, what key components should you consider?
2. In providing nursing care for the dying or bereaved client and family, what cultural considerations should the nurse include in the plan?
3. Compare and contrast the religious beliefs and practices concerning diet, medications, and procedures for five of the religious groups discussed in this chapter.
4. Analyze the contributions of religious organizations to the US and/or Canadian health care delivery system. What effect do health care facilities that are owned and operated by religious groups have on the overall cost and quality of health care in the United States and Canada? Critically analyze concerns about these religiously operated facilities in terms of philosophical, ethical, and legal aspects pertaining to types of services offered to patients.
5. What religious rituals mark significant developmental milestones for children and adolescents? Identify the ritual or ceremony, the approximate age at which the child or adolescent participates in it, and the name of the religion(s) associated with it.

CRITICAL THINKING ACTIVITIES

1. Visit a church or worship center not of your own belief system, and interview a member of the clergy or an official representative about the health-related beliefs of that religion. Discuss with him or her the implications of those beliefs for someone hospitalized for an acute or chronic illness. Inquire about the ways in which nurses can be of most help to hospitalized members of this religion.

2. Interview members of various religions concerning their beliefs about health and illness. Compare these interviews with the published beliefs or official statements from these religions. Discuss the implications of the differences (if any) that you found.

3. Interview fellow students, classmates, or coworkers about what they know of the health beliefs of various religions, especially those religions most often encountered among

the patients with whom you work. Make a poster or prepare a presentation comparing the results of your interviews with the official beliefs of those religions. Share this information with your classmates.

4. Interview four or more members of the same religious group who are of various ages (i.e., children, teenagers, young adults, middle aged, or elderly). Ask them about their religious beliefs and how they affect their health. Compare the results, commenting on similarities and differences.

5. Explore the meaning of various unique items of clothing worn by members of different religions.

6. If you have thought about the above exercises in terms of physical health, consider each of the activities from the perspective of mental health and spiritual health.

REFERENCES

American Jewish Year book. (2017). Springer.com

Amish Customs and Culture for Funerals and Burials, Death and Dying. (2015). Countryfarm lifestyles. Retrieved from http://www.countryfarm-lifestyles.com/amish-customs_funerals.html

Anderson, I. (n.d.). Indigenous perspectives on death and dying. Ian Anderson Education Program in End-of-Life Care. Retrieved from https://www.cpd.utoronto.ca/endoflife/Slides/PPT%20Indigenous%20Perspectives.pdf

Attun, B., & Shamoon, Z. (2018). Culturally competence in the care of Muslim patients and their families. *StatPearls* Retrieved from https://www.ncbi.nlm.nih.gov/books/NBK499933/

Barbosa, D. J., Tosoli, A. M. G., De Oliveira Fleury, M. L., Dib, R. V., De Oliveira Fleury, L. F., & da Silva, A. N. (2018). Social representations of mental disorders. *Journal of Nursing UFPE online, 12*(6), 1813–1816. https: // doi.org/10.5205/1981-8963-V126a235018p1813-1816

Bone, N. Swinton, M., Toledo, F., & Cook, D. (2018). Critical care nurses' experiences with spiritual care: The Spirit Study. *American Journal of Critical Care, 27*(3), 212–219.

Buddhism Canada on-the-move. (n.d.). Retrieved from http://buddhismcanada.com/

Buddhist Churches of America. (2018). Retrieved from http://buddhistchurchesofamerica.org/

Bureau of Indian Affairs (2018). Mission and history of bureau of Indian affairs. Retrieved from https://www.bia.gov/bia

Cates, J. A. (2014). *Serving the amish*. Baltimore, MD: Johns Hopkins University Press.

Catholic Charities USA. (2018). Retrieved from https://www.catholiccharitiesusa.org/

Catholic Health Care in the United States. (2018). Retrieved from https://www.chausa.org/about/about/facts-statistics

Christian Science. Fast Facts. (2017). Retrieved from http://www.religionfacts.com/christian-science

Desilver, D., & Masci, D. (January 31, 2017). World's Muslim population is more widespread than you think. Retrieved from http://www.pewresearch.org/fact-tank/2017/01/31/worlds-muslim-population-more-widespread-than-you-might-think/

Farrar, H. M., Kulig, J. C., & Sullivan-Wilson, J. (2018). Older adult caregiving in the Amish: An integrative review. *Journal of Cultural Diversity, 25*(2), 54–65.

Faulkner, J. E., & DeJong, C. F. (1996). Religiosity in 5D: An empirical analysis. *Social Forces, 45*, 246–254.

Friedman, D. A. (2013). *Jewish pastoral care: A practical handbook from traditional and contemporary sources* (2nd ed.). Woodstock, VT: Jewish Lights Publishing.

Health Principles. (n.d.). Health principles: Adventists follow eight health principles. Retrieved from https://www.seventhdayadventistdiet.com/health-principles/

Hindu funeral customs and rituals. (n.d.). Funeralwise. Retrieved from https://www.funeralwise.com/customs/hindu/

Jeffers, S. L., Nelson, M. E., Barnet, V., & Brannigan, M. C. (Eds.). (2013). *The essential guide to religious traditions and spirituality for health care providers*. London, UK: Radcliffe Publishing Ltd.

Jehovah's Witnesses Around the World: USA. (2018). Retrieved from https://www.jw.org/en/jehovahs-witnesses/worldwide/US/

Jewish Healthcare Foundation. (n.d.). Retrieved from http://www.jhf.org/

Kalish, R. A., & Reynolds, D. K. (1981). *Death and ethnicity: A psychocultural study*. New York, NY: Baywood.

Kelley, D. (October 5, 2013). As US Struggles with Health Care reform, Amish go their own way. Reuters. Retrieved from https://www.reuters.com/article/2013/10/05/usa-healthcare-amish-idUSL1N0HR1IV20131005

Klug, L. A. (n.d.). Jewish funeral customs: Saying goodbye to a loved one. The Jewish Federation. Retrieved from https://jewishfederations.org/jewish-funeral-customs-saying-goodbye-to-a-loved-one

Major Branches of Religions Ranked by Number of Adherents. (2005). Retrieved from http://www.adherents.com/adh_branches.html

Markey, D. (2017). Seventh Day Adventist funeral customs with do's and don'ts. Retrieved from https://classroom.synonym.com/seventh-day-adventist-funeral-customs-with-dos-and-donts-12085006.html

McIntyre, A. J. (2008). *The Tohono O'odham and Pimeria Alta*. Chicago, IL: Arcadia Publishing.

Mental Health and Wellness. (n.d.). Mental health and wellness: Wholeness in our brokenness. Retrieved from https://specialneeds.adventist.org/mental-health-wellness

Mori, M., Kuwama, Y., Ashikaga, T., Henrique, A., & Miyashita, M. (2018). Acculturation and perceptions of a good death among Japanese Americans and Japanese living in the US. *Journal of Pain and Symptom Management, 55*(1), 31–38.

Ohr, S., Jeong, S., & Saul, P. (2017). Culture and religious beliefs and values and their impact on preferences for end-of-life care among four ethnic groups of community-dwelling older persons. *Journal of Clinical Nursing, 26*(11–12), 1681–1689.

Oklevueha: Native American Church. (n.d.). Retrieved from https://nativeamericanchurches.org/

Pattison, S. (2013). Religion, spirituality and health care: Confusions, tensions, opportunities. *Health Care Analysis, 21*, 193–207. doi:10.1007/s10728-013-0245-4

Pew Research Center, Religion and Public Life. (2017). Retrieved from http://pewforum.org/religious-landscape-study/

Rahmwati, I., Wihatstuti, T. A., Rachmawatic, S. D., Kumboyono, K. (2018). Nursing experience in providing spiritual support to patients with acute coronary syndrome at emergency unit: Phenomenological study. *International Journal of Caring Sciences, 11*(2), 1147–1151.

Religious Landscape Study (2017). Retrieved from http://www.pewforum.org/religious-landscape-study/

Religious Literacy Project: Islam. (n.d.). Harvard Divinity School. Retrieved from https://rlp.hds.harvard.edu/religions/islam/beliefs-and-practices

Scammell, J. (2017). Religion, spirituality and belief: Is this the business of nurses? *British Journal of Nursing, 26*(9).

Seventh Day Adventist Statistics. (2018). Retrieved from https://www.adventist.org/en/information/statistics/article/go/-/seventh-day-adventist-world-church-statistics-2016-2017/

Sherwen, E. (2014). Improving end of life care for adults. *Nursing Standard, 28*(32), 51–57.

Sorajjakool, S., Carr, M. F., & Bursey, E. J. (2017). *World religions for healthcare professionals*. (2nd ed.). Padstow, Cornwall, Great Britain: Routledge.

Standard FAQ details. (2008). Retrieved from http://www.jointcommission.org/standards_information/jcfaqdetails.aspx?StandardsFAQId=290

Statistics Canada. (2018). Retrieved from https://www.statcan.gc.ca/eng

Toone, T. (2018). It was a historic year for the Church of Jesus Christ of Latter Day Saints. Retrieved from https://www.deseretnews.com/article/900048112/it-was-a-historic-year-for-the-church-of-jesus-christ-of-latter-day-saints-heres-a-look-back-at-2018s-major-moments-mormon.html

What is the Position of the Catholic Church on Organ Donation. (2016). What is the position of the Catholic Church on organ donation. Institute of Bioethics. Retrieved from https://sites.sju.edu/icb/

Chapter 13

Cultural Competence in Ethical Decision-Making

• Dula F. Pacquiao

Key Terms

Advance directives
Advocacy
Autonomy
Beneficence
Communitarian ethic of care
Compassion
Culturally competent care
Culturally congruent care

Empathy
Empowerment
Ethic of care
Ethical relativism
Fidelity
Health Insurance Portability
    and Accountability Act
Human rights
Informed consent

Medical repatriation
Nonmaleficence
Patient Self-Determination
    Act
Principle-based ethics
Social justice
Veracity/truth telling
Vulnerable population

Learning Objectives

1. Differentiate ethical relativism from universalism.
2. Describe how moral philosophies are socially and culturally constituted.
3. Analyze ethical principles and theories supporting human rights.
4. Differentiate social justice from distributive justice.
5. Describe the model of culturally competent ethical decision-making.
6. Use research findings relevant to ethical decision-making.

Nurses are often confronted by ethical dilemmas in their work. Nurses decide on care priorities and allocate human and material resources for their clients. Ethical decisions are complicated by culturally diverse clients with different socioeconomic capacities within health care organizations that emphasize common standards of care. Nurses need to negotiate with varying values not only of their clients but also of other care providers and the organization where they work. In addition, there is increasing realization of health disparities associated with social inequities in local, national, and global societies. Nurses need to be informed of how social inequalities create differences in health outcomes in populations and develop innovations to prevent vulnerability in individuals and groups. While **culturally competent care** addresses diversity, ethical practice grounded in social justice and human rights prevents **health inequity**. This chapter aims to give an overview of differing moral assumptions and the need for ethical relativism as well as the growing recognition of ethical universalistic approaches. It presents a model linking cultural competence and ethics to promote health equity.

Ethical Relativism

A moral philosophy consists of beliefs and assumptions about what is right and wrong, which is the basis of ethics that prescribes the proper action to take in a given situation. Morals and philosophical beliefs are constituted within the social, historical, and cultural experiences of a society. These beliefs evolve as normative patterns of assumptions that serve as an implicit framework guiding the actions and thoughts of group members, which may or may not be shared by persons outside of the cultural group.

Contrasting conceptualizations of human beings exist in Western and non-Western cultures. There is a pervasive belief that human beings are endowed with the capacity for reason and action in Western cultures. Reason is assumed to be a universal capacity, and it is through reason that all human beings can be expected to make valid and truthful judgments in any situation. Since the era of Enlightenment, the philosophic traditions of universalism and rationalism have shaped the Western concept of the person as the focus of moral reasoning. The person is the basic unit imbued with a universal capacity for reason and action (Guest, 2017). Ethical conflicts are often attributed to individual differences in cognitive skills, motivation, information, and/or linguistic capacity, and thus, by compensating for these deficits, a person can be expected to make a rational decision that is universally regarded as logical and morally acceptable. However, not all human behaviors can be classified as simply rational or irrational. Culture can be arbitrary, and human beings create their own distinctive, symbolic realities. Many of our ideas and practices are beyond logic and experience.

In some groups, religious and spiritual dimensions highly influence behaviors. Among such ethnoreligious groups as devout Muslims, Hindus, and Jews, religion is embedded in everyday life. Orthodox Jewish people may not accept euthanasia because of their belief in the sanctity of life. Jewish people generally consult their rabbi regarding matters pertaining to life and death decisions. Religion increases the awareness of the power and benevolence of God over humans; hence, earthly decisions are left to God, and the attitude is one of acceptance of fate rather than control over one's destiny. Members of Jehovah's Witness oppose blood transfusion as a lifesaving measure, and Christian Scientists may prefer their own religious and spiritually based practices of healing to those of traditional medicine. Among Pakistani women migrants in the United States, Islamic religious beliefs are embedded in their practices during childbirth and postpartum (Qureshi & Pacquiao, 2013).

Organ donation may be considered heroic in the biomedical profession and mainstream American culture. Religious, historical, and cultural influences, however, may prevent individuals from becoming organ donors. African Americans may be hesitant to become organ donors because of past and present experiences that built a collective sense of mistrust of the health care system and health professionals (Skloot, 2010). Cultural practices such as female genital cutting, body piercing and tattooing, and taking home a newborn's afterbirth may appear illogical and without any scientific basis. Yet, these practices are supported by value–belief systems that are deeply entrenched in religious, philosophical, and social structure of certain groups. To professional practitioners, resistance to scientifically proven measures belies common sense, but cultural traditions of some groups transcend rationality and logic. Indeed, common sense is not common after all; it is uniquely constructed within the social and cultural life contexts of human groups.

In the West, the person is viewed as a self-contained entity, fully integrated and self-motivating, independent of social roles and relationships, and distinct from all others (Guest, 2017). In contrast, among collectivistic cultures, there is greater continuity and mutuality among group members. Collective decisions by the extended family represented by the clan, tribe, or village make major decisions about the distribution of human and material resources to provide care for their members. Members of collective cultures expect to be physically present for family members who are dying or seriously ill. Numbers of family members present generally exceed the norm for visitation in most hospitals. Negotiating with the religious leader and/or group leader can effectively arrange numbers of visitors in one room at the same time with the client.

In the West, the concept of the individual being imbued with rational capacity translates to an expectation that one can make the decision and be responsible for himself/herself. Respect for autonomy has become the focal context for health care decisions in the United States and Canada. Ethical principles are applied to ensure and maximize individual autonomy. The autonomy paradigm, which has been institutionalized in health care, underlines interactions with and expectations of clients and families by practitioners. The Patient Self-Determination Act passed by the US Congress in 1991 mandates health care practitioners to provide clients with information about advance directives intended to assure their autonomy in situations when they can no longer make a decision. Individuals' choices are presumably carried out on their behalf in the event that they cannot consciously and competently represent their own will. Although the intent of advance directives is consistent with the Western ethos of self-determination, other cultures subscribe to the belief that the fate of human beings is beyond their control. Some believe that executing advance directives will tempt fate and result in unexpected death (Park & Song, 2016).

The US Congress also passed the Health Insurance Portability and Accountability Act (HIPAA) in 1996 that sets national standards for protecting the privacy, confidentiality, and security of individually identifiable health information by covered entities and business associates. HIPAA ensures confidentiality of an individual's health information. Health care practitioners are required to seek the client's informed consent before any information is shared with others, including family members. This poses difficulty for collectivistic groups where family members decide which information is shared with the client and other family members (Park & Song, 2016). The concept of individual autonomy brings an associated expectation of individual responsibility and accountability. This creates a predilection to reward self-care and label those individuals as noncompliant when they do not adhere to prescribed biomedical regimen. Health professionals often ignore social factors that hinder an individual client's ability to act on health teaching and prescribed regimen. Because the focus of care is on individual responsibility and accountability, vulnerable groups tend to avoid seeking medical help unless they are desperately ill or selectively act on parts of the regimen that they have the capacity and resources to implement.

A consequent expectation of self-reliance associated with individualism demands the use of oneself as an instrument to achieve self-determined goals. The ethical principle of autonomy is closely linked with respect for an individual's free will and includes the right to make choices about issues affecting one's well-being. Truth telling or veracity demands avoidance of lying, deception, misrepresentation, and nondisclosure in interactions with clients by health care providers. The ethical principle of fidelity requires health care providers to maintain therapeutic, trusting, and honest relationships with their clients. Veracity and fidelity uphold the concept of individualism and the fundamental right of individuals to be treated with respect and dignity.

By contrast, collective cultures favor group decisions and role assumptions by individuals based on their status in the established group hierarchy. Family and kinship patterns assign

A cross-sectional study in China of 126 caregivers of parents who suffered stroke using surveys conducted in hospitals or in the homes of patients. The study explored whether mutuality and filial piety have a protective effect on caregiver depression. Four structured questionnaires were used: the 15-item Mutuality Scale, the 4-item Filial Attitude Scale, the 9-item Filial Behavior Scale, and the 10-item Center for Epidemiological Studies Depression Scale. Mutuality is the positive relationship in caregiving dyads characterized by affection, reciprocity, sharing values, and sharing pleasant activities. Filial piety is based on the family-centered cultural value influencing children's attitudes and behaviors toward their aging parents. In Chinese cultures, caring for aging parents is considered filial love and one's responsibility.

The study found that high mutuality and stronger filial attitudes were significantly associated with less caregiver depression. Thus, mutuality and filial attitude may be protective factors against caregiver depression. The study results imply the importance of determining cultural beliefs and assumptions that undergird caring behaviors, which can mitigate the burden of caregiving. Health professionals should identify approaches to strengthen the ability of caregivers to care for their loved ones that are congruent with their valued traditions and moral beliefs about elder care.

Reference: Pan, Y., Jones, P. S., & Winslow, B. W. (2016). The relationship between mutuality, filial piety, and depression in family caregivers in China. *Journal of Transcultural Nursing, 28*(5), 455–463.

different roles, status, and power among group members. The social hierarchy governs decision-making, interactions, roles, and obligations of members. Whereas Western health care providers value the individual's autonomy in decision-making, filial piety and respect for the authority of one's elders are the guiding principles among traditional Asian cultures in making decisions about care. Influenced by the Confucian ethic, the Korean culture accepts inherent social inequality among family members as a condition for achieving collective harmony (see Evidence-Based Practice 13-1). By contrast, the Western value of instrumental individualism prizes the ability of individuals to make choices and rely upon themselves to achieve their purpose in life. Although a traditional Chinese adult relies upon family members and the physician to make decisions, a typical American or Canadian adult expects to be given information so he or she can make a decision.

In some cultures, such as African and Islamic groups, elder males occupy higher status and greater influence in decision-making. They may decide to withhold the truth about hopeless prognosis from the client in order to protect the vulnerable member from the burden of truth and despair. Advance planning to identify potential ethical conflicts should be done so that cultural brokers such as a community or religious leader respected by the family can identify an acceptable resolution. A durable power of attorney or health care proxy may be an acceptable accommodation of their group decision-making using a group-designated decision-maker and spokesperson.

In the United States, the mandate to use a trained interpreter who is not related to the client is another source of potential conflict. Group-oriented cultures tend to trust members of their in-group more than do others. In fact, some clients insist that their next of kin is present during their encounter with health professionals and expect their kin to speak on their behalf. Knowing the norms of the groups that the organization serves and working with community members to negotiate between these norms and the legal mandate in health care could prevent potential problems. Some hospitals have developed an interpreter program using community volunteers and bilingual staff members.

Ethical relativism holds that morality is relative to the norms of a particular culture; hence,

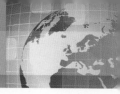

A secondary analysis of a longitudinal study with mixed study design conducted in multisites on Mexican American caregiving families. This secondary analysis involved qualitative analysis of data from the original study. This particular analysis involved 16 Mexican American families who lived along the US border with Mexico, and the sample comprised 22 primary caregivers (individuals who provided care for family members and without any history of mental illness) and 25 care recipients (60 years or older).

The study revealed the centrality of the cultural value of "la familia" in the phenomenon of collective caregiving. Collective caregivers were either a single caregiver providing care to more than one recipient or multiple caregivers providing care to one recipient. Singleton caregivers were family members who made previous commitment to the parent, were available to give the care or expected to take on the caregiver role. When singleton caregivers were unavailable, multiple caregivers shared the tasks and often move into the parental home. Some were involved in repetitive caregiving, moving from one family member to another because of death and emerging illnesses. Collective caregivers took over the tasks when a caregiver was incapacitated.

Recognition and appreciation by the family of caregivers was a protective factor against the burden of caregiving. However, the same family value creates ambivalence toward caregiving and reticence to admit caregiving burden. Health professionals must recognize the significance of family participation in the care of their family members and remain vigilant toward their needs for support and respite.

Reference: Evans, B. C., Coon D. W., Belyea M. J., & Ume, E. (2017). Collective care: Multiple caregivers and multiple care recipients in Mexican American families. *Journal of Transcultural Nursing, 28*(4), 398–407.

there are no universal truths in ethics. It emphasizes the need to examine the context of the decision because sociocultural differences influence whether an act is moral. Ethical relativism is unlike universalistic moral philosophies such as deontology, which upholds the existence of universal truths and unbreakable moral rules applicable to all situations (Kant as cited in Gregor & Timmerman, 2012), and teleology, which judges the morality of an act based on its consequence or outcome. Ethical relativism states that what is right for one group may not be right for another (Wong, 2006).

Feminist theory supports ethical relativism in that it does not support universal truths and requires examination of the context of the situation before making a decision. Drawn from feminist theories, the **ethic of care** emphasizes the need for health care practitioners to develop empathy, compassion, and relationships that promote trust, growth, and the well-being of others (Edwards, 2011). This relationship is significant in caring for the frail and vulnerable individuals who are unable to advocate for themselves, such as disabled, mentally ill, abused, and elderly persons.

Decisions about withdrawal of life support should take into consideration the individual's particular life context (e.g., previous life, current situation, and relationships with significant others). **Communitarian ethic of care** upholds collective decision-making over individual autonomy (see Evidence-Based Practice 13-2). In collectivistic groups such as Nigerians, Haitians, and Filipinos, decisions about care of an individual family member are made by the group and may supersede the individual client's decision, regardless of his/her age or mental capacity to decide.

Principle-based ethics, or principlism, attempts to reconcile the divergence between teleological and deontological models. Ethical principles are derived from ethical theories and commonly used to resolve ethical dilemmas because they link moral decision-making to scientific findings rather than universal rules. Principlism is based on the philosophical pragmatism of William James (Beauchamp & Childress, 2012). The principle of **fidelity** is the obligation to remain faithful to one's commitments. Nurses have an obligation to maintain standards of professional practice as a condition of continuing licensure. The principle of **veracity** upholds the virtues of being honest and telling the truth. **Truth telling** is recognized as a prerequisite to a trusting relationship. **Informed consent** requires veracity of information presented to clients and fidelity of practitioners to professional standards. The principle of **autonomy** upholds the capacity of individuals to act intentionally without controlling influences by others and from personal limitations that prevent meaningful choice. Autonomous persons are allowed to determine their own actions or delegate decision-making to others when they become incapable of making such decisions. **Advance directives** provide specific directions about the course of treatment to be followed by health care providers and caregivers if a client is unable to give informed consent or refuse care because of incapacity. Health care providers are obligated to promote patient autonomy and the right to make informed choices (Entwistle, Carter, Crib, & McCaffery, 2010).

The principles of **nonmaleficence** and **beneficence** require that care providers act in ways that cause no harm and benefit consumers of their care, respectively. Focusing on client safety emphasizes prevention of harm. The goal of using evidence-based practice is to promote the most effective and safe interventions for clients. Beneficence is a much higher-level principle as it not only addresses prevention of harm but also acts to benefit the client. A nurse working with a poor Vietnamese immigrant family affected by tuberculosis (TB) applies the principle of nonmaleficence by using the services of a culturally appropriate interpreter to explain the care regimen to the client and family. The principle of beneficence is applied when, understanding the high incidence of TB among Vietnamese immigrants, the nurse forms a community collaborative consisting of families, vendors, church leaders, and the local schools to work with the Mayor's Office, Department of Health, and the Visiting Nurses to develop policies and programs for prevention and to control the spread of TB in the community.

Ethical Universalism

Globalization has heightened the awareness of health inequities across population groups in local, national, and global contexts (Labonté, 2012; Population Reference Bureau, 2010). Social determinants exist across cultural groups and societies, which result in the social patterning of health vulnerability from differential exposure to life adversities that create cumulative disadvantages in populations. Vulnerable groups exist across societies because of compounded disadvantages that result in poor physical and mental health. A **vulnerable population** is a "subgroup or subpopulation who, because of shared social characteristics, is at a higher risk for [health] risks because of their position in the social strata which exposes them to contextual conditions, creating a higher distribution of risk exposure than the rest of the population" (Frohlich & Potvin, 2008, p. 218). A vulnerable group is a disadvantaged segment of the community requiring utmost considerations because of limited capacity to protect themselves from intended or inherent risks and inability to make informed choices (Shivayogi, 2013). Vulnerability is created by multiple and cumulative risks experienced through the life course that may not be directly related to health such as low socioeconomic status and discrimination. Exposure to multiple risk factors and a greater number of comorbidities are more frequent in vulnerable populations, for example, persons with low income, the less educated, racial and ethnic minorities, aboriginal peoples, those who experienced discrimination, enslavement, oppression and violence, etc.

The existence of global health inequities calls for health professionals to have a worldwide perspective and commitment to the **universalistic ethical principles** of advocacy and empowerment. The nursing profession has maintained its advocacy for providing a safe and caring environment that promotes the patient's health and well-being (Selanders & Crane, 2012). Nurses have the obligation to advocate for equity and social justice in resource allocation, access to health care, and other social and economic services (ICN, 2012). The American Nurses Association Code of Ethics (2015) stipulates that the nurse promotes, advocates for, and strives to protect the health, safety, and rights of an individual, family, community, group, or population (ICN, 2012; Winland-Brown, Lachman, & O'Connor Swanson, 2015).

The World Health Organization (WHO, 2018) has identified the three strategies to promote health and well-being of individuals and populations:

1. advocacy for health achievement through political, social, economic, environmental, behavioral, and biological means
2. enablement/empowerment of all people to access opportunities and resources to achieve their fullest health potential and equity in health outcomes
3. mediation of participation by all sectors (public and private organizations, professionals, media, communities, etc.) in health promotion

Targeting socioeconomic, political, and environmental changes to support health goes beyond individual-based care toward actions with high impact on populations and communities. Such initiatives necessitate multisectoral, multilevel, and interprofessional collaboration.

The universalistic ethical principle of advocacy is rooted in a caring interpersonal relationship and a sense of obligation to care for others. It requires careful attention to the power relationships that influence the individual's well-being, and affirmation of the responsiveness of care by the individual. Advocacy has its roots in the ethics of care emphasizing interpersonal relationships and care or benevolence as central to moral action. This ethical theory, which is also known as care-focused feminism, is based on the assumptions that persons have varying degrees of dependence and interdependence on one another; the vulnerable deserve extra consideration based on their vulnerability; and the need to examine the situational contexts to safeguard and protect the vulnerable (Gilligan, 2008).

Advocacy is also founded on the principle of justice and fairness by ensuring that each person is given his or her due. Justice and fairness are closely related and often used interchangeably. Systemic inequality and social injustices result in health inequity because of unfair distribution of goods, services, and privileges across populations. Equity refers to fairness in the distribution of goods and services based on people's needs. Needs are not necessarily equal; hence, equal access or equal allocation of resources that ignore differences in needs generally fail to achieve equity of outcomes (Bambas & Casas, 2001). According to John Rawls (1971), the stability of a society depends upon the extent to which the members feel that they are being treated justly. Lack of fairness and unequal treatment have led to social unrest, disturbances, and strife.

Rights-based care stems from the principles of human rights emphasizing health as a basic right along with access to quality and safe health care services for all. The Universal Declaration of Human Rights was influential in creating the movement for advocacy across disciplines and institutions. Health promotion should be grounded in social justice, emphasizing a collective societal moral obligation to create equity or fairness in the allocation of risks and rewards to everyone (Braverman, 2014). Social justice must include nondistributive aspects of well-being (Powers & Faden, 2008), which is affected by the nature of a person's social relationships with others. Unjust relationships impose systemic constraints on the development of well-being. People who are victims of social subordination, violence, discrimination, and stigma often experience lack of respect and lack of attachment and determination, which are essential aspects of well-being.

Protection of basic human rights, particularly of the vulnerable, is a fundamental part of health promotion. Health and well-being are achieved when individuals have the capacity and freedom to exercise their rights. While all individuals have the same basic human rights, social justice ensures the rights of the vulnerable. In his *A Theory of Justice*, John Rawls (1971) emphasized that a just society exists when the vulnerable are rendered less vulnerable. Health promotion is grounded in the ethical principle of beneficence that aims to make a positive difference in people's lives. Beneficence is actualized through advocacy and empowerment of individuals and populations for health achievement.

The need for advocacy is inherent among humans whose identities, experiences, and life chances are shaped by the social arrangements of power and statuses. Advocacy is needed as one's ability to compete, negotiate, and secure one's "place" in society is differentially structured by the social structural conditions. Patient advocacy has evolved toward health advocacy to protect people who are vulnerable or discriminated against and empower those who need a stronger voice by enabling them to express their needs and make their own decisions (Carlisle, 2000). According to the World Health Organization (WHO, 1995), advocacy for health is a combination of individual and social actions to gain political commitment, policy support, social acceptance, and systems support for a particular health goal or program. Health advocacy encompasses direct service to the individual or family as well as activities that promote health and access to health care in communities and the larger public. Advocates support and promote the rights of the patient in health care, help build capacity to improve community health, and enhance health policy initiatives focused on available, safe, and quality care.

Empowerment is the process through which an individual and groups gain greater control over decisions and actions affecting their health; it is both an individual and a community process (WHO, 2009). While advocacy tends to be more aligned and driven by others such as health providers or advocates, empowerment is more oriented toward the other's point of view (WHO, 2009), thus more patient-centered. Empowerment is both a process and an outcome; it is considered an outcome of advocacy. Since empowerment involves active engagement and participation by individuals and communities, they achieve greater autonomy, capacity, and

self-efficacy in improving their health and well-being. There is greater likelihood for sustainable outcomes through empowerment because it builds individual and community capacity for health achievement. Empowerment links individual strengths and competencies, support systems, and proactive behaviors to social policy and social change.

Patient empowerment is a process by which patients understand their role and are given the knowledge and skills by their health care provider to perform a task in an environment that recognizes community and cultural differences and encourages patient participation (WHO, 2009). Kaldoudi and Makris (2015) describe patient empowerment as a cognitive process with three levels. At the first level, patients develop awareness of their health status, health-related risks, and measures to stay healthy and prevent illness. The second level is the stage of active participation through active engagement in the health care process, seeking feedback, managing illness and comorbidities, and accessing appropriate resources. At the third level, patients gain control of their health by collaborating in decision-making with health care providers, participating in shared decision-making, and reframing mind-sets to adapt to new situations.

Wallerstein and Bernstein (1994) prefer community empowerment because it is a social-action process that occurs in the social context of human relationships at home and in communities and institutions. Community empowerment is both a process and an outcome in which individuals and groups act to gain mastery over their lives by changing their social and political environment. Institutions and communities are transformed as people who participate in changing them become transformed. Community empowerment is a basis for health care reform as individuals are connected and engaged with others in the community to identify common problems, goals, and strategies for personal and social capacity building to transform their lives (Wallerstein & Bernstein, 1994). The Ottawa Charter for Health Promotion

(WHO, 2018) recognizes the significance of patient and community empowerment in transforming health of individuals and populations.

Model for Culturally Competent Ethical Practice for Health Equity

Leininger first articulated the central purpose of nursing as caring that is grounded in the knowledge of culturally constituted values, beliefs, and practices of the people (McFarland & Wehbe-Alamah, 2015). Transcultural nursing aims to identify the differences and similarities across cultural groups and between professional caregivers and their clients/patients. Leininger defined culturally congruent care as care that is meaningful, supportive, and beneficial from the lens of the people who experience the care. Culturally congruent action modes include cultural preservation, accommodation, and repatterning. One or all three modes of action may be used simultaneously or in a continuum of actions. *Cultural preservation* means maintaining the core values, beliefs, and practices significant to the individual or group. *Cultural accommodation* involves negotiating with existing cultural differences in order to find a meaningful existence of one's cultural lifeways with those of others. *Cultural repatterning* means attempting to help individuals and groups change their way of life to achieve a healthy, safe, and meaningful existence (McFarland & Wehbe-Alamah, 2015). Cultural repatterning enables health practitioners and organizations to promote preservation and accommodate cultural differences. Leininger's culturally congruent decision modes promote bridging of differences applicable with individuals, organizations, and communities. These are significant approaches in bridging cultural differences and finding a common ground among different groups, which are critical in building multisectoral collaboration and partnerships.

More recently, cultural competency has added the notion that the knowledge, skills, and abilities of culturally congruent care can be measured, observed, and validated at any given point using more objective criteria. Culturally congruent and competent care is ethical care that is built upon the delicate balance between ethical relativism and universalism. While culturally congruent/competent care promotes meaningful, supportive, and beneficial care by respectful accommodation of cultural differences, its ultimate aim is achievement of health equity built on an awareness of self and others, valuing diversity and having the capacity to transform differences toward a common, beneficial purpose. Health equity through protection of human rights and promotion of social justice is achieved through culturally competent advocacy and empowerment that integrates diversity within the common aim of health equity and alleviation of vulnerability (see Figure 13-1).

Culturally competent professionals have a global perspective who view themselves within their own values and beliefs and identify themselves as part of an emerging and interlocking world community (Gorman & Womack, 2017). They have the ability to critically examine their own traditions to determine reasonable support for their personal beliefs rather than accept them as absolute truths because of their genuine concern and commitment to the welfare of others. As global citizens, culturally competent individuals have the interconnected capacities for empathy (a profound understanding of others) and compassion (the emotional understanding of others' experiences) (Nussbaum, 2013). Compassionate understanding of the suffering of others compels one to take action on their behalf through advocacy and empowerment (Pacquiao, 2016) as it involves an "awareness, caring, and embracing cultural diversity while promoting social justice and sustainability, coupled with a sense of responsibility to act" (Reysen & Katzarska-Miller, 2013, p. 858).

Vulnerable populations need culturally competent advocacy and empowerment that is built on respect and appreciation of differences and on natural capacities and unique lifeways to achieve individual and group empowerment for health.

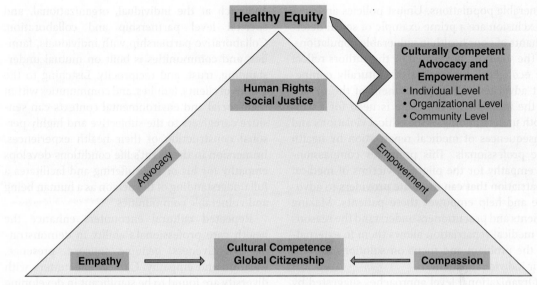

Figure 13-1. Culturally Competent Ethical Care.

Model Application

Achievement of individual and community empowerment requires that culturally competent strategies use multilevel approaches at the individual, organizational/institutional, and community levels. Health promotion needs to shift its focus to building healthy communities beyond disease-based care for patients. Addressing the social determinants of poor health should focus on upstream approaches that transform the capacity of individuals and communities to change their life conditions. As Freire (2000) has noted, individual empowerment is sustainable within an empowered community.

Model Application

Young, Phil, and Lehmann (2014) reported on the practice by US hospitals of transferring undocumented patients in need of subacute medical care to their countries of origin. The practice of medical repatriation is considered by the authors as medical injustice that goes against the ethical obligation of caring for vulnerable patients regardless of their visa or medical insurance status. The authors cited the case of a Mexican undocumented patient who was transferred back to his homeland without his informed consent nor consideration of his medical need.

Medical repatriation is the consequence of the US policy of exclusion of undocumented persons from medical benefits as well as restricting access to medical insurance by legal immigrants. The Emergency Medical Treatment and Active Labor Act (EMTALA) enacted in 1986 requires any hospital that receives Medicare funding to provide emergency care to persons in need. However, EMTALA does not apply outside the emergency department, so once patients are admitted to the hospital and stabilized, there is no clear legal obligation to continue delivering care. The practice of "patient dumping" characterized by denying or limiting medical services to a patient for economic reasons and referring the patient elsewhere has been associated with EMTALA. Although there is some funding for eligible facilities for EMTALA-related services and access to Federally Qualified Health Care, these funds do not cover expensive long-term care for undocumented and uninsured patients. Medical repatriation violates the basic human right to health and access to health care based on laws that create medical and social inequity in vulnerable populations. Unjust policies and laws of exclusion are a prime example of social determinants of poor health in vulnerable populations.

The solutions advocated by the authors reflect the ecological approaches of culturally competent advocacy and empowerment of the model. At the individual level, there is need for an in-depth understanding of the ethical violations and consequences of medical repatriation by health care professionals. This promotes compassionate empathy for the plight of victims of medical repatriation that can motivate providers to advocate and help empower these patients. Making patients and practitioners understand the reasons for medical repatriation allows them to externalize the problem and focus on solutions beyond their individual patient.

Organizational level approaches suggested by the authors include shedding light on these hidden practices to bring deeper and widespread understanding of the problem. In particular, they encourage unraveling of practices by hospitals to determine how different organizations deal with the same issues. They also recommend gathering data regarding medical revenues and surpluses and how these are used. At the community/societal level, there is need for a broad multisectoral and multilevel collaboration to bring different stakeholders together to influence policy. A relevant approach is to publicize the contributions of undocumented persons to the society and its economy. A larger aim is to stir enough public outcry for social justice and putting human lives ahead of profits. There should be a public discourse on whether right to health is a basic human right or a commodity for profit.

Summary

Actions that transform life conditions of vulnerable individuals and populations to achieve health equity begin from compassion and empathy for the least well-off. Culturally competent advocacy and empowerment for social justice and human rights protection are actualized through a multipronged approach at the individual, organizational, and societal level partnership and collaboration. Collaborative partnership with individuals, families, and communities is built on mutual understanding, trust, and reciprocity. Listening to the stories of clients, families, and communities within their social and environmental contexts can sensitize caregivers to the subjective and highly personal construction of their health experiences. Immersion in the client's life conditions develops empathy for his or her suffering and facilitates a full understanding of the person as a human being and vulnerable communities.

Repeated cultural encounters enhance the health care professional's ability in demonstrating attentiveness, genuine concern, presence, warmth, and empathy. Clinical encounters with diversity are found to be significant in developing cultural proficiency and effectiveness (Pacquiao, 2016). Community involvement and immersion in diverse communities create the appropriate context for partnership, collaboration, and compassionate understanding.

Health care providers need experience in caring especially for vulnerable populations locally or abroad. Experience with organizations and advocacy groups such as local churches, the Red Cross, homeless shelters, Doctors Without Borders, and other opportunities can build the skills for culturally competent ethical thinking. Awareness of resources locally, nationally, and globally promotes access to and development of more comprehensive services. Building collaborative partnerships with organizations and communities is important as vulnerable populations have complex, multiple needs that are both simultaneous and evolving.

Partnerships allow sharing of resources, services, and best practices across local, national, and global contexts. Service learning is an excellent opportunity for nursing students to learn about organizations and the communities they serve. Strengthening the community health nursing experience in the curriculum sensitizes students to public health issues and social inequities affecting population health.

REVIEW QUESTIONS

1. Describe ethical dilemmas in achieving health equity for vulnerable populations within the current political milieu in the United States and Canada.
2. Explain how you can promote health for vulnerable populations within the context of your employment.
3. Explain the ethical basis for culturally competent care.

CRITICAL THINKING ACTIVITIES

Identify an example of an ethical dilemma that you have encountered at work or in your community. Identify the particulars of the situation:

1. Who are the people involved?

2. What is the setting?

3. How do different individuals or groups perceive the problem?

4. Identify conflicting values and beliefs at the individual, organizational, and societal levels that influence perceptions.

5. What assessment data about the situation are missing?

6. How can additional information be obtained?

7. What culturally congruent strategies do you recommend?

REFERENCES

ANA. (2015). *Code of ethics for nurses with interpretive statements*. Silver Spring, MD: Nursesbooks.org.

Bambas, A., & Casas, J. A. (2001). Assessing equity in health. Conceptual criteria. In PAHO (Ed.), *Equity and health: Views from the Pan American Sanitary Bureau, Publication 8* (pp. 12–21). Washington, DC: Author.

Beauchamp, T. L., & Childress, J. F. (2012). *Principle of biomedical ethics* (7th ed.). UK: Oxford University Press.

Braverman, P. (2014) What are health disparities and health equity? We need to be clear. *Public Health Reports, 129*(S2), 5–8.

Carlisle, S. (2000). Health promotion, advocacy and health inequalities: A conceptual framework. *Health Promotion International, 15*(4), 369–376.

Edwards, S. D. (2011). Is there a distinctive care ethics? *Nursing Ethics, 18,* 184–191.

Entwistle, V. A., Carter, S. M., Crib, A., & McCaffery K. (2010). Supporting autonomy: The importance of clinician-patient relationships. *Journal of General Internal Medicine, 25*(7), 741–745.

Evans, B. C., Coon, D. W., Belyea, M. J., & Ume, E. (2017). Collective care: Multiple caregivers and multiple care recipients in Mexican American families. *Journal of Transcultural Nursing, 28*(4), 398–407.

Freire, P. (2000). *Pedagogy of the oppressed* (30th ed.). New York, NY: Bloomsbury Academic.

Frohlich, K. L., & Potvin, L. (2008). The inequality paradox: The population approach and vulnerable populations. *American Journal of Public Health, 98,* 216–221.

Gilligan, C. (2008). Moral orientation and moral development. In A. Bailey, C. J. Cuomo (Eds.), *The feminist philosophy reader* (pp. 463–466). Boston, MA: McGraw Hill.

Gorman, D., & Womack, K. (2017). Cultivating humanity with Martha Nussbaum. *Interdisciplinary Literary Studies, 19,* 145–148.

Guest, K. J. (2017). *Essentials of cultural anthropology: A toolkit for global age* (2nd ed.). New York, NY: Norton & Company.

International Council for Nurses/ICN. (2012) *The ICN code of ethics for nurses*. Geneva, Switzerland: Author. Retrieved from http://jimbergmd.com/Way%20of%20Barefoot%20Doctoring/WEB%20way%20of%20bfd/nurses%20code%20of%20ethics.pdf

Kaldoudi, E., & Makris, N. (2015). Patient empowerment as a cognitive process. In C. Verdier, M. Bienkiewicz, & A. Fred, et al. (Eds.), *The proceedings of HealthInf 2015: 8th international conference on health informatics* (pp. 605–610). Lisbon, Portugal. (ISBN: 978-989-758-068-0).

Gregor, M., & Timmerman (Eds.). (2012). Kant: *Groundwork of the metaphysics of morals*. UK: Cambridge University Press.

Labonté, R. (2012). Global action on social determinants of health. *Journal of Public Health Policy, 33*(2):139–147. doi: 10.1057/jphp.2011.61

McFarland, M. R., & Wehbe-Alamah, H. (2015). *Leininger's culture care diversity and universality: A worldwide nursing theory*. Burlington, MA: Jones & Bartlett Learning.

Nussbaum, M. (2013). *Liberal education and global community*. Association of American Colleges and Universities. Retrieved May 16, 2013 from http://uca.edu/liberalarts/files/2013/05/Liberal-Education_Nussbaum.pdf. Accessed on December 1, 2017.

Pacquiao, D. F. (2016). Cultural competence in ethical decision-making. In M. M. Andrews, & J. S. Boyle, (Eds.). *Transcultural concepts in nursing care* (6th ed., pp. 447–464). Philadelphia, PA: Wolters Kluwer.

Pan, Y., Jones, P. S., & Winslow, B. W. (2016). The relationship between mutuality, filial piety, and depression in family caregivers in China. *Journal of Transcultural Nursing, 28*(5), 455–463.

Park, J., & Song, J.-A. (2016). Predictors of agreement with writing advance directives among older Korean adults. *Journal of Transcultural Nursing, 27*(6), 574–582.

Population Reference Bureau. (2010). *2010 World population data sheet*. Washington, DC: Author.

Powers, M., & Faden, R. (2008). *Social justice: The moral foundations of public health and health policy*. New York, NY: Oxford University Press.

Qureshi, R. I., & Pacquiao, D. F. (2013). Ethnographic study of experiences of Pakistani women immigrants with pregnancy, birthing and postpartum care in the United States and Pakistan. *Journal of Transcultural Nursing, 24*(4), 355–362.

Rawls, J. (1971). *A theory of justice*. Cambridge, MA: Harvard University Press.

Reysen, S., & Katzarska-Miller, I. (2013). A model of global citizenship: Antecedents and outcomes. *International Journal of Psychology, 48*(5), 858–870. doi: 10.1080/00207594.2012.701749

Selanders, L. C., & Crane, P. C. (2012). The voice of Florence Nightingale on advocacy. *Online Journal of Issues in Nursing, 17*(1), 1. Retrieved from http://www.nursingworld.org/ MainMenuCategories/ANAMarketplace/ANAPeriodicals/ OJIN/TableofContents/Vol-17-2012/No1-Jan-2012/ Florence-Nightingale-on-Advocacy.html

Shivayogi, S. (2013). Vulnerable population and methods for their safeguard. *Perspectives in Clinical Research, 4*(1), 53–57.

Skloot, R. (2010). *The immortal life of Henrietta Lacks*. New York, NY: Crown Publishing.

Wallerstein, N., & Bernstein, E. (1994). Community empowerment as a basis for healthcare reform. *Health Education Quarterly, 21*(2), 141–148.

WHO. (1995). The world health report 1995—bridging the gaps. Retrieved from http://www.who.int/whr/1995/en/

WHO. (2009). WHO guidelines on hand hygiene in health care: First global patient safety challenge clean care is safer care. Retrieved from https://www.ncbi.nlm.nih.gov/ books/NBK144022/

WHO. (2018). The 1986 Ottawa Charter for Health Promotion. Retrieved August 20, 2018 from http://www.who.int/ healthpromotion/conferences/previous/ottawa/en/

Winland-Brown, J., Lachman, V. D., & O'Connor Swanson, E. (2015). The new 'code of ethics for nurses with interpretive statements' (2015): Practical clinical application part I. *Medsurg Nursing, 24*(4), 268–271.

Wong, D. B. (2006). *Natural moralities: A defense of pluralistic relativism*. New York, NY: Oxford University Press.

Young, M. J., Phil, M., & Lehmann, L. S. (2014). Undocumented injustice? Medical repatriation and the ends of health care. *The New England Journal of Medicine, 37*(7), 669–673.

Appendix A

Transcultural Nursing Assessment Guide for Individuals and Families

- Joyceen S. Boyle and Margaret M. Andrews

Biocultural Variations and Cultural Aspects of the Incidence of Disease

- Does the client and/or family members relate a health history associated with genetic or acquired conditions that are more prevalent for a specific cultural group (e.g., diabetes, hypertension, cardiovascular disease, sickle cell anemia, Tay–Sachs disease, G-6-PD deficiency, lactose intolerance)? Does the client's family relate such a history?
- Are there socioenvironmental conditions more prevalent among a specific cultural group that can be observed in the client or family members (e.g., lead poisoning, alcoholism, HIV/AIDS, drug abuse, ear infections, family violence, fetal alcohol spectrum disorder [FASD], obesity, respiratory diseases)?
- Are there diseases against which the client has an increased resistance (e.g., skin cancer in darkly pigmented individuals, malaria for those with sickle cell anemia)?
- Does the client have distinctive features characteristic of a particular ethnic or cultural group (e.g., skin color, hair texture)? Do his or her family members have such features? Within the family group, are there variations in anatomy characteristic of a particular ethnic or cultural group (e.g., body structure, height, weight, facial shape and structure [nose, eye shape, facial contour], upper and lower extremities)?
- How do anatomic, racial, and ethnic variations affect the physical and mental examination?

Communication

- What language does the client speak at home with family members? In what language would the client prefer to communicate with you? What other languages does the client speak or read? What other languages do the client's family members speak or read?
- What is the fluency level of the client in English—both written and spoken? What is the fluency level of the client's family members?
- Does the client need an interpreter? Do his or her family members need an interpreter? Does the health care setting provide interpreters? Who would the client and his or her family members prefer to assist with interpretation? Is there anyone whom the client would prefer not to serve as an interpreter (e.g., member of the opposite sex, person younger or older than the client, member of a rival tribe, ethnic group, or nationality)?
- If the client is hearing or visually impaired, how does he or she communicate? Are any assistive devices used to foster communication and/or ensure the client's safety?
- What are the rules and style (formal or informal) of communication? If the client is hearing impaired and requires someone who knows sign language, how will arrangements be made? If the client is blind and requires that communications be made available in braille, how will that be accomplished? How much time will it take to provide the resources needed for hearing and visually impaired clients? How does the

client prefer to be addressed? What do his or her family members prefer? What are the preferred terms for greeting?

- How is it necessary to vary the technique and style of communication during the relationship with the client to accommodate his or her cultural background (e.g., tempo of conversation, eye contact, sensitivity to topical taboos, norms of confidentiality, and style of explanation)? How do these factors vary with family members, if at all?
- What are the styles of individual and family members' nonverbal communication?
- How does the client's nonverbal communication compare with that of individuals from other cultural groups? How does the client's style of nonverbal communication differ from the health care provider's style? How does it affect the client's relationships with you and with other members of the health care team? How does communication with the family influence the care environment?
- How do the client and family members feel about health care providers who are not of the same cultural or religious background (e.g., Black, middle-class nurse; Hispanic of a different social class; Muslim or Jewish care provider)? Does the client prefer to receive care from a nurse of the same cultural background, gender, and/or age? How do family members react to care providers of different cultural backgrounds, age, and gender?
- If the client and family members are recent migrants from Central America, Mexico, or Asian countries, do they have a plan in place to deal with the possibility that one or more adults may be detained and not return home after work? To protect family integrity, arrangements should be made in advance for the children's safety.

Cultural Affiliations

- With what cultural group(s) does the client report affiliation (e.g., American, Hispanic, Irish, Black, Navajo, American Indian, or combination)? It is becoming increasingly

common for Americans to identify with two or more groups, such as Native American and African American. Equally important, to what degree does the client identify with the cultural group (e.g., "we" concept of solidarity or as a fringe member)?

- How do the views of other family members coincide with or differ from those of the client regarding cultural affiliations?
- What is the preferred term that the cultural group chooses for itself? What term does the client choose?
- Where was the client born? Where were his or her parents born? What are the generational similarities and differences in regard to cultural identification, language, customs, values, and so on?
- Where has the client lived (country, city, or area within a country) and when (during what years of his or her life)? If the client has recently immigrated to the United States from another country, knowledge of prevalent diseases in his or her country of origin as well as sociopolitical history may be helpful. If the client is a recent immigrant, did he or she live in countries of transit or refugee camps? For how long? Current residence? Occupation? Occupation in home country?

Cultural Sanctions and Restrictions

- How does the client's cultural group regard expression of emotion and feelings, spirituality, and religious beliefs? How are feelings related to dying, death, and grieving expressed in a culturally appropriate manner?
- How do men and women express modesty? Are there culturally defined expectations about male–female relationships, including the nurse–client relationship?
- Does the client or family express any restrictions related to sexuality, exposure of various parts of the body, or certain types of surgery (e.g., vasectomy, hysterectomy, abortion)?
- Are there restrictions against discussion of dead relatives or fears related to the unknown?

Developmental Considerations

- Are there any distinct growth and development characteristics that vary with the cultural background of the client and family (e.g., bone density, psychomotor patterns of development, fat folds)?
- What factors are significant in assessing children of various ages from the newborn period through adolescence (e.g., male circumcision, female genital mutilation [FGM], expected growth on standards grid, culturally acceptable age for toilet training, duration of breastfeeding, introduction of various types of foods, gender differences, discipline, and socialization to adult roles)?
- What are the beliefs and practices associated with developmental life events such as pregnancy, birth, puberty, marriage, and death?
- What is the cultural perception of aging (e.g., is youthfulness or the wisdom of old age more valued)?
- How are elderly persons cared for within the cultural group (e.g., cared for in the home of adult children, placed in institutions for care)? What are culturally accepted roles for the elderly?

Economics

- Who is the principal wage earner in the family and what is the income level? Is there more than one wage earner? Are there other sources of financial support? (*Note:* These may be potentially sensitive questions.)
- What insurance coverage does the client and his or her family have? Does the client and/or family members understand the terms/rates/coverage of their health insurance policies?
- What impact does the economic status have on the client and his or her family's lifestyle and living conditions?
- What has been the client and family's experience with the health care system in terms of reimbursement, costs, and insurance coverage?

Educational Background

- What is the client's highest educational level obtained? What values do the family members express regarding educational achievements?
- Does the client's educational level affect his or her knowledge level concerning his or her health literacy—how to obtain the needed care, teaching related to or learning about health care, and any written material that he or she is given in the health care setting (e.g., insurance forms, educational literature, information about diagnostic procedures and laboratory tests, admission forms, etc.)? Does the client's educational level affect health behavior? As an example, in the United States, cigarette smoking and obesity have been linked to socioeconomic levels.
- What learning style is most comfortable and familiar? Does the client prefer to learn through written materials, oral explanations, videos, and/or demonstrations?
- Does the client access health information via the Internet or use social media as a source of health-related information?
- Do the client and family members prefer intervention settings away from hospitals and other clients, which may have negative connotations for them? Are community sites such as churches, schools, or adult day care centers a good alternate choice for the client and his or her family, considering they are informal settings that may be more conducive for open discussion, demonstrations, and reinforcement of information and skills? Are the client and family more comfortable in their home setting?

Health-Related Beliefs and Practices

- To what cause does the client attribute illness and disease or what factors influence the acquisition of illness and disease (e.g., divine wrath, imbalance in hot/cold, yin/yang, punishment for moral transgressions, a hex, soul loss, pathogenic organism, past behavior, growing older)? Is there congruence within the family on these beliefs?

- What are the client's cultural beliefs about ideal body size and shape? What is the client's self-image in relation to the ideal?

- How does the client describe his or her health-related condition? What names or terms are used? How does the client express pain, discomfort, depression, or anxiety? In some cultures, clients may somaticize their emotional feelings, for example, "My heart hurts" rather than say, "I'm feeling sad or depressed about my physical condition."

- What do the client and family members believe promotes health (e.g., eating certain foods, wearing amulets to bring good luck, sleeping, resting, getting good nutrition, reducing stress, exercising, praying or performing rituals to ancestors, saints, or other deities)?

- What is the client's religious affiliation? How is the client actively involved in the practice of religion? Do other family members have the same religious beliefs and practices? Do the client and/or family members incorporate religious practices, such as healing ceremonies or prayer, into health/illness care?

- Do the client and his or her family rely on cultural healers (e.g., curandero, shaman, spiritualist, priest, medicine man or woman, minister)? Who determines when the client is sick and when he or she is healthy? Who influences the choice or type of healer and treatment that should be sought?

- In what types of cultural healing or health-promoting practices does the client engage (e.g., use of herbal remedies, potions, or massage; wearing of talismans, copper bracelets, or chains to discourage evil spirits; healing rituals; incantations; or prayers)? Do family members share these beliefs and practices?

- How are biomedical health care providers perceived? How do the client and his or her family perceive nurses? What are the expectations of nurses and nursing care workers?

- Who will care for the client at home? What accommodations will family members make to provide caregiving?

- How does the client's family and cultural group view mental disorders? Are there differences in acceptable behaviors for physical versus psychological illnesses?

Kinship and Social Networks

- What is the composition of a "typical family" within the kinship network? What is the composition of the client's family?

- Who makes up the client's social network (family, friends, peers, neighbors)? How do they influence the client's health or illness status?

- How do members of the client's social support network define caring or caregiving? What is the role of various family members during health and illness episodes? Who makes decisions about health and health care?

- How does the client's family participate in the promotion of health (e.g., lifestyle changes in diet, activity level, etc.) and nursing care (e.g., bathing, feeding, touching, being present) of the client?

- Does the cultural family structure influence the client's response to health or illness (e.g., beliefs, strengths, weaknesses, and social class)?

- What influence do ethnic, cultural, and/or religious organizations have on the lifestyle and quality of life of the client (e.g., the National Association for the Advancement of Colored People [NAACP], churches, such as African American, Muslim, Jewish, Catholic, and others, that may provide schools, classes, and/or community-based health care programs)?

- Are there special gender issues within this cultural group? Do the client and family members conform to traditional roles (e.g., women may be viewed as the caretakers of home and children, while men work outside the home and have primary decision-making responsibilities)?

Nutrition

- What nutritional factors are influenced by the client's cultural background? What is the meaning of food and eating to the client and his or her family?

- Does the client have any eating or nutritional disorders (e.g., anorexia, bulimia, obesity, lactose intolerance)? Do the client's family members have any similar disorders? How do the client and family view these conditions?
- With whom does the client usually eat? What types of foods are eaten? What is the timing and sequencing of meals? What are the usual meal patterns?
- What does the client define as food? What does the client believe constitutes a "healthy" versus an "unhealthy" diet? Are these beliefs congruent with what the client actually eats?
- Who shops for and chooses food? Where are the foodstuffs purchased? Who prepares the actual meals? How are the family members involved in nutritional choices, values, and choices about food?
- How are the foods prepared at home (type of food preparation, cooking oil[s] used, length of time foods are cooked [especially vegetables], amount and type of seasoning added to various foods during preparation)? Who does the food preparation?
- Has the client chosen a particular nutritional practice such as gluten-free, vegetarianism or abstinence from red meat or from alcoholic or fermented beverages? Do other family members adhere to these beliefs and practices?
- Do religious beliefs and practices influence the client's or family's diet (e.g., amount, type, preparation, or delineation of acceptable food combinations [e.g., kosher diets])? Does the client or client's family abstain from certain foods at regular intervals, on specific dates determined by the religious calendar, or at other times? Are there other food prohibitions or prescriptions?
- If the client or client's family's religion mandates or encourages fasting, what does the term *fast* mean (e.g., refraining from certain types of foods, eating only during certain times of the day, skipping certain meals)? For what period of time are family members expected to fast? Are there exceptions to fasting (e.g., are pregnant women or children excluded from fasting)?

- Are special utensils used (e.g., chopsticks, cookware, kosher restrictions)?
- Does the client or client's family use home and folk remedies to treat illnesses (e.g., herbal remedies, acupuncture, cupping, or other healing rituals often involving eggs, lemons, candles)? Which over-the-counter medications are used?

Religion and Spirituality

- How does the client or family's religious affiliation affect health and illness (e.g., life events such as death, chronic illness, body image alteration, cause and effect of illness)?
- What is the role of religious beliefs and practices during health and illness? Are there special rites or blessings for those with serious or terminal illnesses?
- Are there healing rituals or practices that the client and family believe can promote well-being or hasten recovery from illness? If so, who performs these? What materials or arrangements are necessary for the nurse to have available for the practice of these rituals?
- What is the role of significant religious representatives during health and illness? Are there recognized religious healers (e.g., Islamic Imams, Christian Scientist practitioners or nurses, Catholic priests, Mormon elders, Buddhist monks)?

Value Orientation

- What are the client's attitudes, values, and beliefs about his or her health and illness status? Do family members have similar values and beliefs?
- How do these influence behaviors in terms of promotion of health and treatment of disease? What are the client's or family's attitudes, values, and beliefs about health care providers?
- Does culture affect the manner in which the client relates to body image change resulting from illness or surgery (e.g., importance of appearance, beauty, strength, and roles in the cultural group)? Is there a cultural stigma associated

with the client's illness (i.e., how is the illness or the manner in which it was contracted viewed by the family and larger culture)?

● How do the client and his or her family view work, leisure, and education?

● How does the client perceive and react to change?

● How do the client and his or her family perceive changes in lifestyle related to current illness or surgery?

● How do the client and his/her family view biomedical health care (e.g., suspiciously, fearfully, acceptingly, unquestioningly, with awe)?

● How does the client value privacy, courtesy, touch, and relationships with others?

● How does the client relate to persons outside of his or her cultural group (e.g., withdrawal, suspicion, curiosity, openness)?

Appendix B

Transcultural Nursing Assessment Guide for Families, Groups, and Communities

- Joyceen S. Boyle and Margaret M. Andrews

Family and Kinship Systems

- Are the families nuclear, extended, or blended? Do family members live in close proximity? What is the role and status of individual family members? By age and gender?
- How do the family and/or group members relate to the larger community or groups?
- Are there distinct neighborhoods or areas of the community where distinct cultural, ethnic, or religious groups, refugees, or immigrants live?
- What are the communication patterns within the distinct community groups?
- If working with a refugee community, ask about names of tribes and/or clans.
- What place do the "ancestors" have in the worldview of the group? How is the belief in the power of the ancestors incorporated in the daily life and rituals of the group?
- Is the group now or has it traditionally been matriarchal or patriarchal? Is there a preference for first cousins to marry? Who is permitted to marry whom among those who are related by blood/genetics?

Social Life and Networks

- What are the daily routines of the group? What are the important life cycle events such as birth, marriage, family bearing, family rearing, and death? How are they celebrated or observed?

- How are the educational systems organized? How do schools receive and accept input from the community? How do they assist students and their families who are new immigrants or refugees?
- What are the social/economic problems experienced by the group within the community or by the community itself?
- Are there special concerns with a particular ethnic or cultural group such as abuse of alcohol, Fetal Alcohol Syndrome Disorder (FASD), gang membership, and polygamy? How does the group view domestic violence and corporal punishment?
- Are newly arrived groups, such as immigrants or refugees, included within the local community or isolated? Who are the group's local leaders?
- Are there centers or organizations that reach out to special groups within the community? What activities or opportunities are available to new community members? For example, are General Educational Development (GED) courses, English as a second language classes, housing assistance, and/or work training available to newcomers?
- How does the social environment contribute to a sense of belonging? Do all members of the group belong to a distinct religious group? What are the ways that the group practices its religion? What are the dominant religious groups within the community?

- What are the group's social interaction patterns? Do all members of the group speak a common language?
- Are ethnic grocery stores, restaurants, and churches located within the community? What foods do members of the cultural group commonly eat? What foods/substances do they commonly avoid (i.e., alcohol, pork products)?
- Are members of the group comfortable moving away from the larger group?
- Where are ethnic groups, immigrants, or refugees located within the larger community?

Political or Government Systems

- Which factors in the political system influence the ways in which the group perceives its status vis-à-vis the dominant culture, that is, laws, justice, and cultural heroes?
- How does the economic system influence control of resources such as land, water, housing, education and technical training, jobs, and opportunities?
- What is the legal status of the group members? Refugee or immigrant visas? Temporary worker permits? Documented or undocumented?
- How does the local government respond to the ethnic and cultural makeup of the group? What are the ways that the local community "embraces its diversity?"

Language and Traditions

- Are there differences in dialects or languages spoken between health care professionals and local groups within the community?
- What is the literacy level of members of the group? Can they read or write in any language(s)?
- Do health care facilities provide educational materials in diverse languages?
- In what ways do the major cultural traditions of history, art, drama, and so on influence the cultural identity of the group?
- How are local cultures or ethnic traditions embraced during holidays or special celebrations?

Worldviews, Value Orientations, and Cultural Norms

- What are the major cultural values about the relationships of cultural groups to nature and to one another? How can the group's ethical beliefs be described?
- What are the norms and standards of behavior (authority, responsibility, dependability, and competition)?
- Is the group communal or individualistic? How different is their worldview from the dominant worldview of the larger society or culture?
- What are the cultural attitudes about time, family, hospitality, family work, and leisure?
- What are the common values of the group, such as education, work, and so on?
- How are the cultural values reflected in factors such as dress? Do the women cover their hair? Do they prefer skirts or dresses over pants or trousers?
- Are there unique cultural practices within the group that might bring wider community censure, such as the role of women, discipline of children, and relationships between husband and wife?

Religious Beliefs and Practices

- What are the major religious beliefs and practices within the community?
- How do they influence daily life? How do they relate to health practices? What are the practices surrounding major life events such as birth, marriage, and death?
- Does the cultural group have particular practices related to grieving or mourning?

Health Beliefs and Practices

- What are the group's attitudes and beliefs regarding health and illness? Does the cultural group seek care from indigenous (folk) practitioners? Are there traditional practitioners (shamans, curanderos, others) within the group?

- Where do group members go to seek care? Who makes the decisions about seeking health care? Accepting treatments? Are there biologic variations that are important to the health of this group? What are the group's expressed health concerns? Are there cultural or ethnic stores in neighborhoods selling medicinal herbs? What are the primary health concerns and/or illnesses in this population/cultural group (e.g., malaria, HIV/AIDS, female genital mutilation [FGM], malnutrition, tuberculosis)? How do the group's concerns align with those of the local and state health care systems?

Health Care Systems

- Do community health care facilities provide interpreters? Do physician offices and other health care facilities offer educational materials in languages other than English? Are health facilities located in accessible locations, that is, in ethnic neighborhoods? Do health care providers incorporate aspects of other health care

systems, for example, acupuncture and referrals to traditional healers?
- Do members of the group have access to health care? Do they have adequate transportation? Are the hours of operation of health care facilities and availability of appointment times appropriate for members of the group?

Economic Factors

- Does the group or community own or operate its own clinic, neighborhood health center, child or adult day care center, long-term care facility, or nursing home? How will the group or community pay for health care services?
- Is there a group health care policy for all members? Will key leaders in the community work with members to collectively pay for health care services? For example, although the Amish religious leaders have no health insurance, members pool their resources and often settle a hospital bill in cash at the time of the client's discharge.

Appendix C

Transcultural Nursing Assessment Guide for Health Care Organizations and Facilities

- Joyceen S. Boyle, Margaret M. Andrews, and Patti A. Ludwig-Beymer

Environmental Context

- What is the general environment of the community that surrounds the health care organization? Where is the facility located in proximity to the population that it serves?
- What is the socioeconomic status of the adjacent community? What are race/ethnicity characteristics of residents? What are the identified health disparities?
- What are the community's views on health and illness?
- Is there appropriate and easy access to the facility? Is the signage to the facility easy to understand and follow? Are there adequate parking facilities? Are bus routes nearby?
- Is there access to social services? Where are residential and business districts located? What are the sources of employment near the facility?
- What is the proximity to other health care facilities? What facilities are available for the disabled?

Language and Ethnohistory

- What languages are spoken within the institution? By employees? By patients?
- How formal or informal are the lines of communication within the organization?
- Is the organizational governance hierarchical? What communication strategies are used within the organization?

- What is the history of the organization? What was the original mission of the organization? How does the history influence the current organization? How has it traditionally responded to change?

Technology

- How is technology used in the organization? Who uses it? Do all work stations have access to computers? Do all employees have access to e-mail? Are electronic medical records being used? Is new technology in place in the emergency department, critical care areas, labor and delivery, laboratory, and x-ray departments?

Religious/Philosophical

- Does the institution have a religious affiliation? How is this shown in the décor of the institution? How does the religious affiliation influence the philosophy, values, and norms of the agency?
- Is the institution public or private? For profit or not-for-profit?
- Are documents such as The Patient's Bill of Rights prominently displayed within the institution? Are such documents displayed in languages other than English, that is, in Spanish? Are patients/family members provided with documents/explanations related to privacy rights?

Social Factors

- What are the working relationships within nursing? Between nursing and ancillary services? Within each nursing unit? Between physicians and nurses? How closely are staff members aligned throughout the organization?
- Is the environment initially "warm and loving?" How do volunteers or staff members at the information desk behave? Do employees get together outside of work?
- Is there a hierarchal distance between ancillary staff, nurses, and administrators?
- How are family members welcomed (or not welcomed) to the unit? Is the waiting room comfortable? Reading materials? Are they appropriate for the visitors?
- Are computers and telephones available for visitors? Vending machines? Dining facilities?
- Is the signage adequate within the institution? Is the signage in languages other than English? Can visitors easily find their way to a specific unit or room?
- What ways has the institution taken to be inclusive to visitors or patients?

Cultural Values

- Are values explicitly stated? What is valued within the institution? What is valued as "good" and "bad?" Is there a gap between stated values and what actually happens on a daily basis?
- Are interpreter services readily available? Translated medical literature and educational materials?
- How does the institution value and institutionalize culturally competent care?
- How does the institution recruit and retain minority staff members? How are personnel trained in cultural competencies?
- Is there coordination with traditional healers, use of community health workers?
- How does the organization respond to the community it serves (clinic hours, locations, physical environment, network memberships, and written materials)?

- How does the interior design, decor, and art work reflect the cultural values of the institution and community at large?

Political/Legal

- Where does the power rest within the institution? With the administration? With the physicians? With the business office? With nursing? Is power shared? How is power divided among competing groups? Is there an active Board of Directors? What are their responsibilities? What types of legal actions have been taken against the institution? On behalf of the institution?
- How do employees or staff have input? How does the institution encourage or value suggestions or contributions from staff?

Economic

- What is the financial viability of the institution? Has this changed over the past 10 years? Who makes financial decisions? What values are the basis of financial decisions? How do the salaries and benefits compare with those of competitors in the immediate environment?

Education

- How is education valued within the institution? What type of assistance (financial, scheduling, flexibility) is provided for staff seeking advanced training or degrees? What opportunities are offered to those staff who are earning advanced degrees? Does the institution pay baccalaureate-prepared nurses more than associate degree nurses?
- Does the institution provide clinical learning experiences for medicine, nursing, and other health professionals? How does the institution demonstrate that it values students?
- Are advanced practice nurses utilized? What is the educational background of staff nurses? Nurse managers? Nursing leaders? How does this compare with the educational levels of staff in competing institutions?

Appendix D

Transcultural Nursing Assessment for Refugees

- Joyceen S. Boyle and Martha B. Baird

Migration Experience

A refugee is a special status of immigrant defined as a person residing outside his or her country of nationality, who is unable to remain in or stay in his/her country because of persecution on account of race, religion, nationality, or membership in a particular social group or political opinion (UNHCR, The UN Refugee Agency, 1992).

According to the UN Refugee Agency (UNHCR) (2017), at the end of 2016, a record high 65.6 million people had been "forcibly displaced worldwide as a result of persecution, conflict, violence, or human rights violations" (p. 2). Both the International Rescue Committee (IRC) (2017) and the UNHCR report that 22.5 million persons are considered to be refugees. Refugees arrive to a host or resettlement country from a variety of cultures and backgrounds. Some refugees are highly educated and held positions of influence in their home country, whereas some arrive from less developed environments and may have little or no formal education. Therefore, it is important to conduct an individual assessment of each arriving refugee.

Refugees may experience symptoms of mental health distress due to circumstances that led to being forced out of their country of origin, in addition to the stressors associated with their migration journey. There are a number of mental health assessments that have been found to be reliable and valid in a variety of cultural groups and languages adapted for use in different refugee groups (Kleijn, Hovens, & Rodenburg, 2001).

Many refugees have spent time (often years) in so-called transit countries, those countries that they first flee to when they leave their country of origin. For example, Greece and Kenya are examples of transit countries for persons fleeing violence in Syria and Somali.

Ask your client how to pronounce his or her name; find out what name he or she wishes to be called. Be sure you're clear on what is the first and last name as in many cultural groups, the children do not share the same surname as their parents. How do they wish to be greeted?

- Ask about the client's primary language and assess his or her ability to communicate in English in both written and oral forms. What other languages does the client speak and write?
- Ask the clients in which language they prefer to receive written health care information.
- How long has your client been in this country?
- Has he or she lived in other US cities?
- How did the client travel here from the home country?
- How many years did the client spend in the diaspora (or the time from leaving the country of origin to the present day)?
- What other countries has the client lived in? What were those circumstances like?
- Did the client come to this country with family members? With others from the same village or from the same clan?

- Can the client describe the migration experience? Ask about the events that happened to the client that he or she believes are important.
- What precipitated the client's leaving his or her country?
- Did the client have any major health events prior to arrival in the host country? If so, what?
- And did the client receive treatment? If so, where, and what were the outcomes?

The US Health Care System

- What were the client's experiences like when seeking health care in the United States?
- Has the client ever experienced discrimination? What was that experience like for his or her family members?
- What barriers might exist to using the US health care system, such as language difficulties, lack of financial resources, and transportation?
- What provisions, if any, are made for refugee health care within your community?
- Are bilingual health care workers readily available?
- Is there distrust, suspicion, or unfamiliarity of health care workers and biomedicine?
- Is there eye contact with the health care professional?
- Are health care professionals genuinely interested in learning about the refugees?
- Does your client or others in the refugee community strongly prefer same sex providers?
- What are the difficulties of accessing health and social services for refugees?
- Who is available in the sponsoring refugee agency to assist with health education, referrals, and continuity of care?

Language and Traditions

- What are the differences in dialects or languages spoken by health care professionals and the refugees?
- Can some of the problems be identified prior to a health care visit?
- What is the literacy level of members of the refugee group?

- Can they read and write in any language? This may vary within specific refugee groups depending on educational level and social status within home country.
- Do the health care facilities provide educational materials in appropriate languages?
- Are there appropriate numbers and appropriate ages and genders of translators and interpreters available in health care agencies?
- Are the interpreters/translators trained and/or certified?
- Is there adequate outreach to individual homes and families?

Traditional Beliefs and Practices of Healing

- What is the client's understanding of his or her health problem? The understanding of how a client views his/her condition is extremely helpful information. It facilitates the health care provider's understanding of the social and cultural construction of illness. This information helps us understand the client's beliefs and behavior, facilitates further discussion of an ailment, and guides the course of treatment. It is always helpful to begin this discussion with a statement of respect such as: "I know different people have very different ways of understanding illness...help me understand how you see things."
- The following nine questions from Kleinman (1980) can be a useful way to gain the client's perspective about the illness or health condition:

  1. What do you think has caused your problems?
  2. What do you call the problem or illness?
  3. Why do you think it started when it did?
  4. What do you think your sickness does to you?
  5. How severe is your sickness? Will it have a long or short course?
  6. What kind of treatment do you think you should receive?
  7. What are the most important results you hope to receive from this treatment?

8. What are the chief problems your sickness has caused for you?
9. What do you fear most about your sickness?

- How do religious beliefs and practices relate to health and illness?
- Do members of the refugee group seek care from indigenous healers and/or folk practitioners?
- Do they use traditional herbs or medicines?
- Are there cultural or ethnic stores in the neighborhood that sell herbs and traditional medicines?
- Does the individual purchase any medicines, herbs, or vitamins from their home country?
- What contemporary health care is available for this refugee group?
- What immunizations has the client received? When?
- What insurance or payment mechanisms are provided? For how long?
- Does the client understand how to access care?
- Which individuals in the family and/or in the refugee group make decisions about seeking health care? About the treatment options?
- What are the primary health concerns and/or illnesses in this refugee group (e.g., female genital mutilation [FGM], malnutrition, mental health/trauma issues)?
- How do the refugees' concerns align with those of the local and state health care systems? For example, FGM can be a significant concern during labor and delivery. In addition, if the procedure is carried out in the United States by relatives of the female child/adolescent, health care providers have ethical and legal reporting obligations.

Family and Kinship Systems

- Are the families extended or nuclear or other?
- Has the structure of the family changed during or since migration?
- Do family members live in close proximity? Do they visit often?
- Where are the members of your client's family?
- What is the role and stature of individual family members?

- How do family members relate to each other?
- How have family roles changed since coming to this country?
- Ask if there are tribes and/or clans in the refugee group.
- Do the parents and/or others make arrangements for marriages?
- Is there a preference for first cousins to marry?
- What is the role of "elders" or "leaders" in this refugee group? How do they function within the community?
- Did the client leave family members behind or lose family members from death in the home country?

Social Life and Networks

- What are the daily routines of this group?
- How do the routines vary by gender?
- How have family roles changed?
- Is the refugee group integrated into the community or fairly isolated?
- Who are the group's leaders?
- How does the refugee group observe important life cycle events?
- What are the educational aspirations of individual/family refugees?
- What are the educational experiences of the children?
- Are there special concerns such as abuse of alcohol, domestic violence, gang membership, polygamy, and child marriage? How does this refugee group view these issues?

Religious Beliefs and Practices

- What are the major religious beliefs and practices within the refugee community?
- Does your client adhere to the predominant beliefs?
- Is there a special church associated with the refugees? (Churches often serve as a site for social life of the refugee community and are comfortable and acceptable places for health educational programs and other forms of outreach.)

- How is social life integrated within the church membership?
- How do the religious beliefs and practices influence everyday life? How are they expressed in everyday life?
- Are there special beliefs and practices surrounding major life events such as birth, marriage, and death?
- Are there special "cultural" occasions, such as circumcision rites and *quince años* parties?
- Are there specific beliefs about gender roles? Are these beliefs tied to religious beliefs?

All refugees resettled to the United States receive a comprehensive physical examination and mental health screening within their first 30 days of their arrival. This is usually conducted in a public health clinic or primary care setting. There are several mental health assessment tools that have been translated and culturally adapted for use with different refugee groups. If a refugee has a positive mental health screening, they should be referred to a mental health care provider for further assessment.

The Refugee Health Screener-15 (RHS-15) is commonly used to asses newly arrived refugees in host countries. The RHS-15 has been translated into 15 languages and is used to measure indicators of mental health symptoms and distress including depression, anxiety, and coping.

The Hopkins Symptoms Checklist-25 (HSCL-25) measures symptoms of anxiety and depression. It consists of 25 items; Part I has 10 items for anxiety symptoms; Part II has 15 items for depression symptoms.

The Harvard Trauma Questionnaire (HTQ) is a checklist that inquires about a variety of traumatic events as well as the emotional symptoms considered to be uniquely associated with trauma and torture.

REFERENCES

International Rescue Committee. (2017, September). The future of refugee wealth in the United States. What's at stake in 2018. Retrieved from https://www.rescue.org/sites/default/files/document/1872/pdpolicybrieffinal2/pdf

Kleijn, W. C., Hovens, J. E., & Rodenburg, J. J. (2001). Posttraumatic stress symptoms in refugees: Assessments with the Harvard Trauma Questionnaire and the Hopkins Symptom Checklist-25 in different languages. *Psychological Reports, 88,* 527–532.

Kleinman, A. (1980). *Patients and healers in the context of culture: An exploration of the borderland between anthropology, medicine and psychiatry.* Berkeley, CA: University of California Press.

United Nations High Commissioner for Refugees (UNHCR) The UN Refugee Agency. (1992). Handbook on procedures and criteria for determining refugee status under the 1951 convention and the 1967 protocol relating to the status of refugees. Retrieved from http://www.unhcr.org/cgi-bin/texis/vtx/search?page=search=&docid=3d58el3b4query=definition%20of%20refugee

The UN Refugee Agency. (2017, June 19). Global trends: Forced displacement in 2016. Retrieved from http://www.unhcr.org/globaltrends2016/

Index

(*Note*: Note: *b* refers to material located in a box; *c* refers to a case study; *e* refers to evidence-based practice; *f* refers to a figure; *r* refers to a research application; *t* refers to a table).

A

AAFP (American Academy of Family Physicians), 143
Ability, 5
Abortion
  Baha'i international community, 388
  Catholicism, 394
  Church of Jesus Christ of Latter-day Saints, 399
  Jehovah's Witnesses, 408
  Seventh-Day Adventists, 412
Acculturation, 312, 346
  concept of, 312
  stress of, 312
Acculturation Rating Scale for Mexican Americans, 159–161
ACNM (American College of Nurse Midwives), 143–144
ACOG (American College of Obstetricians and Gynecologists), 158
Acupuncture, 118
Adaptors, 20
Addison's disease, 87
Administration, 283
Adolescents
  cultural backgrounds, 196
  culturally competent nursing care for
    family belief systems, 196–197
    family, nursing assessment of, 196–198
    family structures, 197–198
    nursing interventions, 198–200
  health care needs of, 193–194
  rapid repeat birth prevention, 195*b*
Adult behavior, chronologic standards for, 211–220
Adulthood, 209–210, 212–213
  cultural influences, overview of
    adult behavior, chronologic standards for, 211–220
    developmental tasks, 214
    developmental transition, 215–216
    physiologic development, 210–211
    psychosocial development, 210–211

health-related situational crises
  African American women, 224
  caregiving, 223–224
  culturally competent nursing care, 228–233
Advance directives, 420–421
Advocacy, 422
Affective displays, 20
African American church functions, 328
African American community
  church, 328
  culture, 317–319
  of HIV/AIDS context and influential factors, 225–228
  prevention challenges, 225
African American family, 167*f*
African American population, health disparities among, 130*b*
African American pregnant woman, 166–167, 166*f*–167*f*
African American women's infant-feeding practices, 161*b*
African Asian American family, 128*f*
African European American family, 128*f*
African-American Heart Failure Trial (A-HeFT), 60
Agency for Healthcare Research and Quality (AHRQ), 270
Aggregates, 334
Aging, perspectives of, 242
A-HeFT (African-American Heart Failure Trial), 60
AHRQ (Agency for Healthcare Research and Quality), 270
Albinism, 87
Allah, 401
Allergies, review of, 64–72
Alternative lifestyle choices, 139–143
Alternative therapies, 118*b*
American Academy of Family Physicians (AAFP), 143
American College of Nurse Midwives (ACNM), 143–144
American College of Obstetricians and Gynecologists (ACOG), 158
American Counseling Association, 322

American Indian Culture, 319–320
American Indian Human Resource Center, 319–320
American Medical Association, 151
American Nurses Association (ANA), cultural competence, 266, 267*b*
American Organization of Nurse Executives (AONE), 267, 284, 284*b*
American Psychiatric Association, 314
American Psychological Association (APA), 306–307
American women, HIV/AIDS cases, 224–228
Amish, 385–387
  considerations, 389–390
  death and dying, 389
  health care practices, 388–389
  medical and surgical interventions, 388
  Old Order Amish, 387
  ordinance, 398
  religious support system for sick, 388–389
  reproduction, 388
  substance use, 388
Amniocentesis, 64, 391–392, 394, 399, 401, 403, 405, 412
Analgesia, racial and ethnic variations, conversion of, 70*b*
ANC (Antenatal Care Model), 144
Andrews/Boyle transcultural interprofessional practice (TIP) model
  assumptions (about humans), 13
  assumptions (about transcultural nursing), 12
  communication, 15–24
    chronemics, 20–21
    effective, 13
    eye contact and facial expressions, 19–20
    gestures, 20
    greetings, 19
    interpreters, 17–19
    interprofessional health care team, 15

Andrews/Boyle transcultural interpro-
    fessional practice (TIP) model
    (*Continued*)
  language, 17
  modesty, 22–23
  posture, 20
  problem-solving process, 24–26,
    25*f*
  proxemics, 21
  silence, 19
  technology-assisted communica-
    tion, 23–24
  cultural context, 14
  goals, assumptions, and compo-
    nents, 11, 12*b*
Andy Weaver Amish, 387
Anglicanism, 411
Anointing of the Sick, 393
Antenatal care, cultural beliefs related
    to, 144–149
  cultural preparation for childbirth, 149
  food taboos and food cravings,
    147–148, 148*b*
  substance use, 149
Antenatal Care Model (ANC), 144
Anthropology, 4–6
Anxiety, 230
AONE (American Organization of
    Nurse Execuitves), 267, 284,
    284*b*
APA (American Psychological
    Association), 306–307
Apocrine sweat glands, 88
Apolipoprotein E (APOE), 61
Arab community organizations, 323
Arab Muslim culture, 323–324
Aromatherapy, 118
Art, cultural groups communication, 24
Asian American core cultural values,
    321
Asian Countries, antenatal, intrapartum,
    and postpartum care in, 150*b*
Asian/Pacific Islander culture, 320–321
Assessment tools, organizational
    culture, 277
Assimilation, 346
Asylees, 342
Autonomy, 418, 420–421
Ayurveda, 245
Ayurvedic medicine, 118

B

Baby-Friendly Hospital Initiative
    (BFHI), 161
Bad nerves, 230

Bed sharing, 184
Behavior, biocultural variations
    in, 83
Beneficence, 421
Bereavement, 382
BFHI (Baby-Friendly Hospital
    Initiative), 161
Bias, 35
Biocultural aspects, of disease,
    74*t*–76*t*
Biocultural variations, 77
  blood pressure, 79
  body proportions, 78
  client's hygiene, 83
  and clinical significance, 95*t*–96*t*
  in head, 89–91
    ears, 90
    eyes, 89
    hair, 89
    leukoedema, 90
    mouth, 90
    teeth, 90–91
  in height, 77–78, 93*t*–94*t*
  in illness, 92
  in mammary venous plexus, 91
  in measurements, 77–79
  in musculoskeletal system, 91–92,
    93*t*–94*t*
  in pain assessment, 80–83
  physical appearance, 83
    Addison's disease, 87
    age-related changes, 87–88
    albinism, 87
    cyanosis, 85
    ecchymoses, 87
    erythema, 86
    hyperpigmentation, 85
    jaundice, 85–86
    melanin, 84
    Mongolian spots, 84
    pallor, 86
    petechiae, 86
    in skin, 84–88
    in sweat glands, 88–89
    uremia, 87
    in vital signs, 79
    vitiligo, 85
  Bioelectromagnetic-based therapies,
    117
  Biofield therapies, complementary
    health approaches, 117
  Biomedical health paradigm,
    107–108
  Biomedical model, 108
  Birth and culture, 149–157

birth positions, 154
  cultural expression of labor, 154
  infant gender, cultural meaning
    attached to, 154–157
Birth control-related mistrust, 132
Birthing plan, 128–129
Blended family, 127–128, 197
Body proportions, biocultural varia-
    tions in measurements, 78
Body structure, biocultural variations
    in, 83
Body-based methods, 117
Bolman and Deal's organizational
    culture perspective,
    273–274
Brahman, 400
Brauche, 388
Breast-feeding
  cultural influences on, 159–161
  promotion, 360
Brit milah, 406–407
Buddha, 390
Buddhism, 390
Buddhist adolescent, end-of-life care
    for, 202
Buddhist Churches of America
  Buddhism, 390
  death and dying, 392
  diet, 391
  general beliefs and religious prac-
    tices, 390–391
  health care practices, 391
  holy days, 390
  medical and surgical interventions,
    391–392
  religious objects, 390
  religious support system for sick,
    392
  reproduction, 391–392
  rites and rituals, 391
Buddhist family, 201

C

Café au lait spots, 87–88
Caida de la mollera (fallen fontanel),
    190–191
Cardiovascular disease (CVD)
  aboriginal women's cardiac prob-
    lems, 355*b*
  health promotion goals, 244, 245*t*
Caregiving, 223–224, 249–250
Caring for people of color, 6–7
Caring hospital, 292
Carrier screening, 61–64
Caste system, 400

Catholic Charities USA, 383–384
Catholicism
  beliefs and religious practices, 392–393
  Catholic, 392
  death and dying, 395
  diet, 392–393
  health care practices, 393–395
  holy days, 392–393
  medical and surgical interventions, 393–394
  religious objects, 392
  religious support system for sick, 394–395
  reproduction, 394
  rites and rituals, 392
  social activities, 393
  substance use, 393
CBS (Central Broadcasting System), 310–312
CCATH (Cultural Competency Assessment Tool for Hospitals), 285–286
Center for Mental Health Services (CMHS), 305
Centering Pregnancy, 145
Central Broadcasting System (CBS), 310–312
Certification in transcultural nursing (CTN-A), 11
Chief complaint, 72–73
Child abuse, 188–189
Child poverty, in United States, 175–176
Child rearing
  culture-universal and culture-specific, 178–189
    child abuse, 188–189
    elimination, 186
    gender differences, 189
    menstruation, 186–187
    model depicting cultural perspectives of, 179f
    nutrition, 180–184
    parent-child relationships and discipline, 187–188
    sleep, 184–186
    values, attitudes, beliefs, and practices of, 178–179
  practices, model of, 174f
Childbearing, 214
Childbearing, transcultural perspectives in
  African American pregnancy, 166–167

African American women's infant-feeding practices, 161b
antenatal, intrapartum, and postpartum care in Asian Countries, 150b
birth and culture, 149–157
  birth positions, 154
  cultural expression of labor, 154
  infant gender, cultural meaning attached to, 154–157
childbirth and postnatal cultural practices, in Nepal and other countries, 152b
clinical implications, 138
  cultural variations influencing pregnancy, 139–144
  cultural belief related to antenatal care, 144–149
  cultural preparation for childbirth, 149
  food taboos and food cravings, 147–148, 148b
  substance use, 149
cultural belief systems and practices, 127–128
culture and postpartum period, 157–161
  cultural influences on breastfeeding and weaning, 159–161
  postpartum depression (PPD), 158
  postpartum dietary prescriptions and activity levels, 158–159
  postpartum rituals, 159
fertility control and culture, 131–137
  continuation of unintended pregnancy, 133–134
  contraceptive methods, 134
  cultural influences on fertility control, 136–137
  global contraception concerns, 134
  refugees and reproductive health, 134–135
  religion and fertility control, 135–136
  unintended pregnancy, 132–133
hispanic pregnant women, 163–164
indigenous peoples/native American pregnant women, 164–166, 165f
intimate partner violence, cultural issues related to, 161–163
positive childbirth experience, intrapartum care for, 155b

pregnancy and childbirth practices in United States, 128–131
pregnancy and culture, 137–144
  biologic variations, 137–139
Childbirth, cultural preparation for, 149
Childhood obesity, racial and ethnic differences in, 181b
Children
  childhood disorders, biocultural influences
    ethnicity, 192
    immunity, 191–192
    intermarriage, 192
    race, 192
  chronic illness, 192–193
  culturally competent nursing care for
    extended family, 197
    family belief systems, 196–197
    family, nursing assessment of, 196–198
    nursing interventions, 198–200
  in culturally diverse society, 173–174
  culture-universal and culture-specific
    child abuse, 188–189
    cosleeping, 184
    cradleboard, 184–185, 185f
    elimination, 186
    gender differences, 189
    menstruation, 186–187
    nutrition, 180–184
    pandanus mat, 184–185
    parent-child relationships and discipline, 187–188
    premasticate, 180
  die from, 184
  disability in, 192–193
  health promotion
    culture-bound syndromes, 191
    illness, 189–190
  as population
    child health status, 176
    crying, 178
    growth and development, 176–177
    infant attachment, 177–178
    poverty, 175–176
    racial/ethnic composition, 174–175
Children's health, impact of poverty on, 175–176
Chiropractic healing, 118

Christian Science, 395
  considerations, 397–398
  death and dying, 397
  general beliefs and religious prac-
    tices, 395–396
  health care practices, 396–397
  holy days, 395
  medical and surgical interventions,
    397
  religious support system for sick,
    397
  reproduction, 397
  rites and rituals, 396
  social activities and substance use,
    396
Christian Science Journal, 396
Chronemics, 20–21
Chronic disease self-management,
    ethnic groups, 113*b*
Chronic illnesses, cause of, 192–193
Chronic pain, 326
Chronic pain management, interdisci-
    plinary team approach to, 82*b*
Chronic traumatic encephalopathy
    (CTE), 60
Church(es). *See also* Black church
  African American, 328, 364
  Buddhist, 390–392
  Native North American, 409–410
Church of Jesus Christ of Latter-day
    Saints, 398
  death and dying, 400
  diet, 398
  general beliefs and religious prac-
    tices, 398–399
  health care practices, 399–400
  holy days, 398
  medical and surgical interventions,
    399
  religious objects, 398
  religious support system for sick,
    399–400
  reproduction, 399
  rites and rituals, 398
  social activities, 398–399
  substance use, 399
Civic responsibilities, 216–218
Clients
  cultural assessment of, 36–42
  with home birth midwife, 131*f*
  with special needs
    communication and language
      assistance, 48–51
    deaf, culture of, 47–48
    health disparities, 46–47

Clinical decision making, 56
Clinical decision making/nursing
    actions, 97–98
  cultural care, 97
    preservation, 97
  evaluation, 97–98
Clothing, 23
CMHS (Center for Mental Health
    Services), 305
Codeine to morphine conversion,
    analgesia, 70*b*
Communication, 13*b*
  transcultural mental health nursing,
    326–327
  transcultural nursing assessment
    guide, 429–430
Communication networks, 342–343
Communitarian ethic of care, 420
Communities
  agencies, 321
  culturally competent organizations,
    290–292
  organizational culture, employees,
    and, 274–277
  transcultural nursing assessment
    guide
    economic factors, 437
    family and kinship systems, 435
    health beliefs and practices,
      436–437
    health care systems, 437
    language and traditions, 436
    political/government systems, 436
    religious beliefs and practices, 436
    social life and networks, 435–436
    worldviews, value orientations,
      and cultural norms, 436
Community assessment example,
    291*b*
Community health nurses, 334–335,
    364–366
Community health, psychiatric, and
    pediatric nurses, 184
Community health representatives
    (CHRs), 352
Community nursing, 334–335
Community nursing practice
  cultural factors within
    demographics and health care,
      339
    diverse cultural groups, access to,
      348–349
    refugee, 340–346
    refugee families, planning nursing
      care for, 343–346

subcultures/diversity within com-
    munities, 339–340
traditional cultural values, main-
    tenance of, 346–348
cultural influences, 338–339
cultural issues in, 337–349
Community settings, 354
culturally competent nursing care,
    overview of, 335–336
transcultural framework, 336–337
subcultures identification, 336
values and cultural norms, identi-
    fying, 337
Community-based collaborative
    action research (CBCAR)
    intervention, 334, 345*b*
Community-based nursing, 334–335
Community-based participatory
    research, 291
Community-based services, 241–242,
    256–259
Community-based settings, 334
Compassion, 424
Competent care, deaf clients, cultur-
    ally congruent and, 49*b*
Competent interpreter services, 289
Complementary health approaches,
    116–119
  bioelectromagnetic-based therapies,
    117
  biofield therapies, 117
  body touch, 117
  efficacy of, 119
  external energy therapies, 117
  mind and body practices, 117
  natural products, 117
  senses, 117
  therapies of, 118*b*
  traditional alternative medicine, 117
Conjugal family, 197
Consequential dimension, 374–375
Consumers, 305–306
  of mental health care, 305–306
Context, 14
Continuing care retirement communi-
    ties (CCRC), 241
Contraceptive methods for fertility
    control, 134
Coping behaviors, cultural compe-
    tence, 353
Copy-number variants, 59–60
Core curriculum, TCN, 10–11
Corporate culture, training, 282
Cosleeping, 184
Cradleboard, 184–185, 185*f*

Credentialed health professionals, 15
Critical care unit nurses, nuclear family members, 274
Cross-cultural communication, 31–32, 204
   interprofessional health care team, 16f
Crying, cultural differences, 178
CTE (chronic traumatic encephalopathy), 60
CTN-A (advanced certification in transcultural nursing), 11
CTN-B (basic certification in transcultural nursing), 11
Cultural accommodation, 424
Cultural affiliations, 430
Cultural assessment, 36–41, 56, 349–350
   basic principles of, 350b
   content of, 57
   diverse communities, 349–366
Cultural baggage, 34–35
Cultural barriers, health disparities, 272b
Cultural belief related to antenatal care, 144–149
   cultural preparation for childbirth, 149
   food taboos and food cravings, 147–148, 148b
   substance use, 149
Cultural belief systems, 106
   metaphor, 106
   and practices, 127–128
   worldview, 106
Cultural blind spot, 325
Cultural care
   accommodation/negotiation, 97
   assessment tools, 277
   preservation/maintenance, 97
   repatterning/restructuring, 97
Cultural competence, 10, 33–34, 266, 324–325
   American Nurses Association recommendations, 267b
   coping behaviors, 353
   education, 130
   family systems, 353
   in health maintenance and health promotion, 350–356
   internal evaluation of adherence to, 285–287
   lifestyle practices, 353–356
   in prevention programs, 359–360
   primary prevention, 356–360
   secondary prevention, 356, 360–363
   tertiary prevention, 356, 364–366

Cultural Competency Assessment Tool for Hospitals (CCATH), 285–286
Cultural context
   depressive disorders, 302b, 313
   influence of, 14f
Cultural differences, 294
   in response to drugs, 71t–72t
Cultural diversity, 42
Cultural explanation, 313
Cultural factors, within community demographics and health care, 339
   diverse cultural groups, access to, 348–349
   refugee, 340–346
   refugee families, planning nursing care for, 343–346
   subcultures/diversity within communities, 339–340
   traditional cultural values, maintenance of, 346–348
Cultural feeding practices, 180
Cultural Formulation Interview (CFI), 313
Cultural idiom, distress, 313
Cultural imposition, 35
Cultural influences
   individuals and families, 338–339
   older adult in community, 242–252
Cultural knowledge, 335
Cultural norms
   behavior of, 436
   concept of, 300
   health history, 73
   history, 73
Cultural pain, 307
Cultural repatterning, 424
Cultural restrictions, 430
Cultural sanctions, 430
Cultural self-assessment, 35
Cultural sensitivity, 352–353
Cultural stereotype, 35
Cultural values, 439
   African American culture, 317–319
   beliefs and practices, 312–313, 317–324
     American Indian Culture, 319–320
     Arab Muslim culture, 323–324
     Asian/Pacific Islander culture, 320–321
     Hispanic/Latino culture, 322–323
   culture care model, 279b
Cultural variations influencing pregnancy, 139–144

Culturally and linguistically appropriate health care services (CLAS), 269b
   Standards, 266–268
Culturally competent care, 24, 334–335, 416–417
   community for, 334–335
   definitions and categories of, 33–46
     clients, cultural assessment of, 36–42
     individual cultural competence, 42–46
     organizational cultural competence, 46
     self-assessment, 35–36
   foundation of, 334
   guidelines for, 33, 34t
   rationale for, 32–33
Culturally competent ethical practice, 424–426
   model application, 425–426
Culturally competent mental health care, 324–326
Culturally competent organizations, 266
   definition of, 266
   Edward Hospital mission, vision, and values, 286f
   need for, 268–272
   role of health care organization leaders, 282b
Culturally congruent action modes, 424
Culturally congruent care, 8, 320–322
   and competent care, deaf clients, 49b
Culturally congruent services and programs, 292
Culturally diverse society, children in, 173–174
Culturally diverse women
   health beliefs, 317
   mental health for, 304
Culturally responsive health care services, 285
Culture, 4–6, 290
   of deaf, 47–48
   fertility control and, 131–137
     continuation of unintended pregnancy, 133–134
     contraceptive methods, 134
     cultural influences on fertility control, 136–137
     global contraception concerns, 134
     refugees and reproductive health, 134–135

Culture (*Continued*)
  religion and fertility control,
    135–136
  unintended pregnancy, 132–133
  and postpartum period, 157–161
    cultural influences on breastfeed-
      ing and weaning, 159–161
    postpartum depression (PPD),
      158
    postpartum dietary prescriptions
      and activity levels, 158–159
    postpartum rituals, 159
Culture care repatterning/restructur-
  ing, 424
Culture shock, 312
Culture-bound syndrome, 313–315,
  315*t*–317*t*
Culture-bound syndromes, 73, 314
Culture-specific nursing care, 4
Culture-specific syndrome, 314
Culture-universal nursing care, 4
Culturologic nursing assessment, 56
Curanderos, 322, 354–356
CVD. *See* Cardiovascular disease (CVD)
Cyanosis, 85

D

Dance, cultural groups communica-
  tion, 24
De novo family, 143
Deafness, prevention of, 50*b*
Death
  bad, 381
  child, 382
  good, 381
Decision making, and mental health
  care, 305–306
Deferred Action for Childhood
  Arrivals (DACA) programs,
  310–312
Demographic barriers, health dispari-
  ties, 272*b*
Depression, 58
  cultural context, 302*b*, 313
Determinism, 107–108
Developmental considerations, 431
Developmental crises, 210
Developmental tasks, 210, 214
Developmental transitions
  in career success, 215–216
  in marriage and raising children, 218
  in roles and relationships, 218–220
  in social and civic responsibility,
    216–218
Diabetes mellitus, 138

Diagnostic Statistical Manual-5
  (DSM-5)
  cultural criteria changes in, 313–314,
    314*t*
Dietary supplements, 110, 118
  decisions and evaluating informa-
    tion, 112*b*
Disability, 5
  cause of, 192–193
Disabling hearing loss, 47
Discrimination, 35–36
Disenfranchised Grieving, 307–309
Disparities
  in mental health care, 306–309
  in mental health treatment, 307
Distress
  cultural idiom, 313
  DSM-V (2013) cultural concepts,
    314*t*
Diverse cultural communities, access
  to, 348–349
Diversity, 42
  within communities, 339–340
Dolor de corazón, 58
Down syndrome, 89
Drug efficacy, genetic screenings, 61
Drug sensitivity, genetic screenings, 61

E

Ears, biocultural variation in, 90
Ecchymoses, 87
Eccrine sweat glands, 88
Economic factors, 279*b*
Economics, 431, 437, 439
Edinburgh Postnatal Depression Scale,
  156–158
Education, 279*b*, 439
Educational background, 431
Elimination, childrearing behaviors,
  186
Emblems, 20
Emergency contraception (EC), 134
The Emergency Medical Treatment
  and Active Labor Act
  (EMTALA), 425–426
Emic, 41
Emigrate, 32
Empathic communication, 326–327
Empathy, 326–327
Employees, organizational culture and
  community, 274–277
Empty nest syndrome, 211
EMTALA (The Emergency Medical
  Treatment and Active Labor
  Act), 425–426

Energy therapies, complementary
  health approaches, 117
Enhancing the Rights of Adolescent
  Girls, 188
Enlightenment, 390
Environmental context, 279*b*
Epigenetics, 58–59
Erythema, 86
Ethic of care, 420
Ethical relativism, 417–421
Ethical universalism, 421–424
Ethnic nursing care, 6–7
Ethnicity, 6, 192, 240
Ethnocentrism, 35, 304
Ethnohistory, 58, 438
Ethnonursing research, 8–10
Ethnoreligion, 374
Etic, 41
Eucharist, 392
Evaluation, care plan, 24
Evil eye (mal ojo), 107, 190
Experiences of pain, 328
Experiential dimension, 374–375
Extended American family, 220*f*
Extended family, 197–198, 201
Eye contact, 19–20
Eyes, biocultural variation in, 89

F

Facial expressions, 19–20
Faith healing, 396
Families
  social unit, 41–42
  transcultural nursing assessment
    guide
      economic factors, 437
      family and kinship systems, 435
      health beliefs and practices,
        436–437
      health care systems, 437
      language and traditions, 436
      political/government systems, 436
      religious beliefs and practices, 436
      social life and networks, 435–436
      worldviews, value orientations,
        and cultural norms, 436
Family belief systems, 196–197
Family systems, 353, 435, 442
Fast-food restaurants, popularity of,
  182–183
Fasting, 392–393
Female genital mutilation and cutting,
  140*b*
Female genital mutilation/cutting
  (FGM/C), 139

Female sterilization, 134
Feminist theory, 420
Fertility control and culture, 131–137
  continuation of unintended pregnancy, 133–134
  contraceptive methods, 134
  cultural influences on fertility control, 136–137
  global contraception concerns, 134
  refugee women and girls, minimum initial service package for, 135*b*
  refugees and reproductive health, 134–135
  religion, 135–136
  unintended pregnancy, 132–133
Fertility-related cultural practices, 131–132
Fidelity, 420–421
First-trimester care, 144
Folk healer, 44–45
Folk healing system, 15, 44–45, 111–116
Folk illnesses, 314
Food cravings, during pregnancy, 147–148, 148*b*
Food taboos, during pregnancy, 147–148, 148*b*
Formal support, 249
Four Noble Truths, 390
Four-visit focused ANC (FANC) model, 144
Francophone community, 336
Friendscraft, 197–198, 388
Funeral, 380

G

Garment, 398
Gender differences, 189
Gender practices, 131–132
Generativity, 213
Genetic(s), 58–59
Genetic diseases, clinical implications, 62*t*–64*t*
Genetic tests, carrier screening, 61–64
Geneva, reproductive health care for migrant women in, 133*b*
Genome, 58–59
Genomics, 58–59
Genotyping, 92–96
Gestures, 20
Ghanaian women's cultural beliefs, 154
Ghasl El Mayyet, 404
Ghost illness, 191

Girls
  menstrual periods, 186–187
  mother, developmental stage, 187*f*
Global Consensus Statement, 134
Global Strategy for Women's Children's and Adolescents' Health, 134
Globalization, 129
God's law of harmony, 396–397
Governance, 283–285
Greetings, 19
Grief, 382
Guided imagery, 118
Guttmacher Institute, 134

H

Hadith, 402
Hair, biocultural variation in, 89
Hajj, 401
Halal, 402
Hard of hearing, 47
Harmony, 108
Harvard Trauma Questionnaire (HTQ), 443
Healers, scope of practice, 114*t*–115*t*
Healing, 396
Healing systems, 110–119
  types of
    complementary, integrative, and alternative health system, 116–119
    folk healing system, 111–116
    professional care systems, 110–111
    self-care, 110
Health and Human Services (HHS), 270
Health and illness behaviors, 110
  socioeconomic status affects and, 240–242
Health behavior, 110, 242–243
Health belief system, 436–437
Health belief systems, 106–109
  and children, 190–191
  holistic paradigm, 108–109
  magico-religious paradigm, 107
  scientific paradigm, 107–108
Health care institutions, 344
Health care provider decisions, clash with parental preference, 199*b*
Health care settings, form/checklist, 57–58
Health care systems, 437
Health disparity, 268–272, 271*b*
  clients with special needs, 46–47
  strategies and tools for reducing, 283*b*

Health education, 362
Health inequity, 416–417
Health Insurance Portability and Accountability Act (HIPAA), 418
Health literacy, 113*b*
Health Ministries, 412
Health professionals, 149
Health promotion, 106
  childhood disorders, biocultural influences on, 191–192
  chronic illnesses, cause of, 192–193
  health belief systems and children, 190–191
  illness, 189–190
Health providers, 137
Health surveys, 136
Health system barriers, health disparities, 272*b*
Health tourism, 32
Health-illness
  behaviors, 110
  situational crisis, 210
  transitions, 218
Health-related beliefs and practices, 431–432
Health-related situational crises, 220–233
  adult development
    adult health transitions and nursing interventions, 231–233
    health promotion interventions, 228–231
  caregiving, 223–224
  context of HIV/AIDS and African American community, 224–228
Healthy communities, 290
Healthy People 2020, 334–335, 335*b*
Height, biocultural variations in measurements, 77–78
The Herald of Christian Science, 396
Herbal remedies, 65*t*–68*t*
  Chinese Americans, 65–69
Herbalists, 322
High blood, 229
Hijab, 22, 22*f*
Hindu, 400
Hinduism, 400–401
  death and dying, 401
  general beliefs and religious practices, 400
  health care practices, 401
  Hindu, 400
  medical and surgical interventions, 401

Hinduism (*Continued*)
  religious objects, 400
  religious support system for sick, 401
  reproduction, 401
  social activities, 400
  substance use, 400
Hispanic pregnant women, 163–164,
  163*f*
Hispanic/Latino culture, 322–323
Hispanics, hypertension prevention
  beliefs, 347*b*
Historical trauma, 307–309
Historical Unresolved Grief, 307–309
HIV/AIDS
  American women, 224–225
  care, 228
  context of, 224–228
  prevention challenges, 225
  preventive efforts, barriers, 225
  treatment, 227
Holistic, 109
  paradigm, 108–109
Home birth midwife, client with, 131*f*
Home birthing pool, client in, 131*f*
Home going, 380
Homeopathic medicine, 118
Homophobia, 227–228
Homosexual behavior, concealment of,
  227–228
Hopkins Symptoms Checklist-25
  (HSCL-25), 443
Hot/cold theory, 109
HTQ. *See* Harvard Trauma
  Questionnaire (HTQ)
Human papillomavirus vaccination, 351*b*
Human resource frame, 273
Human Resource standards, Joint
  Commission standards, 268*b*
Human rights, 422
Human rights barriers, for displaced per-
  sons, in Southern Sudan, 341*b*
Humans, assumptions, 13*b*
Humors, 109
Hyperpigmentation, 85
Hypertension prevention beliefs, 347*b*

I

Illegal alien, 310–312
Illness
  behavior, 110, 244
    health and, 110
    Mechanic's determinants of, 111*t*
  biocultural variations in, 92, 106
  health and health promotion,
    189–190

Illustrators, 20
Immigrant, 32, 340–346
  mental health care, 309–313, 311*b*
Immigrate, 32
Immunity, biocultural influences,
  191–192
Implementation, care plan, 24
In vitro fertilization (IVF), 142
Independent churches, 411
Indian Health Service (IHS), 319–320
Indigenous healers, 15
Indigenous peoples/native American
  pregnant women, 164–166,
  165*f*
Individual cultural competence,
  33–34, 42–46
Individuals residing, in country, 342,
  342*t*
Infant attachment, 177–178
Infant gender, cultural meaning
  attached to, 154–157
Infants, low birth weight, 194*f*
Informal social support, 249
Informal support, 250
Informed consent, 420–421
Institutional racism, barrier of, 294
Integration, 346
Integrative health care, 116
Intellectual dimension, 374–375
Inter-agency Working Group on
  Reproductive Health in Crisis,
  135
Intergenerational transmission of
  trauma, 307–309
Intermarriage, biocultural influences,
  192
International Society for the
  Prevention of Child Abuse and
  Neglect (ISPCAN), 188
Interpersonal communication, 326
Interpreters, 17–19, 289
  overcoming language barriers, 18*b*
Interprofessional collaboration, 15
  practice, 33
Interprofessional health care team,
  14–15
Intimate partner violence (IPV), 323
Intimate partner violence, cultural
  issues related to, 161–163
Intimate space, 21
Intrapersonal reflection, 325–326
Intrauterine insemination, 142–143
Islam
  Allah, 401
  death and dying, 403–404

diet and substance use, 402–403
  general beliefs and religious prac-
    tices, 401–403
  health care practices, 403–404
  holy days, 402
  medical and surgical interventions,
    403
  Pillars of faith, 401
  religious objects, 44–45, 403
  religious support system for sick, 403
  reproduction, 403
Islamic law, 136
Islamic law, blood, 187
Islam's holiest city (salat), 401
ISPCAN (International Society for the
  Prevention of Child Abuse and
  Neglect), 188

J

Jaundice, 85–86
Jehovah, 404
Jehovah's Witnesses, 404
  death and dying, 405
  general beliefs and religious prac-
    tices, 404–405
  health care practices, 405
  holy days, 404–405
  medical and surgical interventions,
    405
  religious support system for sick,
    405
  reproduction, 405
  social activities, 405
  substance use, 405
Joint commission standards, address
  culture, 267*b*
Judaism, 406
  death and dying, 408–409
  diet, 407
  general beliefs and religious prac-
    tices, 406–407
  health care practices, 407–409
  holy days, 406
  medical and surgical interventions,
    408
  religious objects, 407
  religious support system for sick,
    408
  reproduction, 408
  rites and rituals, 406–407
  social activities, 407
  substance use, 407
  Talmud, 406
  Torah, 406
Justice, 422

K

Karma, 400
Kashrut, 407
Khat *(Catha edulis)*, 149
Kinship, 359, 435, 442
  networks, 432
  systems, 279b
Kippot, 407
Korean American women, 146–147
Kosher, 407
Kufungisisa, 313

L

La cuarentena, 360
Labor, cultural expression of, 154
Laboratory tests, biocultural differences in, 92–96
Lactose intolerance, 77
Lamaze childbirth education, 144
Language, 16–17, 279b, 438, 441
Language access services (LAS), 48
Language barriers, 359
Language spoken, 436
LAS (language access services), 48
Latino culture, 323
Lead exposure in pregnant and lactating women, risk factors for, 146b
Leadership standards, Joint Commission standards, 268b
Leininger, Madeleine (foundress of TCN), 5–8
Leininger's culture care model, 274
  example of, 279b
Leininger's Sunrise model, 8
Leininger's Theory of culture care diversity and universality, 8
Lesbian childbearing couples, 141, 142f
Leukoedema, 90
Levels of prevention, 356
Liberal Beachy Amish, 388
Library of Congress, 310–312
Lifestyle practices, cultural competence, 353–356
Limited English proficiency (LEP), 289
Linguistic competence, 289–290
Literature, 24
Long Acting and Reversible Contraception (LARC), 134
Long-term care, 238
Lutheranism, 411

M

Machismo, 360
Magico-religious paradigm, 107

Magnet designation, 279
Magnet research, forces of magnetism, 278b
Major depressive disorder (MDD), 318
Malnutrition, 183–184
Mammary venous plexus, biocultural variations in, 91
Marianismo, 323
Massage therapy, 118
Maternal fetal medicine facts, 130
Maternal morbidity and mortality, 129
Maternal role attainment, 143
Maternal Self-Report Inventory (MSRI), 143
Medications
  plant-derived, 69
  traditional Chinese medicine, 65–69
Meidung. *See* Amish
Melanin, 84
Mennonites, 388
Menopause, perception of, 210–211
Menstruation, 186–187
Mental health care
  concept of, 300
  cultural competence
    developing, 324–325
    intrapersonal reflection, 325–326
  cultural values, beliefs, and practices, 317–324
    African American culture, 317–319
    American Indian Culture, 319–320
    Arab Muslim culture, 323–324
    Asian/Pacific Islander culture, 320–321
    Hispanic/Latino culture, 322–323
  culture-bound syndrome, 313–315, 315t–317t
  decision making, and mental health care, 305–306
  disparities in, 306–309
  DSM-5, 313, 314t
  immigration policy, 309–313, 311b
  intrapersonal reflection, 325–326
  patient's experience of pain, 328
  population trends, 304–305
  stigma, 307, 308b
  transcultural mental health nursing
    definition of, 300–304
    intrapersonal reflection, 325–326
    pain experiences, 328
    spirituality, 327–328
Mental health nurses, 300, 326
  transcultural mental health nursing, 300
  working, 312–313

Mental health treatment, disparities in, 307
Metaphors, 106, 109
Mexican American cultural networks, 359
Microorganisms attack, 108
Middle adult, 212–213
Midlife crisis, 211
Migration experience, 440–441
Minority health care professionals, 130
Mitzvah (a good deed), 408
Mobility, biocultural variations in, 83
Modesty, 22–23
  cultural views, 358
Mohel, 406–407
Mongolian spots, 84
Monochronic culture, 20
Morality, contrasting social constructions, 419–420
Mormon Church, 23. *See also* Church of Jesus Christ of Latter-day Saints
Mormonism, 398–400
Mortality, in United States and Canada, 290
Mother-child relationships, 178
Motherhood, cultural views of, 359
Mothers premasticate, 180
Mourning, 379
Mouth, biocultural variation, 90
MSRI (Maternal Self-Report Inventory), 143
Musculoskeletal system, biocultural variation in, 91–92, 93t–94t
Music, cultural groups communication, 24
Muslim fertility rates, 136
Muslin, 404
Mutual goal setting, 24

N

NAACP (National Association for the Advancement of Colored People), 432
Names, guidelines for, 221t
National Alliance on Mental Illness (NAMI), 301
National Association for the Advancement of Colored People (NAACP), 432
National Center for Complementary and Integrative Health (NCCIH), 65–69, 116, 121

National Center on Minority Health and Health Disparities (NCMHD), 291
National Institute of Drug Abuse (NIDA), 319–320
National Institute of Nursing Research (NINR), 334
National Standards for Culturally and Linguistically Appropriate Services (CLAS) in health care, 268–272, 269*b*
National Survey of Family Growth, 132
National Tribal Behavioral Health Agenda, 320
National Vital Statistics Reports, 144
Native American culture, 320
Native American family system, 362–363
Native American pregnant women, 164–166, 165*f*
Native Americans, beliefs and practices related to diabetes, 362*b*
Natural products, 117
Naturopathy, 118
NCCIH (National Center for Complementary and Integrative Health), 65–69, 116, 121
NCMHD (National Center on Minority Health and Health Disparities), 291
Nepal, childbirth and postnatal cultural practices in, 152*b*
Nerves, 230
New Order Amish, 388
NIDA (National Institute of Drug Abuse), 319–320
NINR (National Institute of Nursing Research), 334
Nirvana, 390
Noble Eightfold Way, 390
Non-English-speaking patients, 289
Nonethnic cultures, 5, 47
Nonmaleficence, 421
Nontraditional support systems, 143–144
Nonverbal communication, 16–17
Nonverbal expressions, 200
Nuclear family, 197
Nurse executive communication, 284*b*
Nursing actions, 97
Nursing assessment, family, 196–198
Nursing care, 106, 229
  application of cultural concepts to, 201–202

factors to consider, 349*b*
hospitalization of Amish child, 202*b*
plan, evaluation of, 201
religion and spiritual, 373–415
transcultural perspectives
  of adults, 209–210
  of older adults, 237–238
Nursing interventions, 198–200
Nursing personnel, 145–146
Nutrition, 180–184, 432–433

O

Objective data, 36–41, 57
Objective materialism, 107–108
Occulistics, 19
Occupational cultures, 5
Older adults
  activity theory, 242
  age in place, 241
  aging, perspectives of, 242
  challenge, 258–259
  clients, guidelines for communicating, 247*b*
  continuity theory, 242
  cultural influences, 242–252
    caregiving, 249–250
    culture change, understanding, 247–249
    intragroup differences, 252
    social support, dimensions of, 250–252
    traditional beliefs/practices, 245–247
  demographics, 239–240
  disengagement theory, 242
  disparities, 239–240
  income level, 240
  individual clients, integrating social/cultural factors
    community-based services for, 256–259
    decisions on continuum of care, 254–256
    faith and spirituality, 254
    purpose of, 253–254
  needs for care, 242
  in nursing care, 237–238
  pain management in, 256*b*
  practices, adoptation, 248
  responses in health care, 239*b*
  retirees enjoy an activity in their residential community, 258*f*
  social roles, assessing, 249*b*
  socioeconomic status, 240–242
Older client treats pain, 248

Ombligero, 360
Oral hyperpigmentation, 90
Organ donation, 417
Organizational cultural competence, 33–34, 46
Organizational cultures, 272–277
  assessment tools, 277
  behavior, 272
  building
    community involvement, 290–292
    culturally congruent services and programs, 292
    governance and administration, 283–285
    health care organization leaders role, 282*b*
    internal evaluation of adherence, 285–287
    linguistic competence, 289–290
    physical environment of care, 288–289
    staff competence, 287–288
  community context, 290–292
  employees and community, 274–277
  theories of, 273–274
    Bolman and Deal's, 273–274
    Schein's, 274
Osteopathic medicine, 118

P

Pain, 80
  assessment of, 80–83
  cultural, 307
  experiences of, 328
  management, older adults, 256*b*
  threshold, 80
Pallor, 86
Pandanus mat, 184–185
Papanicolaou (Pap) test, 343–344
Paradigm, 106
Paralanguage, 16–17
Parent Teacher Association (PTA), 216
Parent-child relationships, 187–188
Parteras, 358
Participatory action research, 291
Participatory women groups (PWG), 145
Patient Self-Determination Act, 418
Personal space, 21
Petechiae, 86
Peyote religion, 409
PGD (Preimplantation genetic diagnosis), 64
Pharmacogenomics, drug efficacy, 61
Phenylketonuria (PKU), 192

Physical appearance, biocultural variations in, 83
Physical environment, 288–289
Physiologic development, 210–211
Pica, 147
Pillars of Faith, 401
Placental burial rituals, 159
Planning care, 24
Political frame, 273
Political/government systems, 436
Political/legal, 279b, 439
Polychronic culture, 20
Polygyny, 136
Population
   child health status, 176
   crying, 178
   growth and development, 176–177
   infant attachment, 177–178
   poverty, 175–176
   racial/ethnic composition, 174–175
Population trends, and mental health, 304–305
Positions of birth, 154
Positive childbirth experience, intrapartum care for, 155b
Postpartum care, Jewish laws, customs, 217b
Postpartum depression (PPD), 158
Postpartum dietary prescriptions and activity levels, 158–159
Postpartum rituals, 159
Posttraumatic stress disorder (PTSD), 343
Posture, 20
Potential demographic, cultural, and health system barriers, 272b
Poverty
   children's health, 176
   in rural African American communities, 364
PPD (Postpartum depression), 158
Pregnancy, 137–144
   beliefs and practices of, 359, 360b
   biologic variations, 137–139
   cultural views of, 359
Pregnant Muslim woman, 136f
Preimplantation genetic diagnosis (PGD), 64
Prejudice, 35–36
Premasticate, 180
Presbycusis, 90
Primary level of culture, 6
Primary prevention, 356–360
   cultural competence in, 356
Principle of totality, 393

Principle-based ethics, 420–421
Problem-solving process, 14, 24–26, 25f, 42
Professional care systems, 110–111
Professional cultures, 5
Promotoras, 352, 358
Protestantism, 410–411
Provision of care, 268b
Proxemics, 21
Psychomotor skills, 43–44
   transcultural nursing, 44b
Psychosocial development, 210–211
PTA (Parent Teacher Association), 216
PTSD (Posttraumatic stress disorder), 343
Public health nursing, 334–335
Public space, 21
Pujos (grunting), 186
PWG (Participatory women groups), 145

Q
Qigong ("chee-GUNG"), 118–119
Quality care, 24
Qur'an (Koran), 402

R
Race, 6, 192
Racism, 35, 37b
Rapid repeat births, 195b
Reasons for seeking care, 72–73
Reductionism, 107–108
Reformed denominations, 411
Refugee Health Screener-15 (RHS-15), 443
Refugee women and girls, minimum initial service package for, 135b
Refugees, 32, 346
   families, characteristics of, 215b
   and reproductive health, 134–135
   transcultural nursing assessment guide for
      family and kinship systems, 442
      language and traditions, 441
      migration experience, 440–441
      religious beliefs and practices, 442–443
      social life and networks, 442
      traditional beliefs and practices of healing, 441–442
      US health care system, 441
   women, 343–344
Regulators, 20

Reiki ("RAY-kee"), 119
Reincarnation, 400
Relationship-building competencies, 284b
The Relief Society, 400. *See also* Church of Jesus Christ of Latter-day Saints
Religions, 323, 327–328, 374, 433
   Amish, 385–387
      considerations, 389–390
      death and dying, 389
      health care practices, 388–389
      medical and surgical interventions, 388
      Old Order Amish, 387
      ordinance, 398
      religious support system for sick, 388–389
      reproduction, 388
      substance use, 388
   Buddhist Churches of America
      Buddhism, 390
      death and dying, 392
      diet, 391
      general beliefs and religious practices, 390–391
      health care practices, 391
      holy days, 390
      medical and surgical interventions, 391–392
      religious objects, 390
      religious support system for sick, 392
      reproduction, 391–392
      rites and rituals, 391
   Catholicism
      Catholic, 392
      death and dying, 395
      diet, 392–393
      general beliefs and religious practices, 392–393
      health care practices, 393–395
      holy days, 392–393
      medical and surgical interventions, 393–394
      religious objects, 392
      religious support system for sick, 394–395
      reproduction, 394
      rites and rituals, 392
      social activities, 393
      substance use, 393
   Christian Science, 395
      considerations, 397–398
      death and dying, 397

Religions (*Continued*)
  general beliefs and religious prac-
    tices, 395–396
  health care practices, 396–397
  holy days, 395
  medical and surgical interven-
    tions, 397
  religious support system for sick,
    397
  reproduction, 397
  rites and rituals, 396
  social activities and substance
    use, 396
Church of Jesus Christ of Latter-day
    Saints, 398
  death and dying, 400
  diet, 398
  general beliefs and religious prac-
    tices, 398–399
  health care practices, 399–400
  holy days, 398
  medical and surgical interven-
    tions, 399
  religious objects, 398
  religious support system for sick,
    399–400
  reproduction, 399
  rites and rituals, 398
  social activities, 398–399
  substance use, 399
consequential dimension, 374–375
contributions of, 383–384
dimensions of, 374–376
and fertility control, 135–136
Hinduism, 400–401
  death and dying, 401
  general beliefs and religious prac-
    tices, 400
  health care practices, 401
  Hindu, 400
  medical and surgical interven-
    tions, 401
  religious objects, 400
  religious support system for sick,
    401
  reproduction, 401
  social activities, 400
  substance use, 400
human behavior, 374–375
ideologic dimension, 374–375
intellectual dimension, 374–375
Islam
  Allah, 401
  death and dying, 403–404
  diet and substance use, 402–403

general beliefs and religious prac-
    tices, 401–403
  health care practices, 403–404
  holy days, 402
  medical and surgical interven-
    tions, 403
  religious objects, 403
  religious support system for sick,
    403
  reproduction, 403
Jehovah's Witnesses, 404
  death and dying, 405
  general beliefs and religious prac-
    tices, 404–405
  health care practices, 405
  holy days, 404–405
  medical and surgical interven-
    tions, 405
  religious support system for sick,
    405
  reproduction, 405
  social activities, 405
  substance use, 405
Judaism, 406
  death and dying, 408–409
  diet, 407
  general beliefs and religious prac-
    tices, 406–407
  health care practices, 407–409
  holy days, 406
  medical and surgical interven-
    tions, 408
  religious objects, 407
  religious support system for sick,
    408
  reproduction, 408
  rites and rituals, 406–407
  social activities, 407
  substance use, 407
Native American and Indigenous
    People's Churches, 409–410
Protestantism, 410–411
relation to health and illness,
    375–376
ritualistic dimension, 374–375
Seventh-Day Adventists
  death and dying, 413
  diet and substance use, 412
  general beliefs and religious prac-
    tices, 411–412
  health care practices, 412–413
  holy days, 411
  religious support system for the
    sick, 413
  reproduction, 412

rites and rituals, 412
  social activities, 412
  surgical interventions, 412
and spiritual nursing care, 376–383
  for dying, 379–383
  ethnoreligious, assessment of, 377
  for ill children, 377–378
  spiritual concerns, 377
  spiritual health, 376–377
studies, health care practices, 385*b*
in United States and Canada, 383,
    384*t*
Religious affiliations, United States
    and Canada, 383, 384*t*
Religious beliefs, 436, 442–443
Religious healers, 15
Religious/nonreligious holidays,
    United States and Canada,
    386*b*
Religious/philosophical, 438
Religious/philosophical factors, 279*b*
Reproductive health care
  for migrant women in Geneva, 133*b*
  refugees and, 134–135
Rights and responsibilities of indi-
    vidual, 268*b*
Ritualistic dimension, 374–375
Roman Catholic tradition, children,
    392, 393*f*
Rural Amish community, 201

S
Salat, 401
Salat El Mayyet, 404
Sandwich generation, 211
Sawa Mahina, Punjabi cultural tradi-
    tion, 157
Sawm, 401
Schein's organizational culture, 274
Scientific paradigm, 107–108
Secondary level of culture, 6
Secondary prevention, 356, 360–363
  cultural competence in, 356
Selective use of technology, 385–387
Self-care, 248
Self-location, 43–44
Sensation threshold, 80
Seventh-Day Adventists
  death and dying, 413
  diet and substance use, 412
  general beliefs and religious prac-
    tices, 411–412
  health care practices, 412–413
  holy days, 411

religious support system for the sick, 413
reproduction, 412
rites and rituals, 412
social activities, 412
surgical interventions, 412
Sexual orientation, 5
Shahada, 401
Shared decision making (SDM), 306
Shema, 406
Sheppard–Towner Act, 151
Shi'a Muslim, 402
Sick role behavior, 110
Sickle cell disease (SCD), 137–138, 138b
Sickle cell trait (SST), 137–138
Siddur, 407
Silence, 19
Single-dose regimen, 134
Single-nucleotide polymorphisms (SNPs), 59–60
Single-parent family, 197
Situational crises, 210, 220–233
Situational transitions, 220–221
Skin
  biocultural variations in, 84–88
  dryness, 200
Sleep, childrearing behaviors, 184–186
Social age, definition of, 212
Social determinants of health (SDH), 37, 130, 421
Social factors, 279b, 439
Social justice, 422, 424
Social life, 435–436, 442
Social networks, 432
Social responsibilities, 216–218
Social roles, 213
Social space, 21
Social support, 249, 353
Social–ecological approach, 336
Society, relation, groups of people, 38b
Sociocultural factors, 211
Socioeconomic status, 5
Southern Sudan, human rights barriers, 341b
Specialized community intervention, 334
Spiritual assessment, 376–377
Spiritual beliefs, 231
Spiritual concerns, 377
Spiritual distress, 377
Spiritual healers, 15
Spiritual health, 377
Spiritual needs, in clients, 378b

Spiritual nursing care, 376–377
  for dying, 379–383
  ethnoreligious, assessment of, 377
  for ill children, 377–378
  spiritual concerns, 377
  spiritual health, 377
Spirituality, 327–328, 376, 433
  faith and, 254
  and religious practices, 328
Staff competence, 287–288
Standards and sources of evidence, address culture, 268b
Steatorrhea, 84
Stereotyping, 129
Stereotyping, of patients, 304
Stress, 230
Stroke belt, 228
Structural frame, 273
Subcultures, 6, 339–340, 389
  identifying, 336
  United States, 340
Subjective data, 57
Sudanese refugee women, CBCAR intervention, 345b
Sunni Muslim, 402
Swartzentruber, 387
Symbolic frame, 273
Symptoms, 73
  client's perception, 73
  of depression, 318
  for psychologic issues, 324

T

Tallit, 407
Talmud, 406
Technology, 279b, 438
Technology-assisted communication, 23–24
Teeth, biocultural variation in, 90–91
Tertiary level of culture, 6
Tertiary prevention, 356, 364–366
  cultural competence in, 356
  goal of, 364
  for traditional African American population, 365b
The Joint Commission (TJC), 376–377
Therapeutic touch, 119
Time orientation, 365b
TIP model. See Transcultural interprofessional practice (TIP) model
To Err is Human, 15
Torah, 406
Traditional African American population, cultural factors, 365b

Traditional beliefs, 339, 348b, 441–442
Traditional Chinese medicine (TCM), 119
Traditional healer, 15, 44–45
Traditional health beliefs and practices, 339
Traditional medicine, 246
Traditional pregnancy-related folk beliefs, 359
Transcultural framework
  subcultures identification, 336
  values and cultural norms, identifying, 337
Transcultural interprofessional practice (TIP) model
  communication, 15–24
    chronemics, 20–21
    cultural context, 14
    eye contact and facial expressions, 19–20
    gestures, 20
    greetings, 19
    interpreters, 17–19
    language, 17
    modesty, 22–23
    posture, 20
    problem-solving process, 24–26, 25f
    proxemics, 21
    silence, 19
    technology-assisted communication, 23–24
  goals, assumptions, and components, 11, 12b
Transcultural mental health nurses, 300, 317, 326–328
  definition of, 300–304
  factors
    communication, 326–327
    pain experiences, 328
    spirituality, 327–328
Transcultural nursing (TCN), 4, 7, 303f, 317
  administration, definition of, 266
  assessment guide
    for groups and communities, 57
    for individuals and families, 57
  biocultural variations, 77
  goal of, 4
  historical and theoretical foundations of, 6–11
    advancements, 10
    core curriculum, 10–11
    Leininger's contributions, 8–10
    psychomotor skills useful in, 44b

Transcultural nursing administration, 284

Transcultural nursing assessment guide

clients
biocultural variations and cultural aspects, 429
communication, 429–430
cultural affiliations, 430
cultural sanctions and restrictions, 430
developmental considerations, 431
economics, 431
educational background, 431
health-related beliefs and practices, 431–432
kinship and social networks, 432
nutrition, 432–433
religion and spirituality, 433
value orientation, 433–434

for families, groups, and communities
economic factors, 437
family and kinship systems, 435
health beliefs and practices, 436–437
health care systems, 437
language and traditions, 436
political/government systems, 436
religious beliefs and practices, 436
social life and networks, 435–436
worldviews, value orientations, and cultural norms, 436

for health care organizations and facilities
cultural values, 439
economic, 439
education, 439
environmental context, 438
language and ethnohistory, 438
political/legal, 439
religious/philosophical, 438
social factors, 439
technology, 438

for refugees
family and kinship systems, 442
language and traditions, 441
migration experience, 440–441
religious beliefs and practices, 442–443
social life and networks, 442
traditional beliefs and practices of healing, 441–442
US health care system, 441

Transcultural Nursing Assessment Guide for Groups and Communities, 57

Transcultural Nursing Assessment Guide for Individuals and Families, 57

Transcultural nursing perspective, mental health, 300–304

Transcultural perspectives
on health history, 57–77
biographic data, 58
culture-bound syndromes, 73
family and social history, 74–77
genetic data, 58–64
past health, 73–74
present health and history of present illness, 73
reason for seeking care, 72–73
review of medications and allergies, 64–72
review of systems, 77

on physical examination, biocultural variations, 83
Addison's disease, 87
age-related changes, 87–88
albinism, 87
body proportions, 78
cyanosis, 85
ecchymoses, 87
erythema, 86
eyes, 89
in general appearance, 83–84
hair, 89
height, 77–78
hyperpigmentation, 85
in illness, 92
jaundice, 85–86
in laboratory tests, 92–96, 95t–96t
leukoedema, 90
in mammary venous plexus, 91
melanin, 84
Mongolian spots, 84
mouth, 90
in musculoskeletal system, 91–92
in pain assessment, 80–83
pallor, 86
petechiae, 86
in skin, 84–88
in sweat glands, 88–89
uremia, 87
in vital signs, 79
vitiligo, 85
weight, 78–79

Transcultural perspectives in childbearing
African American pregnant woman, 166–167
African American women's infant-feeding practices, 161b
antenatal, intrapartum, and postpartum care in Asian Countries, 150b
birth and culture, 149–157
birth positions, 154
cultural expression of labor, 154
infant gender, cultural meaning attached to, 154–157
childbirth and postnatal cultural practices in Nepal and other countries, 152b
clinical implications, 138
cultural variations influencing pregnancy, 139–144
cultural belief systems and practices, 127–128
cultural beliefs related to antenatal care, 144–149
cultural preparation for childbirth, 149
food taboos and food cravings, 147–148, 148b
substance use, 149
culture and the postpartum period, 157–161
cultural influences on breastfeeding and weaning, 159–161
postpartum depression (PPD), 158
postpartum dietary prescriptions and activity levels, 158–159
postpartum rituals, 159
fertility control and culture, 131–137
continuation of unintended pregnancy, 133–134
contraceptive methods, 134
cultural influences on fertility control, 136–137
global contraception concerns, 134
refugees and reproductive health, 134–135
religion and fertility control, 135–136
unintended pregnancy, 132–133
hispanic pregnant women, 163–164
indigenous peoples/native American pregnant women, 164–166, 165f

intimate partner violence, cultural issues related to, 161–163
minimum initial service package for refugee women and girls, 135*b*
positive childbirth experience, intrapartum care for, 155*b*
pregnancy and childbirth practices in United States, 128–131
pregnancy and culture, 137–144
    biologic variations, 137–139
Transcultural Nursing Society (TCNS), 8
Transitions, 210
Trisomy 21, 89
Truth telling, 418
Turnaway Study, 133–134
Type 2 diabetes, 361, 363

U

Undocumented immigrant, 310–312
UNICEF, 139
Unintended pregnancy, 132–134
United States
    pregnancy and childbirth practices in, 128–131
United States, subcultures, 340
Unlawful discrimination, 35–36
Uremia, 87
US health care system, 441

V

Value orientation, 433–434
Value orientations, 436
Vedas, 400
Ventricular septal defects (VSDs), 192
Veracity, 418, 420–421
Verbal communication, 16–17, 200
Vital signs, biocultural variations in measurements, 79
Vitiligo, 85
Vulnerable populations, 32, 421

W

Weaning, cultural influences on, 159–161
Weight, biocultural variations in measurements, 78–79
Western culture, 137
Western health care, 144
White, Anglo-Saxon, Protestant (WASP) views, 214
Womanhood, cultural preparation for, 226*b*
Women, Infants, and Children (WIC), 358
Word of Wisdom, 398
World Health Organization (WHO), 144, 145*b*, 162–163
    positive childbirth experience, intrapartum care for, 155*b*
World Health Organization antenatal care schedule, 145*b*
Worldviews, 34–35, 106, 436

Y

Yarmulkes, 407
Yellow Dirt, 357*b*
Yin and yang, 109
Yoga, 119
Young adult, 212–213

Z

Zakat, 401